In and Out of Harm's Way

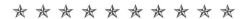

A HISTORY OF
THE NAVY NURSE CORPS

✷ ✷ ✷ ✷ ✷ ✷ ✷ ✷ ✷ ✷

Captain Doris M. Sterner NC USN (Ret.)

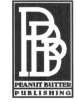

PEANUT BUTTER
PUBLISHING

Seattle, Washington
Portland, Oregon
Denver, Colorado
Vancouver, B.C.

ISBN 0-89716-706-6
LCC 96-072362

Cover Design: David Marty
Editor: Kathleen Markham

10 9 8 7 6 5 4 3 2

Peanut Butter Publishing
226 2nd Avenue West • Seattle, WA 98119
(206) 281-5965
Post Office Bldg. • 510 S.W. 3rd • Portland, OR 97201
Cherry Creek • 50 S. Steel • Suite 850 • Denver, CO 80209
Granville Island • 1333 Johnston Street • Suite 230
Vancouver, B.C. V6H3R9
e mail: PNUTPUB@aol.com
WWW home page: http://www.pbpublishing.com

Printed in the United States of America

Table of Contents

☆ ☆ ☆

INTRODUCTION

☆ ☆ ☆

What is the U.S. Navy Nurse Corps? What is a Navy Nurse, and **who** is a Navy Nurse? Is there a difference between a Navy Nurse and any other registered nurse? Between the leaves of this book is the history of this elite Corps and the answers to those questions. This is the heritage of a proud group. We are patriots. We are professionals. Above all, once a Navy Nurse, always a Navy Nurse.

There are three letters that I believe will introduce this history in the most appropriate manner. The first letter is from Mrs. Mary (Robinson) Godfrey. Mrs. Godfrey was born 12 January 1886. (You will find her story in Chapter 1.) She wrote this letter in 1990 when she was 104 years old and very mentally alert.

"To My Fellow Navy Nurses, Past and Present:

I know you share with me the pride in being a Navy nurse that I have felt since joining the Navy Nurse Corps in 1910. From nursing at a hospital in Canacao, Philippine Islands, to serving as Chief Nurse aboard the troop ship Leviathan at the close of World War I, every assignment the Navy gave me was challenging and fulfilling — and often fraught with adventure. You have bravely and selflessly carried on in the tradition begun so hopefully, so long ago. On behalf of my contemporaries in the early days of the corps, I salute you and wish you well."

Sincerely,
Mary Margaret (Robinson) Godfrey
Navy Nurse Corps, 1910-1919
Ligonier, Pennsylvania
8 November 1990

The second letter is from Rear Admiral Alene B. Duerk NC USN (Ret.). Admiral Duerk carries the honor of being the first Admiral in the Navy Nurse Corps. She was also Director of the Corps from 1970 to 1975.

"Dear Captain Sterner:

When you volunteered to assume the responsibility of compiling the Navy Nurse Corps history, you undertook a long, overdue and arduous task. I want you to know we greatly appreciate your efforts and are as proud of your work as we are of our history.

For decades directors have explored many avenues to accomplish this project, but personnel and financial resources were not available for such a comprehensive undertaking. In the interim some of our members have done limited research projects and written parts of our history, but a complete chronological record has always seemed beyond our reach. Until the Navy Nurse Corps Association adopted as one of its purposes, 'to gather and preserve the history of the Navy Nurse Corps,' the complete story remained untold. Many volunteers have given generously of their time and talents to assist in the research of such a tremendous undertaking. Without the present day technologies, many people could not have contributed their stories and experiences. Hopefully, our successors will record their experiences to the ever changing dynamics of the Navy Nurse Corps.

On behalf of all Nurse Corps Officers, I offer my gratitude for this significant gift which you and your coworkers have prepared for us. We are especially proud that 'one of our own' has recorded our heritage."

Sincerely,
Alene B. Duerk
RADM NC USN Ret.

The third letter is from a good friend of the Nurse Corps and a fine gentleman: Admiral Horace D. Warden of the Medical Corps of the U.S. Navy. I had the good fortune to work in the Operating Room when he was utilizing his skills as a naval surgeon (we were both a little younger then). He has always encouraged and supported Navy Nurses.

"It is a great privilege to have this opportunity to thank the many, many Navy nurses with whom it has been my pleasure to share duty over the majority of my professional years. Not only have I had the pleasure of sharing duty with you, but I also wish to take this opportunity to thank the many of you who taught me much in the art of the practice of medicine. And our patients can be most thankful to all of you who worked so hard with the care of the many patients that were entrusted to us. God bless you all!"

Horace D. Warden
RADM MC USN Ret.

I must claim "artistic license" for some of the manner, and thought, contained in the extrapolation of historic material from the past to the present, as it appears in this book.* It is, I insist, an honest attempt to transport the reader into those events of the era being described.

We all know that time plays havoc with memory and memories. Some people quoted within these pages are already among the elderly (though never old in spirit) and may be forgiven for relating incidents with a few facts lacking or misinterpreted. They do not detract from the main thrust of this history and, indeed, are somehow lovely in the emotionally charged atmosphere of recalling one's own moments in the performance of truly heartfelt patriotic duty.

There are many, many who have contributed to this publication. They have contributed time, effort, memories, emotions, ideas, money and support of all kinds. They are too numerous to name here, but you know who you are. Herein lay the results of your input, as promised. Thank you, one and all.

Doris M. Sterner
Captain NC USN Ret.

---

* The author extends "artistic license" to include the method of capitalizing, abbreviating and punctuating some words.

PROLOGUE

(1798 - 1908)

☆☆☆

And so it begins. Just as every day follows every other day, just as every event brings another event, so it all merges eventually to an illusion of time called history. Even the history of mankind began one day following another. By the time the days of mankind total years and the years become the eighteenth century, particular events begin to take place: events that start yet another history, the history of the U.S. Navy Nurse Corps. And so it begins.

In 1798 Congress passes legislation to begin the Navy Department of the United States. On March 2nd, the President signs the department into being. The President is John Adams who had been the Vice President of the new nation under General George Washington. John Adams holds the honor of being the first President to be elected under the two party system[1] and he has the Honorable Thomas Jefferson as his Vice President. In the elections of 1800, Jefferson defeats Adams and becomes the third President of these United States.

As for medical affairs at this time, there are only about 12 hospitals in the entire United States in 1800. The Charity Hospital of New Orleans was established in 1737, the Pennsylvania General Hospital in 1751, and the New York Hospital in 1781, to name a few. The Philadelphia General Hospital began in 1731 as an Almshouse with a hospital ward. Bellevue Hospital (New York) began as a New York Public Workhouse in 1736 and with only one room as an infirmary. But, there are no Naval Hospitals in 1800.

In the year 1801, Jefferson assumes the presidency and almost immediately faces a declaration of war from Tripoli (in Libya). Libya is one of the Barbary States on the northern coast of Africa: the Barbary States being Tunisia, Algeria, Libya and Morocco. They are centers for the "Barbary Pirates" that are attacking ships and personnel in the Mediterranean. (As a matter of interest, the phrase "to the shores of Tripoli" in the Marine's Hymn of the U.S. Marine Corps, originates here.) The United States conducts several campaigns against the Barbary States in this time of high-seas piracy.[2] From 1795 to 1801 the United States paid immense amounts of money for the protection of American sailors and ships. But, in 1801, under President Thomas Jefferson, the U.S. goes to war to stop these payments and the pirating.[3] Clearly, the Navy and the Navy Department are now all important because of the geographical location of the war.

There are several hospitals established to take care of the sick and injured in the Mediterranean during this war. "The first seems to have been at Syracuse in Sicily, where Dr. Edward Cutbush, then [a Navy] surgeon on [board] the *President*, landed by order of Commodore Samuel Barron to establish a hospital for the sick and wounded of the squadron."[4] Another Commodore in the area uses (for a short time) a small sailing vessel that he specifically designates as a hospital ship.[5] This may be a harbinger for the future and it may be the inspiration for Doctor Cutbush's intense interest and involvement in hospital ships. In 1808, Navy surgeon Cutbush makes suggestions to higher authorities on hospital ships and on hospital management. This naval surgeon needs to be noticed here because in his writings he mentions women for nursing in the Navy: he suggests that wives of the sailors could provide good nursing care.

The next report of a suggestion for using women as nurses in the Navy comes in 1810 when Secretary of the Navy, Paul Hamilton, proposes, "The wives of seamen killed in the service would make nurses and attendants on the sick, and do all the necessary sewing, washing, etc."[6] Nothing ever comes of either of these proposals.

Onto the year 1811. There are, at this point in time, some temporary buildings being used as hospitals in Philadelphia, Washington, New York and Boston, but they are just that — "temporary" and inappropriate. Also proving unsatisfactory is the custom of billeting the sick and injured in private homes under the care of civilian physicians. The Navy does have certain ships designated as dual purpose ships, but there are no hospital ships per se. In these initial days of the U.S. Navy, certain ships called store, supply or depot ships serve a dual purpose, the second purpose is as a health or hospital ship.[7]

It is now that we introduce Dr. William Paul Crillon Barton, a young man and a surgeon in the service of the U.S. Navy. He is serving aboard one of the Navy's ships, the *Essex*. Doctor Barton finds himself rather discouraged in his shipboard duty. The lack of supplies and equipment severely limit his medical and surgical expertise. He cannot take care of his patients as completely as he believes necessary. Doctor Barton, however, is not one to give up easily. He makes what improvements he can and then fills many sheets of paper with notes of those things he would like to change and see happen.

One day, to his surprise, he receives a request from the Secretary of the Navy. It seems that the Secretary must make a report to Congress on how to operate and manage hospitals, and he wants expert information. The doctor is asked to write any recommendations he might have for inclusion in that report. What an opportunity this is for the energetic and outspoken Doctor Barton. Finally, he has the chance to make his voice heard where it counts. He sits and writes his suggestions from all the notes he has been keeping. "The report containing them [the recommendations] . . . was chiefly written during a tempestuous passage from Norfolk to New York, in the *Hornet* sloop-of-war."[8]

After the young surgeon sends his recommendations to the Secretary of the Navy, he decides to elaborate on his ideas for organizing Naval Hospitals. He spends his spare time writing his thoughts and beliefs on the subject. One of Surgeon Barton's ideas is especially noteworthy here, since it concerns nurses. What makes it so different is that the young surgeon mentions "women" as nurses, not sailors' wives, as Doctor Cutbush advised, nor enlisted men (or loblolly boys) as is the usual procedure at this time.

The year is now 1812 and James Madison is President. In June, President Madison asks Congress to declare war on Great Britain. The United States vehemently objects to the British policy of stopping American ships. Especially objectionable is the impressing (forcing) of American sailors of British birth into British service.[9] Britain is also at war with France and adamantly enforcing a blockade. This results in British seizure of any neutral ship running the blockade, and there are several American privateers doing just that. Thus, the United States makes the decision to declare war. What neither the President nor the Congress know is that, "two days before war [is] declared, the British Government had stated it would repeal the laws which were the chief excuse for fighting."[10] Rapid communication could have prevented the whole affair. It is during this War of 1812 that a British warship demolishes an American ship under the command of Captain James Lawrence. The Captain is mortally wounded, but his dying command is, "Don't give up the ship!"[11]

Meanwhile, one of the most daring, handsome and popular officers in the Navy, Captain Stephen Decatur, commands a squadron of three ships that capture a British frigate after a "desperate struggle."[12] He is promoted to Commodore in 1813. This is the year he has women on board his ship as nurses and during wartime.[13] Their names are Mary Allen and Mary Marshall. Both are wives of seamen in Commodore Decatur's squadron. It is not clear how long they served. Quite possibly it is for only a short time in the month of May, 1813.[14]

Now it is 1814 and we return to Navy Doctor Barton. He finally completes and publishes his "A Treatise Containing a Plan for the Internal Organization and Government of Marine Hospitals in the United States together with a Scheme for Amending and Systematizing the Medical Department of the Navy."[15] In this dissertation he writes, "The nurses whose numbers should be proportionate to the extent of the hospital and number of patients, should be women of humane disposition and tender manners; active and healthy. They should be neat and cleanly in their persons; and without vices of any description."[16] More of his comments, "They [the nurses] should obey punctually all orders from their superiors; and should exact a ready acquiescence in their commands, from the attendants under them."[17] Doctor Barton goes even further to recommend that nurses be included in the management and operation of hospitals; an unheard of, extremist point of view.

In his earnest pursuit of medical excellence, Doctor Barton also makes recommendations for patient management that illustrate the attention he gives to specifics and details; i.e., "Every patient in the hospital shall be obliged to wash his face and hands and comb his hair before breakfast. Those patients who are unable to perform this ablution themselves, must be assisted in doing it, or have it done for them, by their neighbor patients or nurses of the ward. Such patients must be washed with lukewarm water. If any convalescents or pensioners neglect or refuse to perform this process, the nurse must deny them their breakfast until it is done."[18]

In 1808, Dr. Edward Cutbush had produced a dissertation comparable to Doctor Barton's Treatise, "but this lacked the breadth and originality of view characteristic of Barton's book."[19] But then, Surgeon Barton is no stranger to the world of writing and publishing. His father had been a well-known lawyer and "a gentleman of substantial literary attainments."[20] (Indeed, the son and young Navy surgeon follows in his father's footsteps to publish many documents during his career and even becomes noted as an author and Professor of Botany.[21])

To return to 1814, even as Doctor Barton is having his treatise published, new Navy regulations are being put into effect. These regulations describe the position of "loblolly boy" for the U.S. Navy. (Loblolly was the name of "a porridge which (is) the standard ship's diet for the sick."[22] According to the dictionary, porridge is, "a soft food made of cereal or meal boiled in water or milk until thick."[23]) These loblolly boys are men chosen from the ship's crew to assist the ship's surgeon, as needed. The new regulations of 1814 state that this position calls for the man to announce sick call by "ringing the bell about the decks, [and further] he will feed, wash and shave the sick and provide a tub of sand to catch the blood during surgical operation to prevent staining of the deck." (In June of 1798 a young man by the name of John Wall had enlisted as a "loblolly boy." His job was to help the naval doctor with recruiting examinations. According to an article in the Hospital Corps Quarterly, this man is on record as the first enlisted hospital corpsman.[24])

In 1818 more Navy rules and regulations come out containing the following: "In addition to the complement of a hospital ship, there shall be borne, as attendants on the sick, a list of supernumeraries for wages and victuals, a surgeon, two, or if necessary three assistant surgeons, six landsmen as nurses, a baker, four washermen, a servant to the hospital surgeon and a servant to the surgeon's mates." The regulation may be in force, but evidently there are still no hospital ships in the U.S. Navy.

Meanwhile, time goes by and we leave Doctor Barton to continue his career in the Navy as other events take place.

It is the year 1827. John Quincy Adams is now the President. He is the one that envisions a naval academy and proposes this to Congress. But, the proposal never materializes in his presidency. (The Naval Academy at Annapolis is founded in 1845.) What does begin to appear is the first permanent U.S. Naval Hospital.

In Portsmouth, Virginia along the shores of the Elizabeth River, construction is beginning. An architect by the name of John Haviland has been hired to build the Naval Hospital (called Norfolk Naval Hospital, even though located in Portsmouth.) The government had first acquired some land as long ago as 1799 and over the years accumulated the rest of the land that is the site of this, the first Naval Hospital. By 1829 it is still only partially complete when all construction comes to a sudden and complete halt. Funds are exhausted. Even so, the hospital is enough of a structure that it is commissioned in 1830 and the senior medical officer is ordered to start admitting patients. The next year (1831) funds become available and construction resumes. The imposing building is finally finished in 1832. Then in 1833 the Naval Hospital at League Island (Philadelphia), Pennsylvania is built. Following in 1834 is yet another at Portsmouth, New Hampshire with the Naval Hospital at Chelsea, Massachusetts in 1836 and in 1838 the Naval Hospital, Brooklyn, New York.[25]

As a point of interest, when the first senior medical officer of the Portsmouth, Virginia Naval Hospital finishes his tour of duty, it is Dr. William Paul Crillon Barton who relieves him. From that position, Doctor Barton's navy career continues and finally peaks in 1842. This is the year when the Act of August 31, 1842 is passed by Congress. It establishes within the Navy an agency to maintain the health of the Navy and the Marine Corps and the care of the sick and injured in peace and war. This Act states, in part, that "be it further enacted, that there shall be attached to the Navy department the following bureaus . . . 5. A Bureau of Medicine and Surgery. And be it further enacted, that the President of the United States, by and with the consent of the Senate, shall appoint . . . from the surgeons of the Navy a Chief of the Bureau of Medicine and Surgery, who shall receive for his services two thousand five hundred dollars per annum."[26] President John Tyler selects and appoints, with the Senate's consent, Dr. William Paul Crillon Barton as the first Chief of the Bureau of Medicine and Surgery of the Navy Department. Perhaps Commodore Barton says to himself, "At last, my treatise on plans and organization can be used to its fullest." Perhaps the very fact that he wrote and published the treatise influences his selection or it may be that political influence plays its part in this instance. Whatever, it **is** a fact that many of his ideas are carried out. Not so his idea for women nurses in the naval medical organization, however. In November of 1842, he writes to a Navy surgeon at the Portsmouth Naval Hospital, "There should be a matron or woman superintendent of nurses and wards in all naval hospitals. For the present everything in this way must remain in status-quo."[27] It is to be many a year before women nurses will ever see the light of day in the U.S. Navy.

It is remarkable that Doctor Barton and Doctor Cutbush both should persevere in their beliefs for women as nurses in the Navy. In this mid-19th century world, hospitals and nurses are unrivalled places and people of wretchedness, pollution and misery. Except for the religious sisters, those taking care of the sick are women of indecent behavior, drunkards and thieves. The English author Charles Dickens produces a characterization of a nurse of that era when he writes his book, Martin Chuzzlewit, in 1843. The introduction of the book points out that the novel comments on, among other things, the state of the nursing profession. The character Dickens creates is named Sarah (or Sairey) Gamp. Dickens says, "She was a fat old woman, this Mrs. Gamp, with a husky voice and a moist eye, which she had a remarkable power of turning up, and only showing the white of."[28] He goes on to write, "The face of Mrs. Gamp - the nose in particular was somewhat red and swollen, and it was difficult to enjoy her society without becoming conscious of a smell of spirits."[29] Later in the book, Mrs. Gamp is speaking to her patient when she states, "If you should turn at all faint, we can soon revive you, sir, I promise you. Bite a person's thumbs, or turn their fingers the wrong way."[30]

It is true that Charles Dickens writes his novel in London and probably bases his "Sairey" entity on his knowledge of nursing in his own country. But, there is evidence that things are equally dismal in the United States. In 1837 a report is written on the nurses in an American hospital. The report comes from the Bellevue Hospital Visiting Committee that is part of the New York State Charities Aid Association. It says that nurses are ill-paid and from the lower portions of society. Further it contends that nurses take bribes and extortions from patients and that nurses cannot be trusted. Then this report turns to the other side of conditions to state, "Their [the nurses] food was poor and there is record that they even had to sleep in barns on bundles of straw."[31] There is a ray of hope here, for in the 1830's and 1840's several Catholic nursing orders come to the U.S., to establish hospitals and "practicing the highest standards of the times."[32] In fact, just before the Civil War several attempts are made to start schools of nursing, but it is the Civil War itself that produces the demand in the United States for modern nursing. And it is Florence Nightingale who gains credit for beginning nursing as a profession, eventually abolishing the 'Sarah Gamp' reputation of this, subsequently, noble profession.

Florence Nightingale. Born of wealthy British parents. Enters into nurses training at the Institute of Protestant Deaconesses in Germany. In 1853, at age 33, she becomes superintendent of a women's hospital in London. In 1854 the British Secretary of War asks her to take over the nursing of the troops in the Crimea when England and France go to war with Russia.[33] Miss Nightingale and 38 of her handpicked nurses sail to the Crimea and find the hospital there to be in an "old Turkish barracks, huge, dirty and unfurnished. The wounded lay on floors, bleeding and uncared for."[34] She cleans, organizes, cajoles and demands until she and her group finally produce a sanitary environment. She wins the grudging respect of the doctors and becomes famous for her herculean efforts and nursing care results. She also becomes known as "The Lady of the Lamp." The name derives from a poem by Henry Wadsworth Longfellow. The poem is called "Santa Filomena." It says, in part:

> The wounded from the battle-plain,
> In dreary hospitals of pain,
> The cheerless corridors,
> The cold and stony floors.
> Lo! in that house of misery
> A lady with a lamp I see
> Pass through the glimmering gloom,
> and flit from room to room.

On England's annals, through the long
Hereafter of her speech and song,
That light its rays shall cast
From portals of the past. [35]

Even the United States is aware of what Florence Nightingale has achieved and asks for her advice during the Civil War, advice concerning the establishment of wartime hospitals.

It is now 1861. The Civil War. The war that tears country and men to pieces. The war of bitterness whose bile lasts down through the generations, particularly in the south. It is the time of Abraham Lincoln, our sixteenth President, and the time of the slavery issues. In April, the state of Virginia secedes from the Union. The Navy surgeon at Portsmouth Naval Hospital is compelled to resign as Confederate troops take over the hospital. The Union almost immediately equips and mans a hospital ship (the *Ben Morgan*) and stations it off the Old Point Comfort area (near Portsmouth, Virginia) with other Union ships.[36] This ship is, however, one of the Navy's dual purpose ships, not specifically a hospital ship. The *Ben Morgan* had been an ordnance storeship prior to refitting and is temporarily a hospital ship "from February to May 1862."[37] After that she (the ship) is returned to her previous duty carrying ordnance. The Navy frequently uses storeships as dual purpose ships. The first ship named *Relief* (commissioned in 1836) was a storeship reputed to have served some time as a hospital ship in Commodore Perry's squadron during the war with Mexico[38] from 1846 to 1848. This same *Relief* is "still in service during the Civil War, and records appear to indicate that on various occasions she (is) performing hospital ship duties."[39] Meanwhile, in 1861, a Naval Hospital is built and opened in Washington, DC,[40] to take care of the casualties from all-too-near battlefields.

There in the nation's capital a firsthand view of nursing the casualties during the beginning of the war is provided by Louisa May Alcott. (Author of Little Women, Little Men, and other books.) In 1863 she publishes her vignettes of her short tour as an Army nurse. She spent six weeks nursing the wounded then caught typhoid fever and nearly died. During her time in DC she writes many letters home and her Hospital Sketches are taken from those letters. Miss Alcott writes of meeting an Army nurse in her hometown and deciding to accept an offer to become one herself. Her trip from her New England home to Washington is lengthy and arduous, but she describes the journey in a delightful manner: "Philadelphia. An old place, full of Dutch women . . . selling vegetables, in long, open markets. Every one seems to be scrubbing their white steps. All the houses look like tidy jails. . . . Baltimore. A big, dirty, shippy, shiftless place, full of goats, geese, colored people, and coal."[41] When she finally arrives in DC, she begins taking care of the wounded from the battle of Fredericksburg. She writes of these patients, "torn and shattered . . . riddled with shot and shell . . . borne suffering for which we have no name."[42] War is ever thus, Miss Alcott. No one, having seen the dreadfully horrifying destruction done to human bodies and beings, can ever forget or forgive man's inhumanity to man, much less attribute any sense of glory to it.

Meanwhile, back to the Navy during this Civil War; several naval vessels are in use, at times, as hospital ships. "These include the *Ben Morgan*, the *Home*, the *A. Houghton*, the *Mohawk*, the *New Hampshire*, the *Red Rover*, and the *Valparaiso*. The latter is a "smallpox ship" assigned as a "lazaretto."[43] (A lazaretto is a quarantine ship.) All these ships return to usual naval duties when not needed as hospitals, but not so one of them, the *Red Rover*. This paddle-wheeler is a Mississippi river ship that was seized from the Confederates and is specifically turned into a Naval Hospital ship by the Union in 1862. A "wood-burning, side-wheeler . . . the first of the naval vessels to be designated, equipped or commissioned as a hospital ship during the Civil War."[44] A letter written to one of the Navy's Commodores on 12 June 1862 says, "I wish that you could see our hospital boat, the *Red Rover*, with all the comforts for the sick and disabled seamen. She is decided to be the most complete thing of the kind that ever floated. . . . The ice box of the steamer holds 300 tons. She has bathrooms, laundry, elevator for the sick . . . amputating room, nine different water closets, gauze blinds to the windows to keep the cinders and smoke from annoying the sick . . . **a regular corps of nurses**, and two water closets for every deck."[45] By "a regular corps of nurses," the writer undoubtedly means men as nurses not women. (In the previous year, 1861, the Navy replaced the loblolly boy title with the rating and title of "nurse."[46])

On 20 June 1862, the flag officer commanding the Western Flotilla for the Union, writes a letter to the Honorable Gideon Wells, the Secretary of the Navy. In this letter he states, "The department will be gratified to learn that the patients are, most of them, doing well. Sister Angela, the Superior of the Sisters of the Holy Cross ... has kindly offered the services of the Sisters for the hospital boat of this squad when needed. I have written ... to make arrangements for their coming."[47]

It is Christmas eve in the year 1862. The *Red Rover* is to be formally commissioned a hospital ship in the U.S. Navy on December 26th. The crew has already been assigned. But, on this special Christmas eve, three more members, for the medical department, board the ship: three trained nurses. They are nuns from the Holy Cross School of Nursing (Saint Mary's, Notre Dame, at South Bend in Indiana.)[48] Their names are, Sister Veronica, Sister Adela and Sister Callista.[49] On 9 February 1863 they [are] joined by Sister M. John [carried on reports as Sister St. John].[50] (Since the *Red Rover* is the Navy's first hospital ship and since the above named nuns are the first female trained nurses working aboard this ship, can we say these are the ancestors or pioneers of our Navy Nurse Corps?) There are also, eventually, five black lay nurses working under the direction of the sisters. Their names are, Alice Kennedy, Sarah Kinno, Ellen Campbell, Betsy Young and Dennis Downs.[51] Evidence further indicates that several "contraband" women are taken aboard the *Red Rover* and employed as nurses or laundresses.[52] (During this Civil War, "contraband" means "a Negro slave, who fled to or was smuggled behind the Union lines or remained in territory captured by the Union Army."[53]) As a matter of further interest, "Muster rolls of *Red Rover* show that nurses, men and women, sister and lay, [are] paid [fifty cents] a day. The rate for Army nurses [is] forty cents."[54]

Mother Angela Gillespie is the founder and administrator of Holy Cross nursing as well as American Provincial of the sisters of the Holy Cross in this period of American history. As such she has the authority to volunteer nurses[55] which she did in the case of the Navy's hospital ship. She also supplies nursing sisters to many of the overburdened hospitals that take care of the multitudes of sick, wounded and disabled resulting from the many Civil War confrontations.

In 1863 permission is granted for the Navy to obtain structures for a hospital in Memphis. General Grant orders that a former Confederate building be turned over to them for this purpose and the Commercial Hotel of Memphis is so selected.[56] Sister St. John leaves the *Red Rover* in September to take charge of the nursing service at this hotel that is now renovated to a hospital for the Navy. Mother Angela provides what nursing sisters she can. Doctors and other personnel arrive and another medical facility begins. Shortly after a battle in Mississippi, just south of Memphis, a young sailor is brought to the Navy's Memphis hospital. He is "in the last stages of malaria contracted on duty along the miasmatic shores of the Red River."[57] The young sailor is semiconscious and the Navy doctors believe his case is hopeless. But, there is a nun taking care of him, by the name of Sister de Sales O'Neill. "She [is] not willing to let him die. She [begins] to nurse him back to health, using all her wonderful skill and persistency."[58] The patient recovers. (In 1890, the Governor of Ohio is requested to speak at the ground breaking for a Catholic hospital addition. The Bishop introduces the Governor to the Sister Superior of the hospital. The Governor is that young sailor and the Sister Superior is Sister de Sales O'Neill.[59])

The *Red Rover* continues her medical missions throughout the Civil War and until November 1865. She is then taken out of Navy service and sold at auction. Her log shows that 2,947[60] patients were cared for during her time as the Navy's first hospital ship.

The Holy Cross Sisters (as recounted above) are not the only trained nurses active in this Civil War. True, most of them are from the Catholic orders, namely: Sisters of Charity, Sisters of Mercy, Sisters of St. Vincent, the Anglican Order and, as related before, the Holy Cross Order.[61] But, to provide more trained nurses, an Army nursing service was begun under the direction of Miss Dorothea Lynde Dix early in the war. "At her own suggestion, Dorothea Dix was appointed ... Superintendent of Women Nurses with the primary job of organizing and recruiting a corps of nurses to serve with the Union Army."[62] (Miss Dix is already renown for her "work for the insane and the improvement of prisons and almshouses."[63]) Mother Angela, of Holy Cross, "In preparation of sister-nurses . . . had certain advantages over . . . Superintendent Dorothea Dix. . . . The Holy Cross Sisters were already organized and disciplined."[64] Undoubtedly, Miss Dix has a job of gigantic frustrations in organization and discipline on the one hand and resistance to female nurses on the other. The Surgeon General of the Army, tries to help Superintendent Dix, as is evident in Circular No. 7 from the Surgeon General's Office in Washington, DC, dated 14 July 1862, "The Army regulations allow one nurse to every 10 patients [beds] in a general hospital. As it is the expressed will of the government that a portion of those nurses shall be women, and as Congress has given to the Surgeon General authority to decide in what numbers women shall be substituted for men, it is ordered that there shall be one woman nurse to two men nurses. Medical officers are hereby required to organize their respective hospitals accordingly. Medical officers requiring women nurses will apply to Miss Dix or to her authorized agent for the place where their hospitals are located. Sisters of Charity will be employed, as at present under special instructions from this office."[65]

Besides the efforts of these educated nurses, much untrained nursing is being attempted by patriotic and caring women such as Clara Barton (who goes on to found the American Red Cross.) Many relatives and friends of the troops and untrained enlisted men (whose names and numbers we will never know) do what they can to ease the suffering around them. "Some women there were doing what they could in home hospitals, taking in food dainties and doing those little extra things that make for comfort and peace of mind. Mrs. Mary Morris Husband was one of these. Both sons were in the Army and it was when one fell ill that Mrs. Husband entered her long career of active nursing service. She was on one of the hospital transports when it was bombarded. . . . [Despite this she continued working and later she went on board another hospital transport for the wounded, making several trips to care for these casualties, too.]"[66] Then, "among the many whose records one would wish to quote more fully [is] Mrs. Tyler [who] was better known as `Sister Tyler' of the Protestant Episcopal Church. She it was who found that the wounded of the Sixth Regiment Massachusetts Volunteers, attacked by the mob in Baltimore . . . as they were hurrying to the protection of the capitol, had been taken to a police station. It is quite a gripping story how she was at first denied admittance and later, after threatening to telegraph the governor, procured the men and took them to the Deaconesses' Home, where their wounds, unattended for eight or ten hours, were cared for. She was superintendent of [a hospital in Baltimore then another in Pennsylvania] . . . and then was placed in charge of the Naval School Hospital in Annapolis, which was receiving the "wrecks of humanity from the Prisons of Andersonville and Belle Isle."[67]

The Civil War ends in 1865. Five days after Lee's surrender, Abraham Lincoln is assassinated.[68]

"The Union Navy [comes] out of the war as the largest and most powerful naval force in the world."[69] Also, as a point of interest, during the war a Rear Admiral David G. Farragut led his squadron into battle in Mobile Bay, Alabama with the command, "Damn the torpedoes! Full steam ahead!"[70]

This Civil War with the resultant frightening numbers of sick, wounded and disabled, causes a tremendous public focus on the conditions of nurses and nursing. In fact, because of all the battle horrors and ravages of disease, changes in nursing are demanded and the trend toward major improvements begin. In 1869, the AMA begins to publicly acknowledge the need for adequate training of nurses and recommends "that schools of nursing be established in connection with hospitals all over the country."[71] There had been several attempts to start such schools before the Civil War, but they were not successful.

New England Hospital had been one of the hospitals making such an attempt. In 1872 this hospital opens its reorganized school of nursing with a mostly practical nursing program. ". . . hours [are] long and time off limited to an afternoon every two weeks. There are no night nurses. Very sick patients might interfere with the nurses' sleep, for their rooms [are] between wards. . . . little formal teaching and no textbooks. Some bedside instruction [is] provided by women interns."[72] 1873 and Bellevue Hospital, in New York, opens the first nursing school in the United States based on the system of Florence Nightingale.[73] For the student nurses, in these years, it is long hours and lowly, subservient duties. ". . . medications dispensed by number in order that their contents remain secret to all, but the initiated - among whom the nurses [are] not."[74] There is the attitude that nurses are being over-educated, that it is a waste to give so much education to the nurse who only needs to know the basics of nursing care.[75] Despite the hazards, a slow, but steady growth begins in nursing and in nursing education.

During this period, the Navy has been making progress of its own. In 1870 a Naval Hospital is constructed at Mare Island, California.[76] December of 1870 and the *Pawnee* (a veteran of Civil War combat) is commissioned as a hospital ship at the Navy Yard in Norfolk, Virginia. In early 1871 she sails for the Gulf of Mexico where she carries out her services as, "hospital, receiving and storeship."[77] In the Far East, the USS *Idaho* is serving as a hospital ship at Nagasaki, Yokosuka and Yokohama.[78] Then, on 3 March 1871, the Navy Medical Corps is established as a Staff Corps of the U.S. Navy. Also, the Chief of the Bureau of Medicine and Surgery is given the title of Surgeon General with the relative rank of Commodore.[79] It is about 1873 when the Navy ends the use of the title "nurse" aboard naval ships "and the title 'bayman' [comes] into use."[80] However, the Naval Hospitals keep and continue to use the designation, "nurse." Then in 1875 the U.S. Naval Hospital at Pensacola, Florida is opened.[81] It might be of interest to note that "attendants on the sick at the various [Navy] hospitals [during this span of time] are male nurses, selected from civil life by the medical officer in charge of the institution. They are paid from $15 to $25 per month, and are subject to instant dismissal for incompetency or misbehavior. The number employed is about one to every eight patients."[82]

Meantime, in the civilian world of nursing of 1879, a young lady by the name of Miss M.E.P. Mahoney graduates. She has finished her nurses training at the New England Hospital for Women. This is a noteworthy event because she is, "probably the first colored woman to graduate from a training-school for nurses."[83] Then in 1886, "the first training-school for colored nurses [is] established . . . at Spelman Seminary, Atlanta, Georgia."[84]

In 1887, the Navy opens a Naval Hospital at Widows Island in the state of Maine.[85] Also, in 1887, a civilian hospital, purportedly, distributes the following instructions to the nurses: (Only some of the instructions are shown here.)

"In addition to caring for your 50 patients, each nurse will:

> 1. Maintain an even temperature in your ward by bringing in a scuttle of coal for the day's business.
> 2. Light is important to observe the patient's condition. Therefore, each day fill kerosene lamps, clean chimneys, and trim wicks. Wash the windows once a week.
> 3. The nurse's notes are important in aiding the physician's work. Make your pens carefully; you may whittle nibs to your individual taste.
> 4. Each nurse on day duty will report every day at 7 a.m. and leave at 8 p.m., except on the Sabbath on which day you will be off from 12 to 2 p.m..
> 5. Any nurse who smokes, uses liquor in any form, gets her hair done at a beauty shop, or frequents dance halls will give the Director of Nurses good reason to suspect her worth, intentions and integrity."[86]

The year is 1888 and the Mills Training School for Men is founded in connection with the Bellevue Hospital of New York City. The school is "made possible by a substantial gift to the city by the philanthropist Darius Ogden Mills."[87] In a letter of presentation, Mr. Mills comments, "The training school for female nurses was a great gain. Personal observation of the good it has done has led me to think that an equal service might be rendered by an institution for the training of male nurses."[88] In 1888 the Mills Training School admits 15 male probationers, but only 4 manage to graduate. In 1889 there are 44 probationers and 18 of them stay to graduate.[89] "As with the female probationers . . . several men learned quickly that nursing duties were not what they had expected. There were cases of men who remained at the school for only one hour, for two hours, and for a fraction of a day. The men who did not graduate either were dismissed by the school or left by choice."[90]

The Provident Hospital of Chicago and Hampton Institute open training schools for colored nurses in 1891 followed by Tuskegee Institute in 1892.[91] Also, in 1891, "matrons [nurses] in the Indian Service are classified under Civil Service."[92] Could it be that the Federal Government is taking note of the profession of nursing and female graduate nurses?

In 1893 the American Association of the Red Cross becomes the American National Red Cross. Clara Barton has spent many years and much effort to bring this multi-national organization into the United States. (The United States became the thirty-second signatory power to the Geneva Red Cross Convention in 1882.)[93]

The first national nursing organization in the United States is established in January 1894. It is called the American Society of Superintendents of Training Schools.[94] The title of the organization defines the membership. (Later, in 1912, this organization becomes known as The National League of Nursing Education.[95])

You might like to know, as a small Navy medical historical aside, in 1895 it is "a court-martial offense to permit a nurse to take a patient's temperature. The use of this new and delicate instrument [assume this to be a thermometer] [is] delegated to the ward medical officer:

"Art. 1120 [Navy regulations] Medical officers in charge of wards will personally take the temperature of patients, and will never allow this duty to be performed by the nurses."[96]

Continuing with the Navy; in 1896 a U.S. Naval Hospital is built in Newport, Rhode Island. In 1898 two other Navy Hospitals are constructed; one in Sitka, Alaska and one in Canacao, the Philippine Islands.[97] In another part of the world, Cuba, a revolution is raging. It has been going on since 1895 between the Spanish rulers and the revolutionary rebels. William McKinley is President of the U.S. in 1898 and Theodore Roosevelt is an Assistant Secretary of the Navy.

On 25 January 1898, the U.S. Navy's battleship *Maine* arrives in Havana Harbor. Its mission is to protect the American citizens in the area. "On February 15, an explosion (blows) up the ship and [kills] 260 persons on board."[98] Americans immediately blame the Spanish and 'Remember the *Maine*' becomes a battle cry. "On April 25, the U.S. formally [declares] that a state of war existed with Spain as of April 21."[99] In May, the first battle of the war takes place in Manila Bay, Philippine Islands. Commodore George Dewey, with his squadron of six ships, destroys the entire Spanish fleet [10 ships] without loss of American personnel or an American ship. Back in the U.S., Theodore Roosevelt resigns as Assistant Secretary of the Navy so that he can fight in Cuba. He joins thousands of American troops who are sent to Cuba. They land and meet little resistance.[100] The efforts of Lieutenant Colonel Theodore Roosevelt with his contingent of men, the "Rough Riders," at San Juan Hill are featured in newspaper articles in the U.S. and they become instant heroes at home. In July, the Spaniards surrender.

During this Spanish-American War, "five colored nurses from Tuskegee [serve] in Cuba; a male negro nurse [is] in the U.S. Army service in the Philippines."[101] "Four young women from the Johns Hopkins Medical School [volunteer] their services as nurses, and are assigned to duty at the Naval Hospital, Brooklyn, New York.[102] Six women nurses from the registered list of the Daughters of the American Revolution and five Sisters of Charity at Norfolk also [volunteer], and [are] assigned to duty at the Naval Hospital, Norfolk, Virginia."[103] "When the [Navy] department [decides] to remove the [Spanish] prisoners from the destroyed Spanish fleet at Santiago [Cuba] to Portsmouth, New Hampshire, immediate preparation [is] necessary to care for the sick. . . . One hundred equipped cots and six trained nurses [are] generously supplied by the Red Cross Society."[104] "Early in May of 1898 four women graduate nurses [leave] Washington for Key West, Florida, under orders from the Surgeon General of the Army."[105]

The first trained nurses in the Navy were a group of women employed at the Naval Hospital, Norfolk, Virginia, also in 1898, to care for the sick and wounded of the Spanish-American War. These nurses were neither enrolled nor enlisted and were not sure of being paid for their services. [See footnote.[106]] A verbal agreement was made that they should be reimbursed for their traveling expenses and receive moderate pay if the means could be found for this reimbursement. Later, they were reimbursed from a fund not appropriated by Congress. They served for a period of fifty days.[107] Nurses in the Spanish-American war received $30.00 a month, plus ration allowances.[108] It seems that female graduate nurses are making the military medical departments "sit up and take notice" of the professional nurse.

About two weeks before war was declared, the Navy purchased a ship (the *Creole*) to outfit as a hospital ship. She was the first U.S. ship to "fly the Geneva Red Cross flag."[109] This ship was the first USS *Solace*. The medical personnel of the ship consisted of four doctors, "three hospital stewards, one of whom was a skilled embalmer, eight trained nurses, a cook, four messmen and two laundrymen."[110] The nurses and pharmacists were recruited from the Mills School of Nursing at New York. The rating of ship's cook-nurse was given to the nurses.[111] The first trip of the *Solace* is to Cuban waters to make rounds of the ships blockading Cuba. She picks up the sick and wounded and takes them to the New York Naval Hospital. Back she sails to Guantanamo to collect the wounded marines from the battle there. In July she collects more patients, delivering "44 Army wounded to Fortress Monroe [Virginia] and 55 Navy sick or wounded and 48 Spanish wounded at the Naval Hospital, Norfolk."[112] Then the *Solace* picks up stores, returns to Cuban waters, delivers stores to the blockade ships and takes their patients. She brings the patients back to Chelsea Naval Hospital in Boston and again to the hospital in New York.[113] Some patients brought back by the *Solace* are victims of yellow fever. The cause of yellow fever is still unknown at this time, but medical personnel are aware of the disease and aware of the hazard of importing it from Cuba. Some cases of it did appear among the marines at Key West, Florida.[114] Colonel William C. Gorgas, "a physician, [gains] fame by wiping out yellow fever in Havana, Cuba, after the Spanish-American War."[115] (This physician later gains further fame in the battle against yellow fever and malaria during the building of the Panama Canal in the early 1900's.[116])

Meanwhile, in May of 1898, the War Department purchases a Long Island steamer to convert to another hospital ship. This is the second USS *Relief*. She is prepared and ready to sail for Cuba on 2 July 1898.[117] On the 1st of July, a female graduate nurse reports aboard for the medical department. She is an Army contract nurse. Her name is Esther V. Hasson. (You might want to remember this name.) The ship sails on the 2nd and makes "regular trips between the West Indies and the Army hospital center at Montauk Point [Long Island]. For some time she [serves] at the latter port as a yellow fever hospital."[118] (Miss Hasson remains aboard until 14 November 1899. She is then transferred to the U.S. Army Transport *Sherman* destined for the Philippines, still as a contract nurse.) The Spanish-American War ends in August, 1898.

In the civilian world of nursing, 1898 sees the question of nurse licensure being debated. Graduate nurses have raised the principles and standards of their profession with their own endeavors and efforts and "it [is] but natural that they should look for official recognition and protection in some form of state licensure. Miss Nightingale's opposition to state registration [has] very little effect on this side of the Atlantic. The opposition in this country [comes] from outside groups. . . . The question [is] opened . . . at a meeting of the New York State Federation of Women's Clubs when Sophia Palmer [demands] state examining boards for nurses. The movement [is] at once started."[119] Thus, begins the system of state board examinations and the licensing of registered nurses.

Meanwhile, the Navy Medical Department has made organizational progress with the creation of a very vital entity, the U.S. Navy Hospital Corps. The Surgeon General of the Navy, Rear Admiral Rixey, reports, "On June 17 the President approved an act of Congress organizing a hospital corps of the Navy. The passage of this act is the culmination of the efforts of the bureau for many years. It will give the service a trained corps of men who will now have some reason for remaining in service, having a hope of promotion and advancement as the result of faithful service, sobriety and attention to duty. Its good results are already manifest; changes are being made as rapidly as practicable, and nearly all of the hospitals are now supplied with trained nurses, and in many of them are apprentices undergoing instruction."[120] (The trained nurses refer to those mentioned previously: the volunteers and the contract nurses.)

The next year, 1899, "The Surgeon General [is] authorized by the Navy department to employ and subsist trained nurses. Their number [is] not to exceed twenty at any one time, nor [is] their pay to exceed $4.00 per day."[121] (Again, these are contract nurses.)

At long last we reach the twentieth century. The country is enjoying prosperity along with the excitement of having won the Spanish-American War. It is a nation of gas lights, the horse and buggy, picnics, family sing-a-longs, and of rapid changes.[122] Also, this is an election year. President McKinley is running for re-election. He chooses Theodore Roosevelt as his vice presidential candidate. Their opponent, the Democratic party's candidate, is William Jennings Bryan. Even Mr. Bryan's famous 'silver-tongued' oratory is no match for the public popularity of the Republican candidates. The two Republicans are easily elected. (By the way, for you readers in the state of Florida, this is the year that "air conditioning" is invented in the U.S.[123]) It is a time of reform and change, and it is needed. "In 1900 unskilled workers - many of them children - [are] earning less than ten cents an hour for a twelve hour day."[124] It is a time of industrial revolution.

As for the nursing profession, it welcomes the new century with the publication of its own magazine, called the American Journal of Nursing. By this time, 1900, the field of nursing has grown in size and is proving itself a genuine profession. "More than 500 schools of nursing (have) graduated about 10,000 nurses.."[125] However, too many of the schools of nursing use the student nurses as nursing labor rather than hire the more expensive graduates. But there are many other varied openings for the female graduate nurses nowadays. The male graduate nurses are smaller in number and have fewer employment prospects. A study of the graduates of the Mills Training School (for male nurses) shows that "their work [is] limited to the fields of private duty and institutional nursing."[126] Of course, the male graduates can join the Army or Navy as nurses while female graduates are only offered duty in the Armed Forces as "contract" nurses. These are fairly limited positions. In 1901 the Congress changes this situation when legislation is passed creating the United States Army Nurse Corps. "The Nurse Corps (female) became a permanent corps of the medical department under the Army Reorganization Act. . . . Nurses were appointed in the Regular Army for a three-year period, although nurses were not actually commissioned as officers in the Regular Army."[127] The Navy did not follow suit, not yet.

On 5 September of 1901, President William McKinley is attending a public reception at the Pan-American Exposition in Buffalo, New York. An American-born anarchist stands in the crowd waiting to shake the President's hand. The assassin covers a pistol in his hand with a handkerchief. When the President draws near, the assassin fires. The President dies nine days later. Americans are stunned at the death of their popular President. (The assassin is caught, tried and, later, electrocuted.) Vice President Theodore Roosevelt takes the oath of office as President.[128]

"Teddy" Roosevelt is now at the helm of the government, a government of some forty-five states. This is the President who's motto in foreign policy is "walk softly and carry a big stick." He is the man of the moment and many believe he is the right man for the moment. The country is in need of a strong, popular decision-maker, as in the person of T. Roosevelt.

It is 1901 and the hem line of women's skirts is going up. A short skirt is now being worn. (". . . a short skirt (is) one that [shows] the shoes."[129]) Women are becoming more active. They are even beginning to take jobs as secretaries since the typewriter has been invented. Teaching and nursing had traditionally been the proper fields of women's work.[130] Female emancipation and suffrage [are] becoming prominent social issues.[131]

In the 1902 Report of the Surgeon General of the Navy is a section entitled, "Women Nurses For Naval Hospitals." In this brief segment he indicates that the general opinion of the Bureau of Medicine and the doctors is that women are the better of the trained nurses and that Naval Hospitals would benefit with their presence. The Surgeon General goes on to write, "It is recommended, therefore, that Congress be asked to provide at its coming session for the establishment of a woman nurse corps for the Navy, to consist at first of 1 superintendent nurse, 8 head nurses, 16 nurses of the first class and 24 of the second class. These numbers to be increased at the discretion of the Secretary [of the Navy] as the needs of the service indicate.[132]

In 1902 a bill [is] introduced in the Senate providing for the establishment or organization of the Navy Nurse Corps.[133] Within this bill, "The range of age [is] from twenty-six to forty years, and nurses [are] to be relieved from active duty after fifteen years of continuous service or sooner if incapacitated from any cause originating in the line of duty. Those relieved from active duty (are) to constitute the reserve of the nurse corps.

. . . The bill also [provides] that the nurses receive the same mileage as provided by law for officers while traveling under orders in the United States. The initial pay period recommended [is] $50 a Month." This bill did not pass Congress.[134]

Meanwhile, down in Portsmouth, Virginia at the Norfolk Naval Hospital, "the first formal course of instruction of members of the [hospital] corps [is] begun."[135] The course is described as a three months course following which the men are given certificates of completion. The men are then sent out to various Naval Hospitals.[136] It is interesting to note that the instructor for the course in "nursing and ward management" is a hospital steward. (According to a bayman of this era, the hospital steward is a Chief Petty Officer, later entitled Chief Pharmacist's Mate. This same source states, "Next to the doctor was an apothecary. He mixed up the medicine. And the bayman, he did [the] other work . . . in the sick bay."[137])

It is 1903 and the Navy has a new Naval Hospital in Bremerton, Washington.[138] And in Washington, DC, Congress appropriates money for the Navy to build a new Naval Hospital on Observatory Hill[139] (where the Navy's Bureau of Medicine and Surgery is now located.) Construction begins the next year. (Interestingly, the architect that designed the Corcoran Gallery in DC is the same one who drew the plans for this Naval Hospital.[140]) This year, 1904, is the year the Navy again tries to obtain a Nurse Corps. A bill is sent to Congress. This one recommends a pay of $40 per month and there is no mention of retirement or disability provisions. Again, the bill does not pass.[141]

1905 and the new President of the United States is the old president. Theodore Roosevelt is elected after finishing McKinley's term in office. Additionally, this year sees a 26-year-old physicist, Albert Einstein, publishes his theory of relativity.[142] Meantime, the Navy has decided to refit and bring back into service the hospital ship *Relief*; the ship had been decommissioned in 1902. "The refitting job [is] considerably hampered by a policy wrangle . . . as to whether it should be commanded by a medical officer or a line officer. Surgeon General Rixey [insists] on a medical officer in command, and the argument [grows] so hot that the [Navy] department finally [refers] the matter to the president for decision."[143] The president eventually decides in favor of the Surgeon General so a medical officer is to be in command of the ship.[144]

This is the year (1905) that Japan wins the Russo-Japanese War. President Roosevelt goes on to win the Nobel Peace Prize, in 1906, for his help in ending that war. 1906 also watches the devastation and loss of 452 lives in the massive San Francisco earthquake and fire.[145] Back in Washington, DC, the first patients are admitted to the new Naval Hospital on Observatory Hill and more new plans are being developed for the site. The plans are for a "contagious disease hospital, quarters for hospital corpsmen, sick officers' quarters, **nurses quarters**, and three houses for junior and senior medical officers."[146]

Nursing education has been growing in leaps and bounds. Now the universities are beginning to take note of the profession and its needs for further education. In 1907 The Teachers College in Columbia University (New York) establishes a chair for a professor in nursing and health. The first nurse to be appointed a full university professor is selected.[147] But where is our Navy Nurse Corps? At this point, it appears to be a militant glint in the eye of the Navy's Surgeon General. In his 1907 Report of Surgeon General, Rear Admiral Rixey says, "The desirability of this addition [women nurses] to our facilities for the efficient care of the sick and injured of the service has been made the subject of careful consideration from all points of view by the bureau, and the oft-asserted merits of the proposed departure from long-established custom, which it entails, can no longer be viewed as merely problematical." (One has to wonder if this can refer to reasons for previous non-passage of bills to create the Nurse Corps.)

The Surgeon General goes on to add, "Moreover, in addition to supplying more efficient medical and surgical nursing than is now obtainable, valuable services could be rendered by the trained women nurses in teaching the men of the hospital corps their special duties in caring for the sick, so that when they come to serve on board ship or at distant stations they will be prepared, with greater surety, to render services in accord with the best usages."

Towards the end of his report, Rear Admiral Rixey forcefully addresses the politicians when he states, "It is impossible to find adequate reason for the difficulty experienced in obtaining favorable congressional consideration of such a meritorious measure of relief. Economy itself dictates this provision. The desirability of trained women nurses in the medical branch of the naval service has for five years been urged upon the department, and. with its permission, upon Congress. The bureaus's representation of this measure, the importance of which it urges, has been persistent and forceful, and it has been explained how the lack of proper nursing means greater suffering. The officers and enlisted men enter the Navy with the assurance that they will be taken care of when disabled by disease or wound or injury. The Government supplies physicians and surgeons, splendidly equipped hospitals, and complete emergency facilities on every ship. The most serious omission in this excellent establishment is the want of that skilled nursing which civil institutions enjoy."[148] (The bill will come up in Congress next year, 1908.)

Meantime, Great Lakes, Illinois sees a Naval Hospital built and the United States Naval Medical Bulletin is first published in 1907. And, not the least of events, the United States Navy proceeds to impress the world with its "Great White Fleet." This is the result of a decision by President Roosevelt to counteract strained relations with Japan. When Roosevelt attended the peace talks between Japan and Russia in 1905, he had angered the Japanese with his opposition to Japanese demands for compensation payments from Russia. The Japanese anger increased when, in 1906, "the San Francisco school board decided to segregate children of Japanese descent."[149] Sixteen new U.S. Navy battleships are painted white and the Commander-in-Chief sends them on a world wide good-will tour for 14 months. "The fleet [receives] enthusiastic welcomes in Japan and other countries. Roosevelt [views] the tour as a part of 'big stick' diplomacy."[150]

Now, 1908. A momentous year. On "February 6, 1908, the *Relief* [is] placed in commission under the command of a medical officer, Surgeon Charles F. Stokes."[151] Then, a very brief bill is placed before Congress. It asks for the establishment of the U.S. Navy Nurse Corps. The bill is passed.

[1]   *200 Years, A Bicentennial Illustrated History of the United States,* Joseph Newman, Directing Editor, Books by U.S. News & World Report, Inc., 2300 N Street, N.W., Washington, DC 20037, 1973, Book 1, p. 317.

[2]   *The Columbia-Viking Desk Encyclopedia,* by staff of the Columbia Encyclopedia, William Bridgwater, Editor-in-chief, The Viking Press, New York, 1953, p. 1003.

[3]   *The World Book Encyclopedia,* Field Enterprises Educational Corporation, Chicago, Volume 12, 1966 edition, p. 235.

[4]   Roddis, Louis H., M.D., Captain MC USN, *A Short History of Nautical Medicine,* Paul B. Hoeber, Inc., Medical Book Dept. of Harper Brothers, 1941, p.263.

[5]   Dixon HC USN, Lt. Ben F., "The "White Lily," *Hospital Corps QUARTERLY,* Hospital Ships Number, July 1945, p. 7.

[6]   Holcomb, Richard C., M.D., F.A.C.S., Captain, Medical Corps, U.S. Navy, *A Century With Norfolk Naval Hospital, 1830-1930,* Printcraft Publishing Co., 1930, p. 370.

[7]   Dixon, op. cit., p. 7.

[8]   Barton, Dr. William Paul Crillon, *A Treatise Containing a Plan for the Internal Organization and Government of Marine Hospitals in the United States together with a Scheme for Amending and Systematizing the Medical Department of the Navy,* Philadelphia, 1814, Preface p. x.

[9]   *The World Book Encyclopedia,* op. cit., Volume 20, p. 26.

[10]   Ibid., p. 26.

[11]   Ibid., Volume 14, p. 80.

[12]   Ibid., Volume 5, p. 59.

[13]   Langley, Harold D., "Women in a Warship, 1813," *Proceedings*, U.S. Naval Institute, Washington, DC, 110:1, p. 124.

[14]   Ibid., p. 125.

[15]   Pleadwell, Frank Lester, Captain MC USN, "William Paul Crillon Barton (1786-1856), Surgeon, United States Navy-A Pioneer in American Naval Medicine," *The Military Surgeon,* Vol.XLVI, Number 3, March, 1920, p. 241.

[16]   Barton, op. cit., p.100.

[17]   Ibid., pp. 100-101.

[18]   Barton, Dr. William Paul Crillon, (as quoted in, "History of Nursing in the Navy" by J. Beatrice Bowman, R.N., *The American Journal of Nursing,* Vol. XXVIII, Number 9, September, 1928, p.6.)

[19]   Pleadwell, op. cit., p. 243.

[20]   Ibid., p. 244.

[21]   Ibid., p. 245.

[22]   "White Task Force - the story of the Nurse Corps United States Navy," (NAV MED 939, Bureau of Medicine and Surgery, United States Navy), U.S. Government Printing Office, 1945, fourth page.

[23]   *Webster's New Universal Unabridged Dictionary (Deluxe Second Edition),* Revised by the Publisher's Editorial Staff Under the General Supervision of Jean L. McKechnie, New World Dictionaries/Simon and Schuster, New York, 1979, p.1403.

[24]   Dixon, op. cit., p. 6.

[25]   Roddis, op. cit., p.262.

[26]   *The Act of August 31, 1842*, Chapter CCLXXXVI, Stat. 5, page 579.

[27]   Holcomb, op. cit., p. 370.

[28]   Dickens, Charles, *Martin Chuzzlewit*, Oxford University Press, Oxford, New York, 1984, p. 269. (Edited with an introduction and notes by Margaret Cardwell.)

[29]   Ibid., p.269.

[30]   Ibid., p. 605.

[31]   Deloughery, Grace L., *History and trends of professional nursing*, The C.V. Mosby Co., 11830 Westline Industrial Drive, St. Louis, Missouri 63141, 1977, p. 69.

[32]   Ibid., p. 68.

[33]   *The World Book Encyclopedia*, op. cit., Volume 14, p. 328.

[34]   Ibid., p. 329.

[35]   Longfellow, Henry Wadsworth, *Longfellow's Poetical Works*, George Routledge and Sons, Limited, London, Author's Copyright Edition (before 1892), p. 459.

[36]   Holcomb, op. cit., p. 376.

[37]   Grupp, George W., "Navy Used First Hospital Ship To Treat Civil War Wounded," *Navy Times*, December 5, 1953, p.13.

[38]   Dixon, op. cit., p. 9.

[39]   Ibid., p. 9.

[40]   Roddis, op. cit., p. 262.

[41]   Alcott, Louisa May, *Hospital Sketches*, Sagamore Press, Inc., New York, 1957, pp. 47, 48.

[42]   Ibid., p. 57.

[43]   Dixon, op. cit., pp. 14-15.

[44]   Ibid., p. 16.

[45]   Ibid., p. 15.

[46]   Holcomb, op. cit., p. 450.

[47]   Jolly, Ellen Ryan, LL.D, *Nuns of The Battlefield*, Providence Visitor Press, Providence, Rhode Island, 1927, p.p. 144-145.

[48]   Sister M. John Francis, C.S.C. of Holy Cross Central School of Nursing in South Bend, Indiana, "Holy Cross Sisters As U.S. Navy Nurses," for the *Jacksonville Journal Courier*, press release mailed 10 December 1962, p.1. (Copy provided by courtesy of Sister Alma Louise of the Archives of St. Mary's College, Indiana. -Author.)

[49]   "Civil War Hospital Ship," *All Hands, (Bureau of Naval Personnel Information Bulletin)*, February, 1962, p.60. (The article is based upon the official ship's history, made available through the courtesy of the Ships' History Section, Naval History Division, Office of the Chief of Naval Operations.)

[50]   Ibid., p.60.

[51]   Sister M. John Francis, C.S.C. of Holy Cross Central School of Nursing in South Bend, Indiana, op. cit., p.3.

[52]   Goble, Dorothy Jones, CDR NC USN, unpublished history research notes indicating this information obtained at the National Archives from the complete descriptive muster roll of the crew of the U.S. Naval Hospital, *Red Rover*.

[53]   Webster's New Universal Unabridged Dictionary, op. cit., p. 396.

[54]   Ibid., p.3.

[55]   Ibid., p.5.

[56]   *All Hands*, February 1962, op. cit., p.62.

[57]   Jolly, op. cit., p.142.

[58]   Ibid., p.143.

[59]   Ibid., p.143.

[60]   *All Hands*, February 1962, op. cit., p.63.

[61]   Hickey, Dermott Vincent, *The First Ladies In The Navy - A History of the Navy Nurse Corps, 1908-1939*, June 1963, p.22. (An unpublished thesis submitted to the Faculty of Columbian College of The George Washington University in partial satisfaction of the requirements for the degree of Master of Arts.)

[62]   Holm, Jeanne Maj. Gen. USAF (Ret.), *Women in the Military*, Presidio Press, 31 Pamaron Way, Novato, CA 94947, 1982, p.8.

[63]   Stimson, Major Julia C.,ANC and Thompson, Miss Ethel C.S., "Women Nurses With The Union Forces During The Civil War," *The Military Surgeon*, Vol. 62, January 1928, No. 1, p.3.

[64]   Sister M. John Francis, C.S.C. of Holy Cross Central School of Nursing in South Bend, Indiana, op. cit., p.6.

[65]   Stimson and Thompson, op. cit., p.228-229. (Directly quoted from CIRCULAR No. 7 as it appears in the APPENDIX of the cited article. -Author.)

[66]   Ibid.,pp.211-212.

[67]   Ibid., p.215. (Stimson and Thompson note as reference for this information; Dr. Brockett and Mrs. Vaughan, *Woman's Work in the Civil War*. -Author.)

[68]   *200 Years, A Bicentennial Illustrated History of the United States*, op. cit., Book 2, p. 306.

[69]   *The World Book Encyclopedia*, op. cit., Volume 14, p. 81.

[70]   Ibid., p. 80.

[71]   Jensen, Deborah MacLurg, R.N., M.A., *A History of Nursing*, The C.V. Mosby Company, St. Louis, 1943, p. 157.

[72]   Ibid., p. 162.

[73]   *Encyclopedia Americana*, Grolier, Inc., Danbury, Connecticut 06816, 1981, Vol. 20.

[74]   Jensen, op. cit., p. 166.

[75]   Ibid., p. 167. (Even in my time, 1954, an intelligent, young Navy surgeon asked, "Why do you want to go off to school again [for a B.S.]? You don't need all that education. We don't want to lose a good nurse." - Author)

[76]   Roddis, op. cit., p. 263.

77 "A 1971 View of The Medical Corps Circa 1871," *U.S. Navy Medicine*, Captain M. T. Lynch MC USN, Editor, U.S. Naval Publications and Forms Center, Phila., PA 19120, U.S. Navy Medicine Volume 57, March 1971, p. 52.

78 Ibid., p. 50.

79 Ibid., p. 49.

80 Holcomb, op. cit., p. 453.

81 Roddis, op. cit., p. 263.

82 Gatewood, J.D., M.D., Passed Assistant Surgeon, United States Navy, *Notes on Naval Hospitals, Medical Schools, and Training School For Nurses, with A Sketch of Hospital History*, Press of the Friedenwald Co., Baltimore, 1893, p. 259.

83 Goodnow, Minnie, *Outlines of Nursing History*, W.B. Saunders and Company, Philadelphia and London, 1916, p. 163.

84 Ibid., p. 163.

85 Roddis, op. cit., p. 263.

86 *Direct Line - a report to Direct Payment Subscribers*, New Jersey Blue Cross Plan and New Jersey Blue Shield Plan, Newark, Trenton, Camden, Morristown, No. 8, Spring 1970, backpage.

87 Roberts, Mary M., *American Nursing: History and Interpretation*, Macmillan Company, New York, 1954, p. 315.

88 Ibid., p. 315.

89 Mottus, Jane E., *New York Nightingales: The Emergence of the Nursing Profession at Bellevue and New York Hospital 1850-1920*, UMI Research Press, 1981, Table 30, "Attrition Rates of the Probationers of the Mills Training School, 1888-1918."

90 Ibid., p. 106.

91 Goodnow, op. cit., p. 163.

92 Vreeland, Ellwynne M., R.N., "Fifty Years of Nursing in the Federal Government Nursing Services," *The American Journal of Nursing*, Vol. 50, No. 10, October 1950, p. 626.

93 Dixon, op. cit., p. 18.

94 Jensen, op. cit., p. 179.

95 Ibid., p. 180.

96 Holcomb, op. cit., p. 454.

97 Roddis, op. cit., pp. 262,263.

98 *The World Book Encyclopedia*, op. cit., Volume 17, p. 590.

99 Ibid., p. 590.

100 Ibid., p. 590.

101 Goodnow, op. cit., p. 163.

102 Goble, CDR Dorothy Jones, NC USN, Unpublished history research notes as follows:

"Those who served at U.S.N.H. New York, N.Y.(.) Reporting Tues(day) next after June 3, 1898, and serving until approximately July 28,1898.

Miss Margaret Long
Miss Dorothy Reed
Miss Mable P. Simis
Miss Mabel F. Austin

103 *Report of the Surgeon-General of the Navy*, Government Printing Office, 1898, p. 6.

104 Ibid., p. 6.

105 Hasson, Esther V., R.N., "The Navy Nurse Corps," *The American Journal Of Nursing*, Volume IX, March, 1909, p. 410.

106 Goble, op. cit., from the same unpublished history research notes:

"Names and length of time volunteer nurses and sisters of charity, who served at U.S. Naval Hosp., Norfolk(Portsmouth), during July, Aug. (and) Sept. 1898.

Name	Time
1. Mrs. Emilyn Mann	63 da.
2. Miss Wilhelmine Geisemann	63 da.
3. " Lula M. Plant	63 da.
4. " Lucy N. White	63 da.
5. " Rebecca Jackson	49 da.
6. " Caroline Patterson	47 da.
7. Sister Magdalen Kelleher	55 nights
8. " Chrysostom Moneyhan	55 "
9. " Cecelia Beck	55 "
10. " Victorine Salazar	55 "
11. " Mary Larkin	55 "

107 Bowman, J. Beatrice, R.N., "History of Nursing in the Navy," The American Journal of Nursing, Vol. XXVIII, Number 9, September, 1928. (Miss Bowman was the third Director of the Navy Nurse Corps; see Chapter III. - Author)

108 Deloughery, op. cit., p. 75.

109 Dixon, op. cit., p. 20.

110 Holcomb, op. cit., p. 329.

111 Dixon, op. cit., p. 20.

112 Holcomb, op. cit., p. 329.

113 Ibid., pp. 329. 330.

114 Ibid., p. 330.

[115]   *The World Book Encyclopedia*, op. cit., Volume 15, p, 106.
[116]   Ibid., pp. 101, 106, 107.
[117]   Dixon, op. cit., p.10.
[118]   Ibid., p.10.
[119]   Jensen, op. cit., p. 198.
[120]   Surgeon General's Report, 1898, op. cit., p. 6.
[121]   "Navy Nurse Corps-A Pictorial Review," *United States Navy Medical Newsletter*, Captain M.T. Lynch MC USN, Editor, op. cit., Volume 55, No. 5, May 1970, p. 6.
[122]   *Great Events of the 20th Century*, Editor: Richard Marshall, The Readers' Digest Association, Inc., 1977, p. 94.
[123]   Ibid., p. 29.
[124]   Ibid., p. 94.
[125]   Deloughery, op. cit., p. 75.
[126]   Mottus, Jane E., op. cit., p. 161.
[127]   *Highlights In The History of the Army Nurse Corps*, edited by Colonel Robert V. Piemonte ANC USAR and Major Cindy Gurney ANC, U.S. Army Center of Military History, Washington, D.C., 1987, p. 6.
[128]   *The World Book Encyclopedia*, op. cit., Volume 13, p. 276.
[129]   *Great Events of the 20th Century*, op. cit., p. 94.
[130]   Ibid..
[131]   Ibid..
[132]   Rixey, Rear Admiral Presley Marion MC USN, *Report of the Surgeon General of the Navy*, 1902, p. 13.
[133]   Bowman, op. cit., p. 887.
[134]   Ibid..
[135]   Holcomb, op. cit., p. 454.
[136]   Ibid., p. 454.
[137]   Cooney, John (Hospital Steward/Chief Pharmacist's Mate), *Oral History Interview Tape Transcript*, Interviewer Irene Smith Matthews, taped in 1971.
[138]   Roddis, op. cit., p. 263.
[139]   Herman, Jan K., Historian at the Naval Medical Command, Department of the Navy, *A Hilltop in Foggy Bottom (Home of the Old Naval Observatory and the Navy Medical Department)*, Reprinted from U.S. Navy Medicine, 1984, p. 68.
[140]   Ibid., p. 71.
[141]   Bowman, op. cit., p. 887.
[142]   *The World Book Encyclopedia*, op. cit., Volume 16, p. 428.
[143]   Dixon, op. cit., p. 10.
[144]   Ibid., p. 10.
[145]   *The World Book Encyclopedia*, op. cit., Volume 16, p. 428.
[146]   Herman, op. cit., p. 71.
[147]   Jensen, op. cit., p. 183.
[148]   Rixey, Rear Admiral Presley Marion MC USN, *Report of Surgeon-General United States Navy*, 1907, pp. 26-28.
[149]   *The World Book Encyclopedia*, op. cit., Volume 16, p. 431.
[150]   Ibid..
[151]   Holcomb, op. cit., p. 380.

"... in 1895 it is 'a court-martial offense to permit a nurse to take a patient's temperature.' ..."

☆ ☆ ☆

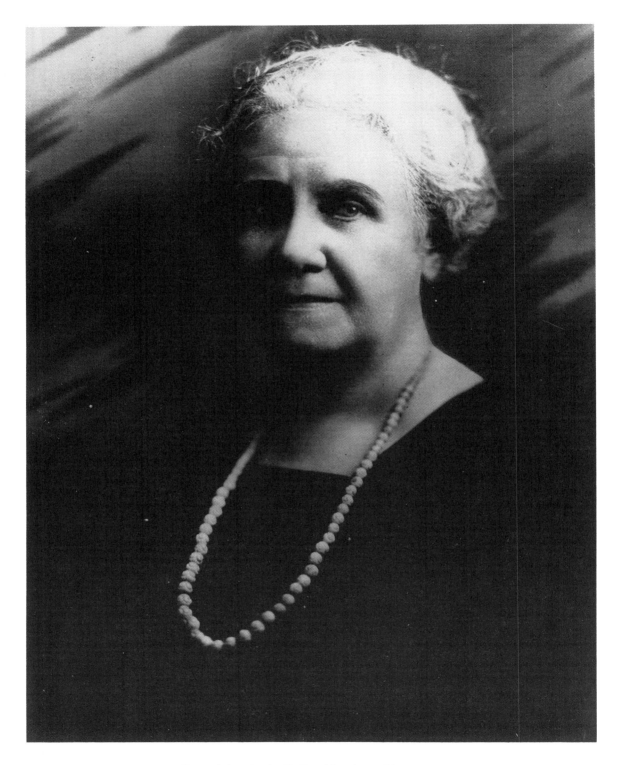

Superintendent - Esther Voorhees Hasson.
(Official U.S. Navy photo courtesy of Nursing Division, Bureau of Medicine and Surgery, Navy Department.)

CHAPTER 1

Superintendent - Esther Voorhees Hasson
(1908 - 1911)

☆☆☆

On 13 May 1908, J. Beatrice Bowman (destined to be the third Superintendent of the Navy Nurse Corps) is practicing her profession of nursing with the Red Cross in the deep South. She is having her first disaster experience in Hattiesburg, Mississippi. "There was a big tornado down there and there were groups from New York and Philadelphia and some place else. . . I met Miss [Hewitt] there in the Washington group and we got to talking . . . I told her I was very anxious to go into the Navy. She said the Bill was being passed upon today! She said she'd learn tomorrow if it was passed and . . . [let me] know. And sure enough, the Bill had passed and we could apply. [Miss Hewitt] said, 'Now as soon as you go home, you put in your application.' Which I did."[1] Miss Bowman goes on to relate, "We had written examinations . . . and no other classes had even gone through what we went through for three days!"[2]

At last, the United States has a Navy Nurse Corps. This is the Bill that Congress passes: "The Nurse Corps (female) of the United States Navy is hereby established, and shall consist of one superintendent, to be appointed by the Secretary of the Navy, who shall be a graduate of a hospital training school having a course of instruction of not less than two years, whose term of office may be terminated at his discretion, and of as many chief nurses, nurses and reserve nurses as may be needed: *Provided*, that all nurses in the Nurse Corps shall be appointed or removed by the Surgeon General, with the approval of the Secretary of the Navy, and that they shall be graduates of hospital training schools having a course of instruction not less than two years. The appointment of superintendent, chief nurses, nurses, and reserve nurses shall be subject to an examination as to their professional, moral, mental, and physical fitness, and that they shall be eligible for duty at naval hospitals and on board of hospital and ambulance ships and for such special duty as may be deemed necessary by the Surgeon General of the Navy. Reserve nurses may be assigned to active duty when the necessities of the service demand, and when on such duty shall receive the pay and allowances of nurses: *Provided*, that they shall receive no compensation except when on active duty. The superintendent, chief nurses, and nurses shall respectively receive the same pay, allowances, emoluments, and privileges as are now or may hereafter be provided by or in pursuance of law for the Nurse Corps (female) of the Army."[3]

The Surgeon General, in his 1908 report, says, "The enactment of authority for the establishment of a corps of female nurses . . . is a source of great gratification to the bureau." Later, in this report, Admiral Rixey writes, "The bureau had inquired into the eligibility of candidates for the position of superintendent, an appointment to this office constituting a prerequisite to the admission of nurses, and on July 21, 1908, the bureau, as a result of the above investigation, recommended . . . a board of medical officers to examine Miss E.V. Hasson as to her qualifications for the position. This candidate was selected on account of her long and meritorious record and experience both in civil and military life [as Army contract nurse, Army nurse, civil service nurse[4]], including service in the Philippines, the hospital ship *Relief*, and on the Isthmus of Panama. In pursuance to orders the above-mentioned board . . . made recommendation . . . that she be appointed. Her appointment was issued on August 18, 1908, and on the following day she reported to the Surgeon General for duty."[5] The indoctrination of the nurses is addressed with these remarks, "The bureau confidently expects that by October 1 a corps of 20 nurses will have been organized. . . . The bureau [proposes] that all recruits in the corps, before being distributed to the various hospitals and other stations, shall be ordered to Washington for a period of from four to six months, where, while at the same time rendering practical services at the Naval Medical School Hospital [the hospital on Observatory Hill] under the guidance of its commanding officer, they will be under the observation of the bureau and superintendent of nurses and will receive such general and special instruction as will familiarize them with the naval service and better fit them to perform their duties in the new environment."[6]

Then the Surgeon General turns to the general plan for the assignments of the nurses, "As regards the initial nucleus of 20 nurses, the bureau intends that a certain number, including a chief nurse, will be at once assigned to permanent duty at the Naval Medical School Hospital, and that the others, including a chief nurse, will be placed under instruction for assignment to one of the other large hospitals (New York) as soon as adjusted to military conditions and other wise prepared to take up practical work in the naval service. And so, as the corps is gradually enlarged, each new group will be assembled in Washington, where they will be critically observed and tutored in the requirements of the naval service, and then ordered wherever they may be needed until all hospitals or other stations have their allotted complement."[7]

At the end of his report, he lists where nurses' duty stations will be, "The hospitals at which it is at present intended female nurses shall be detailed are as follows: Washington [DC], New York, Las Animas [a naval hospital in Colorado which is transferred to the Army in 1922[8]], Mare Island [California], Canacao [Philippines], Norfolk, Chelsea [Massachusetts], Philadelphia, Newport, Annapolis, Puget Sound [Washington], Yokohama [Japan]."[9]

In the Sunday edition of The New York Times on 9 August 1908, an item appears about all this. The item is entitled "Women Nurses For Navy" with a subtitle "Will Be Used in Hospitals-Miss Hassan to be Chief." (They misspelled her name!) The article appears right next to an item of the same length that is titled "Cat Uses The Elevator" with a subtitle of "This is a True Story About Thomas of the Times Building." So much for the importance as seen by The Times' editors. But then on 4 September 1908, The New York Times publishes another article. This one is much shorter and is headlined "Made Chief Woman Nurse" with a subtitle of "Miss Hassan, First to Hold the Office, Has Had War Experience." (They are still misspelling her name.) This time the article is placed directly above an article about "A Monument to Mr. Rockefeller."

Esther Voorhees Hasson was born in Baltimore, Maryland. She was educated in private schools in Washington, DC and Germantown, Pennsylvania. Miss Hasson did her nurses training at the Connecticut Training School for Nurses in New Haven, Connecticut. Her father was a Major (and a surgeon) in the Army during the Civil War. Her brother attended the Naval Academy at Annapolis, serving two years in the Navy until his death in 1903. The military background of her family members, her own military experiences as an Army contract nurse and Army nurse, are to be of great benefit in her new position. The benefit is not only to Miss Hasson, but to the establishment of the Navy Nurse Corps itself. This corps will have a solid foundation.

Miss Hasson is forty-one years old when she executes the oath of office as first Superintendent of the U.S. Navy Nurse Corps, 18 August 1908. Hers is the application selected from the three received by BuMed (Bureau of Medicine and Surgery.) Before being selected she is required to appear before a Board of Examiners in Washington, DC. (The "board" mentioned previously in the 1908 Report of Surgeon General.) (Interesting that the trip has to be made at her own expense.) She is given an "oral examination in nursing, first aid, therapeutics, Materia Medica subjects and general education. She writes an examination consisting of four parts: '1) Give a short account of your life, including education, professional work and any factors bearing on your fitness for Superintendent of a Nurse Corps. 2) Outline the duties of a nurse in military service. 3) Give a scheme for the organization of a female nurse corps of the Navy. 4) Outline a scheme of office organization and records for a corps of female nurses in the Navy."[10] (How would any one of us answer such sweeping and consequential essay questions?)

In March 1909, an article appears in the American Journal of Nursing. It is written by Superintendent Hasson and entitled, "The Navy Nurse Corps." She explains how the corps began, how to apply, how nurses will be chosen, where they will be assigned and, most important, what will be expected of them. This farseeing, innovative lady sets the tone and whole course of the Navy Nurse Corps, for the present and for all time to come when she writes, "Undoubtedly the future status of the Navy corps will rest largely in the hands of its members, and especially is this true of the first nurses. If they are content with low standards either professionally, morally, or socially the status of the corps will be fixed for all time. Future women will accept the standard set by us now without question; if it be high they will rise to it, if it be low they will with equal facility drop to its level.

"We nurses who come into the nursing service of the Navy during this first year of its existence are the pioneers, and it rests with us to make the traditions and to set the pace for those who are to follow."[11] She goes on to say that all nurses selected for the Nurse Corps will spend their probationary period at the Washington Naval Hospital. At that time, the selectees are "expected to inform themselves in regard to the rules, regulations and etiquette of the service, also of the different degrees of rank with insignia of same, not alone of the commissioned officers, but of the warrant and petty officers. . . . Head nurse positions will in all cases be filled by promotions from the grade of nurse."[12] Then she points out, "We hope to make the nursing in our eighteen general hospitals somewhat uniform, so that when ordered from one to the other the nurse will know about the conditions she will encounter in regard to scope of work, hours of duty, duration and frequency of night details, personal privileges, etc."[13]

In the next paragraph of her article, Miss Hasson presents the very core of Navy nursing, "One of the principal duties of the woman nurse in the Navy will be the bedside instruction of the hospital apprentices in the practical essentials of nursing, and for this reason she must be thoroughly conversant with the head nurse routine of a ward. When treatments, baths, or medication come due it is not expected or desired that she will always give these herself, but it will be her duty to see that the apprentices [hospital corpsmen] attached to the ward carry out the orders promptly and intelligently. This arrangement does not, however, absolve the nurse in any way from doing the actual nursing work whenever necessary, but is in a line with the general principle . . . which she is expected to . . . keep uppermost in her mind. I mean the improvement of the apprentices to whom the bulk of the nursing of the Navy afloat will always fall."[14] (For those of you not familiar with Navy nursing, the corpsmen of the Navy must be well trained. This is because, many times, particularly on the smaller Navy ships, the corpsman is the only person aboard with medical knowledge. Additionally, the corpsmen are assigned to U.S. Marine Corps Units and go with the Units in battle and on military exercises. They must be able to care for casualties and emergencies until more expert help is available.)

Next, Miss Hasson speaks of the personal qualities that a Navy Nurse must have. Truly, the spirit, heart and soul of a Navy Nurse is remarkably portrayed by her words; it cannot be written any better: "the cheerful disposition that accepts the ups and downs incidental to changes of station; that adapts itself easily to new environment; that accepts the undesirable detail without complaint and confidently looks forward to the better luck that will surely come next time. Above all she must possess in the highest degree the quiet dignity of bearing which alone can command respect from the apprentices or male nurses whom she must instruct. Although she possesses all else, and yet lacks this one quality, she had best seek another vocation at once as she would be absolutely useless for the work we wish her to do. The ability to get on with others will also be a very valuable adjunct. Ample authority will be given the nurse in all that pertains to the nursing, but we all know that there are women who can produce good results and maintain discipline without keeping things constantly in a state of turmoil. . . . the woman who can inspire the male nurses with a pride in their work and a desire to learn, and who at the same time can reduce to a minimum the friction always incidental to a change in the old order of things, will be the most valuable woman for naval work. Failure to get on harmoniously with co-workers of the corps would be another decided drawback to success. In other words, dignity, self-control and courtesy are the keynotes to the situation. . . . it is my most earnest hope to make it (the Navy Nurse Corps) a dignified, respected body of women, governed largely by that feeling of *esprit de corps* without which no rules ever devised will be of avail to keep us free from all that approaches scandal or disagreeable comment."[15]

Next comes the business of selecting and appointing nineteen more nurses for this new Corps. Out of thirty-three applicants, nineteen are selected.[16] "Considering the period, requirements were high. Applicants were to be graduates of a general hospital school having a course of instruction of not less than two years; clinical experience in medical, surgical, care of men, and contagious diseases. All instruction and experiences must have been in a hospital. Private duty while students [common practice at this time] was not acceptable. If the state had registration, the applicant was to be registered; if no state licensure, she was to be a member in good standing of the Nurses' Associated Alumnae of the United States (now ANA). U.S. citizenship was preferred but was not a requirement."[17] Also, "If accepted and [the applicant's] services were not immediately required, the nurse's name was placed on the eligible list . . . but this was not done unless she agreed to serve in the Nurse Corps . . . for at least three years after appointment. All of the appointments of the Nurse Corps were made by the Surgeon General with the approval of the Secretary of the Navy. Nurses could be discharged from the service for three reasons; 1. at any time upon their services being no longer needed; 2. on account of physical disability interfering, beyond reasonable doubt, with active service in the Navy; 3. for misconduct."[18] It is decided that the Navy Nurse Corps would have positions as nurses and Chief Nurses. "Appointments as chief nurse were not made from civil life, but rather done as a form of promotion from the grade of nurse. A permanent appointment to the grade of chief nurse required the approval of the Surgeon General and the passage of the examination [for] such grade."[19]

On 17 September 1908, Victoria White and Martha E. Pringle are appointed Navy Nurses. Their background and experience qualify them to take the examination for Chief Nurse. They pass all the requirements and they are appointed the first Chief Nurses as of 23 October 1908.

Miss White was born in Sewickly, Pennsylvania and trained as a nurse at St. Luke's Hospital in Bethlehem, Pennsylvania. She was Superintendent at this hospital from 1891 to 1908 when she left to join the Navy. It seems that on 20 July 1908, the Surgeon General of the Navy wrote a letter to Miss White. In his letter he states, "It is my present intention, if possible, to offer you the first position as chief nurse with the view that, should the Superintendent of nurses for any reason prove unsatisfactory, you might have the opportunity to succeed her. As chief nurse you would have compensation . . . of $75.00 per month with allowances and at first could act as assistant to the Superintendent in the work of organizing and later on take charge of the group of female nurses at one of the large hospitals as New York. Should this proposition be agreeable to you, please write and let me know."[20] She accepts and is appointed a Navy Nurse on 17 September 1908. Her age is 49 years at this time. In the latter part of October, Chief Nurse White is assigned to the Naval Medical School, at Observatory Hill, as the Instructor of the new Navy Nurses. (She stays in the Navy until 1913 when she is honorably discharged.)

Miss Martha Pringle was born in Ann Arbor, Michigan. She received her nurses' training at the St. Louis Protestant Hospital in St. Louis, Missouri. She graduated in 1898. She was a "contract nurse" for a year then she joined the Army Nurse Corps in 1901. She was an Army nurse from February 1901 to December 1902 and again from June 1903 to July 1908 when she left to join the Navy. She is appointed a Navy Nurse 17 September 1908.[21] She is 42 years old. (Miss Pringle retires in 1926 due to longevity.)

During October and early November 1908, seventeen other nurses enter the Navy:

1. J. Beatrice Bowman was born in Des Moines, Iowa. She attended the Medico-Chirurgical Training School for Nurses in Philadelphia, Pennsylvania. She graduated in May 1904 and did some work with the American Red Cross. Appointed a Navy Nurse 1 October 1908 at the age of 26 years. (Retires in 1935.)

2. Sara M. Cox was born in Canada, but did her nurses' training at Boston City Hospital in Boston, Massachusetts, graduating in 1890. She was an Army contract nurse, 1898 to 1899, and was one of the first to join the Army Nurse Corps in 1901. She resigned from the Army in 1902 to return to civilian life. Appointed a Navy Nurse 1 October 1908. Miss Cox is 45 years old. (Retires in 1928.)

3. Clare L. DeCeu was born in Ontario, Canada. She graduated in 1902 from Buffalo General Hospital Training School in Buffalo, New York. Appointed a Navy Nurse 1 October 1908 when she is 35 years old. (Honorable discharge in 1912. Reappointed in 1914. Dies of carcinoma in 1933 while still on active duty.)

4.   Mary Hilliard DuBose. Born in Memphis, Tennessee she attended the Lane Hospital Training School in San Francisco, California, graduating in 1902. She had six years experience in nursing at several hospitals in California. Appointed a Navy Nurse 29 September 1908 when 30 years old. (Retires in 1929.)

5.   Elizabeth M. Hewitt was born in Smithport, Pennsylvania and went to Columbia and Children's Hospitals in Washington, DC for her nursing. She graduated in 1895 then went on to serve as an Army contract nurse in 1898 and 1899. She was Assistant Superintendent of Children's Hospital for three years before joining the Navy. Appointed a Navy Nurse 3 October 1908. Her age is 36 years. (Retires with physical disability in 1933.)

6.   Lenah Sutcliffe Higbee was born in Chatham, New Brunswick, Canada. She attended the Margaret Fahnestock Training School of New York Post-Graduate Hospital, New York City in 1899. Mrs. Higbee also took a six-month postgraduate course at Fordham Hospital in New York City. She is the widow of Lt. Colonel John Henley Higbee of the U.S. Marine Corps whom she had married shortly after graduating from nurses training. Appointed a Navy Nurse 1 October 1908 when she is 32 years old. (Honorable discharge at own request in 1922.)

7.   Estelle Hine was born in Osseo, Wisconsin. Graduated from Northwestern Hospital, Minneapolis, Minnesota in 1894. Did private duty nursing then served with the Army: first as a contract nurse then in the Army Nurse Corps until 1906. Then she returned to private duty. Appointment as Navy Nurse 29 September 1908 at the age of 36. (She resigns in 1910 to reenter the Army Nurse Corps.)

8.   Della V. Knight was born in Thompsontown, Pennsylvania. Received nurses' training in German Hospital, Brooklyn, New York and graduated in 1904. She served in the Army Nurse Corps from 1904 to 1907. Appointed a Navy Nurse 29 September 1908. She is 30 years old. (Retires in 1930.)

9.   Elizabeth Leonhardt. Born in Washington, DC. Graduated from Protestant Episcopal Hospital, Philadelphia, Pennsylvania in 1892. She did private duty nursing in Seattle, Washington for six years then returned to DC to work in a sanitarium there. Appointed a Navy Nurse 3 October 1908 at the age of 41. (Retires in 1928 after twenty years of naval service.)

10. Mrs. Florence Taney Milburn (widowed) was born in Maryland. In 1907 she graduated from nurses training at Children's Hospital in Boston, Massachusetts. She was nursing at a hospital in Lexington, Kentucky before joining the Navy. Appointed a Navy Nurse 1 October 1908 when she is 35 years old. (Resigns with honorable discharge in 1915.)

11. Margaret D. Murray was born in Baltimore, Maryland. Received her training at Baltimore City Hospital, Baltimore, Maryland and graduated in 1906. She then did nursing for the government in Panama for two years. Appointed to the Navy 25 October 1908 when she is 26 years old. (Resigns in 1913.)

12. Sara B. Myer was born in Newark, New Jersey. Graduated from Methodist-Episcopal Hospital, Brooklyn, New York in 1902. Miss Myer did private duty nursing in Brooklyn until 1905. She had service in the Army Nurse Corps from 1905 to 1908. Appointed a Navy Nurse 28 October 1908. She is 30 years old. (Retires in 1930.)

13. Ethel Reeder Parsons was born in St. Mary's County, Maryland. Received her nurses' training at St. Joseph's Hospital, Philadelphia, Pennsylvania and graduated in 1904. Appointed a Navy Nurse 28 October 1908 at the age of 27. (Resigns in December 1909. Enrolls in the Reserve in 1917 and honorably discharged in 1918. Appointed to the Navy in 1918 and honorably discharged in 1921. Reappointed in 1922. Retires in 1932.)

14. Adah M. Pendleton was born in Edinburg, Indiana. In 1907 she graduated from the Garfield Memorial Hospital Training School in Washington, DC in 1907. Appointed a Navy Nurse 2 October 1908. She is 26 years old. (Retires with physical disability in 1933.)

15. Isabelle Ross Roy was born in Brooklyn, New York. In 1903 she graduated from a 27-month nurses training course at the Memorial Hospital for Women and Children in Brooklyn, New York. Following graduation she did private duty nursing. The Navy doctor at the New York Navy Yard in 1908 gives this young lady her initial health examination and states on the health certificate, "displays a slight hesitation in speech when embarrassed." Appointed a Navy Nurse 28 October 1908 at the age of 40 years. (She did receive her appointment, but the speech impediment proves to be an obstacle in her naval career. By the end of her three years in the Nurse Corps, her fitness reports show a lack of administrative skills and the disadvantages associated with her speech problem. She is honorably discharged in 1911.)

16. Boniface T. Small was born in Melvale, Maryland. Graduated from Johns Hopkins Hospital, Baltimore, Maryland in 1908. Appointed a Navy Nurse on 1 October 1908 when she is 25. (Honorable discharge in 1911.)

17. Elizabeth J. Wells was born in Park Hill, New Hampshire. Graduated from Garfield Hospital, Washington, DC in 1903. She practiced her nursing at one of the hospitals in DC before joining the Navy. Appointment to Navy dated 1 October 1908 at the age of 29. (Honorable discharge in 1911.)

These then are the first twenty female nurses of the United States Navy Nurse Corps. "The Sacred Twenty." It is important to point out that although the term "The Sacred Twenty" may have been derisive at first, it soon is said with true and sincere respect. (And still is.) It seems that this label is given the group, in a mocking manner, by some Navy men. Mrs. Mary Robinson Godfrey (a Navy Nurse of 1910 to 1918) tells us that the nurses who came after these first twenty named them the "sacred twenty." She says that the original twenty stood and held themselves apart so that the other nurses gave them that name.

A Chief Warrant Officer of the Hospital Corps is asked (in an oral history tape done in 1971) how the men felt about the new Navy Nurses and did they like the idea. His reply was, "They didn't at first. And they [the men] wanted to know what kind of a rating to give them. And the Chief Petty Officer [at the time] said `why give it to them, they don't do anything.'"[22] (Some of the corpsmen were still saying this in the 1960's and 1970's. Some will probably say it ad infinitum. However, many change their minds when they do independent duty and face true emergency situations. Then they know that by instructing, watching and making them do the work, the nurses are training them, in many ways.) Later (in the oral history tape) the same Chief Warrant Officer states, "I thought if they [the Navy nurses] were a Chief Petty Officer, why, it would be a pretty good job for them. And quite a few of the people thought that."[23] Nonetheless, these pioneering nurses receive neither officer ranking nor enlisted rating, though they are **treated**, in many ways, more as officers. Legislation has not designated any ranking or rating, but these nurses are definitely members of the Navy and subject to the discipline of the Navy.

Imagine, if you will, what these ladies are facing and how they must feel. They have entered a military man's world in an era when women's liberation is a generally unknown state of being. They must learn the officers' ranks and enlisted men's ratings. True, some of them have spent time in the Army Nurse Corps and as military contract nurses. However, think about this; a Captain in the Army is equal to a Navy Lieutenant, while a Navy Captain is the same as an Army Colonel. All the other ranks are different as well. The Navy's Hospital Steward is a Chief Petty Officer. Even the language is unlike any other. A ladder is a staircase, a bulkhead is a wall, a "rope-yarn" Sunday is a half-day off duty, and a head is a bathroom. The port side of a hospital ward is the left side and the starboard is the right. These are just a few examples. This must all seem like "Greek" to the Sacred Twenty. Additionally, they have to contend with the attitudes of the doctors and the hospital corpsmen (still called nurses in the Navy hospitals.) The doctors are used to dealing closely with the male "nurses" in the male world of Navy medicine. The Hospital Corps' men look up to the doctors for their instructions and knowledge in a type of male bonding. These men have developed close rapport and now here are unknown females coming between the two. There is bound to be resentment and even bitterness. As one of the Sacred Twenty writes (later on), "These pioneers were no more welcome to most of the personnel of the Navy, than women usually are when invading what man calls his domain. The welfare of the patients was the one object in having nurses and the patients, as a rule, were most grateful to see them. Paradoxical as it may sound, men are men when strong and healthy, but when sick, they are not men, but patients. As few were immune to sickness or injury, the number of patients who reverted to type and became men again, carried quite a different feeling for women, that is, nurse, in the Navy. The knockers became the boosters and Father Time did the rest. It sounds untrue, but some of the older medical men in the Navy were the strongest opponents of the Nurse Corps. Most of these doctors had not worked

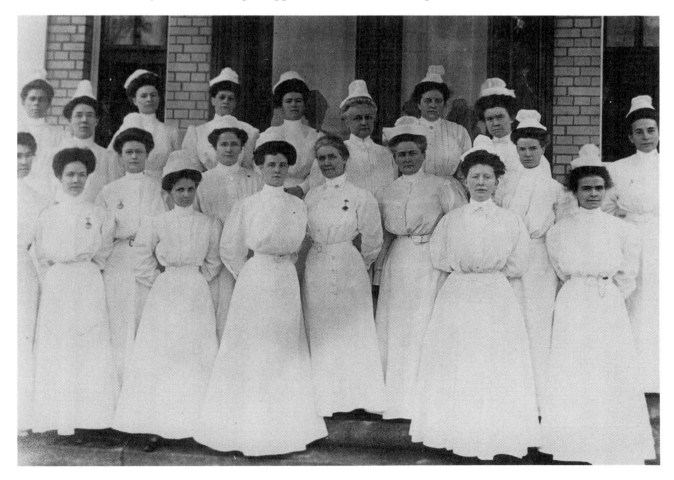

The Sacred Twenty. (Photo courtesy of NNCA Memorabilia Collection.)

with nurses in civilian life and some of them had gone into the medical work of the Navy to get away from women patients and incidentally their nurses. They disliked petticoat government in the wards of the naval hospitals very much."[24]

To return to the newly appointed Navy Nurses and their arrival in Washington, DC in the fall of 1908; there are no government quarters available for them to live in. "Miss Hasson leased, furnished and financed quarters at 511 Twenty-first Street, N.W."[25] for the new Navy Nurses. The Surgeon General of the Navy had written a form letter to all thirty-three of the Nurse Corps applicants on 24 August 1908. In that letter he stated, "All nurses on duty in Washington will be required to live in the Nurses Home, which is under the supervision of the Superintendent of the Navy Nurse Corps, female. The quarters now being fitted up consist of 2 new houses on 21st Street, Washington and will furnish comfortable rooms for each nurse with adequate comfortable reception and dining rooms. The allowance for expenses at the home will [be] $15.00 for rooms and $22.00 for subsistence making the total pay of nurses on duty here $77.50 per month."[26]

The original twenty are "given an allowance for quarters and subsistence . . . and [run] their own mess."[27] (Webster's dictionary describes "mess" as a group of people who regularly have their meals together, as in the Army or Navy.) As for duty, the group reports to the Chief Nurse of the Naval Hospital in DC, Miss Martha Pringle. Their duty hours are for seven days per week in shifts of:

8:00 a.m. — 3:00 p.m.
3:00 p.m. — 10:00 p.m.
10:00 p.m. — 8:00 a.m.

These hours are unusually liberal for the time. Most institutional nurses are working 12-hour days; private duty nurses are working 24-hour duty.[28] The newly developed regulations for the Nurse Corps explain that "No nurse shall be required to take night duty for more than a month consecutively . . . and no nurse will ordinarily be called upon for ward night duty more frequently than one month out of every three." One paragraph later then states, "In hospitals where there is an active operating service a nurse detailed to an operating room may be exempted from night duty on the recommendation of the chief nurse if such exemption is approved by the commanding officer."[29]

The duties of the nurses are detailed in the regulations and show the planning that went into beginning this Nurse Corps. "All nurses on duty in a naval hospital or on board a hospital ship will be under the immediate supervision of the chief nurse and directly responsible to her in all matters relating to duty, conduct, and discipline."[30] Interestingly, the regulations then state that "Women nurses will not be detailed for general duty in venereal wards."[31] Now the details of ward duty, "A nurse detailed for duty in charge of a ward will be responsible for the nursing care of all patients therein, and will at all times maintain quiet, order, and discipline on the part of all patients and others assigned to ward duty under her.

"Upon coming on duty and relieving the night nurse, she will receive the report of the latter, take over her duties, acquaint herself with the condition of the patients, see that the ward is put in order, and the records, charts, requisitions, treatment book, etc., are brought up to date and are prepared for the signature of the ward medical officer, whom she will be prepared to receive and accompany upon his morning rounds.

"The nurse in charge of a ward will keep the treatment book of the ward and will see that all orders regarding treatment are carried out promptly and intelligently.

"It shall be the duty of the ward nurse to see that all hospital apprentices assigned to duty in the ward are instructed in practical nursing and the care of the sick."[32]

Even though there are no Reserve nurses at this time (1908, 1909), the regulations address this subject, "A nurse who serves faithfully and satisfactorily for at least six months and receives an honorable discharge will, if she desires, be placed on the reserve list.

"Reserve nurses must sign an agreement to enter active service whenever needed, and to report by letter to the Surgeon General on the 1st of January and the 1st of July of each year. Reserve nurses will be entitled to wear such device as may be adopted to designate the Navy Nurse Corps, but are not entitled to pay, allowances, or other privileges.

"A nurse will be dropped from the reserve list upon reaching the age of 45 years; or if she ceases for five years to practice her profession; or if she becomes permanently incapacitated from ill health; or if she fails without satisfactory reason, to promptly respond to a call into active service or if she fails to notify the Surgeon General of any change in her permanent address; or for other good and sufficient reason.."[33]

Then there are little tidbits of information such as, "Members of officers' and enlisted men's families are not entitled to the services of Navy Nurses, and they will not be detailed for such duty except with the prior approval of the Surgeon General. If an emergency should require such services in advance of the approval of the Surgeon General, a report . . . shall be made to the Surgeon General."[34] "This matter of diverting nurses from their primary hospital assignments was a difficult problem for the Nurse Corps for many years and is the subject of much correspondence between the Superintendent and chief nurses as well as the Surgeon General and commanding officers at the various hospitals and dispensaries. There were no wards . . . for dependents . . . hence nursing was of necessity in the quarters or homes. While ostensibly a voluntary duty during off hours the local conditions and pressures tended to 'volunteer' the nurses and establish this as a regular expected service."[35]

One other item that refers to the nurses is, "The pay, allowances, and privileges of nurses are specified by law, and they are forbidden to receive presents from patients, or from the relatives or friends of patients, for services rendered when on duty."[36]

As for Chief Nurses, their duties include conferring "with the commanding officer or the executive surgeon regarding all details of duties in which nurses are to be assigned. The chief nurse will be considered as responsible to the commanding officer for prompt compliance on the part of all nurses of all orders issued by proper authority. The chief nurse will also be responsible for the proper conduct of the duties assigned to nurses and for the maintenance of order and discipline among them."[37] Then the "chain of command" for reports is established: "All reports relative to nurses shall be submitted by the chief nurse to the executive surgeon for submission to the commanding officer, and all general directions regarding nursing duties will be transmitted by the executive surgeon or commanding officer through the chief nurse."[38] This chain of command is further defined for all nurses, with "Under proper restrictions and on suitable occasions, nurses shall have the undisputed right to communicate with the commanding officer of the hospital. All such applications shall be made through the chief nurse and executive surgeon, who will first investigate the complaint or request and be able to express their approval or disapproval of the same. A nurse will be held accountable for vexatious, frivolous, or false complaints."[39]

Additionally, the Chief Nurse is placed in charge of the nurses' quarters and held responsible for its condition and cleanliness. She also is held responsible for the linen room and the diet kitchen in the hospital. There are, as well, the many reports she must provide; i.e. "efficiency reports of the nurses serving under her to the commanding officer on the 1st days of January, April, July, and October. Blanks for these reports will be furnished by the Surgeon General. Such reports will include not only an estimate of a nurse's professional work, but will also include, under the head "Remarks," a statement as to her physical fitness and general adaptability for the naval service."[40] In addition, the Chief Nurse must "keep the official register of nurses, in which she shall enter the name, date of reporting, days sick or on leave, efficiency marks, name and address, or any other facts concerning each nurse that it may be important to record, and such register shall be under her charge and available for inspection by the commanding officer or executive surgeon whenever called for.

"The chief nurse shall also keep a daybook, in which the detail of nurses to duty for the day is entered, the nature of the duty, number or hours on duty, etc., of each nurse."[41]

All the Navy Nurses are entitled to Navy medical care when ill and all are granted thirty days leave per year, with pay. All Navy Nurses provide for their own uniforms and the laundering of the uniforms. The working uniform for Navy Nurses is "shirtwaist, skirt, and belt of light weight, white cotton drilling, made according to prescribed patterns and measurements; Bishop collar; cap of white Persian lawn with one inch band of black velvet; on the left sleeve of the uniform, half-way between the shoulder and elbow will be [embroidered] the

Geneva Red Cross'; the pin which will be the special insignia of the corps will be about the size of a silver quarter, made of heavy gold plate with a dull rough surface. The design in blue enamel will be that of an anchor combined with the caduceus, immediately under the design will be the letters USN, also in blue enamel."[42] Nurses are not permitted to wear the pin for the first six months of service while their adaptability to the military is decided.

Let us now return to the Sacred Twenty. We left them as they reported into the Naval Hospital in Washington, DC. In early October 1908, an orientation course is given them. It consists of "demonstrations and lectures on nursing and service conditions both at home and abroad, care of the sick on hospital ships, nursing of tropical diseases, naval hygiene and sanitation, requirements of hospitals and hospital ships, first aid and emergencies, bacteriology of the air and skin in relation to surgical cleanliness, methods of sterilization, etc. This instruction [is] supplemented by practical work in dispensary and laboratory and [is] further supplemented by a course of lectures by the Superintendent of the Nurse Corps on the subjects of military nursing, ethics and etiquette, etc., with a view to making the organization more adaptable to the needs of the naval service and to preparing the members of the corps for professional intercourse and cooperation with the Army nurses and nurses of other countries with whom they might be brought in contact."[43] The orientation period is completed in March of 1909 and the nurses receive their first assignments. Mrs. Milburn makes Chief Nurse and is assigned to the Naval Medical Hospital in DC along with nurses Sara Cox, Della Knight, Sara Myer, and Ethel Parsons. Mrs. Higbee goes as Chief Nurse to Norfolk Naval Hospital in Portsmouth, Virginia as do nurses Boniface Thomasina Small, and Elizabeth Leonhardt. Miss DeCeu is made Chief Nurse at Naval Hospital Annapolis, Maryland with nurses Margaret Murray, and Adah Pendleton. Miss White is sent to the Naval Hospital in Brooklyn, New York as Chief Nurse with nurses Mary DuBose, Elizabeth Hewitt, Estelle Hine, Isabelle Roy, Elizabeth Wells, and J. Beatrice Bowman. Later on in November of 1909 Miss Pringle goes, as Chief Nurse, to the Naval Hospital at Mare Island, California.[44] By the end of 1909 there is a total of 37 Navy Nurses in the Corps and they are assigned to the above named duty stations.

A description of the first Navy Nurses' arrival at the Norfolk Naval Hospital states, "On Saturday morning, April 17, 1909, exactly two months after the new Hospital building was re-occupied, a group of three women entered its portals. The group (was made up of) Mrs. Lenah S. Higbee . . . and two other nurses, Misses Ethel Swann and Mary C. Nelson."[45] The Commanding Officer of the Naval Hospital had asked for "nurses" to be sent, but he was expecting hospital corpsmen.[46] Imagine his chagrin when the three Navy Nurses walk into his office. Since Navy Nurses were unexpected, no quarters were available for the nurses so they found accommodations at the "Waverly Apartment on Court Street, Portsmouth. and [had their meals] from the cafe in the same building."[47] In June of 1909, the Navy Nurses, "were joined by four other nurses, Misses Mary Humphrey, Betty Mayer, Thomasina B. Small and Elizabeth Leonhardt. . . . The introduction of women nurses in the Navy had often been mentioned, but there was always an attitude of doubt as to whether the plan would work in a hospital without a single female patient, distinctly a man's hospital; in fact, made up of sailors who had always done their own laundry, tailoring, and mending, cooking and chambermaid-holy-stoning, and it seemed to the old-timers as if the good old days might be coming to an end."[48]

As stated above, Miss J. Beatrice Bowman was one of the nurses sent to the Naval Hospital in New York. In her oral history tape she says, "And then . . . five of us were sent up to New York and I was one of the five. That was over in Brooklyn, Flatbush. It was a lovely hospital, but those were harrowing days. . . . We had a southern gentleman as a Commanding Officer and he would stand for no nonsense. Captain Smith. He was a delightful man, but he knew what we had to go through and he was right back of us to the end."[49]

Meanwhile, civilian professional nursing is making strides of its own. One of the biggest strides occurs in 1909 with "a full course in nursing under the University of Minnesota. This [is] largely due to the efforts of Dr. Richard Olding Beard, who had always been sympathetic with nurses in their educational aspirations. The school of the university hospital [is] put on a university basis, and . . . [becomes] recognized as the pioneer in this new type of educational affiliation."[50] Also, in 1909, a nurse by the name of Jane A. Delano becomes "President of the

Nurses' Associated Alumnae [ANA], Superintendent of the Army Nurse Corps, and a member of the War Relief Board of the American Red Cross and Chairman of its National Committee on Red Cross Nursing Service. She [stands] in a unique position of leadership, with professional nursing, Red Cross nursing, and Army nursing under her guidance."[51] Miss Delano is in agreement with an idea "to establish Red Cross nurses, beyond question, as the reserve for the Army Nurse Corps"[52] and she is in a unique position to accomplish this. You see, "The Red Cross Nursing Service was planned on a large scale by the voluntary affiliation of the American Nurses Association with the Red Cross officials in a Central Committee on Nursing Service, the nurses' association undertaking the responsibility of supplying the Red Cross on its call with any needed nurses."[53] So all these positions that Miss Delano holds are advantageous to her goal: the use of the Red Cross as the Army Nurse Corps' reserve force. (This subject becomes much more important to the Navy Nurse Corps later in World War I and World War II.) (Miss Delano continues her efforts until 1912 when the work with all the responsibilities becomes too great. She writes to the Army Surgeon General, "my only object in resigning . . . is that I may have the time to devote to the development and maintenance of an efficient reserve of Red Cross nurses for the service of the Army.")[54]

"The relationship of Red Cross Nursing Service with the Navy Nurse Corps, though supposedly the same as with the Army Nurse Corps, was never actually as close. The connection of Red Cross nurses with the Army dated from the Spanish-American War; with the navy there was no similar traditional relationship. . . . The Navy Nurse Corps, not established until 1908, had been less publicized among nurses than the Army Nurse Corps. But the most important fact was that the Navy Nurse Corps was likely to remain small and to need few reserves. In general, the Navy remained more aloof from the Red Cross than the Army and, although it was generally understood that the Red Cross maintained the nurse reserves for both corps, Red Cross Nursing Service was at no time named in a Navy manual as the reserve for the Navy Nurse Corps."[55]

As for 1910 and the rest of the world, William H. Taft is President having been elected to follow in the footsteps of Theodore Roosevelt. Unfortunately, the 350-pound President Taft bears the stigma of being the one to propose the federal income tax.[56] In Germany the first chemotherapeutic drug is invented, while in France the neon lamp is invented.[57] Meanwhile, over in East Wellow, in Hampshire, England in a small, quiet churchyard, Florence Nightingale is laid to rest.[58] She had devoted most of her ninety years of life to the profession of nursing.

Turning to the nursing profession in the United States, there are now 1100 schools of nursing. The types of nursing available to the graduates of these schools fall, generally, into three categories: hospital nursing, private duty, and public health nursing. Public health nursing is **the** growing field for nurses, to the extent that Columbia University decides to start the first university course in this type of nursing.[59] Also, 1910 sees the beginning of the first training for nurse anesthetists.[60]

Remember, back in the early 1900's, President Roosevelt decided in favor of putting a medical officer, rather than a line officer, in command of a hospital ship? Doctor Stokes was the one eventually put in command of a hospital ship: the *Relief.* Now, in 1910, Doctor Stokes leaves the *Relief* and comes to Washington as the new Surgeon General of the Navy. Doctor Stokes starts by immediately provoking the dislike of the outgoing Surgeon General. Then a month after taking office, Doctor Stokes devotes some reproachful attention to the Superintendent of the Navy Nurse Corps. He writes "a memorandum to Miss Hasson asking her and her mother to withdraw [within <u>four</u> days] . . . from the nurses quarters since he [does] not consider this consistent with the dignity of the Superintendent, and that better relations, efficiency and harmony would result. At this time Miss Hasson and her aged mother [reside] in their own home, but [take] their meals in the nurses' mess. Miss Hasson [protests] this arbitrary directive, explaining that she had personally . . . assumed the financial responsibility to the extent of $1100 for the renting and furnishing of the quarters and the establishment of the mess, since no official arrangements had been made for the first group [of Navy nurses]. . . . Furthermore, she [is] aware of no disharmony, but would take her meals in a separate room to preserve the dignity of her position."[61] Admiral Stokes replies to Superintendent Hasson giving "her till 1 June to wind up arrangements, with the admonition . . . that no one except nurses attached to the Washington station were to be admitted to the nurses' mess [obviously meaning Miss Hasson's mother] and that a full accounting was to be submitted to him."[62] After that episode, things go from bad to worse. The Surgeon General takes it upon himself to issue instructions, pertaining to nurses, without conferring with Miss Hasson and without informing her. Then, "on 27 September 1910 Admiral Stokes [asks] that she submit her resignation on 1 October. . . ."[63] She does not resign at this point, but both continue to irritate one another. Meanwhile the Surgeon General decides upon a different system of training for hospital apprentices. In his report of 1910 he mentions using certain Naval Hospitals for their training in bedside nursing: Naval Hospitals New York, Norfolk, Mare Island in California, and Canacao in the Philippine Islands. Specifically, he writes, "At these hospitals they will receive practical training in the care of the sick in the wards - at the bedside under the guidance of the female Nurse Corps."[64] This is probably why Mrs. Florence Milburn and Miss Margaret D. Murray (both of the Sacred Twenty) receive orders to the Naval Hospital, Canacao, Philippine Islands in December of 1910. Mrs. Milburn is sent as the Chief Nurse. Also, in this year on October 31, twenty-four year old Miss Mary Robinson joins the Navy Nurse Corps. (This young lady later marries and becomes Mrs. Mary Godfrey. She is still living, at the age of 107, as this book is being written. You will learn more about this Navy Nurse as we go along and in the episodes about World War I.) She tells us that her pay at this time is "Fifty dollars a month and I sent ten home to my sister."[65] She goes on to tell us about meeting Admiral Dewey while she is stationed at the Naval Hospital in Washington, DC. (Admiral George Dewey USN gained fame and became a hero during the Spanish-American War.) "One day a Captain came in where I had been sent [to work] and he [began] examining [patients'] eyes. He broke something and I quickly gave him another instrument. He looked at me and said, `You're the kind of a nurse we want in the Navy. You're the first one I've seen.' And, it was right then that Admiral Dewey came in. He said, `Oh, you're the first Navy nurse I've seen. I'm so glad.' He made such a fuss over me that the doctor motioned me to get out before Admiral Dewey had a conniption fit. He was so delighted they had gotten nurses in the Navy. When he had wanted them he couldn't get them. The Army had them, but not the Navy. I remember him [Admiral Dewey]. He was a little short fellow."[66]

Also, in 1910, Navy Nurse pay is raised to $50.00, as mentioned above, with a $5.00 increment every three years. And, a different collar is adopted for the Navy Nurses' hot weather uniform: a collar called "Emma."[67]

In January 1911, Miss Hasson finally submits her resignation to the Secretary of the Navy. With the resignation she includes her reasons and specifically states her problems with the Surgeon General. Admiral Stokes "curtly [forwards the resignation], recommending acceptance with the observation that it confirmed his opinion that Miss Hasson was temperamentally unfit to be Superintendent of the Navy Nurse Corps."[68] Mrs. Lenah Sutcliffe Higbee is appointed Superintendent on 20 January 1911.

Note: Miss Hasson transferred to and remained in the U.S. Army Reserve. During World War I she spent some time at U.S.A. Base Hospital #12 in France. In 1924 she wrote to the Superintendent of the Navy Nurse Corps from the Veterans Bureau in Palo Alto, California. She had been living with an elderly woman who had died. Miss Hasson was working for the Veterans Bureau until the woman's estate was settled but she did not stay very long. In her letter she wrote, "As the Tommies overseas used to say, I am fed up with the Veterans Bureau and long to get back to a more refined atmosphere."[69]

[1] Bowman, J. Beatrice (Third Superintendent of the Navy Nurse Corps), *Oral History Interview Tape Transcript*, Interviewer Irene Smith Matthews Lt(jg) Navy Nurse Corps, taped in 1971.

[2] Ibid..

[3] *Public Law 115*, SIXTIETH CONGRESS, Session I, Chapter 166, 1908, p. 146.

[4] Hickey, Dermott Vincent, *The First Ladies In The Navy - A History of the Navy Nurse Corps, 1908-1939*, June 1963, p. 52. (Unpublished thesis, see Prologue.)

[5] Rixey, Rear Admiral Presley Mairon MC USN, *Report of Surgeon-General United States Navy*, 1908, pp. 29-32.

[6] Ibid..

[7] Ibid..

[8] Roddis, Louis H., M.D., Captain MC USN, *A Short History of Nautical Medicine*, Paul B. Hoeber, Inc., Medical Book Dept. of Harper Brothers, 1941, p. 263.

[9] Rixey, Rear Admiral Presley Mairon MC USN, op. cit..

[10] Laird, LCDR Thelma NC USNR, Jones, LCDR Dorothy NC USN, Feeney, LCDR Elizabeth NC USN, Seidl, CDR Elizabeth NC USN (Ret), Blaska, CDR Burdette NC USN, *Chronological History NAVY NURSE CORPS*, Prepared by: Nursing Division, Bureau of Medicine and Surgery,

1 August 1962, pp. 2,3.

[11] Hasson, Esther V., R.N. Superintendent of the Nurse Corps, United States Navy, "The Navy Nurse Corps," *The American Journal of Nursing*, Volume IX, March, 1909, pp. 414,415.

[12] Ibid., p. 412.

[13] Ibid..

[14] Ibid., pp. 412,413.

[15] Ibid., p. 413.

[16] Hickey, op. cit., p. 53.

[17] Laird, Jones, Feeney, Seidl, Blaska, op. cit., p. 3.

[18] Lyons, Barbara A. LCDR NC USN, *Formation, Organization and Growth of the Navy Nurse Corps 1908 - 1933*, 1968, p. 18. (An unpublished manuscript written in response to instructions from Nursing Division, BuMed in 1968.)

[19] Ibid., p. 19.

[20] Goble, CDR Dorothy Jones, NC USN, Unpublished history research notes.

[21] Ibid..

[22] Cooney, John (Navy Service 1893 to 1922. Retired as Chief Warrant Officer.), *Oral History Interview Tape Transcript*, Interviewer Irene Matthews Lt(jg) Navy Nurse Corps, taped in 1971.

[23] Ibid..

[24] Bowman, J. Beatrice, R.N., "History of Nursing In The Navy," *The American Journal of Nursing*, Vol.XXVIII, Number 9, September 1928.

[25] Dock, Lavinia L., R.N., Noyes, Clara D., R.N., Clement, Fannie F., B.A., R.N., Fox, Elizabeth G., B.A., R.N., Van Meter, Anna R., B.A., M.S., *History of American Red Cross Nursing*, The MacMillan Company, New York, 1922, p. 686.

[26] Rixey, Rear Admiral Presley Mairon MC USN, *Circular Letter to Navy Nurse Corps Applicants*, August 24, 1908.

[27] Bowman, AJN, 1928, op. cit..

[28] Laird, Jones, Feeney, Seidl, Blaska, op. cit., p. 3.

[29] *Regulations and Instructions for the Nurse Corps, U. S. Navy*, Authorized by the Secretary of the Navy and Prepared Under the Direction of The Surgeon General, Government Printing Office, Washington, 1909, p. 11.

[30] Ibid., pp. 10, 11.

[31] Ibid., p. 11.

[32] Ibid..

[33] Ibid., p. 12.

[34] Ibid., p. 8.

[35] Hickey, op. cit., p. 57.

[36] Regulations and Instructions for the Nurse Corps, U. S. Navy, 1909, op. cit., p. 8.

[37] Ibid., p. 9.

[38] Ibid..

[39] Ibid., p. 17.

[40] Ibid., p. 10.

[41] Ibid., p. 9.

[42] Hasson, Esther V., "The Navy Nurse Corps," *American Journal of Nursing*, 1909, p. 267. (As quoted in Lyons, Barbara A. LCDR NC USN, op. cit., pp. 26, 27.)

[43] Rixey, Rear Admiral Presley Mairon MC USN, *Report of Surgeon-General United States Navy*, 1909, pp. 30, 21.

[44] Feeney, LCDR Elizabeth NC USN, Unpublished Navy Nurse Corps history research notes.

[45] Holcomb, Richmond C., M.D., F.A.C.S., Captain, Medical Corps, U.S. Navy, *A Century With Norfolk Naval Hospital 1830 - 1930*, Printcraft Publishing Co., Portsmouth, Va., MCMXXX, pp. 369, 370.

[46] Bowman, AJN, 1928, op. cit..

[47] Holcomb, op. cit., p. 375.

[48] Ibid., p. 370.

[49] Bowman, *Oral History Interview Tape Transcript*, op. cit..

[50] Dock, Lavinia L., R.N., Stewart, Isabel M., A.M.,R.N., *A Short History of Nursing*, G.P. Putnam's Sons, New York: London, 1938, p. 179.

[51] Kernodle, Portia B., *The Red Cross Nurse In Action*, Harper and Brothers, New York, 1949, p. 50.

[52] Ibid., p. 51.

[53] Dock, Lavinia L., R.N., Stewart, Isabel M., A.M.,R.N., op. cit., p. 168.

[54] As quoted in Kernodle, Portia B., *The Red Cross Nurse In Action*, op. cit., p. 51.

[55] Kernodle, op. cit., pp. 109, 110.

[56] *200 Years, A Bicentennial Illustrated History of the United States*, Joseph Newman, Directing Editor, Books by U.S. News & World Report, Inc., 2300 N Street, N.W., Washington, D.C. 20037, 1973, Book 2, p. 326.

[57] *Great Events of the 20th Century*, Editor: Richard Marshall, The Readers' Digest Association, Inc., 1977, p. 29.

[58] Ibid., pp. 85, 86.

[59] Goodnow, Minnie, R.N., *Nursing History*, Press of W.B. Saunders Company, Philadelphia, 1948, pp. 182, 184, 185.

[60] Ibid., p. 207.

[61] Hickey, op. cit., pp. 71, 71. (Mr. Hickey notes as reference for this information, Elizabeth Feeney's unpublished Navy Nurse Corps History manuscript which is to be found in the Nursing Division files at the Naval History Museum, Navy Yard, Washington, D.C.. - Author)

[62] Ibid., p. 72.

[63] Ibid..

[64] Holcomb, op. cit., p. 463. (Citation from the Navy Surgeon General's report of 1910.)

[65] Godfrey, Mary Robinson (Navy Service 1910 to 1919), *Oral History Interview Tape Transcript*, Interviewer CDR Virginia Eberharter NC USN (Ret.), taped in 1988.
[66] Ibid.
[67] Laird, Jones, Feeney, Seidl, Blaska, op. cit., p.2 (in the 'Chronological History of Changes in Uniform section.')
[68] Ibid., p. 73.
[69] Goble, op. cit..

"Undoubtedly the future status of the Navy corps will rest
largely in the hands of its members,
and especially is this true of the first nurses.
If they are content with low standards either professionally,
morally, or socially the status of the corps
will be fixed for all time.
Future women will accept the standard set by us now
without question; if it be high they will rise to it,
if it be low they will with equal facility drop to its level."

☆ ☆ ☆

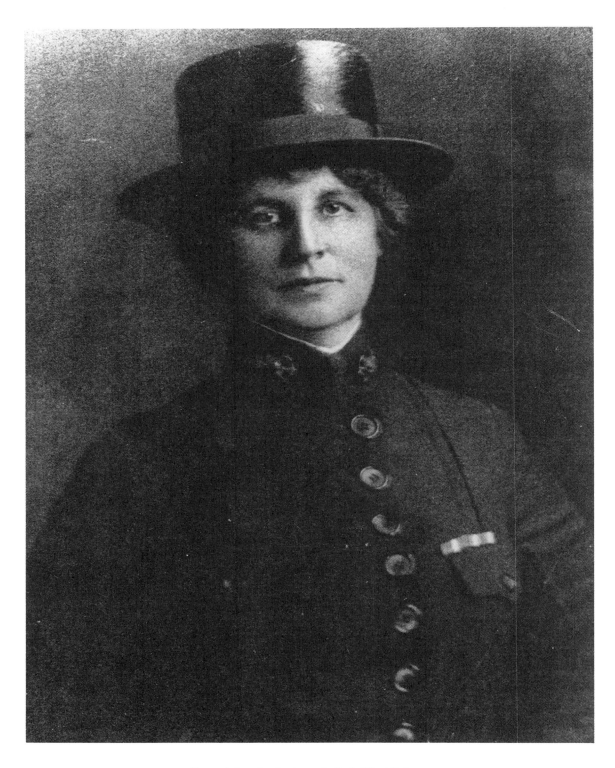

Superintendent - Lenah Sutcliffe Higbee
(Official U.S. Navy photo courtesy of Nursing Division, Bureau of Medicine and Surgery, Navy Department.)

CHAPTER 2

Superintendent - Lenah Sutcliffe Higbee
(1911 - 1922)

It is 20 January 1911. Lenah Sutcliffe Higbee is the Chief Nurse of the Norfolk Naval Hospital in Portsmouth, Virginia. In Portsmouth, on this date, Mrs. Higbee appears before a notary public and takes the required oath for appointment as Superintendent of the Navy Nurse Corps. She had received her appointment orders on the 18th, she executes the oath on the 20th and, on the 23rd, reports in to the Bureau of Medicine and Surgery of the Navy Department in Washington, DC. (She must have packed in a hurry.) The fact that her husband had been an officer in the Marine Corps undoubtedly has provided Mrs. Higbee with a knowledge of Navy protocol and service proprieties. With this and her proven professional background, she manages to develop a peaceful working relationship with the Surgeon General (no doubt, to the relief of both parties.)

In 1911 the census of the Navy Nurse Corps is 86. The number of nurses and duty stations are as follows:

Superintendent	1
Washington, DC	18
Philadelphia, PA	9
Norfolk, VA	16
Annapolis, MD	6
Brooklyn, NY	10
Mare Island, CA	15
Canacao, P.I.	8
Guam, M.I.	3

This is the year that J. Beatrice Bowman is promoted and sent, as Chief Nurse, to the Naval Hospital at League Island, Philadelphia. In addition, another of the Sacred Twenty, Elizabeth Leonhardt, is promoted to Chief Nurse and receives orders to Guam in the Marianas Islands where (in 1909) a Naval Hospital had been constructed after a civilian hospital was destroyed by an earthquake.[1] You see, after the Spanish-American War, "the Navy took over Guam from the Spanish . . . (and) health officers found themselves faced with a serious leprosy problem [among other basic health and sanitation problems.]"[2] In 1901 Rear Admiral Schroeder [U.S. Navy] had helped in the construction of a hospital for the natives. This hospital also provided some sick quarters for the Navy. The hospital was named for the Admiral's wife. Then in 1905 another hospital was "constructed for the care of women and children. . . ."[3] This was the hospital destroyed by the earthquake. "The Navy then [after the quake] provided funds for a naval hospital to be combined with the existing . . . hospital to provide a capacity of 100 beds. The first training of native women as nurses began . . . under the supervision of the wife of "[4] one of the Navy doctors. The Navy doctors did the instructing so that the native women could provide the nursing care of the women and children at the hospital.[5] When (in 1911) the Navy Nurses arrive, they find the living primitive and the food supply rather limited because of the polluted soil. There are cockroaches everywhere as well as lizards and centipedes. There are frequent earth tremors and occasional typhoons for other intermittent excitement. The Medical Department had established general sanitation and, as mentioned, a program to train the native women for nursing care. The Navy Nurses begin a formal nursing program: teaching the selected trainees with the idea of eventually training them to become nurses or health missionaries in their own communities. (Until this time older women with questionable cleanliness had been the midwives.) At the end of two years, the selected girls/women are to be awarded a diploma, a pin, and a midwife certificate.[6] "The duty on Guam [teaches] Navy nurses to treat and understand many illnesses and diseases that they [have] never before been confronted with. Tuberculosis, yaws, hookworm [are] among the diseases . . . prevalent on the island. Strange accidents such as injuries from being gored by caraboas [*sic*] [carabaos are water buffaloes], falls from cocoanut [*sic*] trees [which cause] unusual fracture complications and . . . there [are] serious infections that [develop] from fish bites. . . ."[7] These Navy Nurses are truly pioneering.

Meanwhile, back in Washington, DC, the massive building program for the Naval Hospital complex on Observatory Hill is completed. "Total patient treatment capacity for the hospital [is] 130 beds - 78 beds for the main hospital, 22 beds for the quarters for sick officers, and 30 beds for the contagious disease hospital."[8] In addition there is a corpsmen's quarters and a nurses' quarters. "The nurses' quarters (now Building One) [contains] in the basement a kitchen, storerooms and a bedroom for attendants. The first floor [features] quarters and an office for the head nurse, a reception room, lecture room, and dining room. The second and third floors [have] accommodations for 18 nurses."[9]

Also, in 1911, Navy Nurses are assigned as instructors at the two new facilities for the training of hospital apprentices. One school is at the Naval Training Station at Newport, Rhode Island and the other is at Mare Island, California.[10] Medical officers and chief petty officers also share in the teaching. Following intensive courses at the new facilities, the students are to be sent to various Naval Hospitals where they will learn practical bedside-nursing on the wards under close supervision of Navy Nurses.[11]

In professional nursing, the Nurses' Associated Alumnae of the United States becomes the American Nurses' Association (ANA) in 1911. A year later, the National Organization for Public Health Nursing (visiting nursing) is formed. It is a new association that includes lay people as well as nurses: including, that is, anyone "doing any form of public health nursing."[12] (The name change for the National League of Nursing Education has been mentioned previously in relation to this year.) Also, in 1912, The National Association of Colored Nurses achieves "official recognition by being admitted to the International Council of Nurses."[13]

As for the rest of the country, it is a presidential election year. President Taft decides to run again, but Teddy Roosevelt tosses his hat into the ring and the Republican party is torn in two. "Theodore Roosevelt . . . [while] trying for a comeback . . . [calls] the Republicans' William Howard Taft . . . a 'fathead'; President Taft, who had been picked by Roosevelt as his successor four years before, [labels] T.R. a 'demagogue.'"[14] "Woodrow Wilson, the former President of Princeton and dynamic Governor of New Jersey, [succeeds] in capturing the Democratic nomination"[15] and wins the election easily. President Wilson gets "only 42 percent of the popular vote, but in the electoral college [he receives] an overwhelming 435 out of 531 votes."[16]

Back at the Navy's Bureau of Medicine and Surgery, the Surgeon General is devoting some of his time and energy to problems with quarters for Navy Nurses. In Surgeon General Stokes' Report of 1912, he states that the Naval Hospital in Brooklyn, New York had remodeled and enlarged a building to house ten nurses. Further, Pearl Harbor was constructing quarters for nurses while at the new Naval Hospital at Chelsea, Massachusetts the commanding officer took quarters from one of the doctors to provide quarters for his nurses. The Surgeon General goes on to recommend that quarters also be built for nurses at the Naval Hospitals at Las Animas, Colorado and Puget Sound, Washington.[17] Besides the quarters matter, there is the continuing problem of the nurses being 'volunteered' for home care of dependents. The Naval Hospitals have no wards for sick wives and children of the military men. In too many cases it became "a regular [and] expected service."[18] For many years this matter "is the subject of much correspondence between the superintendent and chief nurses as well as the Surgeon General and commanding officers at the various hospitals and dispensaries."[19] In Surgeon General Stokes' Annual Report, he speaks of this subject and its "abuse and lack of consideration. He [adds that he is] contemplating . . . the establishment of two wards for women and children — one at a Pacific coast hospital and one at an Atlantic coast hospital."[20] Clearly, this man has concern and consideration for the welfare of the members of the Navy Nurse Corps as well as the dependents. However, the Comptroller General did not seem to share such concern when he ruled (in 1912) that nurses are "only entitled to 40 cents per day for commuted subsistence instead of 75 cents, and their pay [is docked] for the difference until the alleged debt [is] satisfied. [Commuted subsistence is allowances for subsistence plus quarters, heat and light when not provided by the Navy.[21]] Twenty-eight nurses [leave] due to this hardship or to accept the better offers available in civilian life."[22] Another problem concerned the Chief Nurses. They did not receive the pay of Chief Nurse while on leave or while traveling.[23] (Evidently there were a number of problems with pay from the very inception of the Nurse Corps. In 1910 Miss Hasson, the first superintendent, made "the plaintive observation that 'The long torturous military channels in the Army were as nothing in comparison to those of the Navy.'"[24]

The Nurse Corps now (1912) has an active duty strength of 110 nurses. The nurses are fulfilling the needs for their profession in most of the Naval Hospitals and in the specialties: Operating Room Technic, Dietetics, Massage, and even X-Ray Technic.[25] Other nurses are being sent overseas to the various naval medical facilities to relieve or augment the nursing staffs. Mary Robinson is one of these and is on her way to the Philippines. (Later she is known as Mrs. Godfrey. Remember mention of her previously?) She states that "I must have gone in 1912 and came back in 1915. . . . It took 28 days to cross the Pacific. We saved our money and we came back by way of the Suez Canal because that's what all the nurses did."[26] She goes on to say, "Oh, I had a wonderful time in the Philippines. A wonderful time. Going over I met an Army officer. He had been promoted to Lieutenant. He later became my brother-in-law. I told him all I wanted over there was a horse and he gave me the dearest horse I ever saw. He gave me this horse with the understanding that it would be given to a friend of his in the Army if I left the Philippines. He [the Lieutenant] left about a year later, but we were always friends during later life and my sister fell in love with him and married him."[27] Then she speaks of making ice cream in the Philippines. "We got a little hand freezer and made ice cream for everybody that was sick. One day one of the Chinese kitchen workers came and asked what that was. I told him it was for making ice cream. He asked what ice cream was so I gave him some and he thought that was wonderful. That made it so I could go in the kitchen any time I wanted. I was just a lucky person. . . . Nobody could say anything about me to those Chinese - no sir. . . . But the food was absolutely marvelous."[28]

In 1913 the strength of the Nurse Corps reached 130. During this year some Navy Nurses found themselves stationed aboard two transport ships for a brief period of time. Mary DuBose (of the Sacred Twenty) is one of these nurses. She went aboard the USS *Mayflower* on 6 March 1913 followed by duty aboard the USS *Dolphin* on 27 March 1913.[29] Also, in 1913, Navy Nurses are introduced to their distinctive Navy Nurse Corps' Pin (Insignia.) It is round and about the size of a quarter. It has a "wreath of oak leaves around the edge, [medium] blue field, fouled [gold] anchor with a red, white and blue shield superimposed on the anchor and U.S.N. [in gold] below the anchor."[30] "The pin [is] worn on [the] white indoor uniform (no out door uniforms at [this] time) and [is] worn at center of neckline (bottom of V at neck.)"[31]

Now we travel out across the Pacific to Samoa. This is an island group "about 4,800 miles southwest of San Francisco"[32] and directly east of Australia. These islands are divided into American Samoa and Western Samoa. In American Samoa, the largest island is Tutuila and it is here that the capital of the American group (Pago Pago) is located. A little history will explain what is to follow: "In January 1872, the United States signed a treaty with the Kingdom of Samoa obtaining rights to establish a naval station at Pago Pago. In 1889, the United States, Britain, and Germany agreed to Samoan neutrality and created a tripartite protectorate over the islands. A convention in 1899 recognized the paramount interests of the United States in the islands east of longitude 171[degrees] W[west] and of the Germans in the islands west of the meridian. By deeds of the high chiefs [of the islands], the eastern group was ceded to the United States in 1904. . . . The islands were placed under the jurisdiction of the U.S. Navy. . . ."[33] This information becomes important because "On 26 August 1913 the Surgeon General [orders], 'A school is hereby directed to be established in American Samoa for the purpose of training native Samoan women in the principles of nursing with a view to their making use of this teaching in their own country, and among their own people. For this purpose, two members of the Nurse Corps, United States Navy, will be ordered to Samoa who, together with the medical officer of the Navy attached to the station, will give the instruction.'"[34] On 6 October 1913, "Acting Chief Nurse Mary H. Humphrey and Nurse Corinne Anderson [report] at Tutuila, Samoa. Initial efforts to inaugurate [a] training school for native girls [encounters] difficulties. By December, disagreements [lead] to a report to the Secretary of [the] Navy by a Board of Investigation. As a result, [the two] nurses [are] admonished by [the] Secretary of [the] Navy, but [are] given further opportunity to work out [the] program. School [opens] 6 February 1914 with 3 pupils."[35] (The two Navy Nurses evidently work through their disagreements and difficulties because the school and program go on to be a success. Consider that this is 1913 and 1914. These ladies are on an island about 3,000 miles from their own country, in the middle of the Pacific Ocean and in the middle of a culture and climate such as they have never known. Who wouldn't have a 'few difficulties?' Let's give these pioneering ladies the credit they are due. And by the way, the school these two Navy Nurses start continues, under Navy Nurses, until 1951 when jurisdiction of American Samoa is placed under the U.S. Department of the Interior.) Meanwhile, the nursing school for natives, on another island, Guam in the Marianas, is expanding. Additional Navy Nurses are reporting aboard this year, 1914, with a course in tuberculosis nursing and a course in massage being added to the curriculum.[36]

Back in the United States, the nursing profession is continuing to improve itself and its members. There are now registration laws in twenty-four states.[37] These laws are much needed. Last year, 1913, a committee of the American Hospital Association "reported that it had surveyed the field and found no less than nine types of workers who were calling themselves nurses. It discovered . . . that the word 'nurse' could mean anything or nothing in the way of preparation for [nursing] practice."[38] (The national nursing organizations discuss the problem and make recommendations to the AHA in 1916, but "no formal action is taken."[39])

As for Navy nursing in 1914, the census of the Navy Nurse Corps is 135. The new 1914 edition of the Manual of the Medical Department (Navy) states that applicants for the Nurse Corps must be citizens of the U.S. and they must be single. They have to be graduates of "reputable training [schools] giving a thorough professional education . . . of at least 2 years in acceptable general [hospitals] of 100 beds or more." The manual goes on to say that applicants must have state registration or eligibility for joining the American Nurses Association. Further they are required to take written professional and mental examinations and no applicants will be accepted unless they agree to serve for three years.

The background and education of students for professional nursing are much on the mind of many nurses as well as the nursing organizations and the military nursing sections. The American Nurses Association meets in April of 1914 and Navy Chief Nurse J. Beatrice Bowman addresses the group on this subject. She states, "The short hours, the certain pay, the rested look of the Navy nurse (the latter acquired by regular hours of rest and duty), these I believe to be the only facts known to superintendents or nurses outside the military service. It is not generally known that she [the Navy nurse] must possess a thorough knowledge of administrative work and must be sufficiently trained in professionalism. It is because of their innate executive ability that our nurses have 'made good,' rather than because of the training in administrative work. Could the nurses be given a course in administration, I feel sure more would qualify for executive work, and the general professional standard would be raised through the efficiency of the individual. Why? Because the nurse comes from the training schools for the most part equipped only for the practical work."[40] This lady tells it like it is: executive experience or in other words, management training and leadership experience are required. Navy Nurse Corps pioneers soon discovered that this area of nursing is essential to the success of nurses in the Navy and that it is not being included in the civilian training of nurses. (Indeed, this can easily be said about later years, as well: at least through the 1960's.)

We leave nursing, momentarily, for there are catastrophic events about to take place in this year and in the societies of this earth. The European world of 1914 is made of a fragile, volatile society. It is the age of industrialization and colonialism and there are conflicts of territory and fiery nationalism running rampant. (Even as now in 1992.) Austria-Hungary and Serbia both believe they have right of ownership to two provinces that provide outlet to the Adriatic Sea. One of the provinces is Bosnia.[41] The situation is emotional and tense. On a Sunday in June, the heir to the thrones of Austria-Hungary, Archduke Francis Ferdinand, and his wife are in their royal car traveling through a welcoming crowd "in Sarajevo, the capital of the Austrian province of Bosnia."[42] A young man (a Bosnian revolutionary) dashes from the crowd, leaps onto the running board of the car, fires two shots at the Archduke and one shot at the wife. Both are killed. Governments and tempers flare. One month later Austria-Hungary declares war on Serbia then three months later (October), "The Central Powers—Austria-Hungary, Germany, and the Ottoman Empire [Turkey]—[are] at war with the Allies—Belgium, France, Great Britain, Russia, and Serbia."[43] World War I has begun.

At the same time, the United States is having its own troubled relationship with the dictator of Mexico (Huerta.) In the spring of 1914, fourteen American sailors are arrested when they go ashore at Tampico, Mexico. President Wilson acts immediately. "He [refuses] to accept Huerta's apology, and [demands] that Huerta publicly salute the American flag in Tampico. When Huerta [refuses], Wilson . . . [orders] American forces to occupy the Mexican port of Veracruz. Eighteen Americans [are] killed in the action."[44] An agreement is finally reached, but then another government faction takes over the Mexican government and a rebel, General 'Pancho' Villa, begins "raiding American settlements across the Rio Grande."[45] Rather than go to war, President Wilson orders General John J. Pershing and some of his troops to patrol the border.[46] (As a matter of interest, a young, vigorous, and athletic Franklin Delano Roosevelt is an Assistant Secretary of the Navy during President Wilson's administration.)

As for the World War and Europe, the majority of the American public opts for neutrality, wishing to stay out of it. President Wilson professes "to be unable to judge the causes and justice of the first World War."[47] So, "for a time, he and America [watch] the conflict."[48] But, one section of the population, the American Red Cross, is unable to stand by and simply watch. The war is causing drastic shortages of medical personnel and supplies in Europe so the American Red Cross prepares to help. The Red Cross gathers supplies and medical personnel aboard a ship, the S.S. *Red Cross*, to send medical units to the war areas. The ship leaves toward the end of 1914. On board are two recently 'honorably discharged' Navy Nurses: J. Beatrice Bowman and Katrina Hertzer. In September, Miss Bowman requested the Navy for an 'honorable discharge' and permission to leave the U.S.. She receives her discharge on 31 October then sails with the Red Cross to England to help in the war efforts. She is assigned as a supervisor of one of the units at a Royal Navy Hospital near Portsmouth, England. From there she is sent to the American Women's War Hospital in South Devon, England. In March of 1915, she writes a letter requesting to "be taken back in the [Navy Nurse Corps'] Active Service List on 1 May. . . . I have not only gotten all the experience possible, but . . . I am needed more at home than here. . . . nothing but convalescent patients . . . for two months . . . come in one week and gone out the next, meaning they come for 'a wash and a shave' and are discharged on furlough."[49] She returns to the United States in April and is reappointed to the Navy Nurse Corps on 7 May. On 10 May she is again reappointed as a Chief Nurse. (Miss Hertzer, who accompanied J. Beatrice Bowman on the Red Cross ship, also returns to the U.S. and re-enters the Navy.) Then, by 1 October 1915, the American Red Cross is forced to withdraw nearly all of its relief efforts from overseas because of a lack of funds.

A nurse-anesthetist, Faye Fulton, is a civilian nurse who also joined the Red Cross in 1914 to help in the overseas crisis. (This nurse later enters the Navy Nurse Corps, in 1917.) In a taped interview, Faye states, "In 1914, I went to France with the American Red Cross."[50] "The ship sailed September 13, 1914, chartered from Hamburg-American Line, 2 stacks on ship, painted white, stacks had large red crosses. There was no one on board but nurses, doctors, and crew (staff of 160). Twelve nurses and three doctors made up a unit. Each unit was named for the city from which it came, namely: New York, Baltimore, Chicago, and Philadelphia. Two units went to each of the following countries: England, France, Germany, and Russia. (Three units had been sent earlier to Servia, now called Serbia). . . . The first stop for our ship was Falmouth, England, where two units left to stay in England. Then we went on to Bordeaux, France, where the Philadelphia and Baltimore units left the ship and were transported by train to Pau, France, 500 miles south of Paris, where the hospital was in a casino. . . . The ship then went on to take units to Germany and Russia. All these units served for one year."[51] "We [arrived at Pau] and we had our hospital. . . . We were at the base of the Pyrenees Mountains. . . . We had but little snow at a time. The flowers were coming up through this little, soft, flaky snow, and the white peacocks were walking around. . . . We would go for our patients . . . down at the railroad. There would be a representative from the French and a representative from the Americans. And the doctors would send so many to the American hospital and so many to the French hospital . . . both in this same building. At that time we had about, I should say, maybe fifty patients and the French would have maybe the same amount. We took care of the patients that came back from the front."[52] Later, in the interview tape, Faye Fulton speaks of her anesthesia experience saying, "In 1914 I used Chloroform entirely for one year. Many people would think that that was rather a long period of time, but I'm glad to say that I didn't have any fatality and I know of but one patient that developed an acute condition due to Chloroform." Miss Fulton's unit left in 1915, as did all the other units, to return to the States.

As for the war situation itself, Americans are shocked when "the British liner *Lusitania* [is] sunk by a German U-boat with the loss of 128 Americans in May, 1915."[53] Further, Germany has started to use poison gas in the war and tried to blockade Great Britain.[54] But, President "Wilson [refuses] to alter his position of strict neutrality in the European war, turning a deaf ear on those who [urge] a tougher policy toward Germany."[55] Then, in October, the world learns of yet another incident. An English nurse by the name of Edith Cavell "had organized the first school for nurses in Brussels, Belgium. Here, following the occurrence of several battles in its vicinity, school and hospital offered care to soldiers of all armies. By the Germans arresting her, however, Miss Cavell [is] charged with another activity, that of complicity in the escape to neutral territory of able-bodied Allied soldiers who had been separated from their companies and were in hiding nearby. Pleading guilty, Edith Cavell [is] sentenced to death, and executed. . . ."[56]

Meantime, in the U.S. Navy Medical Department, "Two Hospital Corps Training Schools [are] again started, one at the Training Station at San Francisco, and one at the Training Station at Newport, RI, and by June 30, 1915, about 159 [corpsmen] [are] under instruction in these schools."[57] (The schools had been halted for a while because of a shortage of hospital corpsmen: those available had been needed to take care of the sick and injured aboard the ships of the Navy.[58]) At the Hospital Corps School in Newport, a Navy Nurse (Mary McCloud) is asked to lecture for one hour each week on nursing.[59] Another step forward for both the Nurse Corps and the Hospital Corps.

In 1916 there are 152 Navy Nurses on active duty. Overseas, in Samoa, the first class of three native nurses graduate and justify the stormy beginnings of the nursing program as well as the efforts of the first Navy Nurses. The three new graduates are given diplomas and gold nursing pins. Over in Guam, uniforms and caps are authorized for the native students in that nursing program. The Chief Nurse at Guam, J. Beatrice Bowman, is assigned additional duty as a member of the faculty of a local normal school. There, she begins to instruct the teachers in public health. Sadly, also at Guam, Nurse Nellie M. Sherzinger, USN, of Columbus, Ohio, is the first nurse to die in service.[60] The cause of death is Tuberculosis.[61]

1916 also finds the U.S. again having recurring problems with the neighbors down south of the border. 'Pancho' Villa is once more raiding across the frontier into New Mexico: "killing and burning as [he goes.]"[62] President Wilson calls on General John J. Pershing and the Army and gives orders to pursue the Mexican raiders deep into Mexico. This does not make for friendly relationships with the Mexican government and a war is narrowly avoided. (Resentments about the intrusion, last for a long time thereafter.) 200,000 United States Army personnel are involved in the chase "and there [are] five base hospitals, five camp hospitals, and one cantonment hospital along the border. [Cantonment means, "the assignment of troops to temporary quarters."[63]] Obviously the Army Nurse Corps [cannot] meet the situation with its 150 members."[64] The Red Cross offers reserve nurses to the Army and eventually 257 Red Cross nurses are "used on the border, most of them for a period of only a few weeks."[65] It is interesting to note that "For the first time a considerable number of reserve nurses [have] a taste of army discipline and [learn] one very important fact: once assigned to the army, they [are] no longer under the direction of the Red Cross."[66] Evidently discipline is a source of complaint for a few of the nurses, but they soon discover that the Red Cross doesn't have jurisdiction in the Army.

The above affair, is an example of the American Red Cross acting as the 'reserve' source for the Army Nurse Corps. As mentioned previously, in 1911, "The American Red Cross was designated as the only volunteer agency authorized to serve with the armed forces in time of war. Enrolled Red Cross nurses, therefore, constitute the reserve of the Army and Navy Nurse Corps."[67] In August of 1916, the 64th Congress creates the U.S. Naval Reserve Force, with provision for nurses. Nurses are to be "enrolled in the U.S. Naval Coast Defense Reserve or the Volunteer Naval Reserve. The difference between the two classes [to be] that members of the Volunteer Reserve [will not] receive the retainer fee of $12.00 a year which the Class 4 N.C.D.R. (or U.S.N.R.F.) [will], in addition to active duty pay when they [are] called into service."[68] The month after this enactment, September, Chief Nurse Katrina Hertzer, USN, is assigned to Nursing Service at Red Cross National Headquarters.[69] (She is the same one who, with J. Beatrice Bowman, was on the Red Cross Ship to Europe in 1914.) Miss Hertzer is appointed to help in the enrollment of nurses and to act as *"liaison* officer between the [Red Cross] Nursing Service and the Navy Nurse Corps."[70] (She remains in this position until 1921.)

The profession of nursing takes a step forward in 1916, with "the conversion of a hospital school into a professional school of nursing at the University of Cincinnati. . . ."[71] Also, taking this step, at the same time, is "Teachers College in cooperation with the Presbyterian Hospital School of Nursing, New York."[72] These are the "first basic programs in nursing education leading to a degree. . . ."[73]

This 1916 is also a presidential election year. President Wilson and his Vice President run on the Democratic ticket against the Republican ticket headed by Supreme Court Justice Charles Evans Hughes. "On election night, the outcome [is] confused because of delays in receiving the election returns. Wilson [goes] to bed believing Hughes [has] won. Many newspapers [carry] stories of Wilson's 'defeat.' But the final count in California [gives] the state to Wilson by 4,000 votes. This [insures] his re-election."[74]

In January of 1917, the Germans announce their "total blockade of the British Isles - anything that [moves will] be sunk."[75] (This threat includes American ships.) President Wilson severs all U.S. diplomatic relations with Germany because of this announcement. Meantime, the British have broken the German communication code so that they (the British) are able to decipher German communiques. They "decipher a particularly important message . . . between Berlin and Washington."[76] It comes from the German foreign secretary and is to the German ambassador in DC. The British send a copy to President Wilson. The message reads, "We [the Germans] intend to begin unrestricted submarine warfare. We shall endeavor to keep the United States neutral. In the event of this not succeeding, we make Mexico a proposal of alliance on the following basis: make war together, make peace together. Generous financial support, and an understanding on our part that Mexico is to reconquer the lost territory in Texas, New Mexico and Arizona."[77] Needless to say, the President is shocked. Between this and a record number of sinkings of U.S. merchant ships, he begins to plan for the U.S. entering World War I. The U.S. Army, under General Pershing, had been pulled out of Mexico (where they'd been chasing after 'Pancho' Villa and his men) so General Pershing feels free to tell the President, "I would like to command the expedition. . . ."[78] Meaning that he would like to command the Armed forces when the U.S. enters World War I. On the 2nd of April President Wilson goes before Congress and asks for a declaration of war. On the 6th of April, the United States declares war on Germany.[79]

Meanwhile, across the ocean, one of the Allies is in deep trouble. Russia is about to collapse. "The Russian common soldiers were sent into battle without guns to support them, without even rifle ammunition; they were wasted by their officers and generals. . . . A profound disgust for the Tsardom was creeping through these armies of betrayed and wasted men."[80] Then the Russian masses revolt, in March of 1917, overthrow their government and force the Tsar to abdicate.[81] A new Tsar takes over and Russia "still [fights] on and [makes] a last desperate offensive effort in July. It [fails] after some preliminary successes and another great slaughtering of Russians. The limit of Russian endurance [is] reached. Mutinies now [break] out in the Russian armies . . . and on November 7th, 1917, . . . [the] government [is] overthrown and power [is] seized by the Soviet Government, dominated by the Bolshevik socialists under Lenin. . . ."[82] In December, Russia signs an armistice with the Germans.

During all of this, America is mobilizing for war. A selective-service act starts the draft of young men, Liberty bonds are promoted, the States ring with the song 'Over There' and people are asked to economize on food.[83] On 26 June the first American troops begin to land in France. One of General Pershing's staff officers, remembering the help of the French during the American Revolution, announces, "Lafayette, we are here!"[84] On the 30th of July, "German saboteurs set off an explosion at . . . [an] ammunition shipping station, near Jersey City,

N.J.."[85] This only serves to increase the American enmity toward the Germans. Then in October of 1917, the first American troops enter the trenches in France and come face to face with WWI.

All of this mobilization effort has effect throughout the U.S. and particularly on the medical community. One organization is admirable for its readiness: the American Red Cross Nursing Service. "Red Cross had started the enrollment [of qualified graduate nurses] in 1905, and from an initial enrollment of 50 nurses the first year, the reserve list had steadily increased in number until in April 1917 it [totals] more than 8,000."[86] "Great numbers of carefully selected nurses had been enrolled and could now be turned over for service with the expanding Army Nurse Corps and Navy Nurse Corps."[87] In total, the Red Cross has "the nurses' organization for twenty-six base hospitals . . . completed — 1,250 nurses and 599 nurse's aides. They had taken their examinations and immunity treatments and were ready to be mobilized. In process of organization were also 31 navy detachments of 20 nurses each. . . ."[88] During WWI, "nursing units [are] furnished the Navy on the same terms as the army. The five base hospitals for the navy had 250 beds each instead of 500, and the personnel [is] smaller than for the army base hospitals, with only 40 nurses [later raised to 50.] Naval station hospital units and navy detachments corresponded to hospital units and emergency detachments for the army. Eventually 339 nurses were assigned to naval hospital units organized by the Red Cross and 540 as members of navy detachments."[89] In a book written in 1922 (History of American Red Cross Nursing), it states, "In three respects the Navy Nurse Corps set up requirements of no little embarrassment to its reserve, the American Red Cross Nursing Service.

"First, it was required that a candidate for the naval services be a woman of the highest professional training and of mature judgment, because she was expected to have entire charge of the nursing education of the hospital apprentices of the Navy. When in the exigency of war the Red Cross Nursing Service let down its enrollment bars to admit young graduates of small institutions, the Navy Nurse Corps refused to accept these nurses, on the ground that they lacked the experience and the years which make for proficient instructors.

"The second point covered physical condition . . . described in a circular letter sent in June 1917 . . . : Perfect physical condition is essential. Overweight or imperfect eyesight, unless corrected by glasses, will debar a nurse from enrollment. . . . The requirement covering eyesight proved particularly troublesome. Miss Noyes [of the Red Cross] once remarked to Mrs. Higbee [Navy Nurse Corps Superintendent]: "Does the Navy contemplate making sharp-shooters out of your nurses?"

"But the most formidable requirement of the Corps was that its members be of American citizenship. However, when the pending shortage of nurses was foreseen in 1917, the Navy lowered this requirement."[90] (Needless to say, the requirements that the above quotation refers to, are those that were set by the first Superintendent of the Navy Nurse Corps. Those requirements helped establish the demeanor and elite 'tone' of the Corps from the very beginning.) Despite this minor controversy, in this same book, the authors state, "As was the case with the Army, the relations of the Red Cross Nursing Service and the Navy Nurse Corps during the war [are] at all times intimate and cordial."[91]

When the U.S. declares war on the 6th of April 1917, there are 160 nurses in the Navy Nurse Corps. On the 15th of April, the Secretary of the Navy authorizes the Surgeon General to appoint Reserve nurses as permitted by the 1908 Act that created the Nurse Corps. Shortly thereafter, the Secretary authorizes enrollment of nurses in Class IV, U.S. Naval Reserve Force (as permitted by an Act of Congress in 1916.) On the 25th of April, the first nurse enrolled in the USNRF reports to the Naval Hospital in the Naval Home, Philadelphia. (Her name is Anna C. Lofving.) Naval Base Hospital Units begin to organize at several civilian hospitals. By the 1st of July there are 190 USN nurses and 155 USNRF nurses on active duty. On the 30th of July, Jessie G. Coon of San Francisco, California reports for duty with Base Hospital #2 (Stanford University Unit.) (This nurse is believed to be the first appointed as a Reserve nurse, USN.) The Hospital Corps instruction programs are increasing and more nurses are being assigned to teaching in the programs. The Manual of the Medical Department is changed so that USN (regular) nurses no longer renew after each three year period; the appointment to USN is continuous until formally ended. Then on the 22nd of September 1917, the first Navy Nurses sail for Brest, France. They are of the Brooklyn Hospital Unit (Naval Base #1.) They sail aboard the USS *Henderson* with their Reserve Chief

Nurse, Frances Ban Ingen, USN. Also, aboard the *Henderson*, is a small group of Naval personnel (no nurses) from the Philadelphia Methodist Hospital Unit (Naval Base #5.) This Philadelphia Unit consists of 7 Medical Officers, 2 Supply Corps Officers "and about 125 enlisted men. . . . These [are] mostly reservists, of a wide variety of ratings, including cooks & [sic] bakers, yeomen and storekeepers, and, of course, many pharmacists mates. Many of these [are] recent college graduates."[92] Ensign Brown (the author of a Base #5 history) goes on to say, "The morning we [are] to sail from Philadelphia, amid the excitement of relatives and friends wishing Godspeed . . . a leading Philadelphia doctor arrived in a large and impressive Locomobile touring car, complete with chauffeur.......evidently overcome by a burst of patriotism, he asked our Dr. Curl [Navy MC and commanding officer of the Unit] if he would like to have his car. Of course Dr. Curl said `Yes.' There [is] no time left for the lengthy preparation of the car for ocean travel, including great detail in the draining of fuel, etc. We merely attached slings to the car's axles, and hoisted her aboard the Henderson. Arriving in France, the car [is] about the first thing off the ship....our lad designated as Dr. Curl's driver [turns] the key, and off she [goes]! This fine car [serves] Base Hospital #5 in many capacities for over a year. The transmission finally [burns] out, ...as I recall, we [give] the engine to the Y.M.C.A., who [uses] it to run an electric light plant in some remote location."[93]

The *Henderson* sails from Philadelphia to New York where it joins the second U.S. convoy to France. The convoy includes transport and cargo ships, as well as, the USS *Antilles* and the USS *Finland*. It takes "three weeks getting to France, mainly dodging German submarines. . . . After a week or so [following debarking] . . . we [receive] orders to proceed to Brest and establish our hospital there. . . . Meanwhile the nurses' unit of the Methodist Hospital [Philadelphia] and a number of its doctors, had sailed from the U.S.A. aboard the British ship SS *St. Louis*."[94] (The Navy Nurses are Alice. M. Garrett (Chief Nurse), Mary Young (Assistant Chief Nurse), Faye Fulton (Anesthetist), Beulah Basler (Operating Room Nurse) and 39 other Navy Nurses.) Faye Fulton and Beulah Basler tell of the trip, "Our unit was headed by Miss Alice Garrett who was Superintendent of the Methodist Hospital. She joined the Navy with us as our Chief Nurse. . . . We left Philadelphia in October of 1917 by train from Philadelphia to New York where we boarded the *St. Louis* ship. We sailed along alone to Europe. We were met two days out of Southampton by two destroyers. . . . We landed in Southampton. . . . We stayed in Southampton, then, two days and two nights before we were able to cross the English Channel. That was a rocky trip, I'll tell you that, because things rolled around. The horses were down below, I guess they balanced the ship. . . . But the Channel was dangerous crossing on account of so many submarines. . . . [In France] we boarded a train for Brest. We were on this train two nights and one day. When we landed in Brest, we were met by the doctors of our hospital."[95]

Meantime, Brest has been busy becoming one of the largest U.S. Navy Bases and the hospital is a necessity, so the small medical group that first arrived, from the USS *Henderson*, goes to work at once. "[They] first [locate] a large residence suitable for a Nurses' home....[they negotiate] a lease for this, and [move] the nurses in. They also [locate] what [seems] to be a good location for our hospital.......a Catholic Convent . . . in partial commission. [They start] proceedings to commandeer it for our use, and [move] in......even building a temporary galley to provide our food. HOWEVER, the Mother Superior of this Convent [prevails].....and we [are] ordered to move out and go elsewhere!"[96] Finally, they find another convent; old and completely abandoned. "It [is] not very promising to see . . . consisting mainly of walls, floor, roof, and windows, and very little else. No plumbing, or water, or wiring, or lighting. . . . So we [move] in .....and immediately set to work to build a modernly-equipped hospital in these antique buildings. . . . The necessary carpenters, plumbers, painters, electricians, etc., we . . . find among our growing enlisted force. . . . A few examples, among many, may be of passing interest:

"We needed a man to take charge of all of our electrical work, which was, of course, very extensive. Lining up the crew, our Captain asked if any one had had any experience in installing electrical wiring. Up stepped one of my 4th class cooks . . . said he had been head of his own wiring contracting firm!!!! Why was he a cook, then? Well, the day he enlisted in the Navy, they were only taking cooks!! In one jump he was made a Chief Electricians Mate. . . .

"We needed a man to serve as Chief Master at Arms....to be, in effect, in charge of the enlisted men. One of our Reserve pharmacists mates . . . seemed right for the job......in one jump he was made Chief Master at Arms....and he proved to be the ideal man for the job.... ["After the War, he went to work for Wyeth and Co., Manufacturing Chemists in Philadelphia, in their shipping room. A few years later he [became] President of Wyeth."]"[97]

"Of course, even with the mountain of hospital equipment and supplies that we . . . brought with us from Philadelphia, there were many needed things that we had not foreseen. Our best friend in these cases was the AMERICAN RED CROSS. Somehow, they seemed able to find or 'salvage' just about anything that we needed.....even to the steam boilers for our sterilizers and for our fine galley which we had built. . . . About the first medical activity to be put into full commission in our hospital [is] the Operating Room....thanks especially to the incredible Faye Fulton, anesthetist, and her assistants, and the surgical group from the Methodist Hospital Unit."[98]

As the growth of U.S. Navy ships and personnel increases in the Brest area, the more the patient load at Base Hospital #5. "We reached the size of several hundred beds...still the demand increased. Finally we [resort] to large tents, set up in what had been the gardens of the former Convent. In all we [reach] a capacity of some 700 beds."[99] Miss Basler reports that "most of our patients were off the ships coming from [the] United States to France. We had constant work. It was more on the order of a civilian hospital. . . . And these patients had to be taken care of until they [are] physically fit to go on duty which [makes] them stay much longer than an ordinary patient in any [civilian] hospital."[100] Miss Fulton (anesthetist) states, "I remember distinctly, a strangulated hernia that had to be brought up [to the operating room] very quickly and at that time . . . we used plenty of Ether . . . a gauze and a can of Ether. . . . We also used some Nitrous Oxide and Oxygen. . . . We would give an induction with a little Ethyl Chloride."[101] Then Miss Basler tells us, "One of the tragic cases we had was from an explosion on a ship. . . . We had five men burned from their heads to their feet. . . . It was before the day of antibiotics, so they were treated entirely locally with paraffin dressing, which was very painful to have applied. It took one nurse and one corpsman to one patient for a half day. I'm glad to say these patients all survived the burn. One man developed pneumonia later and died, but they were cured. They bore not even a scar."[102] The two nurses go on to say, "We had a great deal of work when the flu epidemic broke out in the United States as well as France. We had to put up tents in our yard. We doubled our patient capacity. And by the way, the patients that we had that developed flu came over from America on the ships. And they were much more serious than the flu developed in France. We treated . . . great numbers of them."[103] Of the War itself, Miss Basler says, "During the Marine drive in France, the Army needed help. They notified the Navy and a group of eight doctors, five nurses and four corpsmen went [to help].... We were getting patients eight hours after they were wounded on the front, brought in four at a time in an ambulance by the boys who had trained in Allentown, Pennsylvania. We operated eighteen hours straight until [one of the doctors] decided that we cannot do more than twelve hours at a time. We [are] there for approximately two weeks helping at this Army hospital."[104] (The Armistice is signed 11 November 1918, but the first group of nurses, from Base Hospital #5 [including Miss Basler], do not leave until January 1919. Miss Fulton did not get home until May 1919. Base Hospital #5 is decommissioned in November of 1919.)

To return to the first group of Navy Nurses (Brooklyn Hospital Unit, Base #1) that sailed for France: one of the nurses is Esther Nelson Behr Hunter. This 25 year old nurse had accepted an appointment as a Reserve Navy Nurse on 5 July 1917. On 13 September 1917 she reported for active duty. On the 22nd of September she is aboard the *Henderson* heading for the War. According to a letter that she writes home, the *Henderson* lands the nurses at a small French seaport where they stay for three days. Then they board a French train for a two-day ride to their destination. "Dark, cold, damp and had to walk two miles to our bunks! No lights and many puddles! Starved, homesick & hungry. We landed into a Monastery - a very large place - all stone — was one of the Famous Boys Schools (Catholic). . . . Then the French had it for a [hospital.] Vacated for the [Americans.] No wood, coal, etc. We (40 of us) slept in a big dormitory on real French hospital beds. Ask the Boys what they are like - we have them [the beds] in this [hospital.] Try piling some rocks carelessly on one another & cover it with a handful of straw - then you have a French [hospital] Bed. However, we all slept like the Devil. We remained in this place until December 5th. No, we had no patients. . . . Many nurses got sick as our food gave out & we had bread & water for three days, no heat & beaucoup [much] rain & cold. . . . December 5th at 7 p.m. we went to Brest & landed there at 9 a.m. the next morning. . . . Hard tack & jam makes the 3 meals on the train. . . . Well, we landed into a dark dirty rotten building just vacated by a French [hospital.] `Cooties' had their [headquarters] there. We scrubbed, painted, washed until it looked quite decent, but before we were half finished on December 10th — Troops started to land and it was awful. They kept coming, until they were landing 60,000 a week. You have no idea what work that means. We sure did work. [Then came a] Let up in the sickness about [the] beginning of June [1918.]"[105]

On the 4th of July 1918, she writes, "Yes, we had our 4th of July celebration over here. . . . First the American soldiers marched to their place, then the American sailors, next the French soldiers and sailors, next the Portugese who have round shoulders & carry their guns poorly . . . two bands and the French Naval School for young French boys - ages 13 [to] 18 [years.]

"They all took their places - and then the American Admiral & General - the French Admirals, decorated in their best bib & tucker, walked down the lines, followed by many Officers & silk hat Harrys!! until the French yelled with us. . . . I had the flag that Dad gave me when I left home and I sat up in my hospital uniform - well starched - on the shoulders of two 6 footers and had a real picnic.

"Three large dirigibles flew quite close and airplanes flew up in the air as thick as German prisoners at the Front." Then Nurse Hunter goes on to say, "Have been getting quite a few 'gas' cases in the hospital lately. They sure are wrecks of manhood. They cannot stand any light, cough a great deal, hearing is poor and many lose their voice entirely. Many have been burnt around the abdomen and inside if their hands. Luckier the

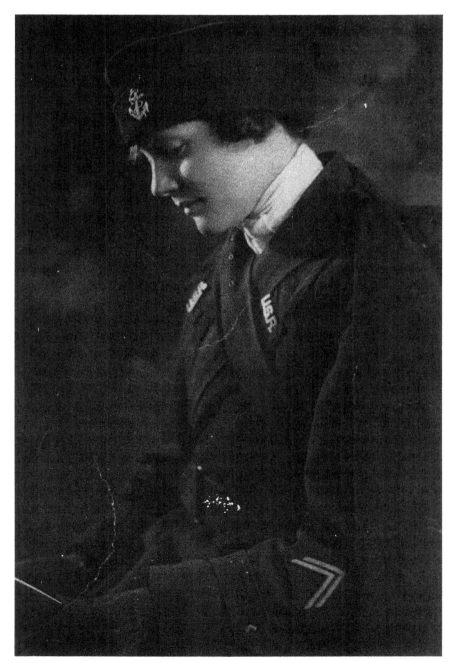

Esther Nelson Behr Hunter. Pictured in uniform designed by her. France 1918. (Photo credit - provided by Joseph N. Hunter, son of Esther Hunter.)

man who loses his legs or arms than be gassed. The Marines have done wonderful work - and the boys that came over to France in our convoy are nearly all killed - many are gassed and crippled. . . . The French & English Officers who come here from the Front talk in a wonderful manner of the bravery & caring of the American soldier."

Then she speaks of "the pretty little French flowered cemetaries [sic] where the soldiers are buried [and] are always well kept up by the French people. Different little Clubs take care of the American graves & watch them carefully. If many Mothers could see the pretty little graves covered with French flowers, that their dear brave sons are buried in, they would gain a great deal of contentment. A very pretty custom is - a bunch of flowers are placed always on the grave to represent the bouquet from the boy's Father & Mother."[106]

In a later letter, Nurse Hunter continues about her tour of duty, "Then July 17th we (22 of us) were rushed up here [outside Paris] on three [hours] notice . . . to take care of the Marines. . . . The Germans were then about 15 miles from Paris. All day and especially the night we could hear the guns. We had some day air raids & a couple of big night air raids. . . . The Big Bertha [largest gun built at this time] . . . went off every 15 or 20 [minutes.] [I] Have a piece of shrapnel from the burst that fell behind our house and 50 feet from the tents. Everything was kept absolutely dark, no lights in the streets etc.. . . .

"[The] wounded we got in every day will never be forgotten. Never did I see such masses of bones & flesh. Never such suffering. We worked 18 [hours] some days. Finally, as they [the Germans] were pushed back, things quieted down, except night air raids!"[107]

"Got a lot of boys in a convoy to-night who were wounded the night of the 10th [of November 1918.] The casualties on that day and night were appalling. God have mercy on the boys who suffered so severely. U.S.A. never will know the long sorrow list until months have passed. . . . Many Mothers have lost four to five sons. The raving of some of the sick at night is terrible. . . . [The] pitiful part is — they smile thru [sic] all their pains & sufferings. No pen could ever tell the terrible pains that the boys have gone thru — and . . . there are so many 16 & 17 [year] old boys in it. When they go thru Fire & Hell — [and] get back here to the [hospital], really they still are kids! . . .

"Needless to say France turned inside out when the Armistice was signed. I was in Brest & the harbor was filled with boats. The noise was deafening & the old Brittons [French] who are always very [staid] paraded with the sailors. Fireworks were set off by all the Ships. Next day a big parade of men who had just landed, etc. Much excitement."[108]

Meanwhile, in Scotland on the Firth of Forth (near Edinburgh), Navy Base Hospital No. 3 has been established. "[This] unit had been organized by the American Red Cross from the personnel of . . . the California Hospital, Los Angeles, California. . . . [The] superintendent of nurses of the California Hospital had organized the nursing staff of Navy Base No. 3, but Miss [Sue Sophia] Dauser, after instruction at the Naval Training Camp at San Diego, led the nursing unit into foreign duty [as its Chief Nurse.]"[109] (Miss Dauser is a 1914 graduate of California Hospital. You might want to keep her name in mind.) The 'History of American Red Cross Nursing' quotes Miss Dauser as writing, "United States Navy Base Hospital No. 3 mobilized at Philadelphia . . . [in] December 1917. Until August 1, 1918, the nurses did temporary duty in and near Philadelphia. On August 1, 1918, we embarked from New York. . . . We arrived at Liverpool [England], August 15, 1918, and by train arrived at Edinburgh, Scotland, early next morning. The hospital we took over had been under the British Admiralty for four years. . . .

"The building in pre-war days was a poorhouse. It was well built and so arranged as to adapt itself most conveniently for a hospital, and afforded ample room for seven hundred and fifty patients. The British hospital equipment was established in the building and all of our own equipment had arrived there before us. We installed our own and accepted enough of the old to enable us to carry about seven hundred and fifty patients. We found our own equipment more convenient. For instance, our beds were the high white hospital beds: the old ones were low black iron cots. We also had enough white paint with us to paint the walls, which had formerly been bright and striking colors. . . .

"The hospital was open to the four military organizations, the British Navy and Army and the American Navy and Army. The majority of Naval patients were influenza cases, but bluejackets were only a small per cent of the number of patients we cared for. Something like seventy-five per cent of the capacity of the hospital was held for the British Army; even this did not seem sufficient and the wounded would overflow this percentage most of the time. These patients came to us in convoy trains. They had been taken off the battlefields about three days before, and had nothing more than First Aid at the field stations."[110]

Yet another Naval Hospital in Great Britain, is the United States Navy Base Hospital No. 4. The personnel are from the Rhode Island Hospital of Providence, Rhode Island. (This is another organization by the American Red Cross for an overseas base hospital as in the foregoing examples.) Grace MacIntyre was the Assistant Superintendent of Nurses of the Rhode Island Hospital and is appointed as Chief Nurse for the Base Hospital No. 4 unit. The nurses of this unit are "mobilized September 12, 1918 in New York."[111] Miss MacIntyre later writes about their journey across the Atlantic, "We sailed September 23 on an English Ship, the *Briton*. The personnel on board consisted of 2200 troops and of 60 women, including our nurses and a group of Red Cross workers. A dirigible balloon and a group of airplanes accompanied us out of the harbor until we met our convoy. . . . On October 2, three submarines were sighted. On October 6, a wireless was received announcing that a submarine was after the *Briton*. While at dinner that evening, we received a terrible shock. One of our own [convoy] ships . . . rammed us, destroying one of our life-boats and tearing away a portion of the rail from one of the decks. When this happened, perfect silence prevailed in the dining saloon. A general paleness was on everyone's face, as we all felt that we had been torpedoed. Our ship soon righted herself and happiness permeated the room again."[112] It wasn't long after this that Spanish Influenza invaded the troops aboard the ship. "The sick report of the troops on board . . . jumped from 6 to 160 in forty-eight hours. Seeing the danger, Miss MacIntyre and her co-workers . . . volunteered their services, with the result that what was chaos (there being practically no accommodations or facilities on board to care for such numbers) was handled in . . . a most admirable manner under the circumstances. They [the nurses] have worked night and day in the cold and damp, on decks that were being washed by seas, without any lights whatsoever, exposed to the dangers of contagion with a deadly malady and they have rendered these services most cheerfully. . . ."[113] They finally dock at Liverpool where seven nurses go to a medical facility in Scotland and four others to another in Cardiff, Wales. The rest of the Navy Nurses go to Whitepoint in Ireland where Base Hospital No. 4 is established. Miss MacIntyre writes of their arrival there, "Our hospital was opened thirty hours after our arrival to meet an emergency caused by . . . [a ship cutting] a destroyer in half. Several men had been killed and about twenty, I think, injured. . . . [Our] commanding officer was much pleased with the manner in which the nurses threw themselves into the work after their strenuous voyages, both across the Atlantic and the Irish Sea. He said: `They all rebounded like rubber balls.'"[114]

Besides base hospitals, the Navy maintains smaller hospitals, dispensaries and sick-bays in Great Britain, France, the Azores, Gibraltar and Italy.[115] Generally, the nurses are not assigned to these smaller units. However, several Navy Nurses, from the base hospitals in France, are assigned to Navy Operating Teams. For instance, Base Hospital No. 5 (the Philadelphia unit) furnishes such operating teams for detached duty at the front and loan to the Army, when needed. A Navy Nurse, Elizabeth Dewey writes of her team duty saying, "As we were going off duty the evening of July 19, 1918, we four nurses, Miss Faye Fulton and Miss Dewey, anesthetizers [sic], and Miss Alice Hurst and Miss Caroline Thompson, were told to be ready to leave for the front at 5 A.M.

"We met the others of the two operating teams at the station the next morning. Drs. George Ross and John Jones were in command; assistants, Drs. Tanner and Lyon, and Chief P.M. [Pharmacists Mate] Shank and P.M. Steel, Diable and Hornsburger were the other members of the teams."[116] The teams make their way to their new assignment at a field hospital. They finally find the hospital located in a hotel of a small French town. Miss Dewey writes that, "In about a half hour both teams were working in the hotel parlor, a medium-sized room reached by a hallway three stretchers long, and wide enough for the stretcher-bearers to walk beside each other. The long French windows of this room were closed; blankets were nailed up outside the shutters to hide the light. The furniture was gone. In its place were two operating-tables and a plank on clothes-horses made a third. . . . A pile of blood-soaked, filthy clothing grew in one corner of the room and millions of flies rose and buzzed when an addition was made to the pile. As a patient was carried out, the stretcher nearest the door was brought in and another shoved in at the far end from the ground outside. The work in that room never stopped day or night, except long enough in the morning to scrape out the filth of the night work, and in the evening to close everything before lights went on; the ground outside was not cleared of stretchers until the fourth day. . . . Only the most urgent cases were operated at No. 12 [the field hospital.] The others were sent on to where facilities were better. Some of the wounds contained maggots and nearly all were gas gangrene cases. . . . The pluck of the men kept us at it. Most of them were conscious and told us they had the Germans on the run. . . . Over 3500 wounded went through No. 12, between July 18 and July 24. About 300 non-transportable cases were operated upon there and the Navy teams performed about 160 of those operations."[117] (Miss Dewey is later commended by the Commander of the U.S. Naval Forces in France. Part of the commendation reads, "She acted as anesthetist during most of her service there, in addition to which, when relieved from that duty, she did extra duty in assisting the nurses in the care of the wounded with their dressings. On one occasion, under extremely unsatisfactory surroundings, she gave anesthetics steadily for fourteen hours without leaving the table, and after this strenuous labor she visited the cases which had been operated upon."[118])

The Base Hospital European Units during World War I are as follows:

"Base Hospital #1, {Brooklyn Hospital) [in] Brest, France. Admitted first patient 14 December 1917. Discharged last patient 21 December 1918. 9035 cases treated; 757 major operations; 2368 operations at front by unit's surgical teams of medical officers, nurses, and hospital corpsmen. Chief Nurse: Frances Van Ingen, Reserve Nurse, USN.

"Base Hospital #2. . . . [Lane Hospital, San Francisco.[119]] Strathpeffer, Scotland. Closed December 1918. Chief Nurse: Elizabeth Hogue, Reserve Nurse, USN.

"Base Hospital #3. (California Hospital, Los Angeles Unit.) Leith, Scotland. Chief Nurse: Sue S. Dauser, Reserve Nurse, USN. August 1918 [to] January 1919. Daily average patients 295.

"Base Hospital #4. (Providence, Rhode Island Hospital Unit.) Queenstown, Ireland. Reserve Chief Nurse: Grace M. McIntyer, USN.

"Base Hospital #5. (Methodist Episcopal, Philadelphia.) Brest, France. Smaller units in London, England and L`Orient, France. Reserve Chief Nurse: Alice Garrett, USN."[120]

Back in the U.S., during the war years, the Navy Medical Department and the Nurse Corps find challenges of a different sort, but none the less important. When war is declared, "the Washington Naval Hospital [is] unprepared to receive the sick and wounded expected from the battlefields of France. . . . At the south end of the reservation carpenters hastily [construct] eight temporary wooden structures to meet the wartime emergency."[121] The same type of construction takes place down at the Naval Hospital in Portsmouth, Virginia, but to a greater extent. Ada McGrath (Navy Nurse 1917 to 1919) describes what happens in April 1917 when a troop ship sails into Norfolk because of an outbreak of contagion aboard: "we had three and four of these long, long rows of tents just for meningitis, `cause we had so many patients. They started building bungalows immediately and it was amazing how rapidly that those buildings were put up. . . . Just a floor and walls and a roof. And just as soon as they got one building done, they'd move the beds with the patients [from the tents] to a bungalow. . . . [They did have the Naval Hospital main building, but] it wasn't equipped for contagion at all. [The tents were all for contagion.] The day after we [the nurses] arrived, a group of young men arrived: corpsmen. . . . [They] had some training as corpsmen . . . and I don't know what we would have done without them. They were wonderful.

"[Over] 700 boys were brought in from that troop ship with spinal meningitis, measles, scarlet fever, [and] diphtheria. . . . I was assigned to the meningitis camp and it was an awful experience. These boys were desperately ill. They were dying . . . day after day, until Rockefeller Center sent serum; one of the first serums for spinal meningitis and a doctor specially trained. . . . He was only one man with two hands to handle that huge number of meningitis cases. It was marvelous what he was able to do; these spinal punctures, one right after another. And these tents, no floors, just beds in these big tents and the beds so close together that you'd have to move a bed out in order to get in to work on the other patient. . . ."[122]

In her interview, Miss McGrath gives us an interesting insight as to how she came to be a Navy Nurse in WWI. When she graduated from nurses training in 1906, she registered with the Red Cross. She states, "they just were asking for volunteers for no specific purpose at that time. . . . Several years went by without any call or any inquiry, then, suddenly, we [some classmates from training] began to get letters for information, where we were and what we were doing and how we could be reached in a hurry. . . . Then, about 1915 [or 1916], we began to organize in units and after a few months were told to keep prepared with a packed suitcase for any emergency call. . . . But, nothing happened until Good Friday of 1917. The day [President] Wilson declared war, the Red Cross notified each of us [presumably, the unit from New Jersey] by telegram to meet at the Newark [New Jersey] Pennsylvania [name of the railroad] Railroad Station . . . which we did, and we were taken [by train] to Norfolk, Virginia." Miss McGrath and the nurses with her remained Red Cross nurses for three months, then in July 1917 they were formally enrolled in the Navy for four years. She states, "we weren't given any choice."[123] Evidently, when nurse McGrath registered with the Red Cross she had been asked which military service she would prefer and she had indicated the Navy. (Remember, the Red Cross was the 'Reserve' for the Army and Navy Nurse Corps.)

After the meningitis outbreak subsided, Miss McGrath tells us "to my great surprise, one day, I was told I was to go as housekeeper for the nurses quarters . . . I knew no more about ordering meals or groceries [the nurses ate their meals in the quarters] . . . never had any experience at all. . . . [The Navy had taken a] house, a double house, which had a number of bedrooms, large rooms, and just put beds and dressers in them and chairs. . . . [There] had been a nurse [as housekeeper] in the quarters from the day it opened. . . . But they changed her and sent her on duty into the main hospital and put me in as housekeeper. Which I hated. . . . And in two or three months they opened up a second nurses quarters and I had two houses. Then after a while they sort of simmered down and I had just one."[124] (A Navy Nurse as head of the nurses Quarters was still in force in the late 1940's and early 50's.)

In 1918, Navy Nurse McGrath is transferred to the Brooklyn Naval Hospital in New York. While she is there the influenza epidemic begins. "[These] two [Navy] nurses developed flu and were terribly ill. And both died . . . in the Navy Hospital and several of us were quarantined immediately. I felt symptoms, I think, well, the day of the funeral. We had a regular military funeral: the Navy Band and the Hearse, the two, and then, I guess, all the nurses they could spare. . . . [Somehow], I don't know who decided it, but I was told that I was the senior of the group so I was the leader. . . . I was feeling wretched. I never will forget that march for several blocks through the Navy grounds out to the street and then several blocks to a main thoroughfare. Then we were led, by the band, back to the hospital and the hearse went on [its way.] You see, one [coffin] was going to Washington and the other to somewhere in Massachusetts. . . . We were in quarantine from then for several days. I wouldn't remember whether it was ten or fourteen or what. . . . I do remember the day we were released. . . . I was notified . . . that I was to go that afternoon to the tailor because my Norfolk jacket [part of uniform] needed alterations. . . . I wore the cape and the blue dress and the velour hat . . . and I carried the Norfolk jacket on my arm. I took the subway and I remember going across the Brooklyn Bridge in that train. There seemed to be an awful lot of people on the streets and everywhere that I could see coming out of the subway and then onto the bridge. And there was such a racket. Whistles were blowing, bells were ringing. . . . [Sitting] next to me was an elderly man. And at first I didn't notice him until he put his hand on my knee and rubbed it over the cloth of the cape. Well, I recognized immediately what he was doing. He was feeling the quality of the material. Then I looked up and he said, 'Don't mind me, I'm Rector of Grace Church.' . . . Grace Church, you know, is very near Astor Place [subway stop] in New York. And the next stop is Astor Place and I change there for a Sixth Avenue subway. He got out there too. He got out and walked right behind me. As we got onto the platform, there was this awesome noise and such a terrible crowd; flags were flying, bells were ringing, whistles were blowing. It was deafening. And this elderly man kept talking in my ear and he said, 'Show me where can I buy a cape like this. I want it for my niece.' I said, 'But you can't. It's government property.' He said, 'Then I can buy the material and tell her about it. How much will I need?' I said, 'Well, I wouldn't know.' And with that he reached down and picked up the edge. . . . He picked up that cape at the very hem and held it out straight. It had a seam down the back. Held it out straight and he tried to measure the length of that seam. . . . And people who were doing all this howling began looking at me. And I said, 'But what's it about?' And he said, 'Oh, didn't you know? It's the Armistice.'"[125]

The influenza that Miss McGrath mentions, is pandemic (worldwide) in 1918 and 1919. Twenty million deaths are caused by the disease, partly because of complications.[126] Because of the tremendous patient loads in the Navy Medical facilities, the Navy Department takes an unprecedented action: the employment of civilian nurses is authorized during the influenza crisis. Also, "Navy nurses [are] transferred from details as dieticians to meet the crisis and some 30 civilian dietitians [are] substituted at 13 hospitals."[127] To give you an example of the extent of the situation; at the Naval Hospital, Great Lakes, Illinois, this hospital of 2800 beds is unable to handle their influx of 'flu' patients. A nearby detention camp is taken over with barracks to accommodate one thousand additional beds. The Chief Nurse of the hospital (J. Beatrice Bowman) has to provide nurses as each new ward is opened. Miss Bowman notes that "it was a terrible time."[128] She says, "I looked out from my office window and there'd be seventy to ninety caskets out there. . . . A terrible experience. . . . And oh, we needed nurses. My nurses didn't stop to get orders to do double duty. They [did] the duty assigned them and then when they came off [that duty] they immediately went to wards where they knew they were needed and that was their gift to the war. But, they worked like Trojans. . . . They were wonderful women."[129]

At the Naval Hospital in Philadelphia, the war precipitated a tremendous expansion in patient load and in personnel. A newly recruited Navy Nurse writes of it all, "At this hospital we had trying days and the memory of them will last as long as life. The work in itself was hard, and the difficulties seemed harder because the work was so strange. . . . At the outbreak of the war this hospital was the only Naval base in Philadelphia and we saw this base of less than one hundred patients grow, in a few days, to one with more than six hundred patients. Many of these men were, like ourselves, new in the service. Add to this, the naval discipline which insisted upon sick call at 9 A.M., all medications, nourishments and treatments on time and everything in readiness for inspection at 10 A.M.[sic] This was usually made by the executive officer accompanied by the chief nurse. Captain's inspection with all its details occurred every Saturday morning."[130] Then this nurse writes more about the differences between civilian nursing and nursing in the Navy, "We were employed not so much as nurses, but as instructors and supervisors of the hospital corpsmen. These men were to serve aboard ship. They were to be the nurses in time of distress, and we had to work with this thought always in mind. Often when haste was imperative it would have expedited matters to have done the work ourselves; for example, to give a hypodermic. But no, we had to supervise the corpsman while he gave it; otherwise present expediency, we knew, might interfere with a terrible future contingency. This reminds me that as yet no pen has been so facile as to describe in true worth the hospital corpsman. . . . They came from every walk of life. At one time I had two lawyers, a seminarian and a registered pharmacist working with me."[131]

Another nurse new to the Navy writes of her experiences, "Early in May, 1917, sixteen of us nurses received orders to report to the U.S. Naval Hospital at Newport, Rhode Island. We found a warm welcome awaiting us. The hospital was then overcrowded with very sick boys and there were not enough nurses to care for them. I was assigned to Ward D Medical for duty; I found seventy-six patients, most of whom were very ill with measles. A number of these patients had already developed pneumonia, while others had developed ear complications. One nurse had the supervision of this ward and the nursing care of these patients. She had as her assistants six hospital corpsmen. These hospital corpsmen had been carefully trained in the care of the sick and it was really wonderful to see how well most of them performed their duties and how kind they were to their 'sick buddies,' as they called them. . . . Miss Hoag was later assigned to Ward C, the 'pus surgical' division. She wrote: Here we had fifty-six bed patients, suffering from empyema, gangrenous appendices, infected arms and legs and crushed hands and feet. Some of these patients had been in the hospital for months and had grown thin and pale, but still seemed happy and cheerful."[132]

Even in 1917 the Navy Nurse Corps recognized the necessity for the continuing education of Navy nurses, as the following indicates: "Early in July, 1917, a group of nurses from the Naval hospital at Newport was sent to the City Hospital at Providence to take a two weeks' course in the technique of caring for contagious cases. Minnette Butler, a reserve nurse at Newport, wrote:

"This course was a great help during the months of epidemics which followed. In July a hundred cases of diphtheria developed within one week among the civilian population at Newport. Fearing that the contagion might spread to the training station, our commanding officer offered to assist the city health department. These officials furnished cars and a past assistant surgeon, a nurse and a corpsman were detailed to visit every hotel, bakery, ice cream parlor, restaurant and dairy in the city and take cultures of all people handling milk. The authorities had reason to suspect that the trouble was coming from the milk supply.

"After the city had been 'cultured' in this way, they made the rounds of farms outside the city and visited ninety families. In a Portuguese cottage, a seventeen-year-old boy, with a heavy membrane in his throat, was found ill in bed with diphtheria. His mother was caring for him; she also milked the cows and was sending a supply of contaminated milk to many city houses. A constable was placed on the grounds to see that all milk was buried. No new cases developed, but had it not been for the prompt and efficient work of the Naval culture squad, an epidemic might have developed which would have proven to be a real crisis.

"Fate, however, could not let Newport rest, it seemed, because a terrific explosion occurred soon afterwards at the Torpedo Station. It caused many deaths and maimed, burned and blinded many others."[133] It is not only the war zone that is hazardous duty during WWI.

At the Chelsea Naval Hospital in Massachusetts, a new Navy Nurse writes that "One of my first troubles was with Navy regulations and parlance. . . . The Navy 'paper work' was a new and difficult task and the language bewildered us. How were we to know that 'squil gee the deck' meant to polish the ward floor?"[134] Miss McQuade goes on to write, "One day toward the last of August [1918] we were told an epidemic had broken out among the men of the receiving ship [in Boston Harbor.] It was influenza, they said. The word did not mean much to us that lovely August afternoon as those of us off duty made beds in an empty ward. That night, during which sixty-seven sick men came in, was the beginning of the influenza epidemic that has become history. We worked as we never worked before. The influx of patients, the calls for extra nurses, the illnesses of the staff, the deaths, all were repeated later in other hospitals, but to those of us who experienced the initial outbreak when the disease and its treatment were unfamiliar to all, this trying period has left a memory that will not fade for many years."[135]

The influenza hit the Marine Base at Parris Island, South Carolina in 1918 and in November Navy Nurses are assigned there to help during the crisis. One of these ladies writes, "The Naval hospital, which was a rambling, white, two-storied building on the water's edge, had had only corpsmen in attendance upon the patients and medical officers to direct their work. Being the first nurses ordered to this Post, we naturally felt it was quite an adventure and tackled the work with enthusiasm.

"Our first patients were suffering from influenza. After some weeks the epidemic abated and we than had many surgical cases. . . .

"During the spring [1919] a large addition to the hospital was built; across the street the nurses' new quarters was completed and it was a joyous day when we moved in. Instead of sharing a dormitory, each nurse had a delightful room to herself."[136]

In 1918 there are, all together, twenty-five Naval Hospitals in the continental United States at this time for Navy Nurses.

The hospitals are:

> "Annapolis, Maryland
> Brooklyn, New York
> Cape May, New Jersey
> Charleston, South Carolina
> Chelsea, Massachusetts

Fort Lyon, Colorado
Georgetown University Hospital, Wash., DC
Great Lakes, Illinois
Gulfport, Mississippi
Key West, Florida
League Island, Pennsylvania
Mare Island, California
New London, Connecticut
New Orleans, Louisiana
Newport, Rhode Island
Pensacola, Florida
Pelham Bay Park, New York
Philadelphia, Pennsylvania
Portsmouth, New Hampshire
Portsmouth, Virginia
Puget Sound, Washington
Quantico, Virginia
San Diego, California
Washington, DC
Hampton Roads, Virginia"[137]

There are five other stations where Navy Nurses are assigned during WWI. All five are on foreign soil and far from the war zone. However, the Navy Nurses at these medical facilities find that they, too, face challenges and changes, but of a far different type. Two of those stations are Canacao, Philippine Islands, and Guam, Marianas Islands. A third station is the one in Tutuila, Samoa. In 1918, in Samoa, Chief Nurse Hannah Workman, USN, begins classes in public health for the pastors' wives.[138]

The fourth station is in the Caribbean. You see, in 1917 the United States pays twenty-five million dollars for the territory to be called The Virgin Islands of the United States. (An area of islands formerly a part of the Danish West Indies.)[139] Then, in September of 1917, two Navy Nurses arrive in the Virgin Islands: Acting Chief Nurse Alice M. Gillett, USN, and Nurse Eva R. Dunlap, USN. Nine more nurses report in within a few months. The nurses are stationed at St. Thomas and at St. Croix. One Navy Nurse is detailed as welfare nurse for the Christianated District, in St. Croix. This nurse also has duty as Supervising Nurse for the Richmond Insane and Leper Asylums. Also, a school of nursing for native women is started by the Navy Nurses at the Municipal Hospital in St. Thomas in November of 1917 (with 13 students.) A month later, in December of 1917, a school of nursing is founded by the Navy Nurses at St. Croix.[140] The fifth foreign station is in Port au Prince, Haiti (also in the Caribbean area.) On 25 July 1918, Chief Nurse Lucia D. Jordan, USN and Nurse Josephine Y. Raymond, USN land in Port au Prince. ("These two nurses are loaned, by the Navy, to the State Department which in turn [loans] them to the Republic of Haiti."[141]) They are there to instruct and to assist the Catholic Sisters in developing a training school for the native women. The first session of this school begins on 15 October 1918. The classes at the school, have to be given in French since this is the language of the educated Haitians.[142] There are fifty applications received for the first class; forty-nine are eligible; twenty-three are accepted since there are only twenty-three openings. The course is two years long and the first three months are probationary. A diploma is to be awarded to those who complete the course.[143]

At all five of these overseas stations, "Navy nurses have done little less than wonders. For, under direction of the medical officers, the nurses have developed dispensary and social service at Cavite and Canacao [both in the Philippines]; have trained the Chamorro nurses and midwives of Guam; have taught Samoan women to nurse, especially to do district nursing, and recently they have undertaken to make trained attendants out of native women of the Virgin Isles. This pioneer work of fighting ignorance and dirt afar from home and friends is not easy or at all romantic - at least, not while you're in the midst of it. But it's a beautiful victory, none the less, and one well worthy of the best traditions both of the Navy and of the nursing profession."[144] (This accolade is written in February 1918. It is written by Anita McGee, M.D. who had been an Acting Assistant Surgeon, U.S. Army, in Charge Army Nurse Corps, 1898-1901 and a Supervisor of Nurses, Imperial Japanese Army, in the Russo-Japanese War.)

To return to the War, the Navy data book for 1918[145] lists several hospital ships that are functioning during this time. There is a *Repose* listed as a floating dispensary with the Asiatic Fleet. A *Comfort*, *Mercy*, and a *Solace* are listed as serving with the Atlantic Fleet. A *Relief* is listed as a hospital ship, but it is in the process of being built at the Philadelphia Navy Yard.[146] The *Mercy* and the *Comfort* were formerly the *Havana* and *Saratoga*. At the beginning of WWI, these two ships were purchased and converted to hospital ships.[147] All three of the active hospital ships are "commanded by naval medical officers."[148] There are no Navy Nurses aboard these ships; that duty assignment will come later.

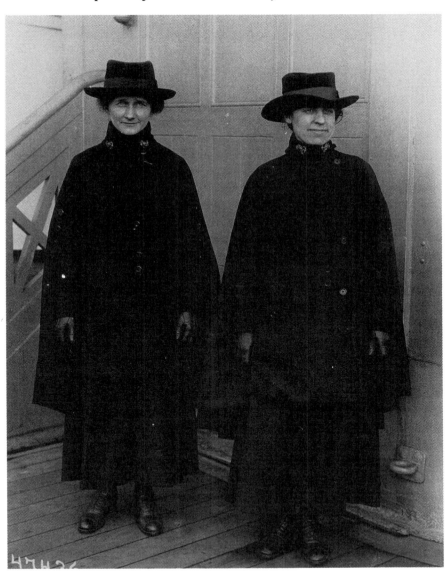

Navy Nurses aboard USS *George Washington* 1918. (Photo Courtesy of Navy Bureau of Medicine and Surgery.)

On 22 September 1918, the first Navy Nurse is interred at Arlington National Cemetery: Maude Coleman, USN (who succumbed to 'Influenza.'[149]) A few days later, on the 28th of September, a section of the Arlington National Cemetery is set aside for Army and Navy Nurses.[150]

In October 1918, across the sea in Germany, this month is "a story of defeat and retreat along the entire Western front. . . . Frenchmen and Englishmen [can] not believe their newspapers as day after day they [announce] the capture of more hundreds of guns and more thousands of prisoners. . . . There [is] an attempt to bring out the German fleet for the last fight, but the sailors [mutiny] (November 7th). The Kaiser and the Crown Prince [bolt] hastily, and without a scrap of dignity, into Holland. On November 11th an armistice [is] signed and the war [is] at an end."[151]

On the 2nd of December 1918, the first Navy Nurses assigned to transport duty (transporting American troops home from the war) report aboard the USS *George Washington*. The Chief Nurse is Sophia V. Kiel, USN. (On the ship's first trip, the President of the United States, Woodrow Wilson, travels with them on his way to the Paris Peace Conference. He is "the first President to cross the Atlantic Ocean while in office."[152]) Also, on 2 December, Chief Nurse Mary Robinson (Godfrey) reports aboard the USS *Leviathan*.[153] The *Leviathan* is one of the largest ships afloat, at this time, and Mrs. Godfrey tells us that it takes "two thousand men to operate that ship. . . . [The ship left] from Hoboken, New Jersey and went to Brest [France] but it was so large and took up so much water, they had to dock three miles out. There were only two places in the world that that ship could dock . . . someplace near the Suez Canal and Hoboken . . . Because it drew so much water."[154] Mrs. Godfrey says that on their last trip back, with the troops from overseas, General Pershing sailed with them. (General John Joseph Pershing commanded the American Expeditionary Forces in Europe during WWI.[155]) Mrs. Godfrey states that she and her nurses were at dinner on the ship one night when the General came in. She told her nurses if the General looked their way they should "just bow our heads and keep on eating. So he came in, he stopped and looked until he found us and then he bowed and we just bowed back. . . . I said to the nurses, 'That's for all nurses, not just us.'"[156]

During the war years, nurses learned about the horror of war, the results of battle and armament on human bodies, the consequences of mustard gas, pandemic 'Spanish flu' and so much more concerning their profession and themselves. Navy Nurses came to understand other matters as well. One most important matter brought to their attention is their position as, not only professional nurses, but as members of the military. As members of the Armed Forces, they are governed by all the laws and regulations of that organization, especially during wartime. "In 1918 [during the war] this matter came to a head when two nurses who were ordered to the naval hospitals at Canacao and Guam refused to carry out their orders and submitted their resignations. The handling of previous cases had apparently been to simply separate the nurses. . . . [In] 1918 under war time conditions and the great need for nurses a [stern] view was taken. The Bureau of Medicine and Surgery wrote the Secretary [of the Navy] stating that the nurses were part of the military establishment and were expected to conform to regulations; [the] nurses had left the service without waiting for official action; they went absent without leave and had refused to obey orders. Heretofore, said the Bureau, official action was to discharge them from the service, but the nurses did not regard this as serious and it had no restraining effect. Accordingly, the Bureau recommended the two nurses be tried by court martial and they were discharged after a Summary Court Martial on 4 November 1918."[157] (They are lucky they weren't shot.)

Yet another change due to the war, is the instruction of the hospital corpsmen. The course for the men, at the training stations, had been six months long, but wartime needs causes the time to be decreased. The course "is condensed into three months of intensive study . . . supplemented by additional experience, bedside teaching and class work in the hospitals."[158] Navy Nurses continue to be deeply involved in the training and in the practical hospital experience of the corpsmen; this being "one of the most important reasons for the existence of the Navy Nurse Corps [especially in war-time]."[159]

During the war, four Hospital Corps Schools are taxed to their capacities as they carry out their teaching mission. The oneat Great Lakes has a normal capacity of three hundred students and at one point, during WWI, has twenty-two hundred registered students.[160] The other three schools are at Newport, R.I., San Francisco, California, and Norfolk, Virginia.[161] "The Bureau of Medicine and Surgery [receives] offers of assistance in the training of hospital corpsmen from various universities and three of these [are] accepted. A four months' course for one hundred men at the Medical and Dental Schools, University of Minnesota; a six-weeks course for three hundred men at the College of Pharmacy, University of New York, and a three-months course for one hundred and fifty men at the Philadelphia College of Pharmacy."[162]

A review of the statistics for World War I shows that 1,551 Navy Nurses serve from 6 April 1917 to 11 November 1918. For the period between 6 April 1917 to 3 March 1921 (official war period) a total of 1,835 serve; 327 of these nurses are on duty outside the USA.[163] Nineteen Navy Nurses die during 6 April 1917 to 11 November 1918: Influenza causes ten deaths, Pneumonia causes five deaths, Meningitis causes two deaths, one nurse dies of Carcinoma, and one nurse dies of Acute Bright's Disease. Eight of the nineteen are Reserve nurses, eight others are USNRF nurses and three are Regular Navy. Only one of the nurses dies overseas. She is one who succumbs to Pneumonia at Base Hospital #3 Leith, Scotland. Seventeen more Navy Nurses die from 11 November 1918 to 3 March 1921 (official war end.) Eight Reserve, seven USNRF and two Regular Navy Nurses. No Navy Nurses die as the result of enemy action.

Four Navy Nurses receive the Navy Cross for their WWI service. Lenah S. Higbee, Superintendent of the Navy Nurse Corps is one of the recipients. Her citation reads, "For distinguished service in the line of her profession and unusual and conspicuous devotion to duty as Superintendent of the Navy Nurse Corps." (The Navy Cross and Citation are presented to her on 11 November 1920.) The other Navy Crosses are awarded posthumously to three Navy Nurses who died from Influenza. They are:

> Reserve Nurse Marie Louise Hidell, USN
> Reserve Nurse Lillian Mary Murphy, USN
> Reserve Nurse Edna Elizabeth Place, USN

Two nurses receive Navy Letters of Commendation (both ladies are of the Sacred Twenty): Chief Nurse Elizabeth Leonhardt, USN and Chief Nurse Martha E. Pringle, USN. Two other Navy Nurses receive Army Letters of Commendation. These are Reserve Nurse Mary Elderkin, USN and Reserve Nurse Jeannette McClellan, USN. These two nurses, along with a group of Army nurses, receive their awards for "Extraordinary service in connection with military operations against an armed enemy of the U.S., under the following circumstances:

> For eight consecutive days the above named nurses were on duty with a field hospital company operating a tent hospital in the open fields north of . . ., France, not withstanding nightly enemy air raids upon the town and harassing shell fire during the daytime they repeatedly refused to retire further to the rear and continued to administer to the needs of the wounded, exhibiting at all times a splendid spirit of self-sacrifice, courage and devotion to duty which largely contributed to the welfare and rapid convalescence of the wounded officers and soldiers entrusted to their care."[164]

Also, receiving an award from the Army (a Certificate for especially meritorious service) is Reserve Chief Nurse Frances Van Ingen, USN of Base Hospital #1 at Brest, France.[165]

Meantime, Congress has been passing a few laws that directly affect Navy Nurses. On 15 June 1917, an Appropriation Act is passed that "[provides] that Navy nurses should be paid the same commutation allowances given Army nurses."[166] Then on 6 October 1917 a law is passed that provides "compensation for death or disability and [for] government insurance benefits."[167] In July of 1918, Congress amends "the 'War Risk Insurance Act' pertaining to compensation for death or disability in line of duty, including nurses."[168] The insurance called War Risk Insurance is for "Only nurses who had been militarized, that is, had become members of the Army or Navy Nurse Corps were eligible. Non-militarized nurses, of whom there were about 1000 who served directly under the ARC [American Red Cross] were not eligible. Nurses who might have been militarized (there were some who, in their eagerness to serve overseas, had accepted Red Cross appointments rather than risk assignment by the [Army Nurse Corps] to cantonment hospitals [hospitals at Army training bases] in the US) had reason to regret their decision."[169] On 9 July 1918 a law passes that increases pay for the Army and Navy Nurses. Some of the pay rates are:

	Per Year
Superintendent	$ 2,400
Chief Nurse (plus pay as nurse)	120
Nurse (first three years)	720
Nurse (three to six years)	780
Nurse (six to nine years)	840
Nurse (nine to twelve years)	900
Nurse (after twelve years)	960
Extra pay for overseas	120
(not Puerto Rico or Hawaii)	

Also included in the legislation is "Cumulative leave at the rate of thirty days for each calendar year of service not to exceed 120 days at any one time and sick leave not exceeding 30 days in one calendar year. . . . Allowances for quarters and subsistence and provision for medical care [are] also covered."[170] There is just one problem with this law. The Chief Nurses had been receiving $360 a year in addition to regular nurse pay. This law decreases that pay to $120 per year plus the regular nurse pay. Imagine the blow that would be, especially to a Chief Nurse overseas in the war zone. On the 22nd of November 1918, Navy Nurse Corps Superintendent, Mrs. Higbee, writes a letter to the Chief Nurse at Great Lakes, J. Beatrice Bowman. In her letter, Mrs Higbee states, "I am working very hard to have the pay of the Chief Nurse restored and also to have the grade of Assistant Chief Nurse with one-half the pay of Chief Nurse and if this gets through, I believe that we will get better results from our Assistant Chief Nurses."[171] On 28 February 1919, a Bill (Public No. 241 - H.R. 15947) is passed that results in returning the additional pay of Chief Nurses to $360 per year[172], but it contains no provisions regarding Assistant Chief Nurses. Also, in February, Legislation passes to give a "bonus of $60 for World War I service to nurses and others."[173] In March, Congress passes a law providing "full pay and allowances to nurses while prisoners of war."[174] There are no Navy Nurse prisoners of war in WWI.

There is one piece of legislation (H.R. 10469) that is not approved. It is introduced by the Honorable F.C. Hicks on 5 March 1918. A most significant passage of the Bill states, "for [the] purpose of defining status of members of [the Nurse Corps] . . . that nurses be classed as officers."[175] It is not passed. It will be twenty-four years and another World War later before the status of Navy Nurses is finally specified by law.

As for the uniform of the Navy Nurses, in an article dated February 1918, Dr. Anita McGee, M.D. writes that the Navy Nurse "has a uniform now. For the street there is a suit, with long overcoat, detachable cape and soft felt hat; the whole of dark blue except for red in the cape lining. The corps badge on the coat, which is also worn with the white ward uniform, is the medical acorn and leaf superimposed on the Navy anchor. The cap of the chief nurse in the hospital has a band of gold for distinction, but the street uniform has no emblem of rank."[176]

"When the United States entered the European War, the Navy Nurse Corps, like that of the Army, had no distinctive outdoor uniform for its nurses."[177] However, in September 1917 when the first Navy Nurses to go overseas arrive in New York, "they [are] furnished with the blue serge dress, the ulster, the velour hat and other articles of equipment which the American Red Cross [is] . . . issuing to Army base hospitals assigned to foreign service."[178] Then on 16 November 1917, the Surgeon General issues the following instructions which Mrs. Higbee sends to the Red Cross:

"Outdoor Uniform for Members of the Navy Nurse Corps
Skirt and coat of heavy dark blue serge. . . .
Wash waists, cotton cheviot, dark blue flannel, dark blue silk. . . .
Top coat: dark blue heavy coating, smooth finish, similar to Navy 'cap cloth.' . . .
Cape: [optional for overseas] heavy long cape of cap cloth.. . . Light cape, navy blue serge lined with flannel.
Sweater of any weight desired; color, dark or navy blue or gray.
Rain coat: Coat of tan cravenette [a finish for making fabric waterproof, according to Webster's Dictionary], or rubber, and rubber hat.
Hat: Navy blue velour. . . .
Boots or shoes: Black, heels not higher than 'Cuban;' heavy soles; under certain conditions the Surgeon General may authorize tan boots for heavy walking.
Hosiery: black with black boots or shoes; tan with tan boots or shoes; white with white boots or shoes.
Rubber overshoes.
High rubber boots.
Corps Insignia: to be worn on duty always with wash uniforms and on waists of outdoor uniform, when such uniform is ordered. Collar device for outdoor uniform:- The letters U.S. for members of the

Regular Nurse Corps, and U.S.R. for the reserve nurses and Nurses' Force; to be worn 3/4 inch from collar openings on collar of coat or suit, top coat or heavy cape; Corps device to be worn 3/4 inch from letters U.S. or U.S.R.; collar devices shall not be worn except when in full outdoor uniform or when top coat and heavy cape are worn over wash uniform in hospital reservation.

'Nurses in the United States are not obliged to obtain the entire outdoor uniform except when so ordered by the Surgeon General. No part of this uniform shall be worn on duty in hospital or hospital reservation, unless so ordered by the Surgeon General, except that the top coat, heavy cape or light cape or rain coat or authorized sweater, shall be worn over wash uniform for protection and warmth; and no other garment shall be worn with uniform."[179]

On 21 November 1917, Mrs. Higbee sends to the Red Cross the following:

"*White uniform:* for members of the Navy Corps, Navy Reserve Force and Reserve nurses, U.S. Navy, who are not already equipped with uniforms, shall consist of a one-piece dress . . . with attached soft collar and attached belt."[180]

In August of 1918, a change is made in the Corps device worn by the Navy Nurses. "The pin [is] 1 1/2 inches long by 7/8 inches wide at its widest point. . . . It [is] the fouled anchor with oak leaf and acorn. Superimposed on the leaf [is] NNC. The nurses . . . call them 'Battleships' - they [are] so large and rather heavy. The pins [are] worn (2) one on each side of the collar."[181] At this same time the letters, USN and USR are discontinued and the Corps device is used instead. Also, in 1918, the "dress uniform [is] designated 'Navy Blue Norfolk suit with Kitchener pockets, tan gloves, black shoes or tan boots, sailor hat".[sic] [Sailor hat at this time is a stiff felt wide brimmed hat with black ribbon.[182]] Cape, Navy blue, belted in front, lined with scarlet flannel for wear with white ward uniform."[183] "Three hundred and thirty-four (334) members of the Navy Nurse Corps [are] furnished full equipment to foreign service [during WWI] by the American Red Cross through the Bureau of Nurses' Equipment . . . [in] New York City, at a total cost of $60,120,000. . . . Navy nurses in foreign service [are] allowed to replace worn out articles of wearing apparel by purchases made at cost from the Nurses' Equipment Shop, which [is] maintained at Paris [France] by the Red Cross."[184] Evidently the uniform regulations for Navy Nurses are not very strict during WWI, especially for the nurses in the war zone. One of the Navy Nurses, Esther Nelson Behr (Hunter), at Base #1 Hospital in France, writes a letter to her sister on 21 February 1918. In the letter she says, "Will send you all a snapshot of the new gray uniforms that I had made. They are my own design - plain waist - rather tight long sleeves - deep cuffs of white duck high & low collars of white duck - wide waist band and full skirt with two little gathered pockets in the front. . . . Those uniforms were horrible that they gave us. Mine cost $6.00 apiece. . . ."[185] In another letter written 22 August 1918, Mrs. Hunter comments on pay and on costs overseas, "Heard that the Bill for more pay to [military] nurses passed. We will then make $75 [a month.] However, our laundry costs about $2.00 per week, the nurses who have to get shoes over here, and there are very many, pay from $16 to $24 for a pair of ordinary shoes. . . . The kind hearted Red Cross give everything to their own nurses while the Navy can go sail a boat. We had to pay $7.00 for a straw sailor [hat] that I could buy in N.Y. for the extreme price [of] $3.00."[186]

Meanwhile, civilian professional nursing finds its ranks devastated by the wartime needs for nurses in the military and further depleted by the nurses perishing from the 1918 influenza, pneumonia and other diseases. "To aid in the supply . . .[of nurses], the *Army School of Nursing* [is] organized in 1918. . . . The course . . . [covers] three years, with a special credit of nine months to college graduates. Army hospitals and affiliating civilian hospitals [offer] their facilities for instruction. Applications [pour] in from thousands of enthusiastic women who [want] to make use of this opportunity to give service to their country. [The Army School of Nursing continues until 1931 when it is closed.]

"Another opportunity for a selected group of women [is] offered by the American Red Cross and Vassar College when the *Vassar Training Camp* [is] formed. It [gives] a special three months' course of preliminary instruction in nursing to four hundred and eighteen college graduates, one hundred and sixty-nine of whom [graduate] from cooperating hospitals."[187] "On November 11, 1918, the Armistice [becomes] effective and actual fighting [ceases] but the ills of war [continue] and new ones [arise.]"[188] The sick and injured of the war must receive needed care and the health needs of the rest of the population must be met. "At the same time, the field of nursing [suffers] several setbacks. While new demands [are] being created, its ranks [are] greatly depleted by departure from nursing schools of those who [lose] interest as the war [closes.]"[189] "Greatly influencing the general trend in nursing . . . [has been] the demand for students to carry the nursing load of a rapidly increasing number of hospitals. This demand, which culminated during the war activity, resulted in less careful selection of applicants. Emphasis was placed on getting the work done rather than on nursing education."[190] (In 1917 there were sixteen hundred schools of nursing with forty-three thousand students.[191])

After the war, President Wilson sails to Europe for the Paris Peace Conference. "With him [sails] the First Lady . . . a sprightly widow who could beat him at golf and whom he had married but a year after the death of his first wife. . . . He [is] indeed the best read, the best informed, and the hardest working of the heads of state who [gather] at Versailles. He [is] also the most applauded by the European peoples, hailed as the 'savior,' invited to ride under the Arc de Triomphe, cheered as the spokesman for all mankind.

"But the premiers and presidents with whom he [deals are] not to be lectured at-they [have] their own views of what peace [means]. . . ."[192] President Wilson went to Paris with his 'Fourteen Points' for peace. He has to bargain away most of his 'points' "to save the vital one that [embodies] the League of Nations, and [then he comes] home to violent opposition."[193] Congress refuses to go along with him so he takes his case to the people in a nationwide campaign. He becomes ill in Colorado and returns to Washington, DC where he suffers a paralyzing stroke. He lives out the rest of his term in "the seclusion of the White House, guarded by the First Lady. . . ."[194] (He receives the Nobel Peace Prize for his efforts and lingers, at his home, in ill health until he succumbs in 1924.[195])

On 11 November 1918, the census of the Navy Nurse Corps is 1386 with a breakdown of 278 USN nurses, 503 USN Reserve nurses and 603 USNRF nurses. On 1 December the census is 1403. (Quite a change from the 1908 cadre of 20.) In 1919, without the needs of the battlefields, the Nurse Corps census begins to drop. The year begins with a Nurse Corps strength of 1371 and by 1 November 1919 the number of Navy Nurses is 880.[196] But this is another busy year for Navy Nurses with new duty station assignments and new challenges to meet.

In July of 1918, a young Navy Nurse, Mary Moffett, is stationed at Mare Island, California. She has just received orders to go to Guam. She travels "on an Army transport."[197] She tells us that they call these ships 'the old cattle boats' but that the trip is "very placid. [A] very nice trip."[198] Her Chief Nurse on Guam is Miss Mollie Detweiler. "It [is] a small hospital. There [are] never any more than six nurses. We [work on] a native ward and [with] native nurses."[199] The military patients are sick or injured sailors from the ships and from the few sailors and Marines stationed at Guam. Until the influenza strikes, the military patients are taken care of by the "corpsmen and the chief [on the] enlisted men's ward. . . . All we [the Navy Nurses] [have] to do with [is] the native ward: women. . . ."[200] Influenza hits the island when "the Captain of [a] ship wired in to see whether he [could] stop. He had a patient who lived on Guam and she had the flu and he didn't know whether, since we hadn't had it [the flu], to come in [to harbor] or take them on to Honolulu. So they had [a] conference with the doctors and all. Nobody [at Guam] knew anything about the flu, and they said, 'why, bring her in.' So they brought her in and they put up a tent [on] the grounds [probably for isolation.] Well, almost overnight, every tent was filled. Every [person], male personnel, went down with the flu with the exception of the medical officer. . . . But everyone else was out, every corpsman. . . . There was no room in the hospital. . . . [The flu] went through like wild fire. One day we had no patients and the next we had ten and the next day the place was overrunning. . . . Not any of [the nurses got the flu.]"[201]

In 1919 the Chief Nurse at Guam receives her orders to Japan. Chief Nurse Mollie Detweiler, USN, is the first Navy Nurse to report to the U.S. Naval Hospital Yokohama, Japan. She reports aboard on 5 April 1919.[202] Shortly thereafter Navy Nurse Moffett receives her orders to the Philippines. She travels to her new duty station aboard a 'collier' which she describes as a large ship carrying nothing but coal.[203] She states that the Naval Hospital, Canacao is much larger and "more established in every way [than Guam.]"[204]

Back in the States, in May of 1919, more Navy Nurses are being assigned aboard transport ships. Navy Nurse Mary Hand is Chief Nurse aboard the USS *Imperator.* Several others are assigned briefly aboard other transports in order to help in the returning of "prisoners and internees back to Europe."[205] Chief Nurse Frida Krook is aboard the USS *Martha Washington*;[206] one of her nurses is a young Navy Nurse by the name of Nellie Jane Dewitt.[207] Chief Nurse Grace Kline is assigned to the USS *Princess Matoika*, Chief Nurse of the USS *Powhattan* is Lena Coleman, and on the USS *Pocohantas* is Chief Nurse Martha Pringle (one of the 'sacred twenty.')[208]

July 1919 and no further nurses are enrolled in the USNRF. Since the Nurse Corps is reducing its strength, this route for applicants is closed.[209] Despite the reductions, new duty stations open for Navy Nurses: Ward Island, New York and Key West, Florida. Also, some Navy Nurses are assigned to help the overburdened nursing service at Georgetown University Hospital, Washington, DC. They take care of the Navy patients admitted to this hospital.[210] The influenza pandemic is still taking its toll.

In the civilian medical world, the "American College of Surgeons, after several years of careful preparation, [releases] its first list of approved hospitals in 1919."[211] (The college had begun a hospital standardization program in 1918 and this is, in essence, the beginning of hospital accreditation. "In time, accreditation of a hospital by the college [becomes] one of the criteria for the evaluation of schools of nursing.[212]) Also in 1919, "Nursing Service [in the] Hospital Division [of the] US Public Health Service [is] established."[213] Then in 1920 the National Organization For Public Health Nursing (NOPHN) organizes Industrial and School Nursing Sections.[214]

The world of 1920 celebrates the establishment of the League of Nations with hope that WWI was the war to end all wars. But, the United States does not join the league because of congressional opposition. Also, in 1920, the Panama Canal opens to world shipping. ("Work on the 50.72 mile-long canal began in 1906."[215])

And, "The first commercial radio broadcasts [are] made from Detroit and Pittsburgh. . . ."[216]

You might like to know that this is year the U.S. Navy prepares to switch to the 24-hour clock. United States Navy Regulation, 1920, Article 1032 (effective 15 July 1921), states, "The use of the 24-hour day, with the time expressed as a four-figure group, the first two figures denoting the hour and the second two figures denoting the minutes, is authorized for the naval service in correspondence as well as dispatch, using the civil day commencing at

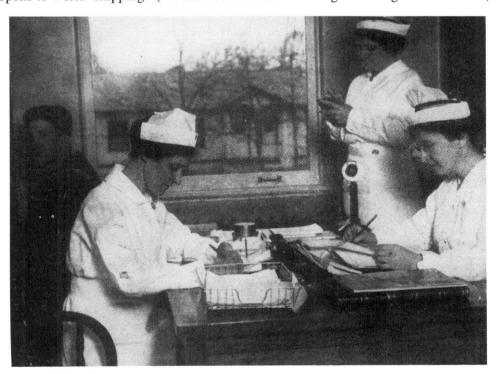

Chief Nurse's office Naval Hospital, Great Lakes, Illinois. Circa 1919
(Photo courtesy of Irene Matthews, former Navy Nurse.)

midnight, expressed as 0000." (Imagine that; in one long, complex sentence, it is all explained, forevermore.)

In January of 1920, several USNRF nurses are recalled to active duty. They are needed to help with all the influenza patients. (A total of thirty-one nurses are recalled during 1920 and 1921.)[217] Also, in January, "the Navy Department issued a booklet `Regulations Governing the Organization and Administration of the Naval Reserve Forces,' which . . . superseded those of October 31, 1918. In this 1920 booklet the following reference to nurses [is] made:

> 'The enrollment of nurses (female) in the Naval Reserve Forces shall be carried on by the Bureau of Medicine and Surgery, under such authority as may be delegated from time to time by the Bureau of Navigation.'"[218]

(Previously, nurses were enrolled in the U.S. Naval Coast Defense Reserve or the Volunteer Naval Reserve.)

Congress passes legislation (May 1920) for military nurses to receive a twenty percent pay raise for the period of 1 January 1920 to 30 June 1922. Then in June, Congress passes legislation that authorizes relative rank for Army nurses. (The rank is relative but the base pay is not.) The Superintendent of the Army Nurse Corps is to be a Major; the assistant superintendents, directors, and assistant directors to be Captains; chief nurses will be First Lieutenants; head nurses and nurses will be Second Lieutenants.[219] Since Congress had previously passed statutes that pertained to both the Army and Navy Nurses, this obvious omission means that the exclusion of Navy Nurses is deliberate. Does Congress wish to withhold rank from the Navy Nurses or, perhaps, was it 'not recommended' to Congress? Whatever the reason, Navy Nurses do not receive relative rank and their position is still neither officer nor enlisted; this, despite their pioneering and outstanding contributions to the Navy and to Navy Medicine.

The next legislation passes Congress in July. This law includes "the Regular Nurse Corps among those whose dependent relatives [will] receive 6 months pay in case of death in line of duty."[220] (This statute would, presumably, apply to both branches of the Service.)

On a more cheerful note, an event of significance is taking place at the Navy Yard in Philadelphia, Pennsylvania. The third USS *Relief* is being prepared for commissioning. The Bureau of Medicine and Surgery had plans for a hospital ship in 1911 but it wasn't until 1916 that Congress allowed for the building of the ship. "The ship was launched 23 December 1919, and was sponsored by . . . [the] wife of the Surgeon General."[221] This is the first hospital ship to be built, as such, from the keel up. (All others are ships refitted as hospital ships.) This new ship is given the catalog number AH-1. Of the other still active hospital ships, the *Solace* is AH-2, the *Comfort* is AH-3, and the *Mercy* is AH-4.[222] Prior to the commissioning of the *Relief*, and before there are nurses aboard any of the hospital ships, there is a saying "in the fleet . . .: 'No mercy on the *Comfort*; no comfort on the *Mercy*; and no *Solace* on either.'"[223] Maybe now the fleet will have some *Relief* because the Navy Nurses are on their way.

From May 22, 1920 to July 2, 1920, Elizabeth Leonhardt (one of the 'Sacred Twenty' has TAD orders aboard the USS *Mercy*. Then comes the commissioning of the USS *Relief* on 28 December 1920. She is commissioned in the presence of the first Navy Nurses ever to be permanently assigned to a hospital ship. The Chief Nurse is J. Beatrice Bowman. The commanding officer of the ship is "a medical officer of the Navy, Commander R.C. Holcomb, who had also served as the inspector representing the Bureau of Medicine and Surgery during her [the ship's] construction."[224] (All hospital ships, at this time, have medical officers in command.)

Another first for the year 1920 is the assignment of the first Navy Nurse to physical therapy. Down in the Virgin Islands, the first class of three native women graduate from the Frederikstad Municipal Hospital Training School at St. Croix: the Training School started by Navy Nurses. Meantime, Navy Nurses are removed from the Training School at Haiti and the work is taken over by American Red Cross nurses.[225] The nurses are removed because they are needed for the Naval Hospitals.

As for the civilian nursing field, by "1920, all states except Nevada [have] passed laws providing for the registration of nurses."[226] Also, it is now being recognized that it is not just the patient, but also the family and even the community who need medical help. As outgrowths of this knowledge is the new field of Medical Social

Service[227] and even more emphasis on public health nursing. It is also 1920 when the ANA establishes its national headquarters in New York City. "All national nursing organizations are now in the same [city and in the same] building."[228]

This is the year that sees Republican Warren G. Harding elected as President along with Calvin Coolidge as Vice President. They win the election against Democrat James M. Cox and his running mate, Franklin D. Roosevelt. During his campaign, Harding "had struck a responsive popular chord when he asserted that 'America's present need is not heroism but healing, not nostrums but normalcy, not revolution but restoration.'... The irony is that what Harding-Coolidge really stood for was the precise opposite of a return to the old rural America ... [because], as the 1920 census [reveals], more people [live] in cities and towns than on farms and in villages of fewer than 2,500 people."[229] Nostalgic or not, America can't turn back. Plus, shock of all shocks, this year (1920), is the implementation of the National Prohibition Enforcement Act.[230] Alcoholic beverages are outlawed. Speakeasies are in. Jazz is in. Al Capone is strongly influencing Chicago. Women are given the right to vote. It is the beginning of the Roaring Twenties.

In 1921, President Harding is busy appointing "his friends to office, qualified or not.... Yet there [are] some outstanding appointments.... [He] put Charles Evans Hughes in charge of an international conference on naval disarmament. Probably the administration's most successful venture...."[231] However, the limitations set by the conference causes the U.S. Navy to enter "a period of decline.... [The limitations on armament cause the scrapping, sinking, or demilitarizing of] about 2,000,000 tons of ships, including 31 major warships...."[232]

At least the disarmament did not affect the new hospital ship as she prepares to join the Atlantic Fleet in early 1921. (Probably to replace the *Solace* which is being decommissioned after service as a hospital ship since 1909.[233]) Chief Nurse J. Beatrice Bowman writes about the *Relief*: "On February 15, 1921 we left the dock for the first time ... anchored in the Delaware [River] for 24 hrs. in order to have our compasses adjusted and at daylight February 16 steamed down the Delaware. Such happiness that at last the great day had arrived and we were off! But much to our sorrow, after reaching the Delaware Breakwater we had to return for repairs to the armature. That took another week, but we found many many things to keep us busy for, did we not have a 500 bed Hospital to equip? ... To a nurse who cares for organizing I know this means much. Supplies of every kind had been placed aboard and the joy of setting up and equipping the beautiful wards, operating rooms, eye, ear, nose & throat room, diet kitchen, etc. will be remembered by the first lucky nurses on the USS *Relief*.... All on board thought we would be seasick and we were watched closely. Bulletins carried by mouth to all parts of the ship if some one or more looked pale. Aside from three having a slight touch of mal-de-mer all proved themselves as good sailors as could be found. Even those who felt badly were plucky enough to report on duty every day and tried to throw off all ill feeling.

"But to describe to you this 'Master Hospital Ship.' She is 485 ft. long, 64 ft. beam, has 64 water tight compartments, and is so safe that could her funnels be plugged she could in safety go under like a submarine or she could be rolled over and would always right herself. A ship of about 10,000 ton displacement and painted white with a green stripe from stem to stern. This green stripe is the uniform of a military ship. Were she a Red Cross Hospital Ship, according to the provisions of the Geneva conventions, she would have a red band instead of the green band. Painted on the side of her hull and on the side of her stack is a large red cross."[234]

Miss Bowman then goes on to describe the interior of the ship: "In the arrangement of the largest wards you will find the quiet room, linen room and pantry or diet kitchen, in one [end] and the dressing room and toilets at the other. ...

"But let us go into the pantry, or as you 'land lubbers' call it, the diet kitchen. Yes I know you envy us those little electric ranges—and they work beautifully too. A spacious wall table of galvanized iron extends along two bulkheads & a deep porcelain sink is in the one table while over the other are dish racks with compartments for plates, bowls, saucers, and cups, so constructed that they are packed securely and safe in a rolling sea. Hot, cold and refrigerated water are over the sink, and all pantries have refrigerators in which the coil system is used. Ice for ice caps may be obtained from the plant and the ice chamber is large enough for that also.

"From the wards I would take you to the hydrotherapy room, beautifully tiled and completely outfitted; to the endoscopic room and then to the diet kitchen. Now in the latter place I would give you an ice cold drink of fresh milk made today . . . or maybe the ice cream is finished. . . .

"Before we go to the main deck let me show you the hold [of the ship] in which is stored a complete field hospital equipment needed even to an ambulance. . . .

"Now we return to the main deck. You remember that you came aboard here. Had you been a Navy Nurse you would have saluted the Flag as you came over the side. We are proud of this honor and I have not yet grown so old in years or in the Service, but that to look upon the Stars and Stripes makes little thrills run up and down my spine, and in my heart I have always saluted 'Our Flag.' That the time has come when we are a part of the military forces and are expected to carry out that military recognition makes us feel more than ever the love of country and its emblem. . . .

"[On the upper deck] we have reached the sick officers' quarters. [The] large chests on the deck contain steamer chairs for convalescing patients. As we enter the sick officers quarters you are impressed with the large ward room with white curtains hanging at every door and port, the chairs with their linen covers, the soft restful green in the color scheme, and the metal furniture which you take to be mahogany. We have eleven private rooms, each furnished with a crib bed [with sides], chair, secretary bureau, ward-robe, washstand with fresh running water over which is a toilet cabinet. A telephone is in every room, a portable light over every bed and with the silent call system could any hospital be more complete? . . .

"On the superstructure deck let me show you not only where the Captain and the Master of the Ship live, but our delightful quarters. Our ward room runs across the ship giving us air and view from both sides—that is we get the view when we are at anchor and the boats are down. Five staterooms open into the ward room and in each live two nurses. These rooms are fitted with two berths, upper and lower, two secretary bureaus, two toilet lockers, a good sized ward-robe and wash-stand with running fresh water. Opening into the ward room also, is our pantry, or you would call it a kitchenette, and down a small passage is the Chief Nurse's stateroom, then come the baths and toilets."[235] Miss Bowman goes on to describe the operating rooms, the mess hall, the storerooms, the bag room and other areas. This is truly a modern ship. (It is reported that "in the 1920's and 1930's, 'White Lily' [is] the nickname for one well-known ship, the USS *Relief*."[236]) Miss Bowman also tells us that "we went out on our first trial up to Rockland, Maine. Then from there we went to Guantanamo Bay [where they probably join the fleet.]"[237]

In 1921 the census of the Navy Nurse Corps is 470 and the Nurse Corps is moving along although, at times, it seems as though the movement is in inches. The Bureau of Medicine and Surgery, on 11 June, puts out a directive stating that "hereafter Nurse Corps members should not be designated in hospitals records as 'Supernumeraries,' but as naval personnel."[238] No rank or rating, but no longer 'supernumeraries.'

August 1921 and The American Journal of Nursing publishes a five page article by Lenah S. Higbee, Superintendent, Navy Nurse Corps. (The article preceding Mrs. Higbee's is on the Army Nurse Corps and is signed Julia C. Stimson, Major, Superintendent, Army Nurse Corps, and Dean, Army School of Nursing. Not only does Mrs. Higbee have no military rank, but her name is misspelled at the end of her article: Higbie. However, at least Mrs. Higbee can no longer be a 'supernumerary.') The article is a summary of the Navy Nurse Corps; how to apply, requirements of eligibility and procedures once one is accepted. For instance, when a nurse receives her first set of orders to report for active duty, she "receives transportation requests entitling her to first class travel, together with a request giving her chair or Pullman accommodation according to the length of her journey. She is also reimbursed for the incidental expenses incurred on this journey and for the transportation of her baggage. Her pay as nurse in the Navy begins from the date she travels in obedience to orders."[239] Then the article goes on to say, "The period of duty at the different stations varies from a year in isolated stations; eighteen months for tropical duty; and two years at stations in the environment of a city. . . . The number of hospitals, hospital ships, and stations in the Navy to which nurses are attached is 43. . . . The unit of duty required of nurses in the Navy is eight hours for day duty and ten hours when on night duty. The night duty is given in rotation and, in the larger stations, may not be more often than once in twelve months; but is more frequent in the smaller stations."[240] The white nurses uniform is discussed stating that the hospitals will launder them. Then Mrs. Higbee writes of the duties of the Navy Nurse as well as pay, leave time, medical care and sick leave. The article could be for recruiting, but it is for information, as well. One of the last paragraphs says, "A form of application for the Victory Medal and button will be issued by the Bureau of Medicine and Surgery, Navy Department, to each nurse, released from active service, who served honorably in the Navy between April 6.1917, and November 11, 1918."[241] After that are listed the names and assignments of recently appointed Navy Nurses then follows the listing of all Navy Nurses recently transferred. Among the orders for transfer, it is interesting to note that two nurses received orders for temporary duty aboard the transport USS *Henderson* and two nurses to the USS *Hancock*. Also, one nurse is ordered to the USS *Mercy*. The latter part of the article is devoted to the new Hospital Ship, USS *Relief*, and lists the names of all eleven of the Navy Nurses assigned aboard.

September of 1921 sees the disenrollment of all nurses on inactive status, USNRF.[242] Also, in September, the Secretary of the Navy, "with the approval of President Harding . . . [relieves] medical officers from the command of hospital ships and [places] them [the hospital ships] under the command of line officers."[243]

This is the year that Navy Nurses are again ordered into Port au Prince, Haiti. But this time they are ordered into the Field Hospital there and not into the training of native nurses.[244] In the Virgin Islands, the first class of native students graduate from the training school set up by Navy Nurses.[245]

On the day after Christmas, 26 December 1921, the Office of the Judge Advocate General of the Navy writes a reply to two letters written to the Secretary of the Navy by the Chief of the Bureau of Medicine and Surgery. The Surgeon General had written asking the Secretary of the Navy if the Navy Nurse Corps was entitled to relative rank as given the Army Nurse Corps by legislation the previous year. Three pages are used to explain the law, define terms, cite cases, but the final paragraph of the document says it all: "Therefore, since the act approved May 13, 1908, establishing the Navy Nurse Corps, makes no reference whatever to rank or relative rank, it does not appear that Congress intended that nurses in the Navy were to have any rank or relative rank, or that there should be any assimilation in that respect with nurses in the Army. You are accordingly advised that, in the opinion of this office, members of the Navy Nurse Corps are not entitled to relative rank, as provided for nurses of the Army by section 10 of the act approved June 4, 1920." It is signed by J.L. Latimer and approved 3 January 1922 by the Secretary of the Navy. (It will be twenty more years before relative rank for Navy Nurses.) Also, on this subject, is a letter by Jas. T. Begg, dated 7 January 1922, and written on stationary of the Congress of the United States, House of Representatives. The letter is written to a gentleman in Ohio. It states, in part: "You will find enclosed a copy of the decision of the Judge Advocate General of the Navy on the granting of relative rank to the members of the Navy Nurse Corps. I am sorry this is unfavorable. I do not think there is any doubt, but what Congress intended to give the same rank and privileges to the Navy Corps as it did to the Army Corps, and hope that in the near future legislation will be proposed to correct this inequality."

In 1922 the Veterans Bureau establishes a hospital division and the Mills School for Male Nurses reopens.[246] (Remember mention of this school much earlier?) For the past ten years, the Mills school "was replaced by a course for the preparation of orderlies as attendants presumably because it was difficult to secure adequate numbers of desirable [male nursing] candidates. Nursing, as a vocation for men, had no prestige. When reopened, the school [is] again . . . placed on the approved list of the New York State Examining Board."[247]

Returning to the Navy Nurse Corps, the census for this year (1922) is 479. In January there is a disaster at the Knickerbocker Theatre of Washington, DC. The theatre is open and well attended despite a recent heavy snowfall. All of a sudden the roof of the theatre caves in because of the weight of the snow. Ninety-seven people are killed and many are injured. Two Chief Nurses (Anne Katherine Harkins, USN and Florence Margaret Vevia, USN) from the Navy Dispensary in DC each receive a Letter of Commendation from the Secretary of the Navy for their work during this catastrophe.[248] In February of 1922, Chief Nurse J. Beatrice Bowman sends a request to the Secretary of the Navy via the Bureau of Medicine and Surgery. (Miss Bowman writes from the USS *Relief* in Guantanamo Bay.) She requests permission to take the examination for the position of Superintendent of the

Navy Nurse Corps. In her letter she states, "In making this request I wish it clearly understood that while there is the slightest hope of keeping Mrs. Higbee, I have no desire whatsoever for the position." For her part, Mrs. Higbee recommends that the request be given favorable consideration. Mrs. Higbee writes, "She [Miss Bowman] has given loyal service, meeting vicissitudes with cheerful optimism and has at all times accepted the duty to which she was detailed without complaint and protest. Her example has been an inspiration to the nurses who served with her and if given this appointment, I believe she will guide and direct members of the Navy Nurse Corps loyally and efficiently."[249] The request is filed for reference. Later on the *Relief* sails up to New York and, on 2 August, Chief Nurse Bowman leaves the ship with TAD (temporary additional duty orders) to the Bureau of Medicine and Surgery, Washington, DC.[250] The groundwork has now been laid for events to come.

In June of this 1922, Congress passes legislation that affects both Army and Navy Nurses. This law gives the nurses a Rental Allowance of forty dollars each month and a Subsistence Allowance of sixty cents per day. (This is what seems so incongruous. Legislation passed for pay or allowances, as in this case, pertains to both the Army and Navy, but when it comes to Relative Rank, it is interpreted as only applying to the Army. It is a 'puzzlement.') It is in November when all USNRF nurses are disenrolled. Eighty-six of these nurses transfer to Nurse, USN and forty-three transfer to Reserve Nurse, USN.[251] Also in 1922, the Naval Medical Bulletin first establishes a Nurse Corps section within its format. This is "devoted to professional and military subjects of interest to members of the Nurse Corps."[252]

Meantime, in October, it is possible for nurses to apply for further education in dietetics, laboratory techniques, anesthesia, physiotherapy, tuberculosis nursing and instructing. Further, "nurses are encouraged to attend nursing conventions whenever possible. . . ."[253] In a short time "six nurses [are] assigned [to] a course in laboratory work . . . at the U.S. Naval Medical School, four [attend] physiotherapy classes at the Naval Hospital, Brooklyn, eight [take] courses in dietetics at Fanny Farmer's School of Cooking in Boston and two [go] to Stanford University for a special course for nurse instructors."[254] (Even in 1922 Navy Nurses are being encouraged to grow in their profession through further education and attendance at civilian professional functions.) Chief Nurse Della V. Knight, USN writes an article about her attendance at "a Course of Lectures on Tuberculosis held at the U.S. Veterans' Hospital, Oteen, North Carolina, during the month of June, 1922. These lectures were given by physicians who have made a very extensive study of tuberculosis and by members of the Nursing Profession who had specialized in caring for tuberculosis patients." She goes on to mention that it had been found that treating the patient at home is much more conducive to recovery versus separating and isolating the patient from his family by sending him to a sanatorium. She stresses the importance of the mental state of the patient in treatment of this disease. She writes, "[all] personal affairs must be looked into, the psychic life of the patient, personality, social status, etc.. The mind must be treated as well as the body." (In light of today's resurgence of this disease, it is interesting to note this nurse's views on the disease and the treatment of 1922.) Also this year, out in Guam, Navy Nurses are being "assigned in public health work . . . as visiting nurses . . . for follow-up care of patients with tuberculosis. . . ."[255]

Any other Nurse Corps events for this year are secondary to the news of 30 November when Mrs. Lenah S. Higbee, Superintendent of the U.S. Navy Nurse Corps, is honorably discharged at her own request. She had submitted her resignation the 23rd of November to be effective on the 30th. She stated, "I now desire a different occupation."[256]

Note: Mrs. Higbee died in 1941, just three years before a U.S. Destroyer was named for her. The USS *Higbee* was launched at Bath, Maine on 12 November 1944. This was the first combatant ship to be named after a woman of the service. The ship was commissioned on 27 January 1945. After the Japanese surrender, the Commanding Officer, Commander Lindsey Williamson, USN, presented the Battle Flag to the Nurse Corps with the following letter:

"You may tell all the nurses that their ship [the USS *Higbee*] earned her keep in fine style by downing 6 Jap planes (four of them in 22 minutes) without suffering a scratch or getting a soul on board hurt, and that is my idea of the way a war should be fought—get rid of the enemy as quickly as possible, and above all, don't forget to dodge the right way at the right time.

Under separate cover I am returning the flag [the battle ensign] to you. The sight of that flag flying on August 15, was something no one on the *Higbee* will forget. Engineers and lower deck ratings got permission to come topside, and the spontaneous cheer each one of them gave upon seeing it waving in the stiff breeze made a chill run up and down my spine. I don't think the United States has anything to worry about as long as we have men like the *Higbee's* crew sailing the seas for us. Thank you very much for the help and consideration the nurses have given us. We hope the battle flag will find a prominent resting place."

Mrs. Higbee would have liked that.

[1]   Hickey, Dermott Vincent, *The First Ladies In The Navy - A History of the Navy Nurse Corps, 1908-1939*, June 1963, p. 62. (Unpublished thesis, see Prologue.)

[2]   "`Women in White' Help Guard Your Health," *All Hands, (Bureau of Naval Personnel Information Bulletin)*, February, 1953, p. 11.

[3]   Hickey, op. cit., p. 62.

[4]   Ibid., p. 62.

[5]   Ibid., p. 62.

[6]   Goble, CDR Dorothy Jones, NC USN (Ret.), Unpublished history research notes.

[7]   Lyons, Barbara A. LCDR NC USN, *Formation, Organization and Growth of the Navy Nurse Corps 1908 - 1933*, 1968, pp. 47, 48. (An unpublished manuscript written in response to instructions from Nursing Division, BuMed in 1968.)

[8]   Herman, Jan K., Historian at the Naval Medical Command, Department of the Navy, *A Hilltop in Foggy Bottom (Home of the Old Naval Observatory and the Navy Medical Department)*, Reprinted from U.S. Navy Medicine, 1984, p. 73.

[9]   Ibid., pp. 72, 73.

[10]   Lyons, op. cit., p. 40.

[11]   Ibid., p. 41.

[12]   Goodnow, Minnie, R.N., *Nursing History*, W.B. Saunders Company, Philadelphia and London, 1948, p. 215.

[13]   Jensen, Deborah MacLurg, R.N., M.A., *A History of Nursing*, The C.V. Mosby Company, St. Louis, 1943, p. 181.

[14]   *200 Years, A Bicentennial Illustrated History of the United States*, Joseph Newman, Directing Editor, Books by U.S. News & World Report, Inc., 2300 N Street, N.W., Washington, DC 20037, 1973, Book 2, p. 119.

[15]   Ibid., pp. 115-117.

[16]   Ibid., p. 328.

[17]   Lyons, op. cit., p. 34.

[18]   Hickey, op. cit., p. 57.

[19]   Ibid., p. 57.

[20]   Ibid., p. 58.

[21]   Ibid., Appendix C, Pay and Allowances of the Navy Nurse Corps, p. 157.

[22]   Ibid., p. 66.

[23]   Ibid., p. 66.

[24]   Ibid., p. 67.

[25]   Laird, LCDR Thelma NC USNR, Jones, LCDR Dorothy NC USN, Feeney, LCDR Elizabeth NC USN, Seidl, CDR Elizabeth NC USN (Ret), Blaska, CDR Burdette NC USN, *Chronological History NAVY NURSE CORPS*, Prepared by: Nursing Division, Bureau of Medicine and Surgery, 1 August 1962, p. 8.

[26]   Godfrey, Mary Robinson (Navy Service 1910 to 1919), *Oral History Interview Tape Transcript*, Interviewer CDR Virginia Eberharter NC USN (Ret.), taped in 1988.

[27]   Ibid.

[28]   Ibid.

[29]   Goble, op. cit.. (Unpublished history research notes.)

[30]   Feeney, Capt. Elizabeth NC USN, *Notes on Nurse Corps Insignia*. (Capt. Feeney used these notes in her slide presentations on Navy Nurse Corps Pins. Used with her permission.)

[31]   Goble, op. cit.. (Unpublished history research notes.)

[32]   *The World Book Encyclopedia*, Field Enterprises Educational Corporation, Chicago, Volume 17, 1966 edition, p. 79.

[33]   *The New Encyclopaedia Britannica*, Robert McHenry, General Editor, Encyclopedia Britannica, Inc., Chicago, Published with editorial advise of the faculties of the University of Chicago, 1992, p. 335.

[34]   Lyons, op. cit., pp. 39, 40. (Citation from the Surgeon General's Report of 1913.)

[35]   Laird, LCDR Thelma NC USNR, Jones, LCDR Dorothy NC USN, Feeney, LCDR Elizabeth NC USN, Seidl, CDR Elizabeth NC USN (Ret), Blaska, CDR Burdette NC USN, op. cit., p. 8.

[36]   Ibid., p. 8.

[37]   Goodnow, op. cit., p. 220.

[38]   Roberts, Mary M., R.N., *American Nursing History and Interpretation*, The MacMillan Company, New York, 1963, p. 109.

[39]   Ibid., p. 111.

[40]   Bowman, Beatrice, "Comments on Navy Nursing," *American Journal of Nursing*, April, 1914, p. 837. (This is part of the American Nurses'

Association's report on the Afternoon Session of their meeting on Saturday, April 25.)

[41]   *The World Book Encyclopedia*, Field Enterprises Educational Corporation, Chicago, Volume 20, 1966 edition, p. 369.

[42]   Ibid., p. 364.

[43]   Ibid., pp. 364, 365.

[44]   Ibid., p. 271.

[45]   Ibid., p. 271.

[46]   Ibid., p. 272.

[47]   Wells, H.G., *The Outline of History*, Revised and brought up to date by Raymond Postgate, Garden City Books, Garden City, New York, Volume II, 1961, p. 872.

[48]   Ibid., p. 872.

[49]   Goble, op. cit.. (Unpublished history research notes.)

[50]   Fulton, Faye and Baster, Beuhla, *Oral History Interview Tape Transcript*, Interviewer Irene Smith Matthews Lt(jg) Navy Nurse Corps, taped in 1970.

[51]   Fulton, Faye, Personal Letter written by Faye Fulton, dated April 10, 1968.

[52]   Fulton, Faye and Baster, Beuhla, *Oral History Interview Tape Transcript*, op. cit..

[53]   200 Years, A Bicentennial Illustrated History of the United States, op. cit..

[54]   The World Book Encyclopedia, op. cit., p. 366.

[55]   Ibid..

[56]   Jamieson, Elizabeth M., B.A., R.N., Sewall, Mary F., B.S., R.N., *Trends In Nursing History*, W.B. Saunders Company, Philadelphia, 1949, p. 461.

[57]   Holcomb, Richard C., M.D., F.A.C.S., Captain, Medical Corps, U.S. Navy, *A Century With Norfolk Naval Hospital, 1830-1930*, Printcraft Publishing Co., 1930, p. 463.

[58]   Ibid..

[59]   Laird, LCDR Thelma NC USNR, Jones, LCDR Dorothy NC USN, Feeney, LCDR Elizabeth NC USN, Seidl, CDR Elizabeth NC USN (Ret), Blaska, CDR Burdette NC USN, op. cit., p. 9.

[60]   Ibid..

[61]   Information obtained from the file card of Miss Sherzinger's assignments, Bureau of Medicine and Surgery, Navy Department, Washington, DC.

[62]   *200 Years, A Bicentennial Illustrated History of the United States*, op. cit., p. 120.

[63]   *Webster's New Universal Unabridged Dictionary (Deluxe Second Edition)*, Revised by the Publisher's Editorial Staff Under the General Supervision of Jean L. McKechnie, New World Dictionaries/Simon and Schuster, New York, 1979, p. 266.

[64]   Kernodle, Portia B., *The Red Cross Nurse in Action 1882-1948*, Harper & Brothers, Publishers, New York, 1949, p. 110.

[65]   Ibid..

[66]   Ibid..

[67]   Gaeddert, G.R., Historical Division, *The History of The American National Red Cross*, Volume IV, The American National Red Cross in World War I, 1917-1918, The American National Red Cross, Washington, DC, 1950, p. 35.

[68]   DeWitt, Nellie Jane, Lt.Comdr. (NC) USN, Acting Superintendent, Nurse Corps, *BuMed Memorandum to Colonel Blanchfield*, dated 5 December 1945, p. 1.

[69]   Laird, LCDR Thelma NC USNR, Jones, LCDR Dorothy NC USN, Feeney, LCDR Elizabeth NC USN, Seidl, CDR Elizabeth NC USN (Ret), Blaska, CDR Burdette NC USN, op. cit., p. 9.

[70]   Dock, Lavinia L., R.N., Pickett, Sarah Elizabeth, B.A., Noyes, Clara D., R.N., Clement, Fannie F., B.A., R.N., Fox, Elizabeth G., B.A., R.N., Van Meter, Anna R., B.A., M.S., *History of American Red Cross Nursing*, The MacMillan Company, New York, 1922, p. 689.

[71]   Roberts, Mary M., R.N., op. cit., p. 115.

[72]   Dock, Lavinia L., R.N., Stewart, Isabel M., A.M., R.N., *A Short History of Nursing*, G.P. Putnam's Sons, New York: London, 1938, p. 179.

[73]   Ibid..

[74]   *The World Book Encyclopedia*, op. cit., p. 273.

[75]   *200 Years, A Bicentennial Illustrated History of the United States*, op. cit., p. 120.

[76]   Ibid..

[77]   Ibid..

[78]   Ibid., p. 121.

[79]   *The World Book Encyclopedia*, op. cit., pp. 374, 375.

[80]   Wells, H.G., op. cit., p. 861.

[81]   *The World Book Encyclopedia*, op. cit., p. 374.

[82]   Wells, H.G., op. cit., p. 862.

[83]   *The World Book Encyclopedia*, op. cit., p. 375.

[84]   Ibid..

[85]   Ibid..

[86]   Gaeddert, G.R., Historical Division, op. cit., p. 37.

[87]   Jamieson, Elizabeth M., B.A., R.N., Sewall, Mary F., B.S., R.N., op. cit., p. 463.

[88]   Gaeddert, G.R., Historical Division, op. cit..

[89]   Kernodle, Portia B., op. cit., p. 110.

[90]   Dock, Lavinia L., R.N., Pickett, Sarah Elizabeth, B.A., Noyes, Clara D., R.N., Clement, Fannie F., B.A., R.N., Fox, Elizabeth G., B.A., R.N., Van Meter, Anna R., B.A., M.S., op. cit., pp. 688, 689.

[91]   Ibid., p. 689.

[92]   Brown, Willard C., (Navy Supply Corps Officer during WWI), *A Brief History of Navy Base Hospital #5 Brest, France, During World War I*,

(written from memory 54 years after), approximately 1972, p. 1. (Copy and permission obtained from donor Irene Matthews Lt(jg) Navy Nurse Corps.)

93   Ibid., p. 3.

94   Ibid., pp. 4,5.

95   Basler, Beulah, (Navy Nurse WWI), Fulton, Faye (Navy Nurse WWI), *Oral History Interview Tape Transcript*, Interviewer Irene Matthews Lt(jg) Navy Nurse Corps, taped in 1970.

96   Brown, Willard C., (Navy Supply Corps Officer during WWI), op. cit., p. 7.

97   Ibid., pp. 7,8.

98   Ibid., p. 9.

99   Ibid..

100   Basler, Beulah, (Navy Nurse WWI), Fulton, Faye (Navy Nurse WWI), *Oral History Interview Tape Transcript*, op. cit..

101   Ibid..

102   Ibid..

103   Ibid..

104   Ibid..

105   Hunter, Esther Nelson Behr, *Personal Letter to her Sister*, dated 21 November 1918.

106   Hunter, Esther Nelson Behr, *Personal Letter to her Sister*, dated 4th of July 1918.

107   Hunter, Esther Nelson Behr, *Personal Letter to her Sister*, dated 21 November 1918, op. cit..

108   Hunter, Esther Nelson Behr, *Personal Letter to her Sister*, dated 18 November 1918.

109   Dock, Lavinia L., R.N., Pickett, Sarah Elizabeth, B.A., Noyes, Clara D., R.N., Clement, Fannie F., B.A., R.N., Fox, Elizabeth G., B.A., R.N., Van Meter, Anna R., B.A., M.S., op. cit., p. 722.

110   Ibid., pp. 722, 723.

111   Ibid., p. 725.

112   Ibid., pp. 725, 726.

113   Report written October 7, 1918, by C.W. Otwell, Commanding Troops on Board H.M.T. *Briton*,to the Commanding Officer, U.S. Navy Base Hospital, No. 4, Queenstown, Ireland, as quoted in Dock, Lavinia L., R.N., Pickett, Sarah Elizabeth, B.A., Noyes, Clara D., R.N., Clement, Fannie F., B.A., R.N., Fox, Elizabeth G., B.A., R.N., Van Meter, Anna R., B.A., M.S., op. cit., pp. 726.

114   Dock, Lavinia L., R.N., Pickett, Sarah Elizabeth, B.A., Noyes, Clara D., R.N., Clement, Fannie F., B.A., R.N., Fox, Elizabeth G., B.A., R.N., Van Meter, Anna R., B.A., M.S., op. cit., pp. 727.

115   Ibid., p. 720.

116   Ibid., p. 748.

117   Ibid., pp. 749, 750.

118   Ibid., pp. 751, 752.

119   Ibid., p. 721.

120   Laird, LCDR Thelma NC USNR, Jones, LCDR Dorothy NC USN, Feeney, LCDR Elizabeth NC USN, Seidl, CDR Elizabeth NC USN (Ret), Blaska, CDR Burdette NC USN, op. cit., p. 12.

121   Herman, Jan K., op. cit., p. 76.

122   McGrath, Ada (Navy Nurse 1917 to 1919), *Oral History Interview Tape Transcript*, Interviewer Irene Matthews Lt(jg) Navy Nurse Corps, taped in 1971.

123   Ibid..

124   Ibid..

125   Ibid..

126   *The World Book Encyclopedia*, Field Enterprises Educational Corporation, Chicago, Volume 10, 1966 edition, p. 207.

127   Hickey, op. cit., p. 86.

128   Bowman, J. Beatrice, *Oral History Interview Tape Transcript*, Interviewer Irene Matthews, taped in 1971.

129   Ibid..

130   Dock, Lavinia L., R.N., Pickett, Sarah Elizabeth, B.A., Noyes, Clara D., R.N., Clement, Fannie F., B.A., R.N., Fox, Elizabeth G., B.A., R.N., Van Meter, Anna R., B.A., M.S., op. cit., pp. 701, 702. (Quotation from a letter by Mary C. McNelis, Navy Nurse.)

131   Ibid., p. 702.

132   Ibid., p. 704. (Quotation attributed to Elizabeth Hoag, Navy Nurse.)

133   Ibid., pp. 705, 706. (Quotation attributed to Minnette Butler, Navy Nurse.)

134   Ibid., p. 707. (Quotation attributed to Nora M. McQuade, Navy Nurse.)

135   Ibid., p. 708. (Quotation attributed to Nora M. McQuade, Navy Nurse.)

136   Ibid., p. 708. (Quotation attributed to Myrtle Gilmore Chandler, Navy Nurse.)

137   Laird, LCDR Thelma NC USNR, Jones, LCDR Dorothy NC USN, Feeney, LCDR Elizabeth NC USN, Seidl, CDR Elizabeth NC USN (Ret), Blaska, CDR Burdette NC USN, op. cit., p. 12.

138   Ibid., p. 11.

139   *The Columbia-Viking Desk Encyclopedia*, by staff of the Columbia Encyclopedia, William Bridgwater, Editor-in-chief, The Viking Press, New York, 1953, p. 1038.

140   Laird, LCDR Thelma NC USNR, Jones, LCDR Dorothy NC USN, Feeney, LCDR Elizabeth NC USN, Seidl, CDR Elizabeth NC USN (Ret), Blaska, CDR Burdette NC USN, op. cit., p. 10.

141   Goble, op. cit.. (Unpublished history research notes.)

142   Lyons, op. cit., pp. 54,55.

143   Goble, op. cit.. (Unpublished history research notes.)

144   McGee, Anita Newcomb, M.D., "The Navy Nurse Corps," *Sea Power*, February 1918, p. 123.

[145] As quoted in: Dixon HC USN, Lt. Ben F., "The "White Lily," *Hospital Corps QUARTERLY,* Hospital Ships Number, July 1945, p. 21.

[146] Ibid., p. 11.

[147] Holcomb, Richard C., M.D., F.A.C.S., Captain, Medical Corps, U.S. Navy, op. cit., p. 381.

[148] Ibid..

[149] Information obtained from the file card of Miss Coleman's assignments, Bureau of Medicine and Surgery, Navy Department, Washington, DC.

[150] Laird, LCDR Thelma NC USNR, Jones, LCDR Dorothy NC USN, Feeney, LCDR Elizabeth NC USN, Seidl, CDR Elizabeth NC USN (Ret), Blaska, CDR Burdette NC USN, op. cit., p. 11.

[151] Wells, H.G., op. cit., p. 865.

[152] *The World Book Encyclopedia,* op. cit., Vol. 20, p. 274.

[153] Laird, LCDR Thelma NC USNR, Jones, LCDR Dorothy NC USN, Feeney, LCDR Elizabeth NC USN, Seidl, CDR Elizabeth NC USN (Ret), Blaska, CDR Burdette NC USN, op. cit., p. 11.

[154] Godfrey, Mary Robinson (Navy Service 1910 to 1919), *Oral History Interview Tape Transcript,* op. cit..

[155] The World Book Encyclopedia, op. cit., Vol. 15, p. 262.

[156] Godfrey, Mary Robinson (Navy Service 1910 to 1919), *Oral History Interview Tape Transcript,* op. cit..

[157] Hickey, op. cit., p. 122.

[158] McGee, Anita Newcomb, M.D., op. cit., p. 124.

[159] Ibid..

[160] Dock, Lavinia L., R.N., Pickett, Sarah Elizabeth, B.A., Noyes, Clara D., R.N., Clement, Fannie F., B.A., R.N., Fox, Elizabeth G., B.A., R.N., Van Meter, Anna R., B.A., M.S., op. cit., p. 712.

[161] Ibid..

[162] Ibid..

[163] DeWitt, Nellie Jane, Captain (NC) USN, Superintedent, Nurse Corps, *Letter to Miss Genevieve McDonald, Commander Jean Templeman Post, No. 162, St. Paul, Minnesota,* dated 15 November 1946.

[164] Goble, op. cit.. (Unpublished history research notes that quote the citation of the award.)

[165] Ibid..

[166] Hickey, op. cit., p. 162.

[167] Ibid..

[168] Ibid..

[169] Roberts, Mary M., R.N., op. cit., pp. 149-150.

[170] Hickey, op. cit., p. 158.

[171] Goble, op. cit..

[172] Hickey, op. cit., pp. 162, 163.

[173] Ibid., p. 163.

[174] Ibid., p. 163.

[175] Goble, op. cit..

[176] McGee, Anita Newcomb, M.D., op. cit., pp. 123, 124.

[177] Dock, Lavinia L., R.N., Pickett, Sarah Elizabeth, B.A., Noyes, Clara D., R.N., Clement, Fannie F., B.A., R.N., Fox, Elizabeth G., B.A., R.N., Van Meter, Anna R., B.A., M.S., op. cit., p. 694.

[178] Ibid..

[179] The Surgeon General as quoted in: Dock, Lavinia L., R.N., Pickett, Sarah Elizabeth, B.A., Noyes, Clara D., R.N., Clement, Fannie F., B.A., R.N., Fox, Elizabeth G., B.A., R.N., Van Meter, Anna R., B.A., M.S., op. cit., p. 695.

[180] Superintendent of the Navy Nurse Corps, Mrs. Higbee, as quoted in: Dock, Lavinia L., R.N., Pickett, Sarah Elizabeth, B.A., Noyes, Clara D., R.N., Clement, Fannie F., B.A., R.N., Fox, Elizabeth G., B.A., R.N., Van Meter, Anna R., B.A., M.S., op. cit., p. 696.

[181] Feeney, Elizabeth Capt. NC USN (Ret.), unpublished notes for her speech, with slides, on the *History of the Insignias of the Navy Nurse Corps,* used with permission.

[182] *Uniforms of the United States Navy 1900-1967,* text accompanying this set of color lithographs written by Captain James C. Tily, CEC, USN (Ret.) in coordination with office of Director of Naval History and Curator for the Department of the Navy, U.S. Government Printing Office, Washington, DC 20402. (See section 'Uniforms of the United States Navy 1918-1919.')

[183] Laird, LCDR Thelma NC USNR, Jones, LCDR Dorothy NC USN, Feeney, LCDR Elizabeth NC USN, Seidl, CDR Elizabeth NC USN (Ret), Blaska, CDR Burdette NC USN, op. cit., p. 13.

[184] Dock, Lavinia L., R.N., Pickett, Sarah Elizabeth, B.A., Noyes, Clara D., R.N., Clement, Fannie F., B.A., R.N., Fox, Elizabeth G., B.A., R.N., Van Meter, Anna R., B.A., M.S., op. cit., p. 698.

[185] Hunter, Esther Nelson Behr, *Personal Letter to her Sister,* dated 21 February 1918.

[186] Hunter, Esther Nelson Behr, *Personal Letter to her Sister,* dated 22 August 1918.

[187] Jamieson, Elizabeth M., B.A., R.N., Sewall, Mary F., B.S., R.N., *Trends In Nursing History,* W.B. Saunders Company, Philadelphia, 1944, p. 488.

[188] Ibid., pp. 490, 491.

[189] Ibid., p. 491.

[190] Ibid., p. 506.

[191] Goodnow, op. cit., p. 182.

[192] *200 Years, A Bicentennial Illustrated History of the United States,* op. cit., p. 133.

[193] Ibid., p. 328.

[194] Ibid., p. 134.

[195] Ibid., p. 328.

196 Figures obtained from personnel report published by the Navy Department.
197 Moffett, Mary, (Navy Nurse 1912-1933), *Oral History Interview Tape Transcript*, Interviewer Irene Matthews, taped 3 October 1970.
198 Ibid..
199 Ibid..
200 Ibid..
201 Ibid..
202 Laird, LCDR Thelma NC USNR, Jones, LCDR Dorothy NC USN, Feeney, LCDR Elizabeth NC USN, Seidl, CDR Elizabeth NC USN (Ret), Blaska, CDR Burdette NC USN, op. cit., p. 14.
203 Moffett, Mary, (Navy Nurse), op. cit..
204 Ibid..
205 DeWitt, Evelyn E., (niece of Capt. Nellie Jane DeWitt NC USN, Director of the Navy Nurse Corps 1945-1950), a short biography of Capt. DeWitt. Used with permission.
206 Laird, LCDR Thelma NC USNR, Jones, LCDR Dorothy NC USN, Feeney, LCDR Elizabeth NC USN, Seidl, CDR Elizabeth NC USN (Ret), Blaska, CDR Burdette NC USN, op. cit., p. 14.
207 DeWitt, Evelyn E., op. cit..
208 Laird, LCDR Thelma NC USNR, Jones, LCDR Dorothy NC USN, Feeney, LCDR Elizabeth NC USN, Seidl, CDR Elizabeth NC USN (Ret), Blaska, CDR Burdette NC USN, op. cit., p. 14.
209 Goble, op. cit..
210 Ibid..
211 Roberts, Mary M., R.N., op. cit., p. 166.
212 Ibid..
213 Ibid., p. 662.
214 Ibid., p. 662.
215 *The World Book Encyclopedia*, op. cit., Vol. 20, p. 275.
216 Ibid..
217 Laird, LCDR Thelma NC USNR, Jones, LCDR Dorothy NC USN, Feeney, LCDR Elizabeth NC USN, Seidl, CDR Elizabeth NC USN (Ret), Blaska, CDR Burdette NC USN, op. cit., p. 14.
218 DeWitt, Nellie Jane, LCDR (NC) USN, Acting Superintendent, Nurse Corps, Navy Memorandum to Colonel Blanchfield, 5 December 1945.
219 Hickey, op. cit., p. 163.
220 Laird, LCDR Thelma NC USNR, Jones, LCDR Dorothy NC USN, Feeney, LCDR Elizabeth NC USN, Seidl, CDR Elizabeth NC USN (Ret), Blaska, CDR Burdette NC USN, op. cit., p. 15.
221 Dixon HC USN, Lt. Ben F., op. cit., p. 11.
222 Ibid., p. 21.
223 Ibid..
224 Holcomb, Richard C., M.D., F.A.C.S., Captain, Medical Corps, U.S. Navy, op. cit., p. 381.
225 Laird, LCDR Thelma NC USNR, Jones, LCDR Dorothy NC USN, Feeney, LCDR Elizabeth NC USN, Seidl, CDR Elizabeth NC USN (Ret), Blaska, CDR Burdette NC USN, op. cit., pp. 14, 15.
226 Jamieson, Elizabeth M., B.A., R.N., Sewall, Mary F., B.S., R.N., *1949, op. cit., p. 472.*
227 Ibid., p. 473.
228 Goodnow, op. cit., p. 215.
229 *200 Years, A Bicentennial Illustrated History of the United States*, op. cit., pp. 138,139.
230 Ibid., p. 144.
231 Ibid., p. 331.
232 *The World Book Encyclopedia*, op. cit., Vol. 14, p. 81.
233 Holcomb, Richard C., M.D., F.A.C.S., Captain, Medical Corps, U.S. Navy, op. cit., p. 380.
234 Bowman, J. Beatrice, Chief Nurse USS *Relief*, Open Letter entitled "The Master Hospital Ship," written at Guantanamo Bay, Cuba, dated March 1921.
235 Ibid..
236 Dixon HC USN, Lt. Ben F., op. cit., p. 2.
237 Bowman, J. Beatrice, *Oral History Interview Tape Transcript*, op. cit..
238 Laird, LCDR Thelma NC USNR, Jones, LCDR Dorothy NC USN, Feeney, LCDR Elizabeth NC USN, Seidl, CDR Elizabeth NC USN (Ret), Blaska, CDR Burdette NC USN, op. cit., p. 15.
239 Higbie [Higbee], Lenah S., Superintendent, Navy Nurse Corps, "Navy Nurse Corps," *The American Journal of Nursing*, August, 1921, pp. 410, 411.
240 Ibid., p. 411.
241 Ibid., p. 413.
242 Goble, op. cit..
243 Holcomb, Richard C., M.D., F.A.C.S., Captain, Medical Corps, U.S. Navy, op. cit., p. 381.
244 Goble, op. cit..
245 Ibid..
246 Roberts, Mary M., R.N., op. cit., pp. 170 and 315.
247 Ibid., pp. 315, 316.
248 Laird, LCDR Thelma NC USNR, Jones, LCDR Dorothy NC USN, Feeney, LCDR Elizabeth NC USN, Seidl, CDR Elizabeth NC USN (Ret), Blaska, CDR Burdette NC USN, op. cit., p. 15.

[249]   Goble, <u>op. cit.</u>.

[250]   <u>Ibid.</u>.

[251]   Laird, LCDR Thelma NC USNR, Jones, LCDR Dorothy NC USN, Feeney, LCDR Elizabeth NC USN, Seidl, CDR Elizabeth NC USN (Ret), Blaska, CDR Burdette NC USN, <u>op. cit.</u>, p. 16.

[252]   <u>Ibid.</u>.

[253]   Bowman, J. Beatrice, R.N., "History of Nursing in the Navy," *The American Journal of Nursing*, September 1928.

[254]   Hickey, <u>op. cit.</u>, p. 132.

[255]   Laird, LCDR Thelma NC USNR, Jones, LCDR Dorothy NC USN, Feeney, LCDR Elizabeth NC USN, Seidl, CDR Elizabeth NC USN (Ret), Blaska, CDR Burdette NC USN, <u>op. cit.</u>, p. 16.

[256]   Goble, <u>op. cit.</u>.

"... as yet no pen has been so facile as to
describe in true worth the hospital corpsman....
They came from every walk of life.
At one time I had two lawyers, a seminarian and
a registered pharmacist working with me."

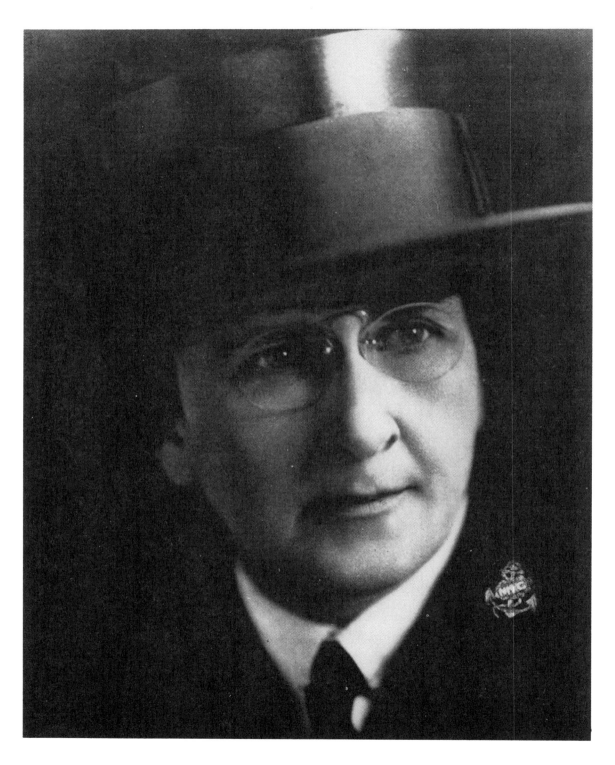

Superintendent - J. Beatrice Bowman
(Official U.S. Navy photo courtesy of Nursing Division, Bureau of Medicine and Surgery, Navy Department.)

CHAPTER 3

Superintendent - J. Beatrice Bowman
(1922 - 1935)

☆☆☆

It is 1 December 1922. Today, J. Beatrice Bowman, one of the 'Sacred Twenty,' is appointed Superintendent of the Navy Nurse Corps. Her orders had been written on 29 November saying, "Upon being appointed Superintendent, Navy Nurse Corps on 1 December 1922 you will regard yourself detached from duty in the Medical Department of the USS Relief and will continue duty in the Bureau of Medicine and Surgery."[1] (Miss Bowman had been stationed at BuMed since 2 August under TAD orders from her permanent assignment aboard the *Relief*.[2]) Within two weeks of her appointment, she is traveling and touring naval stations in the eastern United States.[3]

A Naval Appropriation Act is passed on 22 January 1923. For the first time it authorizes an initial uniform allotment for Navy Nurses. "The new uniform allotment [consists] of six white indoor uniforms of light weight drill, a Navy blue sweater of Spaulding make, a blue silk [velour] and a rough white straw-Knox sailors [hat.] All Chief Nurses and nurses on hospital ships [are] issued blue serge, and white drill outdoor uniforms, these with the capes conform in style with those of the commissioned officers of the United States Navy. These uniforms [are] issued to all nurses, Regular or Reserve, after they . . . [complete] their first six months and [prove] their aptitude and fitness for the service. Reserve nurses [are] required, upon applying for the uniform outfit, to give a written statement as to their intention to remain in the corps for two years, or until such time as the emergency no longer [requires] their assistance.

"The street uniform [is] to have stripes that [will] designate the various grades. Stripes of fine black silk braid [are] worn on the sleeves of the blue coat and lustre braided white linen stripes on the white coat sleeves. The Superintendent [wears] two [one half inch] stripes with a [one quarter inch] stripe between them. The Assistant Superintendent [wears] two [one half inch] stripes; all Chief Nurses [have] one [one half inch] stripe on their sleeve with the [one quarter inch] on top and nurses [wear] one [one half inch] stripe. These stripes [correspond] to the officer grades of ensign to lieutenant commander. . . ."[4] In addition, "for the first time, [the] uniform insignia of [the] Nurse Corps [is] officially endorsed by the Bureau of Navigation [later to become the Bureau of Naval Personnel,] approved by the Secretary of the Navy and incorporated in [the] manual of [the] USN Uniform Regulations."[5] The uniform insignia referred to is the same design as the one issued in 1918 but this one is "reduced in size to [one and one sixteenth inches in] length and [seven eighths of an inch in width.] Two [are] worn, one on each side of the collar."[6]

The January Appropriation Act also includes authorization for three Assistant Superintendents. Therefore, in July, Chief Nurse Clare DeCeu and Chief Nurse Anna G. Davis receive the initial appointments as Assistant Superintendents in the Nurse Corps, Their assignments are to visit schools of nursing for recruiting purposes. They begin giving their procurement talks and utilize lantern slides to enliven their presentations. Miss Davis is especially active in this assignment.[7] Back in March, Superintendent Bowman had "visited Great Lakes and . . . Chicago to bring the work [job description] and need for nurses in the Navy Nurse Corps to the attention of the Superintendents of civilian hospitals in that city."[8] Now, the Superintendent is not alone in her efforts to introduce the civilian nursing community to the Navy Nurse Corps. (The third Assistant Superintendent is assigned to Superintendent Bowman's office at BUMED.[9])

In the latter part of the year, "a new field [is] opened in connection with the duties of Assistant Superintendent. . . . One Assistant Superintendent [is] stationed on the west coast, in the office of the Medical Inspector of Hospitals, and one on the east coast in the Bureau of Medicine and Surgery."[10] Their job is to "study the problems of the Nursing Service of the Navy in order that the military procedure of handling the Corps may be more uniform throughout the naval hospitals."[11] In meeting and talking with the Navy Nurses they are to try and provide the nurses with a better understanding of the ideals and standards of the Corps and the wishes of the Bureau of Medicine and Surgery.[12]

In July of 1923, the census of the Navy Nurse Corps is 495. Also, in this year, three Navy Nurses prepare and write the Nursing Section of the Hospital Corps Handbook: Chief Nurse Sophia Kiel and Navy Nurses Ada Chew and Viola M. Visel.[13]

Down in the Virgin Islands some interesting things are going on with the Navy Nurses stationed there. Reserve Nurse Elsie Jarvis, USN, receives a commendation for her work from the local Chief of the Department of Health. She has been working as the Supervisor of the Insane and Leper Asylums and as Welfare Nurse for one of the Districts in St. Croix.[14] There is a Navy Nurse anesthetist also stationed there in St. Croix. Her name is Helen Rein. This lady had joined the Nurse Corps in 1921. When she applied for information in order to join, Superintendent Lenah Higbee had written her a personal letter. In the letter, dated 22 December 1920, Mrs. Higbee stated, "A notation has been made of your special training in the work of an anaethetist [sic] and of your desire to serve, if possible, in that capacity. As you have noted, nurses are appointed in the Navy for general duty; however, an effort is made to assign them to naval hospitals where their special qualifications can be utilized." Miss Rein is now in the Virgin Islands practicing her specialty and evidently writing letters to the Bureau about her experiences there. On May 17, 1923, Superintendent J. Beatrice Bowman writes a letter to Miss Rein saying, "Your two delightful letters are greatly appreciated, not only in this office but in the Bureau. . . .

"What a happy land you must have, down there among the palms, no one wants to return. Do not stay too long as I notice that those who have stayed their full time show the effects of the tropics. Having had tropical experience, and knowing its effect I am a wee bit worried about the nurses stationed so far. I hope Miss Pingel is well and not sorry that she asked to stay longer. If you see any such signs you will let your chief nurse know about it won't you? Just because she has requested to stay until October is no reason for her being determined to `stick it out.' You see I understand the nurses pretty well and know them to be proud and determined. We must look after one another and not let pride ride us too hard to our fall, especially when there is no need of it.

"With kindest regards to all and many thanks for the picture and the letter."

Navy Nurse anesthetist Rein is detached from the Islands in November. The Chief Municipal Physician, St. Croix, writes a memo to the Commanding Officer, Naval Hospital, St. Thomas, concerning Miss Rein. In it he says, "Since her assignment here she has served at Christiansted Municipal Hospital, Richmond Insane and Leper Asylums, and as District Welfare nurse. In each of these positions her work has been highly satisfactory and because of the unusual nature of the duty to one in the Naval Service, this special report is made.

"As an anesthetist she is unusually well qualified by reason of previous training and experience in the Navy and at Lakeside Hospital, Cleveland. We have found her worthy of every confidence even in the most difficult cases which she has anesthetized in St. Croix." Once again, Navy Nurses are highly appreciated and doing outstanding work in vastly different areas of nursing.

Speaking of different areas of nursing, at the end of June 1923, two Navy Nurses are given TAD ('temporary additional duty' orders) aboard a transport for a voyage to Alaska and return. The ship is the USS *Henderson* and the purpose of the voyage is to take the President and the presidential party to Alaska. President Harding is the first President of the U.S. to visit Alaska during his term in office. The two Navy Nurses assigned this duty are Chief Nurse Sue S. Dauser and Nurse Ruth Powderly.[15]

The President's purpose for the trip is for a "ceremonial visit and vacation in Alaska."[16] President Harding wanted to leave Washington, DC for awhile to avoid the commotion caused by the resignation of his appointee to the Veterans' Bureau and the resultant Senate Investigation and a suicide of one of the Bureau's legal officers. Plus, another suicide of a Presidential insider had taken place in the Attorney General's apartment. Hints of scandal were growing and the troubled President is anxious to get away for awhile.[17] He makes the tour through Alaska and returns to the U.S. towards the end of July. The tired President has what is diagnosed as acute

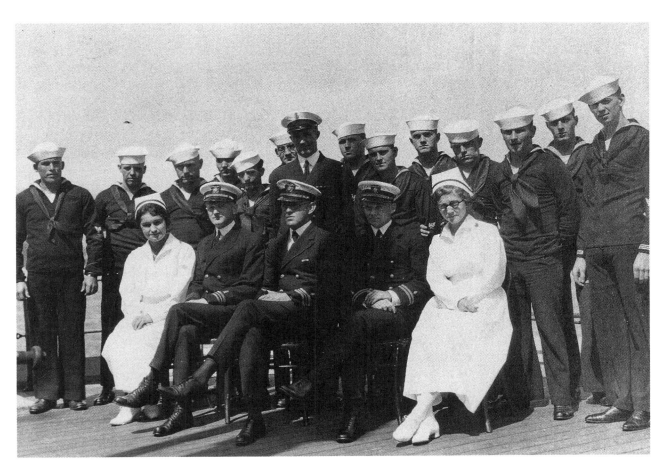

USS *Henderson* Medical Department Personnel, 1923. (Photo courtesy of Navy Bureau of Medicine and Surgery.)

indigestion the night of arrival. "Speaking dates [are] cancelled. The train [from Seattle] [sets] out for San Francisco. . . . After rallying from the Seattle attack, the patient [believes] that he [is] out of the woods."[18] But the "last pictures, taken as he [goes from the train] to the Palace Hotel, [in San Francisco] show a face beginning to sag, to lose its firm outline. . . . He [is] an old, drawn man . . . with a painful, determined smile."[19] At the hotel the two Navy Nurses, Miss Dauser and Miss Powderly, attend to the President[20] as he seems to rally but then develops pneumonia. Again, he seems to recover. In attendance with the nurses are the President's own doctor and a Navy Medical Officer named Joel Boone.[21] (Captain Boone was awarded the Medal of Honor in WWI and holds the prestige of being the most highly decorated Medical Officer in the Navy.) In a 1966 newspaper clip, Miss Dauser is quoted as saying, "I can remember that Harding didn't eat. . . . He was all worn out. His death came between 6 and 7 o'clock in the evening. I had just come into his room to relieve Ruth Powderly on the night shift. Death came suddenly. He was seized by a convulsion and it was all over."[22] The President died of a brain embolism.[23]

Vice President Calvin Coolidge takes over the Presidency but for months the Nation is bombarded with the many exposures of corruption in Harding's administration.[24] It all culminates in what is called the 'Teapot Dome' scandal. Teapot Dome is a naval oil reserve near Casper, Wyoming. It is revealed that the Secretary of the Interior leased this oil reserve and one in California with no competitive bids. The Senate holds an investigation and criminal prosecutions are the result.[25] But, the scandals have very little effect on President Calvin Coolidge who is seen as a prim and proper individual.[26] In fact, Mr. Coolidge runs in the Presidential election of 1924 and is elected. Evidently, the Nation does not see him as tainted by the scandals. Under the four years of Coolidge, the country indulges itself in fads, jazz, sensationalism and the quest for pleasure: the 'roaring twenties.'

Meantime, 1923 sees the publication of 'Nursing and Nursing Education in the United States.' This is the result of an investigation and survey financed by the Rockefeller Foundation. The efforts to produce this study had begun in December 1918 and covers "public health groups, private duty nursing, and twenty-three representative schools connected with hospitals, large and small, public and private, over a wide territory. . . . Findings in the *public health field* [make] clear the need for teaching hygiene in the home. . . . Investigation of the *field of private duty* [reveals] a number of interesting facts. . . . Her [the nurse's} opportunity for teaching principles of hygiene is . . . limited to [the patient] and his immediate family. It is necessary, therefore, that she be a skilled bedside nurse rather than a health teacher. . . . Nurses themselves [are] failing to recognize the need for a subsidiary type of worker [for the care of routine or non-critical cases] whose preparation could be regulated by a system of grading comparable to registration."[27] The "study of *nursing schools* [brings] to light the fact that courses of instruction had received meager attention during the period of rapid expansion. Nearly one-half of such schools [are] connected with hospitals of less than fifty beds. . . . Ancient traditions of asceticism and unquestioning obedience [savor] of the Middle Ages. Ideals emphasizing sacrifice of personal desires and the blind acceptance of authority [have] been carried over from the monasteries and military nursing orders. Moreover, many nurses in responsible positions [have] little preparation beyond that of the basic course. Senior students [are] often used as head nurses, or [are] kept for long periods on night duty. They [are] sent out on private cases, and the financial return [is] made to the hospital. . . . Full-time instructors [are] little known. . . . [Courses are] often based on ward needs, and frequently modified to comply with pressure of work in the hospital."[28]

These are just a few excerpts to give a feeling for the nursing environment of this period of time. The report of the survey of nursing in the U.S., not only indicated the short-comings that were found but made meaningful recommendations, as well. "As an immediate answer to the recommendation that nursing schools be independent of hospitals and on a college level, two endowed university schools of nursing [are] developed, one in connection with Yale University, New Haven, Connecticut, and the other with Western Reserve University, Cleveland, Ohio."[29] In 1924, "The Rockefeller Foundation [finances] a five-year experiment in methods of educating nurses at Yale University."[30] ("*Yale University*, more than two hundred years old and always [till now] a school for men only."[31]) As for Western Reserve, the idea for a collegiate nursing course had been thought of prior to the publication of the Rockefeller report. "The report of the survey [causes] interested lay women to press for further action, and Mrs. Frances Payne Bolton [notifies] the university of her readiness to contribute one-half of the million dollars required by the university for the establishment of a [nursing] school on a parity with other professional schools."[32] (The school becomes a reality and is a success. Eventually, the school is named the Frances Payne Bolton School of Nursing.[33])

On 2 June 1924, at the 24th Annual ANA Convention, a Government Nursing Section of the ANA is established.[34] Also, this year, a nursing service is formed within the government's Indian Bureau. (This, despite the fact that in 1923 the US Civil Service Commission classified nurses as subprofessional.)[35] Further, "by 1924 the schools for hospital corpsmen at Norfolk, Virginia, and Mare Island, California, [have] been accredited by the boards of nurse examiners of [these] states."[36] In July, Navy Nurses are "assigned as Clinical Instructors in [Naval Hospitals] to supervise the training of hospital corpsmen more closely."[37] Then in November, the Bureau of Navigation (later to be BUPERS) issues a directive saying, "When members of the Navy Nurse Corps are embarked in a transport, either for passage or for duty . . . they are to be regarded as of the status of officers in the assignment of quarters, mess et cetera."[38]

September of 1924 and the Surgeon General issues a directive stating that whenever Nurse Corps personnel are on duty, wearing of the prescribed indoor uniform is mandatory.[39] And, this is the year that the Navy Department pays detailed attention to the official wardrobe of the Navy Nurse Corps. An itemized description of all required uniforms and accessaries for Navy Nurses is written into the Navy's Regulations. (As far as can be confirmed, this is the first set of 'Navy Department' regulations for the Nurse Corps.) These regulations set out the requirements in the minutest detail: i.e. the material, the buttons, the placement of pockets, the stitching, the threads, the sizing, etc.. (Undoubtedly, this is done to give exactness to any contract with civilian companies for manufacturing the uniforms but it does make interesting reading.) The regulations speak of the white indoor uniform which is to be of good quality, lightweight drill and the uniform is "To come to 7 inches from the floor and to have a 4-inch hem. . . . [The Belt is to be a] Loose belt 3 inches wide and fastening with two buttons (30 ligne) and buttonholes. Edges of belt single stitched all around 1/8 inch wide."[40] Then the nurse's cap is to "be made of white wash goods of fine quality lawn or handkerchief linen. . . . Across the front fold is placed a black velvet band. . . . The cap of the Navy Nurse Corps shall always be worn on duty, excepting when a member of the corps is in outdoor uniform. It shall be worn in such a manner that the edge will come to the top of the forehead, covering well the hair. The peak of the cap shall be worn as nearly perpendicular as is possible."[41] The regulations state that the "Superintendent of the Nurse Corps shall wear [on her cap] two 1/4-inch gold bands with 1/8-inch band, with equal spacing between, on a black velvet band 1 1/2 inches in width.

"[The] Assistant Superintendent shall wear two 1/4-inch gold bands placed, with equal spacing, on a black velvet band of 1 1/4 inches in width.

"[The] Principal chief nurse shall wear two bands of gold braid 1/4 inch and 1/8 inch in width, respectively, placed with equal spacing on a black velvet band 1 inch in width.

"Assistant chief nurse shall wear one band of gold braid 1/4 inch in width, placed in center of black band, 1 inch in width.

"Nurses who have completed their probationary period and have been accepted, shall wear a black velvet band 1/2 inch in width, in the center of which is sewn a gold band 1/8 inch in width.

"Nurses who have been appointed, but have not completed their probationary period, shall wear a black band 1/2 inch in width."[42]

As for the outdoor blue uniform, it is to be "Dark blue (blue black) 14-ounce serge of Navy standard . . . . [The coat is to be a] Double breasted, semifitting sack coat. . . . Body and sleeves to be lined with gray silk . . . [with] Corps devices to be sewn on ends of collar about 1/2 inch from seam joining collar to lapel and 1/2 inch from end of collar. Oak leaf to be vertical to seam. . . . *Sleeve markings of outdoor uniform.*—Stripes encircle the sleeve. . . .

Superintendent.—Two 1/2 inch stripes with 1/4 inch stripe between.

Assistant Superintendent.—Two 1/2 inch stripes.

All chief nurses.—One 1/2 inch stripe with one 1/4 inch stripe above.

Nurses.—One 1/2 inch stripe.

Material for stripes.—On blue: Fine black silk luster braided braid. On white: White linen braid."[43]

As to the skirt for the outdoor blues, "Material to be made from same material as coat. . . . Length to extend to 7 inches from floor; 4-inch hem."[44] The outdoor white uniform is generally the same except the material is standard Navy drill and the buttons are detachable, white pearl ones. The cape is of 18-ounce standard Navy cloth and is "To be cut to come 13 inches from floor. . . . [The collar is to be] Black velvet, made with stand and fall. Stand to be as high as is consistent with length of neck."[45] There is a raincoat to be of the 14-ounce standard Navy serge. It's "Double-breasted, loose fitting, drawn in to waist by a belt going all around coat. Belt fastening with buckle."[46] And the length of the coat is to be "9 inches from the floor."[47] Since the skirt of the white or blue outdoor uniform is 7 inches from the floor, the bottom 2 inches of the skirt under a raincoat must get rather damp in rain or snow.

Shoes are to be "Black high shoes or oxfords [that] shall be laced . . . and shall be worn with the street uniform. Heels shall not be higher than cuban and shall be fitted with rubber; soles heavy.

"Black patent leather or black suede shoes, conventional style, may be worn when the uniform is worn in the evening. . . . White shoes of canvas or skin, of the same style as the black leather shoes, shall be worn at all times with the white indoor uniform or white street uniform. . . . [Stockings to be] Plain black with blue uniform. Plain white with white uniforms. . . . Gray service gloves shall be worn with blue street uniform or raincoat except upon dress occasions when white gloves shall be worn. White gloves shall be worn with white street uniform, also on dress occasions with blue street uniform."[48]

Two types of Corps Device are described in the regulations: an embroidered one and a metal one. The embroidered consists of "An anchor made in pairs 1 1/8 inches overall. . . . The anchor to have superimposed thereon an oak leaf and acorn with the letters N. N. C.. . . . Anchor and chain, bright gold [finish]. . . . Oak leaf, matte gold [finish]. . . . Letters, fancy silver [finish.]"[49] This device is for wearing with the blue outdoor uniform. The metal device is "An anchor made in pairs 1 1/8 inches overall. . . . The anchor to have superimposed thereon, and integral with it, an oak leaf and acorn with the letters N. N. C. raised . . . above the surface of the leaf. . . . Anchor and chain, bright gold; leaf and acorn, rose gold; letters, N. N. C., bright silver."[50] The metal device is for wearing with the white outdoor uniform and the ward uniform. From there the regulations cover the uniform sweater and the outdoor uniform hats and hat covers; the hat is the one with the two and one-half inch wide all around brim and flat top.

This 1924 publication of Nurse Corps Uniform Regulations, consists of three chapters. Chapter III contains photos that illustrate the various uniforms, the sleeve stripes, the nurse's cap with the different stripes, and the metal corps device. Chapter II is entitled "Specifications of Uniforms and the Wearing Thereof." This is the chapter that is the source of the information presented above. Chapter I is only two pages long and is called "General Regulations." It is indeed a product of the times and well worth a few quotes. For instance; "nurses will be required to have their watches in order and the watch is to be regarded as a necessary part of the uniform to be worn always on duty." Here is an interesting one: "Nurses will be required to arrange their hair neatly and as plainly as is consistent with a pleasing appearance. The bobbing of hair is unapproved as it does not lend to a dignified appearance. Those having bobbed hair will be required to wear it confined in a hair net at all times to give the appearance of neatly dressed hair." This one addresses footwear: "Fancy accessories, slippers, pumps, openwork stockings, or any departure from plain footwear shall not be worn on duty." Here is another: "The nurses shall not roll back the sleeves of their uniforms except when in the act of administering some unusual treatment which shall justify such action." (This one about the sleeves haunted some of us still during the 1950's and early 60's. Some of the senior nurses, of that time, allowed junior nurses NO exceptions to the rolled sleeves regulation.) Here is another: "During cold weather the nurses shall be directed to wear underclothing of sufficient warmth, in order to avoid the necessity of additional outer garments, such as sweaters, capes, etc., while on duty in the hospital." And yet another; "When not on active duty and when remaining within their quarters, nurses may be permitted to wear an approved demitoilet." (Presume this to mean `appropriate leisure-wear or a bathrobe.')

1925. In Lancaster, Pennsylvania a young nurse, Mary Benner, has been doing private duty nursing after graduating from Lancaster General Hospital in 1923. She says, "I read an article written by J. Beatrice Bowman, who was . . . the Superintendent of the Navy Nurse Corps, and it appealed to me so much that I wrote to Washington and was immediately accepted [into the Nurse Corps.] I knew nothing whatsoever about service in either [the] Army or [the] Navy. I was assigned to the . . . Naval Hospital in Brooklyn, New York. . . . It was about six months we were considered, I guess I might use the word, probationers. We were indoctrinated and then we were on our own."[51] About status and pay, Miss Benner goes on to say, "We were appointed and we had all the privileges of an officer except the pay. We were entitled to use the officers' club and we were treated as officers but we did not have the rank. When I came into the service, [the pay] was $70 a month for the first three years [and] $90 for the next three years."[52] The Navy Nurses do not have the rank but are expected to adhere to the rules and regulations as they apply to officers. One of those rules that causes problems involves what is called 'fraternization.' "A ruling that members of the Navy and the Army Nurse Corps should not associate with enlisted men - a regulation issued in the interest of discipline - was the cause of many complaints."[53] Back in 1914, the American Journal of Nursing carried an article by a Chief Nurse in the Navy. The article was one of the presentations at the seventeenth annual convention of the ANA. The Chief Nurse states, "Familiarity with subordinates and co-workers always proves inimical to the efficiency of a nurse and lowers the standard of her discipline and adversely affects the prestige of the entire nurse corps. The effects of such lack of dignity are infinitely more disastrous and far-reaching in a military hospital than in a civil institution."[54] Then in 1922, another Navy Nurse writes of the dilemma, "The status of the nurse, officially, is that of a head nurse in a civil hospital. Professionally and socially she is rated as an officer, It is difficult for the nurse to understand the justice of this ruling at first, when some of the finest timber of our young manhood is of the enlisted personnel. Her own brother, friend and sweetheart may be among them, and why, when she has no rank, should she be subjected to officer's regulations? When she considers that the mere restriction is a recognition of rank, though ever so meager, she usually realizes that it is of too much professional value to treat lightly. In civil life an intimate friendship is not desirable with one's patients; so in military circles, reserve is a safeguard."[55] Many Navy Nurses face this predicament, both from the senior nurse's and the younger nurse's viewpoint. It is never easy but then discipline never is, whether it is self-discipline or imposed discipline.

June 1925 finds two Navy Nurses being tried in a General Court Martial. This is a first for the Nurse Corps. The trial is held at the U.S. Navy Yard in Washington, DC. The charge is 'importing liquor.' (Remember, this is Prohibition time.) The nurses had been detached from the naval facility in Guantanamo Bay, Cuba for duty at the Navy Dispensary in Washington, DC. In the case against one of the nurses, the customs inspector reportedly found three bottles of Scotch and one bottle of Vermouth in a pillow inside a cedar chest consigned to her.

On 18 August, a boiler explosion rips open an excursion steamship in Narragansett Bay about two miles from the U.S. Naval Hospital in Newport, Rhode Island.[56] The ship is the *Mackinac* with six-hundred men, women and children aboard. Fifty-two people die and one-hundred and fifty are burned and injured.[57] Providentially, ships from the U.S. Scouting Fleet are nearby when the explosion occurs. "Boats from these ships [reach] the steamer within minutes and [begin] removing the injured and bringing them to shore. The chief nurse at Newport [Naval Hospital], Esther L. James, [organizes] the nursing staff immediately . . . [and obtains] volunteers from the Red Cross and [from nearby] civilian hospitals."[58] The 'Mackinac Disaster' might have had many more casualties without the doctors, nurses and corpsmen of the Newport Naval Hospital that summer day.

In civilian nursing, this year sees "a critical examination of nursing schools . . . under auspices of the National League of Nursing Education. . . . As a result of the information disclosed, several hundred of the poorer [nursing] schools [close] their doors, and in many others educational standards [are] improved."[59] Then in 1926 the Committee for Grading of Nursing Schools is organized. This committee came about when "the Education Committee of the National League of Nursing Education met with a committee which the American Medical Association had recently appointed for study of nursing education."[60] In 1926, the Committee on the Grading of Nursing Schools develops a five-year program for the following projects:

"1. Supply and demand for nursing service

2. Job analysis of nursing and nurse teaching

3. Actual grading of nursing schools

"Nurses following with interest the proceedings of the group were desirous that the Committee publish a list of schools, graded according to their respective standards of education. . . . Experts in the field of higher education, however, argued drawbacks to an actual grading at this time. Unless each school could be visited personally, the value of the rating would be questionable, and for this the cost would be too great."[61] Many are disappointed when it is decided to drop the grading project. But, the Committee retains its name and concentrates on the other two projects.[62]

On 13 May 1926, the Navy Nurse Corps has its own excitement when President Coolidge signs into law the bill providing retirement for members of the Army and Navy Nurse Corps. The new law allows retirement for thirty years of service or for fifty years of age with twenty years of service. Navy Nurse retired pay is to be "3% times the number of years of service to a maximum of 75%; in addition chief nurses [are] to receive $18, Assistant Superintendents $45, and Superintendents $75 for each year served in such grades."[63] The pen the President uses to sign the Bill is presented to Assistant Superintendent of the Navy Nurse Corps, Anna G. Davis. And, the first Navy Nurse to take advantage of the new law is Chief Nurse Martha E. Pringle, USN, age sixty, with a total of Army and Navy service of twenty-six years and twenty-four days. She retires on 25 November 1926.[64] (She was one of the Sacred Twenty.)

The census of the Nurse Corps is 473 and in June, Reserve nurses, USN are no longer appointed or ordered to active duty. The total of Reserve nurses appointed from 6 April 1917 to June 1926 is 1017.[65]

Sunday, 19 September. Pensacola, Florida is in the direct path of a vicious hurricane. Just nine miles outside the city are the Pensacola Naval Air Station and the Naval Hospital. Navy Nurse M.J. McCloud tells us that the "hospital reservation is on two levels; one enters the gate [to the hospital area] at Sea-level; ascends thirty-two steps to reach a plateau, on which the wards and quarters are built, in a pavillion [sic] style . . . [with] wards being connected by a covered runway. Many large live oak trees adorn the grounds. The reservation is surrounded by a brick wall twelve feet high."[66] Miss McCloud goes on to say that they listened to the radio and learned of the destruction in Miami and other areas of the Florida east coast. "Of course, we hoped for the best and kept on with our usual duties. . . . The sunset at five o'clock was ominous. . . . The Meteorologist at Pensacola kept notifying the public . . . of the approach of the storm. . . . [He stopped at] two o'clock A.M. Monday; [sic] when all electrical wires were blown down, bridges swept away and we were cut off from the outside world; then the news was broadcast from New Orleans that Pensacola was destroyed; `blown off the map.'"[67]

Shortly thereafter, the nurses try to get some sleep in order to be ready for duty or when needed. Navy Nurse L.A. MacFarland states, "in the early morning, having become dimly conscious of a raging wind and heavy rain, I dressed in uniform. I saw that the sky was ominously dark. . . . One couldn't tell whether the clouds came down to the water or the spray, lashed by the ferocious wind, reached up to the sky. The trees were twisting and bending to the fury of the terrific gale, giving up their leaves, twigs, and occasionally, with a protesting roar, their limbs. The air was filled with debris of all sorts - grass, paper, sticks, roofing, etc. The wind seemed to be able to lift and tear whatever it could get under, and was roaring in its work. Every crash, and they were many, told of tree, window, or building unable to stand against such fury."[68] Miss McCloud tells us that at this time the "waves of the Gulf were dashing over Barancas' dock, sweeping everything before it; where once were store houses and a dwelling house, now, nothing could be seen, all having been washed out to Sea. The Bathing Beach was cleaned of bath houses and rafts, by the tidal wave, which dashed its spray to a height of fifteen feet over the Sea-wall, deluging the Navy Yard, the Aviation Station and Warrenton to a depth of five feet."

"The people in Warrenton, a village situated between the Hospital Reservation and the Navy Yard, were warned to move out of their homes as quickly as possible and seek refuge in the [Naval] hospital."[69]

"Captain Odell came by our quarters [nurses' quarters] about seven thirty with a pitcher of hot coffee [made from rain water] for us and forbade us going outside on account of the danger. About eight [A.M.] the people of Warrington [sic] . . . began coming. . . . They `poured' through our gates, mothers with three weeks old babies, children, dogs and puppies, old men and women, men in bathing suits staggering with children in their arms. . . . [About four hundred in all and there are only five Navy nurses.] Empty wards were opened, dry pajamas, sheets and blankets were provided. One of the nurses coming over to our quarters to get some of her dry clothes for the refugees was picked up by the wind and pitched head foremost into a rose bush. [The wind was up to 120 miles per hour.] Fortunately some men were passing and they had to make a regular foot-ball tackle to pull her out. Another nurse was picked up off our front steps and carried some distance away but she managed to land on her feet. Another one was blown all the way around a building before she could get hold of something to hang on and gradually get back inside the ward."[70] Miss MacFarland says that at "sick call, instead of the `Florence Nightingale Lamp,' the doctor and I used a U.S.N. flashlight and visited every patient." About five P.M. the barometer dropped and the wind subsided. However, contact with the outside world did not take place for several days. Miss MacFarland notes that, "During the time we were shut off from the outside world, a good neighbor, an Army Aviator, flying over from Montgomery, Alabama, to convey messages, unfortunately zoomed too low, the plane striking the radio tower and falling in the Commandant's front yard. The plane took fire and in a few minutes pilot and passenger were in our morgue. . . . That was the only fatality connected with the hurricane here."

In early December, 1926, the Commandant of the 11th Naval District, San Diego makes an inspection of the Naval Hospital in San Diego. He comes away quite impressed with the nurses quarters there at the hospital compound. In his report to the Secretary of the Navy, he says, "the nurses quarters at the Naval Hospital, San

Diego, in quality and completeness of furnishings, surpass those assigned to any officer of the service, except, possibly, some Commandant's quarters. The Commandant is in favor of raising the standard in furnishing officers quarters throughout the service to at least the standard of the nurses' quarters.

"In this connection, the Commandant has for a number of years given considerable thought to the question of the Nurse Corps as maintained in the Navy. During this time, the employment of nurses on shore stations and on hospital ships has come under his observation and he has come to the conclusion that there is no real need for the Nurse Corps in the Navy at present; he believes that the Navy would be better without the Nurse Corps. If in the future Congressional authority is obtained to care for the families of commisssioned and enlisted personnel at naval hospitals, there will, of course, be a real need for female nurses; but he believes that their service should be exclusively devoted to dependent wives and children of the personnel of the Navy."[71] [And all females should be married, barefoot and pregnant, I would assume. - the Author.]

The Commandant's report continues, "As a corollary to the above, the hospital corpsmen should be given a higher class of training as nurses."[72]

J. Beatrice Bowman, Superintendent of the Nurse Corps, found out about this report. She replies, "If [the Commandant] would study the quarters provided for nurses in the large civilian hospitals throughout the United States, he would find that quarters for nurses provided by the Navy compare favorably with them, but do not excel."[73] She goes on to explain that the luxuries the Commandant saw, such as "pianos, paintings, ornaments, etc., are bought by the nurses themselves or as gifts from their friends . . . [and these luxuries do] try to give the nurse, who leaves family and friends to be sent to any of the United States possessions or to sea, whenever needed, as pleasant home conditions as possible. The nurses of the country appreciate this and we have it as one of our greatest inducements in recruiting, for certainly the pay alone would not attract the type of woman needed in the service."[74] Then Miss Bowman comes to the heart of the Commandant's problem, "As to the need of the Nurse Corps in the Navy, the Corps stands on its merit and I believe there is not a man in the entire United States Navy, who has at any time been ill, who would be willing to dispense with the care of the Navy Nurse Corps.

"The nurses make the training of the hospital corpsmen their first responsibility next to the care of the sick and it, no doubt, is because the men are so well trained that Admiral . . . feels that the Nurse Corps can be abolished. I feel Admiral . . . has paid us a great compliment and because of it we will renew our hopes for even better results." The Superintendent does have a way with words.

1927. The time of Babe Ruth, the 'Sultan of Swat.' (Baseball, to the uninitiated.) This year he has a total of 60 home runs for the season. It is a record. Then there is the excitement of Charles Lindberg making the first solo flight across the Atlantic Ocean in a single engine plane: *Spirit of St. Louis*.[75] The first talking moving-picture is made and transatlantic telephone service begins between the U.S. and Great Britain.[76] And, installment buying runs rampant across the States.[77]

In May, the Navy Nurse Corps learns, once again, that the Navy's Judge Advocate General has given an opinion that states "nurses are neither officers nor entitled to relative rank."[78] Then in December the Surgeon General of the Navy has one of his requests turned down. He had requested "that the record of members of the Nurse Corps be added to the Register of Commissioned and Warrant officers of the U.S. Navy, and to the Navy Directory."[79] Despite this, Navy Nurses (496 of them) go about their appointed rounds and continue making Nurse Corps' history. For instance, the Assistant Superintendent of the Corps prepares and uses 'Lantern' slides showing the work of Navy Nurses when she makes her recruiting calls at schools of nursing.[80]

When the Navy's 1927 edition of the Manual of the Medical Department is published, the requirements for admission say that applicants for the Nurse Corps must be registered nurses and graduates of schools approved by the Surgeon General. Additionally, the term 'training school' is changed to school of nursing. The Manual also gives age requirements for applicants to the regular Navy as 22 to 35 years, with reserve applicant requirements as 22 to 40 years.

In early 1928, Helen Gavin is on her way for duty aboard the hospital ship *Relief*. She had joined the Navy Nurse Corps in 1924 and was stationed at Great Lakes for three years then for one year at the Naval

Hospital in Washington, DC. Of her work at Great Lakes she says, "we had all these training stations there and we had all these recruits and they were always having epidemics, you know, flu and things of that sort - measles. . . . [It] was different for me because I was put in charge of a ward and before that I was in nursing school and I was always one of the peons."[81] She is referring to the fact that at Great Lakes she was put in charge of a ward and had corpsmen to work with on that ward. As for the *Relief*, it is docked at San Pedro in California. She is sent aboard an Army transport to join her ship. The transport sails to California by way of the Panama Canal (which must have been astounding to a young nurse from a farm family in Wisconsin.) Miss Gavin (later to become Mrs. Whitehead) tells us that after she joins the *Relief*, their first trip is to Hawaii. "We went with the fleet when they went on maneuvers. . . . [Then] we went up to Seattle. . . . And the next year we went to Panama. We went down there for maneuvers. . . . [There were twelve Navy nurses staffing the ship.] We had patients, quite a few of them most of the time. We had a lot of emergencies."[82]

A nurse, by the name of Norma Buttke, joins the Navy Nurse Corps in 1928. She tells us that her "mother wasn't too thrilled about it [her joining the Navy] but later on [her mother] met one of the [Navy] nurses when . . . she drove down to my home and she decided that the girls must be pretty good."[83] When asked what status the nurses had, Norma states, "You're not a commissioned officer and you are not enlisted. You rank below an Ensign. . . . We used to think we were neither fish nor fowl."[84] Her first duty station is at the Naval Hospital, Mare Island, California. When asked about the hours of work she says, "We worked eight to three and three to ten and then night duty was ten to eight. It might vary in different hospitals, just a little. We had a month of night duty at a time in the colder climates and in the tropics we only had two weeks at a time. It was a little harder on you, I think."[85]

The census of the Nurse Corps in 1928 is 503 and in the Congress, the first Bill to provide Retirement benefits for nurses physically disabled in the line of duty is introduced. The Bill fails to pass.[86]

The American Journal of Nursing publishes a comprehensive article by J. Beatrice Bowman in September of 1928.[87] The title of her article is "History of Nursing in the Navy." It is a thorough summary of events leading to the establishment of the Corps and the development of the Corps through 1928. It makes very interesting reading.

Even though the Assistant Superintendents and the Superintendent herself, try to attract and recruit nurses to the Navy, the American Red Cross is still "regarded as the official procurement agency for nursing personnel. At a meeting of the National Committee on Red Cross Nursing Service in December, 1928, J. Beatrice Bowman . . . [declares] that the Red Cross [is] neglecting its obligation to the navy by failing to supply nurses. [The Corps is about fifty nurses below its quota.[88]] Taken aback, Miss Noyes [says] that she had not realized there was great need . . . and had received no special appeal. Miss Bowman [replies] with a definite request and [is] satisfied with the steps that [are] taken - chiefly, publicity through the *Red Cross Courier* and the department devoted to the Red Cross in the *American Journal of Nursing*."[89]

1928 is also the year for a Presidential election. Calvin Coolidge has had enough of the Presidency and states, "I do not choose to run."[90] The Republicans decide to nominate Herbert C. Hoover while the Democrats nominate Governor Alfred E. Smith of New York. Mr. Hoover wins easily and assumes office in 1929. The economy seems to be doing well and the "prices on the New York Stock Exchange that had been steeply rising since the preceding March . . . [continue to rise] through the spring and summer" of 1929.[91]

In January of 1929, the 70th Congress authorizes "the care and treatment of naval patients (active or retired) in other government hospitals when facilities of naval hospitals [are] not available."[92] This includes Navy Nurses. On 3 February, Chief Nurse Mary DuBose, one of the 'Sacred Twenty,' retires after twenty years, four months and three days of active service. In July the census of the Corps is 488.

Out in the Pacific on the island of Guam, Navy Nurses are at work, especially with the native women nursing students. By 1929 a total of fifty students have graduated from the school. (In 1928 the course was changed from a two year course to a three year course.) A nearby Tuberculosis Hospital is staffed with graduates of the nursing school under the supervision of Navy Nurses. Two other graduates of the school are acting as school nurses. One of the school nurses (who works in two of the most distant villages) also does some visiting nurse work and occasional obstetric care. Infant mortality on the island, is now down to less than 2%. In addition, twice a year the Naval Medical Officer, who is also Sanitation Officer, does the 'de-worming' of the 2200 island school children.[93]

The Nurse Corps uniform regulations are reprinted in 1929 but very few revisions are made. One change concerns the skirts: they are now allowed to be 12 inches above the floor. "The major change [is] in the style of the outdoor hat. The wide-brimmed hat of 1924 [is] replaced by a tight-fitting headpiece similar to the cloche worn by women in the 20's. The hat [is] blue for wear with both blue and white uniforms, and [employs] the Nurse Corps device as a cap device."[94]

In September 1929, the stock market becomes extremely inconsistent. In October it drops sharply but collapse is avoided. In November the bottom drops out and there is collapse and disaster. It is the beginning of the great 'Depression.'[95] The immediate effect on the Nurse Corps is that the financial crash wipes out a Memorial Fund started in 1923 by Army and Navy Nurses. The fund's purpose was to place a memorial in the Nurses' Section of the Arlington National Cemetery. (The fund later receives ten cents on the dollar and is resumed in 1935.)[96] The effect on the rest of the country is much more devastating. "Unemployment [mounts] steadily all through 1930 as the Depression [feeds] upon itself in [an] endless downward spiral."[97] Factories close, banks fail, farmers abandon their farms, and the unemployment can "no longer be denied even by the White House."[98] And, "despite vehement protests . . . [President Hoover signs] a tariff measure . . . which [raises] the highest tariff walls in American history. It [amounts] to a declaration of economic war upon the rest of the world, and it [becomes] a major incitement of the world economic collapse which [follows] the onset of the American Depression."[99]

In 1930 the census of the Navy Nurse Corps is 502. Down in the Caribbean, the Virgin Islands' administration is taken over from the U.S. Navy by the U.S. Interior Department. All Navy Nurses stationed there are immediately recalled and sent to other duty stations.[100] In Washington, DC, Superintendent Bowman is busily conducting Nurse Corps business. She attends many of the numerous nursing conferences and meetings in a continuous campaign to publicize and recruit for the Navy Nurse Corps. Sometimes she has a struggle to obtain reimbursement for her expenses associated with the trips. But, she is a determined woman and, at times, pays her own expenses such as the trip to the Massachusetts State Nurses Association in May of 1930 and in October to a meeting of nurses in Allentown, Pennsylvania. Further, Miss Bowman even joins various women's associations in order to foster certain legislation that she feels is in the interest of the Corps. For instance, in 1930 she applies for membership in the Women's Overseas Service League. But, before accepting the membership, she writes to ask if anyone was aware of the "Disability Bill-HR3400." This is a piece of legislation that is in the hands of a Military Affairs Committee in the halls of Congress. She goes on to say that she feels pressure should be brought to bear in order to get a hearing and have it placed on the calendar. She also tells the League that the Secretary of the Navy has forbidden `lobbying' (to Navy personnel) so it's not possible for her to do any active work such as calling on members of Congress to ask for their sympathy and support. She ends with a plea for the League's interest and support.[101]

In June of 1930 the 'Disability Bill' is passed. It provides "for retirement with pay for members of [the] Regular Nurse Corps incurring physical disability in line of duty. The amount of disability pay is 75% of the retiree's active service pay.[102] (From 1908 to [20 June 1930], 51 [Navy nurses] had been surveyed for physical disability without retirement benefits.)"[103] The American Journal of Nursing publishes an article on the Bill in its August 1930 edition. The article is written by J. Beatrice Bowman and is entitled "Disability Bill for Army and Navy nurses." She tells about the Bill itself but also explains the machinations necessary to help get Bills passed or as she writes, " the privilege, or, to put it more accurately, the anxiety of helping to engineer a bill through the Congress."[104]

Interesting to note that in August, the Comptroller-General rules that extra pay for grades above nurse can not be included in computation of active service pay upon which retirement pay for physically disabled nurses is based.[105] In other words, any nurse retired for disability receives retirement pay based on the pay of 'Nurse' even if she is a Chief Nurse or higher.

Also, in 1930, the few remaining Reserve nurses, USN that remain on inactive duty are terminated. The reason for this is probably economics because of the depression. The Naval Reserve Act had been passed in 1925 but was never enforced. It had eliminated nurses in the Navy Reserve simply by using the word 'male' for the Navy Reserves.[106] Therefore, all that is required to release the nurses in 1930 is to simply enforce the 1925 Reserve Act, which is done.

In the civilian sector of professional nursing, 1930 finds the American Nurses Association 100,000 members[107] strong and revising its bylaws to allow "properly qualified men nurses"[108] to join the organization for the first time. (Four years prior to this, the New York State Nurses Association had already organized their Men Nurses' section.[109]) The men nurses are still a small group but they are beginning to play a part in the growing profession.

Overall there are now 213,000 graduate nurses and 80,000 nursing students in 1900 accredited nursing schools.[110] Some of these schools are still inadequate[111] but the weeding out process is a continuing practice at this time.

6 February 1931 and a young graduate nurse from Georgia joins the Navy Nurse Corps and reports for duty at the Naval Hospital, Washington, DC. Her name is Alberta Reeves (her married name later becomes Lamborn.) Her first six months are probationary then she becomes a full fledged 'Nurse' in the Navy. She states, "we wore [our] own white uniforms for the first six months and then they made up tailored uniforms for us, six of those. We had the Navy [nurse's] cap. It wasn't fancy or anything but I think [it was] attractive. We had a black band [on the cap]; I can't remember if we had the black band to start with or not. I know we did, later on, have the black band and had the long gold stripe on top of the black band. . . . We did have a navy blue cape, a long, heavy cape, it was lined with a dark red, and we had an overseas cap. . . . In the winter time I once . . . attended a funeral, over at the Arlington National Cemetery, and I remember wearing [the] cape and [a little] hat [probably the 'cloche'] and we did not know the nurse [being interred]; she was not on duty at Washington."[112] As for social activities, Alberta says that the hospital "was close enough so we could even walk into the city in Washington. It was just a delight to see [the city] and at one time we walked to this National Cathedral which was beautiful, but it was not finished and the gardens were beautiful then, too, and the Washington Monument. But, I didn't walk up there [the Monument] like so many people did. We [the hospital] were real close to the Lincoln Memorial and the Reflection Pool and they had these cherry blossoms all around."[113]

Another young nurse by the name of Bertha Evans (later on her married name becomes St. Pierre) joins the Navy in November of 1931. She says, "That was during the depression. Work was scarce. I wasn't getting much work and my brother was a doctor in the Navy and he wrote me that he didn't know much about the Nurse Corps but it [sounded] like a good deal, why [didn't I] try? So that's why I went in; to get a job. . . . [My] mother wasn't too happy. I asked her why. She said, `all those sailors out there' and I said, `yes, and I want to take care of them.'. . . I went down [to the recruiting station] and signed my name on the dotted line, promised to uphold the Constitution of the United States and to defend my country and all that jazz."[114] (Little does Bertha know that 'all that jazz' will eventually include imprisonment as a prisoner of war [POW].)

Actually, these young Navy Nurses are fortunate in having been accepted into the Nurse Corps since the American Journal of Nursing reports that only 43 new appointments are made from January through June of 1931 and only 20 appointments during the rest of the year. The Nurse Corps census (1 July) is 529.[115]

On 1 March, nurse Anna E. Mears, USN is the first nurse to be retired under the Physical Disability Bill (passed just the previous year.) Then on March 3 the Congress passes an Amendment to the Disability Bill. The amendment provides "for computation of retired pay upon the basis of the entire amount of active service pay **in all grades**[116] not just the pay of 'Nurse.' Later in March, the Judge Advocate General (Navy) issues an opinion "that Reserve nurses are eligible to be retired under provisions of the laws for retirement of Regular Navy (and Army) nurses: both regular retirement and physical disability retirement. But, in November, the Comptroller

General makes a decision that Reserve nurses are not eligible for retirement benefits. This serves to reverse the previous JAG opinion. It hardly matters at this point because on 30 December all 29 Reserve Navy Nurses, on active duty, transfer to the Regular Navy Nurse Corps![117]

During the 1920's and 30's, letters are received from black nurses asking about eligibility for appointment in the Nurse Corps. Generally, a type of form letter answer would go out saying something to the effect that there are no positions available in which they would be happy or adaptable. "During the 20's when J. Beatrice Bowman was Superintendent, she had one assistant . . . that in the replies she sent out [to letters from the black nurses] . . . [the assistant] attempted to give help and guidance. If the nurse was a graduate, she referred her to [the] Civil Service Commission and/or [as the assistant writes] to `Providen Hospital in Chicago, Illinois, which has a school for colored nurses. I would advise that you communicate . . . for information as to opportunities in that hospital or elsewhere in Chicago.'"[118] However, in 1931, in response to inquiries, the answer about 'no positions' is resumed.

The American Association of Nurse Anesthetists is organized in 1931 and also, in this year, the Army suspends its School of Nursing.[119]

As for the Depression and the country in general, things worsen in 1931 and in 1932 become "far worse. By 1932 industrial production [is] approximately half what it had been in '29, with the automobile industry operating at a fifth of its '29 capacity and steel plants . . . at a mere 12 percent of capacity. . . . As every index of production and distribution [goes] down, unemployment, having doubled in '30, at least doubled again in '31, and [doubles] yet again in '32, [as] between 15 million and 17 million workers - a fourth of the national labor force - [are] out of work."[120] Jobless war veterans descend on Washington, DC. "Some of them [take] over unoccupied Buildings; others [scatter] through twenty makeshift camps in and around the city."[121] They come to 'lobby' for legislation for a veterans' bonus but the bill is defeated. President "Hoover [refuses] to acknowledge publicly that the bonus marchers [exist] until some of them [become] involved in a riot in which two [are] killed by police gunfire. He then [orders] the army to remove the marchers from the capital, whereupon six tanks and a thousand troops under the command of the chief of staff, General Douglas MacArthur, [march] against a crowd of unarmed men, women, and children, injuring scores while evicting all from the shacks they had erected."[122]

Meantime, in the early 1930's, a 'drought' is choking the middle of the country. From Canada to Texas the country is a 'dust bowl' with dust storms ruining the crops and rotting the grain. The banks are foreclosing on loans and dispossessing the farmers. Bands of farmers (Okies) join together and head west to California to look for work.[123] ("In 1934, great curtains of dust [are] carried clear across the continent to the Atlantic Coast and far out into the Gulf of Mexico."[124] It isn't until the late 1930's that sufficient rain begins to fall to start ending the drought.) Not only the farmers but thousands of others take "to the road. Often jailed as vagrants, always forced to move on by local authorities, they [`bum'] their way around the country aimlessly."[125] Soup kitchens and breadlines are seen in the cities. On 5th Avenue in New York, well-dressed men are selling apples for five cents each.[126] "Hundreds of thousands [are] driven by hunger to become scavengers. . . . In every city there [spring] up beside the dumps and on other wasteland, collections of shacks made of old boards, flattened tin cans, and sheets of corrugated iron, where jobless men, some with their wives and children, [live] in misery. . . . [These areas are] called Hoovervilles. For by 1932 Herbert Hoover [is] hated by masses of Americans as perhaps no other President [has] ever been."[127]

This Depression does have its effect on the Nurse Corps; in fact, on all government personnel. A law is passed in 1932 to reduce government spending. As a result there is a 15% reduction in base pay for all naval personnel. Also, longevity increases are halted and there is a requirement for a "'legislative' furlough of 30 days leave without pay to be taken during [the] year."[128] As reported in the American Journal of Nursing issues in 1932, from January to June only 12 new Nurse Corps appointments are made and 14 appointments from July to December. The census of the Nurse Corps on 1 July is 504.[129] The May issue of the American Journal of Nursing reports on the biennial ANA convention held in April in San Antonio, Texas. J. Beatrice Bowman is there as the President of the Government Section of the organization and one of the Navy's Chief Nurses, Virginia Rau, gives a speech at the luncheon meeting. The Journal report quotes Chief Nurse Rau as saying, "Navy nursing has its own peculiar appeal. . . . By reason of periodic rotation of the different naval activities, which are located on both coasts as well as in tropical parts, one cannot but acquire the increased knowledge and broader vision which travel brings." (Miss Rau will become more important to Nurse Corps' history in a few more years.) One more item in 1932 again reaffirms the status of nurses in the Navy. In November the Bureau of Navigation sends a message in answer to a request from the Commanding officer of the USS *Relief*. "Since members of [the] Navy Nurse Corps are in no sense officers, rules for precedence have not been, nor will they be, formulated."[130]

On a more positive note and despite the Depression, a vaccine for Yellow Fever is developed in the U.S., as well as the Artificial Cardiac Pacemaker. In Germany the first Sulfa drug is reported.[131] Speaking of drugs, there are no antibiotics in these days and as one Navy Nurse tells us, there is "just the old way of taking care of things, like hot soaks and hot pads and different solutions for infections."[132] These are the years of mustard plasters and turpentine packs. Mustard plasters for chest colds and turpentine packs for infections. On an upbeat note, the first Navy Nurses are selected and given orders to the New Haven School of Physical Therapy[133] and in the civilian world of nursing, the Association of Collegiate Schools of Nursing is organized.[134]

1932 and the presidential election. The Republicans nominate President Hoover and the Democrats nominate Franklin D. Roosevelt. Roosevelt wins in a landslide. He is inaugurated on 4 March 1933. In his inaugural address, with his mellifluous voice and silver tongued oratory he gives depression weary Americans the one thing they need the most, 'hope.' In his address he says, "This great nation will endure as it has endured, will revive, and will prosper. So, first of all, let me assert my firm belief that the only thing we have to fear is fear itself."[135] "Over and over again he [promises] `action . . . direct, vigorous action.'"[136] And he does make things happen. He begins "to submit recovery and reform laws for congressional approval. Congress [passes] nearly all the important bills that he [requests], most of them by large majorities."[137] Roosevelt calls what he is doing, the 'New Deal.' He labels the new laws with names soon known by their initials:

NRA - National Recovery Administration
AAA - Agricultural Adjustment Act
CCC - Civilian Conservation Corps
TVA - Tennessee Valley Authority

(In 1935 he adds the WPA [Works Progress Administration], the SEC [Security Exchange Commission], the REA [Rural Electrification Administration], plus several others.) And the regime slowly begins to show results.

Navy Nurse Alberta Lamborn, stationed in DC at this time, tells us about her meeting with President Roosevelt, "it was [a gathering] for the patients and it was on the lawn [of the White House] in the backyard . . . I can't remember if we had refreshments or not, but I'm sure we had music from the band playing, the Navy band or Marine, but they did play a lot at the many functions they had. And the President rolled out. President Roosevelt rolled out in his wheelchair and he chatted around and shook hands with us and we all felt like we were something, because we got to shake hands with the President."[138]

Navy Nurse Mary Benner is one of two nurses aboard a Navy Transport in 1933. She tells us she boards the transport in San Francisco and they sail to Honolulu, Guam, and the Philippines. She says the two of them (the other Navy Nurse aboard and herself) "visited the [Navy] nurses in both Guam and the Philippines."[139] Then the transport sails to China. They stop at several ports there, "to deliver some people and to pick up some navy people and marines."[140] She tells of going to see the 'Great Wall' of China while the ship is in port for several days. They are able to travel a part of the way to the 'Wall' by car but the rest of the way is made on the backs of donkeys. Then, "While we were in Shanghai I visited two nurses [at an Episcopal Hospital] who had trained with me in the Lancaster [Pennsylvania] General Hospital and they had me to lunch and one of the officers aboard ship got a rickshaw for me to go over and he told the rickshaw driver he wasn't to leave 'Missy' for one minute. But as it happened I stayed there a long, long time. [I] had lunch with the girls and I'll never forget we had celery and it was pink because it was soaked in potassium permanganate, [as] all their fresh vegetables were, of course.

[This was a health precaution used on fresh produce in many foreign countries.] So the girls said they'd give anything for good celery, so I took them back to the ship with me. Incidentally, my rickshaw boy was still sitting, waiting for 'Missy.' We dismissed him and went back in their car and I took them and introduced them to the Commissary Officer and he gave them quite a few bunches of fresh celery [no soaking necessary]."[141] At another port Miss Benner says that the ship is "tied up in the . . . River. We were between, as I recall, a French warship and an English ship. The current was very high and the [river] is filthy and we watched them [the Chinese river people] scooping the garbage from our [the ship's] slop chute onto their sampans. . . . They ate it."[142]

In March of 1933, the Veteran's Administration allows a $75 reimbursement of burial expenses for World War I veterans, including nurses. (Increased to $100 in 1934.)[143] In October there is a "Comptroller General's Decision (A-50986) that members of [the] Navy Nurse Corps are not officers of [the] Navy and thus [are] not entitled to mileage allowances provided for officers."[144] It seems as though almost every year something is promulgated to remind Navy Nurses that they are not officers; interesting. Also interesting is that for years the ANA has supported and favored rank for Navy Nurses. At the 1933 annual "meeting of the Board of Directors of the American Nurses' Association they accepted a proposal that a letter be sent by that Association to the Surgeon General of the Navy . . . [urging] such legislation as could be carried out to improve the status of the Navy nurse."[145]

In December, eight nurses are sent to George Washington University for a four-month course in dietetics. Heretofore, if Navy Nurses were at duty stations where no nurse dieticians were aboard, one Navy Nurse would be assigned that duty. Navy Nurses are expected to be professionally versatile and competent.

In 1933 when Long Beach, California experiences a severe earthquake, the field hospital is taken off the hospital ship *Relief*, set up on shore and plays an important part in the relief efforts. (Back in 1931 when "Managua, Nicaragua was leveled by an earthquake . . . the *Relief* was in Panama. The field hospital was taken off her, loaded onto planes and flown to Managua where it proved invaluable in rescuing victims."[146] So the *Relief*, has had experience with the field hospital prior to the Long Beach catastrophe.)

Also, during the 30's, the "first *U.S.S. Mercy* [ends] a useful career tied up at Philadelphia, Pa., where she [serves] as a shelter for victims of the depression."[147]

The first conference of the newly organized Association of Collegiate Schools of Nursing is held this year. Representatives of 21 institutions set up the standards and objectives "for the permanent organization which [takes] place in 1935. The objectives . . . are:

1. To develop nursing education on a professional and
   collegiate level.
2. To promote and strengthen relationships between
   schools of nursing and institutions of higher education.
3. To promote study and experimentation in nursing
   service and nursing education."[148]

The New York State Nurses' Association's "1933 convention program [is] devoted to the several aspects of [men nurses'] preparation and employment, It [is] reported that only four of the universities in the US [now] offering courses for graduate nurses [will] accept men nurses. One hospital school offering postgraduate courses [will] accept men but only for work in hospital administration. Despite the limited opportunities for advanced work, a few men [are now] holding positions on nursing school faculties."[149]

The Depression is not without its consequences on the nursing profession. The government addresses this situation in 1933 with the Federal Emergency Relief Administration. Under FERA, employment and salaries are provided for unemployed nurses.[150]

In 1932, the Committee on the Grading of Nursing Schools had begun a second study of the surviving Nursing Schools of the first study. The final report of this second study, "along with specific suggestions for improvement, [appears] in book form in 1934. This volume, *Nursing Schools Today and Tomorrow*, [shows] that the chief purpose of hospitals was the care of their patients, that nursing schools had been operated as paying service departments, with student nurses regarded in the same light as employees. . . . It criticized the existent form of apprenticeship teaching [for the student nurses], and emphasized the need for instruction on a college level."[151] In fact, this second study shows that 22% of the schools have no instructor, but this is down from the 42% having no instructor in the 1929 first study.[152] There has been improvement but, as the study shows, more is needed. And speaking of nursing schools, there are twenty-five of them that accept black students; most of these schools being in the south.[153] Also, in 1934, The National Association of Colored Graduate Nurses establishes "a national headquarters in New York with a full-time executive secretary."[154]

The first public health nurse is appointed by the U.S. Public Health Service in 1934 and the ANA begins a national campaign to establish the eight-hour working day for nurses.[155]

Over in Great Britain, in 1934, they develop the 'catseye' studs for highways while the first public launderette appears in the U.S..[156] This country's 'Great Depression' is slightly improved but continues to hold a firm grip on the nation while President Roosevelt forges ahead with his 'New Deal' administration and his radio 'fireside' chats with the American people.

The Navy Nurse Corps is feeling the results of governmental austerity in 1934. In the June edition of the American Journal of Nursing an article by J. Beatrice Bowman and concerning the Navy Nurse Corps states, "On March 11, 1934, orders were received to release 54 nurses either by discharge or retirement. In complying, the request was made that these nurses be placed in the Civil Service list, subject to examination. No new appointment [to the Nurse Corps] has been made in the biennium." On 1 July the census of the Navy Nurse Corps is 349. Applicants for the Navy Nurse Corps are told that the outlook for assignment to the Corps is not very encouraging. Not only are new appointments not being made, nurses already in the Corps are being released.[157] "In 1934 I wrote the Director, [Navy Nurse Corps], BuMed, for information re Navy nursing. The reply [was] the Navy is not accepting applications at this time and they have a long waiting list."[158]

Down in the Caribbean, the U.S. Marine detachment stationed there leaves in August and with them leave the Navy Nurses stationed there. American troops had been there since 1915 when the President of Haiti was murdered and the troops were sent in to protect American interests in the area.[159] The only good news this year is that 10% of the 15% pay cut made in 1932, is restored. (The rest [5%] is restored in 1935.)

In March of 1934, Chief Nurse Myn Hoffman is promoted to Assistant Superintendent of the Nurse Corps and arrives in Washington, DC on assignment to Superintendent Bowman's staff at the Bureau of Medicine and Surgery. On 4 May 1934, J. Beatrice Bowman submitted the following to the Secretary of the Navy through the Surgeon General:

> "Having served in the Navy Nurse Corps for more than twenty-five years and having reached the age of fifty years, I request that I be released from active duty at the expiration of my present year as Superintendent of the Navy Nurse Corps and be transferred to the Retired List on January 1, 1935."[160]

"She [is] the last of the Sacred Twenty on active duty and with her departure the era of the Sacred Twenty [comes] to an end."[161]

But, they will not and should not be forgotten. They forged the foundations of this Navy Nurse Corps and Superintendent Bowman was a dynamic administrator and a progressive professional nurse in the true tradition of those first twenty Navy Nurses. "During her term of office as Superintendent of the Navy Nurse Corps, Miss Bowman was a member of the National Committee on American Red Cross Nursing Service, of the Advisory Committee of Nurses to the Medical Director and to the Medical Council of the U. S. Veterans Bureau, of the American Public Health Association, and of the American Association for the Advancement of Science. She was Chairman of the Government Section of the American Nurses' Association 1930-32, and President of the Graduate Nurses' Association of the District of Columbia 1931-34. She also held active membership in the American Nurses' Association, the National League of Nursing Education, the Army and Navy Country Club, and the National Travel Club."[162]

J. (Josephine) Beatrice Bowman goes on leave 1 September and is retired 1 January 1935. "She served a total of 25 years, 8 months, [and] 23 days with 12 years and 1 month as Superintendent."[163]

1   Goble, CDR Dorothy Jones, NC USN (Ret.), as quoted in her unpublished history research notes.
2   Information obtained from the file card of Miss Bowman's assignments, Bureau of Medicine and Surgery, Washington, DC.
3   Goble, op. cit., .
4   Lyons, Barbara A. LCDR NC USN, *Formation, Organization and Growth of the Navy Nurse Corps 1908 - 1933*, pp. 89, 90.
5   Laird, LCDR Thelma NC USNR, Jones, LCDR Dorothy NC USN, Feeney, LCDR Elizabeth NC USN, Seidl, CDR Elizabeth NC USN (Ret.), Blaska, CDR Burdette NC USN, *Chronological History NAVY NURSE CORPS*, Prepared by: Nursing Division, Bureau of Medicine and Surgery, 1 August 1962, p. 16.
6   Feeney, Capt. Elizabeth NC USN, *Notes on Nurse Corps Insignia*.
7   Laird, LCDR Thelma NC USNR, Jones, LCDR Dorothy NC USN, Feeney, LCDR Elizabeth NC USN, Seidl, CDR Elizabeth NC USN (Ret.), Blaska, CDR Burdette NC USN, op. cit., p. 17.
8   Goble, op. cit..
9   Lyons, op. cit., p. 89.
10   Ibid., p. 88.
11   Ibid..
12   Ibid..
13   Laird, LCDR Thelma NC USNR, Jones, LCDR Dorothy NC USN, Feeney, LCDR Elizabeth NC USN, Seidl, CDR Elizabeth NC USN (Ret.), Blaska, CDR Burdette NC USN, op. cit., p. 16.
14   Ibid..
15   Ibid., p. 17.
16   *200 Years, A Bicentennial Illustrated History of the United States*, Joseph Newman, Directing Editor, Books by U.S. News & World Report, Inc., 2300 N Street, N.W., Washington, DC 20037, 1973, Book 2, p. 140.
17   Ibid..
18   Adams, Samuel Hopkins, *Incredible Era - The Life and Times of Warren Gamaliel Harding*, Octagon Books, A Division of Farrar, Straus and Giroux, New York, 1979, pp. 373, 374.
19   Ibid., p. 374.
20   Rhoades, Frank, "Frank Rhoades [column]," The San Diego Union, 13 May 1966.
21   Ibid..
22   Ibid..
23   Adams, op. cit., pp. 374, 375, 377.
24   *200 Years, A Bicentennial Illustrated History of the United States*, op. cit..
25   *The Columbia-Viking Desk Encyclopedia*, by staff of the Columbia Encyclopedia, William Bridgwater, Editor-in-chief, The Viking Press, New York, 1933, p. 976.
26   *200 Years, A Bicentennial Illustrated History of the United States*, op. cit..
27   Jamieson, Elizabeth M., B.A., R.N., Sewall, Mary F., B.S., R.N., *Trends In Nursing History*, W.B. Saunders Company, Philadelphia, 1949, pp. 510, 511.
28   Ibid., pp. 511, 512.
29   Ibid., p. 513.
30   Roberts, Mary M., R.N., *American Nursing History and Interpretation*, The MacMillan Company, New York, 1963, p. 180.
31   Goodnow, Minnie, R.N., *Nursing History*, W.B. Saunders Company, Philadelphia and London, 1948, p. 272.
32   Roberts, Mary M., R.N., op. cit., pp. 181, 182.
33   Ibid..
34   Laird, LCDR Thelma NC USNR, Jones, LCDR Dorothy NC USN, Feeney, LCDR Elizabeth NC USN, Seidl, CDR Elizabeth NC USN (Ret.), Blaska, CDR Burdette NC USN, op. cit..
35   Roberts, Mary M., R.N., op. cit., pp. 170, 662.
36   Ibid., p. 171.
37   Laird, LCDR Thelma NC USNR, Jones, LCDR Dorothy NC USN, Feeney, LCDR Elizabeth NC USN, Seidl, CDR Elizabeth NC USN (Ret.), Blaska, CDR Burdette NC USN, op. cit..
38   As quoted in Laird, LCDR Thelma NC USNR, et al, Ibid., p. 18.
39   Ibid., p. 17.
40   *Uniform Regulations, United States Navy Nurse Corps*, Navy Department: 1924, Government Printing Office, Washington, DC, 1925, p. 3.
41   Ibid., pp. 4, 5.
42   Ibid., p. 8.
43   Ibid., p. 5.
44   Ibid..
45   Ibid., p. 6.
46   Ibid., p. 7.
47   Ibid..
48   Ibid..
49   Ibid., p. 8.
50   Ibid., pp. 8, 9.
51   Benner, Mary CDR. NC USN (Ret.), *Oral History Interview Tape Transcript*, Interviewer Irene Smith Matthews Lt(jg) Navy Nurse Corps, taped in 1970.
52   Ibid..
53   Dock, Lavinia L., R.N., Pickett, Sarah Elizabeth, B.A., Noyes, Clara D., R.N., Clement, Fannie F., B.A., R.N., Fox, Elizabeth G., B.A., R.N.,

Van Meter, Anna R., B.A., M.S., *History of American Red Cross Nursing*, The MacMillan Company, New York, 1922, p. 716.

54   Hertzer, J., "Comments on Navy Nursing," *American Journal of Nursing*, April, 1914, P. 840.

55   Dock, op. cit., p. 717.

56   Lyons, op. cit., p. 90.

57   Copic, CDR Kathryn M., NC USN (Ret.), from her unpublished research notes.

58   Lyons, op. cit., p. 90.

59   Jamieson, op. cit., pp. 506, 507.

60   Ibid., p. 514.

61   Ibid., pp. 515, 516.

62   Ibid.

63   Hickey, Dermott Vincent, *The First Ladies In The Navy - A History of the Navy Nurse Corps, 1908-1939*, June 1963, pp. 164, 165.

64   Laird, LCDR Thelma NC USNR, et al, op. cit., p. 18.

65   Ibid.

66   McCloud, M.J. Navy Nurse, report of the Pensacola hurricane, Records of the Office of the Director, Navy Nurse Corps, Box 10, #15, Disasters (1925-1961) (2 folders), Operational Archives, Naval Historical Center, Washington Navy Yard, Washington, DC.

67   Ibid.

68   MacFarland, L.A., Navy Nurse, ibid.

69   McCloud, ibid.

70   Wells, Ellen E., Navy Nurse, ibid.

71   As quoted in: Goble, CDR Dorothy Jones, NC USN (Ret.), op. cit.

72   Ibid.

73   Ibid.

74   Ibid.

75   *The World Book Encyclopedia*, Field Enterprises Educational Corporation, Chicago, Volume 12, 1966 edition, p. 290.

76   Great Events of the 20th Century, Editor: Richard Marshall, The Readers' Digest Association, Inc., 1977, p. 165.

77   Ibid., p. 198.

78   Laird, LCDR Thelma NC USNR, et al, op. cit., p. 18.

79   Ibid.

80   Ibid.

81   Whitehead, Helen Gavin CDR USN (Ret.), *Oral History Interview Tape Transcript*, Interviewer CDR Jean Davis USN (Ret.), taped on 24 April 1990.

82   Ibid.

83   Buttke, Norma L. LCdr (Ret.), *Oral History Interview Tape Transcript*, Interviewer LCdr Margaret (Linn) Larson (former Navy Nurse,) taped on 13 May 1988.

84   Ibid.

85   Ibid.

86   Laird, LCDR Thelma NC USNR, et al, op. cit., p. 19.

87   *American Journal of Nursing*, Vol. XXVIII, Number 9, September, 1928.

88   Lyons, op. cit., p. 92.

89   Kernodle, Portia B., *The Red Cross Nurse in Action*, Harper and Brothers, New York, 1947, p. 333.

90   *200 Years, A Bicentennial Illustrated History of the United States*, op. cit., p. 333.

91   Ibid., p. 144.

92   Hickey, op. cit., p. 165.

93   Goble, op. cit.

94   Tily, James C., *The Uniforms of the United States Navy*, Thomas Yoseloff, Publisher, 8 East 36th Street, New York, New York, 1964, p. 256.

95   *200 Years, A Bicentennial Illustrated History of the United States*, op. cit., pp. 145, 147.

96   *Program for the 60th Anniversary of the Navy Nurse Corps*, Brochure prepared by LCdr H. Walker and CDR E. Feeney, 13 May 1968.

97   *200 Years, A Bicentennial Illustrated History of the United States*, op. cit., p. 147.

98   Ibid.

99   Ibid., p. 150.

100   Laird, LCDR Thelma NC USNR, et al, op. cit., p. 19.

101   Goble, op. cit.

102   Bowman, J. Beatrice, R.N., "Disability Bill for Army and Navy Nurses," *American Journal of Nursing*, August, 1930, p. 1016.

103   Laird, LCDR Thelma NC USNR, et al, op. cit., p. 19.

104   Bowman, op. cit.

105   Laird, LCDR Thelma NC USNR, et al, op. cit., p. 19.

106   Goble, op. cit.

107   Goodnow, op. cit., p. 214.

108   Roberts, Mary M., R.N., op. cit., p. 318.

109   Ibid., p. 319.

110   Goodnow, op. cit., p. 182.

111   Ibid., p. 267.

112   Lamborn, Alberta Reeves, Navy Nurse, *Oral History Interview Tape Transcript*, Interviewer LCdr Adelaide Stilwell NC USN (Ret.), taped on 9 March 1990.

113   Ibid.

[114] St. Pierre, Bertha Evans, Capt. NC USN (Ret), *Oral History Interview Tape Transcript*, Interviewer LCdr Margaret Larson NC USN (Ret.), taped on 17 June 1988.

[115] Laird, LCDR Thelma NC USNR, et al, op. cit., p. 19.

[116] Ibid..

[117] Ibid., p. 20.

[118] Goble, op. cit..

[119] Roberts, op. cit., p. 663.

[120] *200 Years, A Bicentennial Illustrated History of the United States*, op. cit., p. 147.

[121] Ibid., p. 150.

[122] Ibid..

[123] *Great Events of the 20th Century*, Editor: Richard Marshall, The Readers' Digest Association, Inc., 1977, p. 266.

[124] *The World Book Encyclopedia*, Field Enterprises Educational Corporation, Chicago, Volume 5, 1966 edition, p. 316.

[125] *200 Years, A Bicentennial Illustrated History of the United States*, op. cit., p. 147.

[126] *Great Events of the 20th Century*, Editor: Richard Marshall, The Readers' Digest Association, Inc., op. cit..

[127] *200 Years, A Bicentennial Illustrated History of the United States*, op. cit., pp. 147, 150.

[128] Laird, LCDR Thelma NC USNR, et al, op. cit., p. 20.

[129] Ibid..

[130] As quoted in: Laird, LCDR Thelma NC USNR, et al, Ibid., p. 20.

[131] *Great Events of the 20th Century*, Editor: Richard Marshall, The Readers' Digest Association, Inc., op. cit., p. 228.

[132] Lamborn, Alberta Reeves, Navy Nurse, *Oral History Interview Tape Transcript*, op. cit..

[133] Laird, LCDR Thelma NC USNR, et al, op. cit., p. 20.

[134] Roberts, op. cit., p. 664.

[135] As quoted in: *200 Years, A Bicentennial Illustrated History of the United States*, op. cit., p. 152.

[136] Ibid..

[137] *The World Book Encyclopedia*, Field Enterprises Educational Corporation, Chicago, Volume 16, op. cit., p. 416.

[138] Lamborn, Alberta Reeves, Navy Nurse, *Oral History Interview Tape Transcript*, op. cit..

[139] Benner, Mary CDR. NC USN (Ret.), *Oral History Interview Tape Transcript*, op. cit..

[140] Ibid..

[141] Ibid..

[142] Ibid..

[143] Laird, LCDR Thelma NC USNR, et al, op. cit., p. 20.

[144] Ibid..

[145] Lyons, op. cit., p. 82.

[146] McCann, Dick Sp(X)1c, "Our Growing Mercy Fleet," *All Hands, (Bureau of naval Personnel Information Bulletin)*, August 1945, p. 9.

[147] Dixon HC USN, Lt. Ben F., "The `White Lily'," *Hospital Corps QUARTERLY*, Hospital Ships Number, July 1945, p. 21.

[148] Jensen, R.N., M.A., Deborah MacLurg, *A History of Nursing*, The C.V. Mosby Company, St. Louis, 1943, pp. 196, 197.

[149] Roberts, op. cit., p. 319.

[150] Ibid., p. 664.

[151] Jamieson, op. cit., pp. 520-522.

[152] Ibid., p. 521.

[153] Goodnow, op. cit., p. 198.

[154] Ibid., p. 200.

[155] Roberts, op. cit., p. 664.

[156] *Great Events of the 20th Century*, Editor: Richard Marshall, The Readers' Digest Association, Inc., op. cit., p. 228.

[157] Feeney, Elizabeth Capt. NC USN, *History of the Navy Nurse Corps/Manuscript Collection*, Box 24, Series V, Vol. III (1922-1935), Naval Historical Center, Washington Navy Yard, Wash., DC.

[158] Quebbeman, Frances, Navy Nurse, *Written Personal History*, 13 May 1991.

[159] *The World Book Encyclopedia*, Field Enterprises Educational Corporation, Chicago, Volume 9, op. cit., p. 17.

[160] Goble, op. cit., as quoted in her unpublished history research notes.

[161] Hickey, op. cit., p. 140.

[162] Prepared by members of the staff of the Navy Nurse Corps for The National League of Nursing Education, year unknown.

[163] Goble, op. cit..

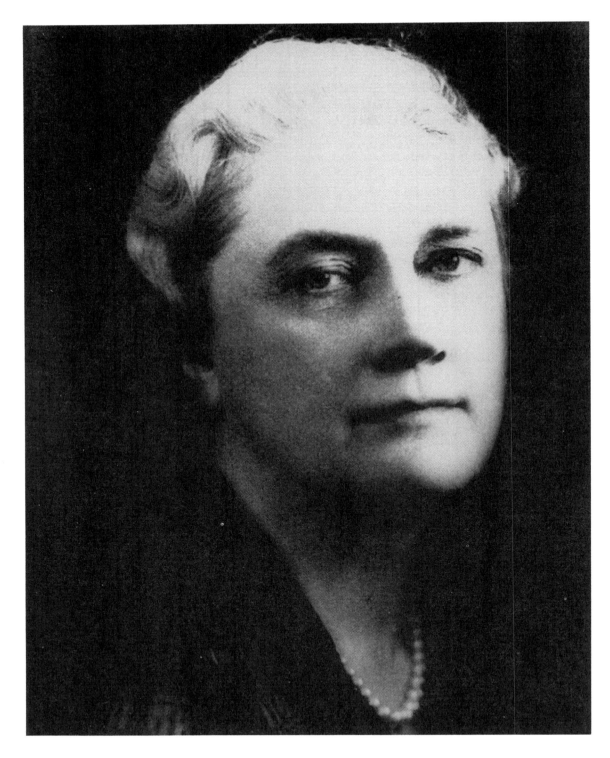

Superintendent - Myn Hoffman
(Official U.S. Navy photo courtesy of Nursing Division, Bureau of Medicine and Surgery, Navy Department.)

CHAPTER 4

Superintendent - Myn Hoffman
Acting Superintendent - Virginia Rau
(1935 - 1939)

It is 1 January 1935. Assistant Superintendent Myn Hoffman becomes the fourth Superintendent of the Navy Nurse Corps. She was born in 1883 in Bradford, Illinois. She attended the Illinois' State Normal School and then taught in the schools there for several years. In 1915 she graduated from nurses' training at St. Joseph's Hospital School of Nursing in Denver, Colorado.[1] Miss Hoffman then worked as a Charge Nurse at Union Hospital, Silverton, Colorado[2] and also practiced nursing for a time in Illinois. Just before the U.S. entered WWI, on 26 February 1917, Miss Hoffman joined the Navy Nurse Corps. The Norfolk Naval Hospital, in Portsmouth, Virginia, was her first duty station. She was promoted to Chief Nurse in September 1919.[3] She then had assignments at several Naval Hospitals including a tour at St. Thomas in the Virgin Islands from 4 September 1928 to 20 February 1930.[4] She had been promoted to Assistant Superintendent and was already in BuMed on the staff of the Superintendent when she is appointed and takes the oath of office as Superintendent of the Navy Nurse Corps.[5]

1935 is the year that the Nurse Corps reaches its lowest census level. On 1 July there are 339 Navy Nurses but at one time this year, the number goes down to 332. However, the Corps still forges ahead. In January the first Navy Nurse is assigned to a post-graduate course in operating room nursing at Johns Hopkins Hospital in Baltimore, Maryland.[6] In February, the Comptroller General's decision is promulgated saying "that Reserve nurses retired under the Act of 20 June 1930 while in the active service of the U.S. are entitled to the retired pay provided therein for regular Corps members."[7] Then in July a Navy Judge Advocate General opinion comes out, "that, since members of [the] Navy Nurse Corps are not officers and thus not entitled to officers allowances for heat, light, and water for quarters, but nevertheless are acknowledged members of naval service, `the practice should continue of furnishing Navy nurses with gas, electricity, fuel and water in the manner prescribed for enlisted men.'"[8]

If you'll remember, back in 1913 the first two Navy Nurses were sent out in the Pacific to the island of Samoa. Here it is 1935 and Navy Nurse Mary Benner receives her orders to Pango-Pango on the island of Samoa. She says, "The only way you could get there was on the Mattson Line [civilian shipping line], no planes went in. The Mattson Line went down once a month. There were four of us there; one chief nurse and three staff nurses and we had a training school for the native nurses. We had about forty little nurses. Well, originally Pango-Pango was nothing more than a coaling station for [the] Navy when they used to coal their ships. . . . That was a very small community and we had this hospital that was one building. There was a nice building that was our nurses quarters. Then there was a building that had a make-shift operating room and delivery room and a couple [of] private rooms, and the rest were all the native huts. . . . And we had these little bare-footed native nurses that we taught. Our [objective] was to teach them so they could go out to the various villages and teach their own people.

"[We] were [in] Eastern Samoa and there was [a] Western Samoa and on the fourth of July the New Zealand nurses, who were stationed over in Western Samoa, called on us [came to visit]. . . . When we went over to visit them [on the King's birthday] . . . we had a very interesting experience. The governor had us come to his home and his home had been the home of Robert Louis Stevenson. So [while there] we got up early one morning and we climbed the hill to his [Robert Louis Stevenson's] grave. . . . [It] was a terrific climb, about 600 feet. . . . [There] are flat stones there [and] there is engraved . . . `Home is the sailor, home from the sea and the hunter home from the hill.' And that was a very interesting experience.

"So, while I was in Samoa we went through one terrific hurricane that we had to evacuate the hospital. We had two concrete buildings down in the town and we evacuated all our patients except our lepers. (We had lepers we were taking care of. They were in a . . . hut above the nurses quarters.) So we grabbed everything and ran and when we came back the next day, we crawled over trees and what have you and found our lunch still on the table. [We] got our patients back, but somehow or other, we'd forgotten our lepers. So later on in the day, we saw them wandering up the road visiting with everybody along the way. They were having a wonderful time. [It was] the first they'd been out for years.

"We had one leper by the name of Maggie that had a little house right as you came up the walk to the hospital. . . . [When] the ship would come in, it would dock for four hours; the Mattson line. And the men [off the ship] would get to talking to her and when I'd go by, I'd just say, 'You know, she's a leper' and they'd run like fury when I would say that to them.

"[These] nurses that we were teaching had an equivalent of a sixth-grade education. . . . They made their own uniforms and they had their own caps and we had a graduation for them. And we sent to [a jeweller] in Philadelphia for their little school pin when they graduated. [Their training was for three years.] And they loved to do the practical work. You couldn't get too far with them in theory because they just didn't have it. But they loved to give baths and enemas and any kind of treatment at all. . . . But [the Samoans] never wanted anybody to die in the hospital and they'd come at night, if somebody was dying, and you couldn't get them to even sign a release [form] and they'd have these torches and they'd be chanting and they'd carry this person [patient] out in the middle of the night, 'cause they didn't want them to die there. [They wanted them to die at home.] And then, of course, we always had our deworming sessions where they had all the children come in to deworm them on the front porch of the hospital."[9]

Back stateside, the historically first Naval Hospital at Portsmouth, Virginia is riding out the drought of Navy Nurses with some twenty-two nurses aboard. There are three Chief Nurses: one is the Principal Chief Nurse, one is Assistant to the Principal Chief Nurse and one is an Anesthetist. The others are: one Physiotherapist, two Dietitians, two Operating Room nurses and thirteen other Navy Nurses plus one Navy Nurse as Instructor in Nursing at the Hospital Corps School on the hospital compound.[10]

On the civilian side of nursing, there are now 1500 accredited Schools of Nursing which is 400 less than five years ago. In addition there are 68,000 student nurses, down from 80,000 in 1930.[11] These decreases are the result of the Committee that is grading and checking the nursing schools.

With the depression and "millions of people on relief or economically dependent, it [is] not surprising that the existing means for providing medical and nursing care [prove] hopelessly inadequate. Studies on the cost of medical care [show] that even under normal conditions most people [are] unable to pay for minimal health services. At the same time thousands of nurses and doctors [have] little or no work. Plans for health insurance and group medical and hospital service [are] greatly stimulated by the depression, and public health agencies [are] compelled to extend their services to much larger groups. The Social Security Act, which [becomes] a law in 1935 [marks] a definite trend in the direction of governmental support for health and welfare activities.

"Nurses [are] directly affected by these changes and a noticeable shift [is] observed from free lance to organized nursing services, from private to public health and hospital nursing."[12] "After 1935, the federal government [is] to have an increasingly potent influence on the evolution of American nursing."[13]

Over in Europe, Germany has been busily rehabilitating itself after WWI and one Adolf Hitler has been busy inserting himself and his National Socialist Party into the government's infrastructure. President Hindenburg made Hitler Imperial Chancellor and Germany resigned from the League of Nations, in 1933. In 1935 Hitler declares that the Peace Treaty of WWI no longer exists and he begins conscription and the rearming of Germany.[14] In October of 1935, Italy, under dictator Mussolini, "invades and conquers Abyssinia ["The grievances alleged [are] trivial border disputes."[15]]; [the] League of Nations fails to act."[16] In 1936, "Franco rebels against [the] Spanish republic, with [the] aid of Nazis and Fascists [Germans and Italians]."[17] All of Europe seems to be seething and simmering with unrest.

It is election time again in the U.S. in 1936. The Republicans nominate Governor Alfred M. Landon of Kansas while the Democrats renominate Franklin D. Roosevelt. President Roosevelt wins in a landslide.[18]

On 1 July 1936 the census of the Navy Nurse Corps is 399. It is beginning to rise from last year's low point. Applicants are, once again, being accepted. But still not accepting from within one group: the black graduate nurses. Under Superintendent Hoffman, the attitude seems to remain as it had been. She receives one letter from a black nurse in Valdosta, Georgia who had, evidently, written once before to the previous administration, "please look over your colored list and find a . . . space for one and let me know pretty soon."[19] Miss Hoffman answers, "you are advised that no encouragement can be offered you regarding an assignment with the Nurse Corps, U.S. Navy as there are no openings for colored nurses. If you will recall the Bureau's letter of Sept. 1, 1932, you were informed at that time that when your services could be utilized the Bureau would get in touch with you. Your name is still retained in the files and it will not be necessary for you to write again."[20] "Other letters [get] the same old routine answer about 'no duties in which (they) would be happy or adaptable.'"[21]

In Pennsylvania, a young graduate nurse applies to the Navy Nurse Corps. Her name is Ann Bernatitis. She had graduated from a School of Nursing in 1934. As she states, "Immediately after graduating, those being depression days, jobs for nurses were non-existent. So I enrolled in a course for Operating Room Technique and Management at the University of Pennsylvania Graduate Hospital in Philadelphia. . . . [While] I was taking the course in Operating Room Technique, two Navy nurses were there enrolled in a course in anesthesia. One [of them] was Winnie Gibson [who is destined to head the Nurse Corps in 1950]. . . and I was so impressed with their dress, their uniform but especially the insignia they wore on their collars. . . . The big anchor. We wore one on either side of our collar lapel."[22]

Ann practices her profession for a year or so then sends an application to the Navy Nurse Corps. On "the first of September in 1936, I received word that my application had been received and [it] requested that I come to Philadelphia to the naval hospital for a physical. I arrived, [and] spent the whole day at the hospital having a physical. [I] went back home and shortly thereafter, about two weeks after that, I received word that I was accepted into the Nurse Corps and that I was to report to duty on the 25th of September 1936 at the U.S. Naval Hospital in Chelsea [Massachusetts]."[23] Ann reports in to Chelsea and finds the nurses quarters "very comfortable. [The Quarters'] building [is] approximately 100 years old, so the rooms were enormous. . . . We all lived in the one building, but each [nurse] had a roommate. The rooms were large enough to accommodate really three or four people but there was not that need for it. There were so few of us there at the time. As I recall, there were only about fourteen of us on duty [with a patient census of about 300]. . . . [The] indoctrination into the Navy was really an on-the-job training. You were assigned to a ward with an older nurse and she in turn indoctrinated you into the routine of the ward. . . . You were given an opportunity to do ward supervision, 'cause after several weeks of indoctrination with an older nurse, you were assigned a ward of your own. Our wards in those days averaged approximately 30 to 40 patients. To this ward were assigned, maybe four hospital corpsmen and you were in charge. Some of these hospital corpsmen had just come from Corps School, so had had instruction in procedures and techniques, but hadn't actually had the opportunity to apply these. So it was my job to teach these corpsmen to apply all the theory they had in Corps School. You were responsible for the teaching of the corpsmen. You were responsible for seeing that the nursing care was done. You were responsible for ordering all the supplies necessary for the ward. . . . You were in charge of all the housekeeping of the ward. . . . The navy was paying me $70 a month plus . . . subsistence in [the] quarters. That was furnished. Your uniforms were furnished to you at that time, the original issue. After that you furnished them yourself."[24] (You might want to remember this lady's name, Ann Bernatitis, for you will meet her again during World War II.)

Yet another Pennsylvania nurse enters the Navy in 1936. Her name is Margaret Nash and she went to nursing school at Mercy Hospital in Wilkes-Barre, Pennsylvania and graduated in 1932. She too practiced her profession for a few years before applying to the Navy Nurse Corps. During those few years she "went up to the Catskill Mountains to a private sanitarium to take a course in tuberculosis because the hospital where I trained . . . did not have tuberculosis, so I wanted to know more about the disease. . . . When I returned from the Catskill

Mountains (my course was supposed to be six months but I loved it up there so I stayed 18 months) there was a flood in Pennsylvania in 1936 and the Sisters had called my mother to request that we all come and help out in the flood. And so I think that was my first experience as far as the Navy was concerned; not exactly with the Navy but part of it [the Coast Guard]. I worked with the Coast Guard . . . out in the boats taking the people from the roofs of the houses. Some of them tried to get their cattle in [the boats]. I remember that we also delivered a baby in the boat. . . . I was working for three days and nights around the clock; I never went home except to get a sandwich from the Salvation Army occasionally. In the meantime, my uncle, who was a congressman in Washington, returned to Pennsylvania to survey the flood situation. He came down [to] the house to visit and asked me what I planned on doing. I said, `Well, right now I'm going to continue doing private duty until I can get something that I like better.' He said, `How would you like to go in the Navy?' Well, of course, I jumped at that and I said, `Do they have nurses in the Navy Nurse Corps?' And so he said, `When I return to Washington, I'll go up and talk with the Superintendent of Nurses [Navy Nurse Corps].' And I said that would be wonderful. And he said, `I'll have her send you out an application.' The only thing I said to my uncle was, `Please, don't tell my mother, because she'll be very upset.' So in three weeks my application arrived; I had the necessary physicals that I had to take care of and in three weeks I was sent to Portsmouth, Virginia. . . . I remember signing my oath on April the 18th 1936."[25] Margaret tells us that she finally told her mother about joining the Navy when she took her physical and "my mother at dinner, every evening, for three weeks, there was nothing but tears."[26] (It isn't until Miss Nash's second duty station, Newport, Rhode Island 1937 to 1938, that her "mother came up and stayed for a week . . . and therefore was convinced that the Navy was all right for her daughter."[27]) (You will also meet this Navy nurse again in World War II.)

Another graduate nurse, Sylvia Lavache (later to become Mrs. Barnes), joins the Navy in 1936. Her reasons for joining give a graphic description of the difficulties facing nurses during the depression. "I graduated from Boston City Hospital in Boston, Massachusetts [in] 1933. I found there were no jobs available for me. I started out doing private duty for a Directory of Nurses in downtown Boston. I lived in a suburb in the southwestern part of the city and was often called at 3 a.m. to go to work - probably for a patient breathing their last breath. The longest job I had during my two and one-half years [that] I served in this way was probably a few days. I made fifty cents an hour or six dollars for a twelve hour day. After about six months, the law was changed by Congress to an eight hour day. This helped but I still resented the many days I spent at home. Discouraged yet stirred by a desire to work <u>everyday,</u> I decided to write a few letters to find other employment. . . . In 1935, I was working WPA or part-time help at the U.S. Marine Hospital in Chelsea, Massachusetts (today known as the U.S. Public Health Service.) . . . The Chelsea Naval Hospital was surrounded by a fence next door."[28] Sylvia had written to the Navy for an application to the Nurse Corps. She applied, took her physical at the Chelsea Naval Hospital and was accepted. She receives orders to the naval hospital at Portsmouth, Virginia. She tells us, "my salary was seventy dollars a month with board, room and laundry. . . . We lived in a pleasant H-shaped building two stories high [the nurses' quarters]. Each nurse had an individual room with a single bed, dresser and small desk and chair. The floors and window sills were dusted each week by [the] help and the rest we did ourselves. We had our own mess and dining room where the chief nurse prepared the weekly menus for the cook. The meals were hearty, nourishing and attractive. We sat at round tables seating about a dozen persons with dishes decorated in blue and gold and sterling silver with a U.S.N. engraving."[29] The Chief Nurse at Portsmouth is Anne K. Harkins. Miss Harkins has issued a set of instructions called 'nurses quarters.' Among the instructions are:

> Breakfast - 7:20 and 8 a.m.
> Lunch - 12:20 p.m.
> Dinner - 6 p.m.

> "1. Nurses must always report for duty at least 10 minutes before the hour; a.m. nurses by 7:50; p.m. nurses by 2:50; and night nurses by 9:50 p.m.

"2. Morning nurses to leave wards or special departments at 12 noon and <u>not sooner</u>, and be back on duty by 1 p.m. Afternoon nurses to leave wards for supper at 5:45 p.m., and are to be back on duty at 6:45.

"3. On Sundays and holidays, the a.m. nurses will leave wards at 12:45 p.m. for dinner, and do not return afterwards, the p.m. nurses going on duty early instead. . . . Food and ice can always be obtained in the refrigerator in the kitchen. Anyone except the relief nurse, who is too late to eat meal at regular time, must wash and put away her own dishes, and leave everything in order. . . . It is forbidden to remove Officers' Mess Silver from the Dining Room. . . .

"4. The p.m. nurse on S.O.Q. [Sick Officers' Quarters] is to turn off the following lights in the Nurses' Qts. at 10 O'clock: Switch #7, South Hall, 1st floor, laundry lights, front door light, and all in the Living Room except center table lamp. Also to make sure that all entrances are securely locked.

"5. Anyone staying out over night must obtain permission from the chief nurse, and leave her address and phone number. It is not intended that nurses time off duty be restricted but they must return to the nurses quarters at a reasonable hour at night. . . .

"9. Nurses are requested (a) to keep entrances locked - keys are always procurable, (b) not to reprimand servants; any difficulties arising should be reported to the chief nurse.

"10. Electrical sewing machine, mangle and other electrical equipment is for the convenience of the nurses and must be left in good condition after use."[30]

Out on the west coast, another graduate nurse joins the Navy in 1936. Her name is May J. Lindner and she reports in to the Naval Hospital, San Diego for duty. "At that time there were 60 nurses on duty at the naval hospital in San Diego, and we usually averaged about 1500 to 1800 patients and we were on probation for the first six months. We wore our own duty caps from our own hospital and then after six months, why we got the Navy Cap (the nurses cap) and our sweaters and our capes and they gave us out little hat [cloche] which I never wore. . . . The white duty uniform was the only uniform we had. . . . Then, after six months I was accepted [probation was over] and we were given classes by one of the nurses on what the Navy was all about and what to expect. We lived in the nurses' quarters there at the hospital and we each had our own room. Beautiful dining room and the meals were prepared beautifully . . . there [were] about twelve tables in the dining room and the senior nurse sat at the head of the table, serving. . . . We did not have rank at that time, neither fish nor fowl, as we used to say, but we had our pay when we first come into the Navy of $70 a month. . . . We went on duty about seven-thirty in the morning until about three in the afternoon and then in the afternoon the nurse would work from three to about ten; the night nurse until seven-thirty in the morning. . . . And every two weeks we got a day and a half off. And the night duty; we had night duty for thirty days . . . and when you came off night duty, you came off on Saturday morning, so you had Saturday morning off and Sunday all day and usually you went back on duty on Monday on P.M. duty. . . . There usually [were] only two nurses on night duty. One of the nurses would cover the SOQ area and the medical wards and the other nurse would cover all the rest of the wards. The nurse who worked in the diet kitchen also had to go and serve breakfast to the SOQ patients and then serve them at lunchtime and also at dinnertime, which meant cooking special eggs and making toast for [the] officers."[31] Miss Lindner also tells us she "did all types of nursing when I first went into the service. I worked in orthopedic wards and medical words and contagious wards and diet kitchen. One of the nurses got sick, [one who] worked in the diet kitchen, so they selected me to go work in the diet kitchen, which I didn't like that much because I was always on duty when everybody else was off duty. And that meant getting up at five-thirty in the morning and doing diet kitchen to get the special diets prepared for the patients."[32]

The 1936 Christmas Menu for the staff and patients at the Naval Hospital, Washington, D.C., lists a bountiful holiday meal with: tomato juice cocktail, roast turkey, cranberry jelly, giblet gravy, apple and celery dressing, spiced baked ham, scalloped pineapple and sweet potatoes, mashed potatoes, buttered asparagus cuts, queen olives, sweet mixed pickles, celery stuffed with cottage cheese, mince pie, pound cake, tutti frutti ice cream, hot Parker House rolls, mixed nuts, candy, fruit, coffee, milk, cigars. Presumably, Nellie Jane DeWitt, dietitian at this hospital, planned this special meal. (Navy Nurse DeWitt is destined to become Director of the Nurse Corps in 1945.) Another Navy Nurse stationed at this hospital as Physiotherapist is Laura M. Cobb.[33] (She is destined to become a prisoner of war.)

The census of the Nurse Corps remains the same in 1937: 427 Navy Nurses. Some nurses leave and new applicants enter the Corps to maintain its strength. One of the new nurses is Nell Williams Hill. "I had an older sister in the Army Nurse Corps and she did not want me to go into the Army because she thought the Navy had more to offer than the Army. . . . At that time, [in order to apply], we wrote directly to the Superintendent of [Navy] nurses . . . at the Department of Medicine and Surgery, Department of the Navy, Washington, D.C.. We were not commissioned, we were appointed for a period of six months: probationary period. . . . [After six months] you were interviewed by the chief nurse of the hospital you were in which [for me] happened to be in Washington, D.C.. [Having passed probation, we] signed a statement agreeing not to resign for a period of three years. Then we were given six ward uniforms and a cape and the cap and a sweater."[34]

Up in Chelsea Naval Hospital, Navy Nurse Ann Bernatitis says, "We had dependents in Chelsea. Because, while I was in Chelsea, they renovated one of the World War I buildings for a dependent unit. Formerly, they [the Navy] didn't have in-patient care for Navy dependents. . . . About a year after I got to Chelsea [1937] they converted one of the old . . . buildings that was still standing, into a dependent unit. I recall that when the building was opened, they staffed it with civilian nurses. And they [the civilian nurses] were having some difficulty in grasping the routine of the Navy. I remember coming down to lunch one day and finding a note on the bulletin board addressed to me from the chief nurse saying, `I want to see you in my suite after lunch.' Of course, the first thing I thought of was what did I do or what didn't I do. . . . When I walked in, she said, `We had a meeting.' Of course, I didn't know who the `we' were. She said, `Tomorrow morning I want you to go to the dependents hospital.' I looked at her in amazement. I said, `But . . . I don't know anything about dependents. I don't know anything about obstetrics [or] pediatrics.' Well, she said, `That's fine. Tomorrow morning you go.' And the next morning I went. . . . So I learned something about obstetrics and pediatrics and all the others. But that [Chelsea] was one of the first places that had started in-patient care for Navy dependents."[35]

Down in Portsmouth, Virginia at the Naval Hospital, Navy Nurse Sylvia Barnes relates what she terms a 'remarkable incident in 1937.' She says that the Chief Nurse Anne Harkins tells them "she [is] going to teach us how 'to open up a ward.' We ordered the necessary supplies, cleaned the furniture and ward and prepared for the admission of crews of blue jackets [sailors] from the various ships then in port. All of these patients had 'catarrhal fever' or the common head cold. Each patient was given sulpha drugs and a pitcher of water after temperature, pulse, [and] respiration were taken and recorded. Almost all had fever. At 10 a.m. the next day, all were discharged as their temperatures were normal and there were no complaints. To me, this was like a miracle because in the past, patients with catarrhal fever usually stayed in the hospital for a week or ten days. At 10:30 a.m. we admitted another ship's crew and the treatment was repeated. Each day the same treatment went on until we must have nursed the whole Navy personnel of the Norfolk Naval Base. [Also,] by this time I had learned to use words like galley, head, deck, bulkhead, overhead, bunk and other nautical terms."[36]

On 6 May 1937 the largest airship ever built (the German *Hindenburg*) is flying over the Lakehurst, New Jersey area in preparation for landing. A Navy Nurse stationed at the Naval Hospital in Philadelphia (about 45 miles from Lakehurst) tells us, "We watched the German airship circle the area for several hours around sunset. When the news came that the *Hindenburg* had exploded, a team of medical officers and nurses made the trip to Lakehurst, N.J. under police escort. German authorities had restricted the area to all others. We brought back a member of the ground crew hit with flying debris. I have a small piece of the fuselage as a memento."[37] Thirty-six people are killed in the crash of the airship as it tried to land at Lakehurst. The scene is broadcast over the radio to the nation by a newsman who's voice keeps breaking as he tries to describe the flaming horror he is seeing. "This tragedy [ends] regular airship service from Germany."[38]

Navy Nurse Norma Heuple Buttke is stationed at the U.S. Navy Hospital Canacao, Philippine Islands in 1937. "It [the hospital] was on the island of Luzon. . . . We had 12 nurses there. The main building had two floors. The sick officers quarters [were] in a separate building right close over the water. It was right at the edge of the water. That was Manila Bay and [leading into it] was . . . Bay. And . . . Bay happened to be where the Pan Am planes, they were hydroplanes you know, they landed on the water. And we could see them. When you were on night duty you could see the ship. [When the Pan Am prepared to take off] they had a pilot ship go ahead with a search light and spot out fishing boats or anything like that so they didn't run into them. When they got out in Manila Bay at the crack of dawn, they took off."[39] Norma is talking about the Pan American Clipper of 1937 that carries air mail at the rate of seventy-five cents for a letter. Then during September and October of 1937, Norma has TAD (temporary additional duty) aboard the transport ship *USS Canapus*. The purpose of the duty is to help repatriate women and children from China (Japan has made a full-scale invasion of China.[40])

Navy Nurse Buttke had joined the Navy in 1928, one year after graduation from nurses' training. She was stationed at Mare Island, California until she resigned in 1930. "I resigned and thought that I would try something else. I decided to come back in because I really missed the personnel, the people you worked with."[41] When she came back she was stationed at San Diego until 1933 when she went aboard the Navy Transport, *USS Henderson*, for a month, through the Panama Canal and arrived at Annapolis for two years of duty. In 1935 she receives orders to Great Lakes, Illinois and drives there in her car. In Great Lakes "It got down to 27 degrees below zero in that winter. . . . Great Lakes had been closed in 1933, I think it was, [because these] were the depression years, and so there weren't any nurses there."[42] But, by the time Norma arrived there were 12 nurses there and they all prepared for the re-opening and re-establishment of the Naval Hospital. After Great Lakes is when she gets her orders to the Philippines. (You will hear more from Navy Nurse Buttke during WWII.)

In the civilian world of Nursing, the school of nursing at Yale University in 1936 had become "entirely a graduate school. Its degree of Bachelor of Nursing (given from 1926 to 1936) [becomes] in 1937 that of Master of Nursing. It has become one of the most conspicuous and influential schools of the country."[43]

As for the rest of the world, not only did Japan invade China in 1937, but the 'Rising Sun' country joins with Germany and Italy (later also Franco's Spain joins) to form a consortium called the 'Axis.'[44] In the U.S., the country is beginning to see the end of the depression but President F.D. Roosevelt is worried about the simmering world agitation. He tries to awaken the people and Congress to the dangers arising in the rest of the world with little success. F.D.R. refuses "to recognize the Japanese puppet state . . . in northern China. He [believes] Japan should respect American rights in the Pacific and Far East. The President [demands] that Japan apologize and pay for the sinking of the American gunboat *Panay* in 1937. The Japanese [meet] his demands at once."[45] Then in " March 1938 the Nazi troops [occupy] Austria and [start] the usual massacres and imprisonments of Jews and anti-Fascists. In September 1938 Hitler [announces] that the `oppression' of Germans in Czechoslovakia [is] intolerable; war [appears] to be near."[46]

Meanwhile, the 75th U.S. Congress passes Public Law #732 on 25 June 1938. It is called the 'Naval Reserve Act.' What it does is to do away with "existing Reserve provisions and [establishes] a new Naval Reserve as a component part of the U.S. Navy."[47] Most importantly, a section of this Act authorizes the appointment of 'female registered nurses.'[48]

On 1 July the strength of the Navy Nurse Corps is 427. And on 1 October 1938, though her term has been less than three years, Superintendent Myn M. Hoffman is given a physical disability retirement. (In 1951 Miss Hoffman dies of a heart attack in her home at Bronxville, New York. She is buried in Arlington National Cemetery with full military honors; six Navy nurses act as honorary pall-bearers.) Assistant Superintendent Virginia A. Rau is appointed 'Acting Superintendent.'

Acting Superintendent Rau had attended Buffalo General Hospital in Buffalo, New York for her nurses' training where she graduated in 1906. She served with the American Red Cross in Europe during WWI[49] then joined the Navy Nurse Corps in March of 1917. She had received a special commendation for her services during the Long Beach, California earthquake in 1933.[50] Miss Rau had been promoted to Assistant Superintendent in 1935 and served on the Superintendent Hoffman's staff since that time. Her first duty station was Naval Hospital, Newport, Rhode Island. She went on to become a Chief Nurse and eventually to her promotion and job in the Nurse Corps section of the Department of Medicine and Surgery, in Washington, D.C..

On 8 November 1938 at Arlington National Cemetery, a ceremony is held for the unveiling of the Army and Navy Nurse Statue in the nurses' section of the cemetery. The monument had been sculpted by Francis Rich who is the daughter of the actress Irene Rich. Both the sculptress and her mother attend the ceremony. Miss J. Beatrice Bowman, Retired Navy Nurse Corps Superintendent makes the Introductory Remarks of the ceremony while the Retired Superintendent of the Army Nurse Corps, Major Julia C. Stimson, makes the Presentation Remarks. The Address speech is given by the Surgeon General of the Army and the Acceptance speech by the Surgeon General of the Navy. The unveiling of the statue is carried out by six Army nurses and six Navy nurses.[51] All twelve nurses wear white shoes, white hose, white ward uniforms. The Army nurses wear their Army capes (fastened at the neck) and cloche-type hats of the Army Nurse Corps and the Navy nurses wear the longer Navy capes (fastened at the neck) and cloche-type hats of the Navy Nurse Corps. The statue is dedicated to the memory of Army and Navy nurses who gave their lives in the service of their country. For those who have not seen the statue, it is a tall, imposing and most dignified symbol of a nurse looking over her shoulder and wearing a ward-type uniform with a cape. Also present at the ceremony are Navy Nurse Hazel V. Bennett and Navy Nurses 'under instruction' in the Dietetics Class at nearby George Washington University.[52] The Memorial has been made possible through contributions of Army and Navy Nurses.[53]

Miss Virginia Rau remains 'Acting Superintendent' until 30 January 1939. On that date Chief Nurse Sue S. Dauser is appointed Superintendent of the Navy Nurse Corps. Miss Rau remains on duty in BUMED until 1 October 1939 when she retires on a physical disability, having served 22 years in the Nurse Corps. (Miss Rau "lived in Bronxville, N.Y. after her retirement and had returned to the Washington area in 1965. She died in 1971."[54])

[1]   Information prepared by the Navy Nurse Corps Officers on the staff of the Director of the Navy Nurse Corps, 1991.

[2]   Information obtained from the file card of Miss Hoffman's assignments, Bureau of Medicine and Surgery, Washington, D.C..

[3]   Information prepared by the Navy Nurse Corps Officers on the staff of the Director of the Navy Nurse Corps, 1991.

[4]   Information obtained from the file card of Miss Hoffman's assignments, Bureau of Medicine and Surgery, Washington, D.C..

[5]   Information prepared by the Navy Nurse Corps Officers on the staff of the Director of the Navy Nurse Corps, 1991.

[6]   Laird, LCDR Thelma NC USNR, Jones, LCDR Dorothy NC USN, Feeney, LCDR Elizabeth NC USN, Seidl, CDR Elizabeth NC USN (Ret.), Blaska, CDR Burdette NC USN, *Chronological History NAVY NURSE CORPS*, Prepared by: Nursing Division, Bureau of Medicine and Surgery, 1 August 1962, pp. 20, 21.

[7]   Ibid., Comptroller General Decision (A-44927), p. 21.

[8]   Ibid., noted as BuMed File: OG/L16-7(350618).

[9]   Benner, Mary CDR NC USN (Ret.), *Oral History Interview Tape Transcript*, Interviewer Irene Smith Matthews Lt(jg)Navy Nurse Corps, taped in 1970.

[10]   *Christmas Menu*, Norfolk Naval Hospital, Portsmouth, Virginia, Christmas 1935. Courtesy of LCDR Hazel Bennett NC USN (Ret.).

[11]   Goodnow, Minnie R.N., *Nursing History*, W.B. Saunders Company, Philadelphia, London, 1948, p. 182.

[12]   Dock, Lavinia L. R.N., Stewart, Isabel M. A.M., R.N., *A Short History of Nursing*, G.P. Putnam's Sons, New York: London, 1938, p. 184.

[13]   Roberts, Mary M. R.N., *American Nursing History and Interpretation*, The MacMillan Company, New York, 1963, p. 279.

[14]   Wells, H.G., *The Outline of History*, Revised and brought up to date by Raymond Postgate, Garden City Books, Garden City, New York, Volume II, 1961, pp. 920, 923.

[15]   Ibid., p. 923.

[16]   Ibid., p. 978.

[17]   Ibid..

[18]   *The World Book Encyclopedia*, Field Enterprises Educational Corporation, Chicago, Volume 16, 1966 edition, p. 418.

[19]   Goble, CDR Dorothy Jones, NC USN (Ret.), as quoted in her unpublished history research notes.

[20]   Ibid., for this letter quote, the Goble notes cite N:ILS-(OG/P12-1).

[21]   Goble, op. cit..

[22]   Bernatitis, Ann Capt. NC USN (Ret.), *Oral History Interview Tape Transcript*, Interviewer Capt. Doris M. Sterner NC USN (Ret.), 7 May 1990.

23   Bernatitis, Ann Capt. NC USN (Ret.), *Oral History Interview Tape Transcript*, Interviewer Irene Matthews Lt(jg) Navy Nurse Corps, taped 19 May 1971.
24   Ibid..
25   Nash, Margaret CDR NC USN, *Oral History Interview Tape Transcript*, Interviewer CDR Florence Twyman NC USN (Ret.), taped 28 September 1990.
26   Ibid..
27   Ibid..
28   Barnes, Sylvia Lavache Navy Nurse, *Written Self Interview*, 31 May 1991.
29   Ibid..
30   *Nurses Quarters*, Listing of ten instructions signed by Chief Nurse Anne K. Harkins, U.S.N., this paper has hand written date of 1936-37.
31   Lindner, Mary J. CDR NC USN (Ret.), *Oral History Interview Tape Transcript*, Interviewer CDR Jean Davis NC USN (Ret.), taped 19 July 1989.
32   Ibid..
33   *Christmas Menu*, Naval Hospital, Washington, D.C., Christmas 1936. Courtesy of LCDR Hazel Bennett NC USN (Ret.).
34   Hill, Nell Williams CDR. NC USN (Ret.), *Oral History Interview Tape Transcript*, Interviewer LCDR Kathleen Donnelly NC USN (Ret.), taped 10 May 1990.
35   Bernatitis, Interviewer Irene Matthews, op. cit..
36   Barnes, op. cit..
37   Quebbeman, Frances, CDR Navy Nurse Corps, *Written Personal History*, 13 May 1991.
38   *The World Book Encyclopedia*, Field Enterprises Educational Corporation, Chicago, Volume 1, 1966 edition, p. 242.
39   Buttke, Norma LCDR NC USN (Ret.), *Oral History Interview Tape Transcript*, Interviewer LCDR Margaret (Linn) Larson NC USN (Ret.), taped 13 May 1988.
40   Wells, H.G., op. cit., p. 978.
41   Buttke, op. cit..
42   Ibid..
43   Goodnow, op. cit., p. 273.
44   Wells, H.G., op. cit..
45   *The World Book Encyclopedia*, op. cit..
46   Wells, H.G., op. cit., p. 924.
47   Laird, et al, op. cit., p. 21.
48   Ibid..
49   American Red Cross Memo dated 26 June 1989. Courtesy of Jan Herman, Editor of Navy Medicine and Historian, BUMED, Navy Department, Washington, D.C..
50   "Obituary, Virginia A. Rau, Navy Nurse Corps," *Washington Post* (newspaper), Washington, D.C., 7 April 1971.
51   Information obtained from an original Program for the ceremony, dated November 8, 1938, 3:00 P.M.. Courtesy of LCDR Hazel Bennett NC USN (Ret.).
52   Information courtesy of LCDR Hazel Bennett NC USN (Ret.).
53   Laird, et al, op. cit., p. 21.
54   *Washington Post* (newspaper), op. cit..

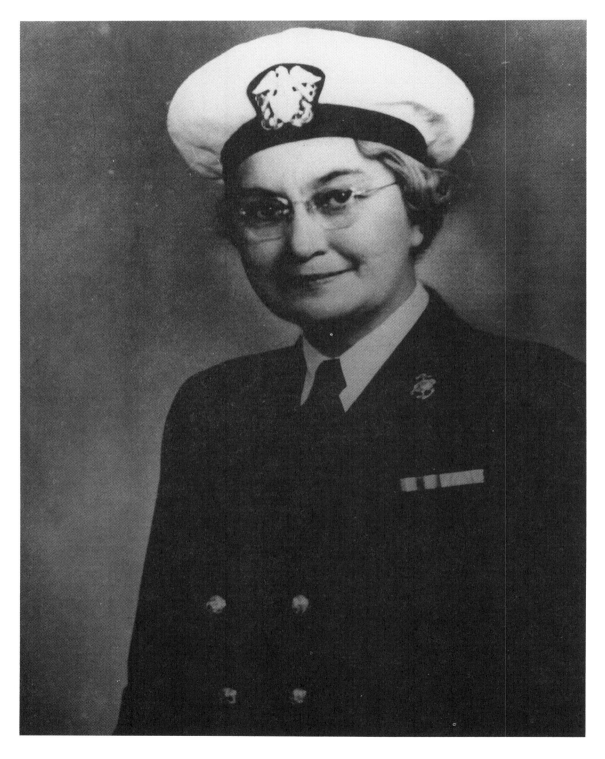

Superintendent - Captain Sue S. Dauser
(Official U.S. Navy photo courtesy of Nursing Division, Bureau of Medicine and Surgery, Navy Department.)

CHAPTER 5

Superintendent - Captain Sue S. Dauser
(1939 - 1943)

It is 30 January 1939. Chief Nurse Sue S. Dauser becomes the fifth Superintendent of the Navy Nurse Corps. She was born in Anaheim, California in 1888, went to Fullerton High School in California and on to Stanford University from 1907 to 1909. At that time she was interested in teaching mathematics, but she changed her mind and interest to nursing. So Miss Dauser attended the California School of Nursing in Los Angeles, graduating in 1914.[1] Then she became an Operating Room Supervisor, at the same hospital, for nearly three years. In the fall of 1917 she was appointed a nurse in the Naval Reserve. She reported to the Naval Hospital, San Diego for a month of instruction and orientation to the Navy then returned to her home by 21 November 1917. On 28 November the Surgeon General appointed her Chief Nurse of Naval Base Hospital #3. The Base Hospital was organized in Los Angeles and then mobilized on 17 December in Philadelphia, Pennsylvania.[2] She was discharged as a Reserve nurse on 10 July 1918 and appointed a Nurse, USN on 11 July and appointed a Chief Nurse the same date. So the only time Miss Dauser served as 'nurse' in the Navy was when she was under training; until the time she makes Superintendent she has served as 'Chief Nurse.' She served with Base Hospital #3 overseas during WWI (as mentioned previously) then spent two different tours at the San Diego Naval Hospital, two different tours at Mare Island, California, one tour at Bremerton, Washington, one tour at Guam, Marianas Islands and one tour at Canacao, Philippine Islands.[3] As for shipboard duty, she had one tour aboard the USS *Relief* when the hospital ship cruised with the Pacific Fleet to Australia and New Zealand, touching Samoa on returning to American waters. Also, there was duty on two transports for short periods of time: the USS *Argonne* (transport service from the west coast to the east through the Panama Canal) and the USS *Henderson* (with President Harding.) Just prior to becoming Superintendent, she had been Chief Nurse at the U.S. Naval Dispensary, Long Beach, California.[4] This lady has a tremendous background for Navy nursing administration; she is going to need all of it and more.

On 1 July 1939 there are 427 Navy Nurses on active service. The 7th of July sees Chief Nurse Elizabeth Marguerite O'Brien, USN assigned to the staff of Superintendent Dauser to administer the Nurse Corps' branch of the U.S. Naval Reserve.[5] Under the regulations of the 1938 Naval Reserve Act, a vigorous recruitment program begins in order to have a Reserve force of Navy Nurses readily available for active duty when needed.[6] By September 1939 the first appointments to the Nurse Corps U.S. Naval Reserve are made when nine nurses take the oath of office. December 26 and 434 Navy nurses are stationed at the Naval Medical facilities as follows:

Canacao, Philippine Islands	16 nurses
Guam	7 nurses
Cuba	3 nurses
Pearl Harbor	12 nurses
Samoa	4 nurses
USS *Relief*	12 nurses
Coco Solo, Panama Canal Zone	3 nurses
15 U.S. Naval Hospitals	332 nurses
U.S. Naval Dispensaries	45 nurses[7]

"[These] 434 nurses [are] the nucleus [that will] have to expand into a corps adequate in numbers and effective in operation to care for the Navy in"[8] the war soon to come.

The nursing profession, as a whole, takes another step forward in 1939 when the National League of Nursing Education begins the accrediting of schools of nursing. Fifty schools are accredited this year and serve as "a basis for further study of values."[9] Also, last year (1938) New York state passed "a law providing for the *licensing* of both professional and practical nurses. It thus made illegal the employment of any who [are] not so licensed. . . . [In 1939] the Joint Boards of Directors of the three national associations of nurses [go] on record as approving a recommendation for a national program to license all who nurse for hire."[10]

On the 1939 world scene, the Nazis occupy all of Czechoslovakia in March. In April, Italy invades and conquers Albania while Hitler cancels Germany's non-aggression pact with Poland. August; Germany and Russia sign a non-aggression pact. September; German troops invade Poland while Russia invades Poland from the east.[11] Great Britain and France declare war on Germany. In the U.S., Congress passes "the Neutrality Act of 1939. This law [makes] it possible for a nation fighting the Axis to buy war supplies from the United States. But [the nation has] to furnish its own ships to carry the weapons."[12] Meantime, Poland is defeated in three weeks. In November, Russia attacks Finland and bombs the capital city, Helsinki. The only world-wide optimistic event of this year is in Great Britain with their production of the wonderdrug 'penicillin.'[13]

1940 and there is no let up of the Nazi Germany 'blitzkrieg.' In March the Russians defeat Finland. In April the Prime Minister of England makes apathetic statements about the war and Hitler answers by invading and defeating Denmark and Norway. In May, Winston Churchill becomes the Prime Minister of England. The same day that Churchill takes office, Germany invades Belgium and Holland. Allied troops trying to come to the aid of Belgium and Holland, flounder in the masses of refugees and the overwhelming onslaught of the Germans. The Allies retreat along the coast to Dunkirk, France. The Germans march over France to surround the troops at Dunkirk.[14] The Allied troops are "extracted from Dunkirk between May 28th and June 2nd by a suddenly assembled fleet of about 666 private boats and 222 naval vessels."[15] This fleet comes from England where an enormous outpouring of civilian 'sailors' volunteer themselves and their boats in this dangerous and heroic endeavor: rescuing the troops from the beaches at Dunkirk. On June 10th Italy declares war on Britain and France. On the 22nd France gives up the struggle with Germany and surrenders. The Soviet Union annexes Estonia, Latvia and Lithuania. In August the Italians invade British Somaliland. Also in August, the German Luftwaffe (Air Force) sends wave after wave of bombers and fighter planes over Great Britain in the attempt to destroy the much smaller British Air Force and to pound the British to their knees. Despite the huge forces against them, the Royal Air Force drives the Luftwaffe from the daytime skies of Britain by September. As the "Prime Minister, Winston Churchill, whose speeches [are] in themselves part of the [defenses] of Britain, [says] of the pilots, 'never, in the field of human conflict, [is] so much owed by so many, to so few.'"[16] The Germans then change their technique to nightly bombing raids in October and through the long winter.[17] This is the Battle of Britain. Meantime, in September, Japan occupies French Indonesia and in late October, Italian troops enter Greece. In November, Hungary and Romania join with the Axis.[18]

In the United States of 1940, the country gets ready for another presidential election. The Republicans nominate Wendell Willkie, a corporate president, against the Democratic nominee, President Franklin Roosevelt. In his campaign speeches F.D.R. promises to try to keep the U.S. out of the war (but at the same time, a few steps are being taken in case the U.S. is forced into it: i.e. the first peacetime draft in American History.[19]) President Roosevelt wins the election for his third term in the White House by carrying "38 of the 48 states, and [winning] 449 electoral votes to 82 for Willkie."[20] On a lighter note, the U.S. produces its first 'Jeep' this year and nylon stockings come out in 1940; 72,000 nylons are sold in the first eight hours.

Meanwhile, the American Nurses Association at long last organizes a Men's Nurses' Section. And, most of the leading organizations of professional nursing join together this year, to form the National Nursing Council on Defense (later on to become the National Nursing Council for War Service.) This 1940 Council formulates plans "to (a) promote a national inventory of registered nurses, (b) expand facilities of existing accredited schools of nursing and (c) supply supplementary nursing services to hospitals and public health agencies."[21] (When the

U.S. does finally enter the war, this Council acts as consultant to the wartime Federal Agency 'Procurement and Assignment Service for Physicians, Dentists, Veterinarians, Sanitary Engineers, and Nurses' which will be responsible "for equable distribution of professional personnel in accordance with military and civilian needs."[22])

On 31 July 1940 there are 458 Navy nurses on active duty and all of them regular Navy. There are no Reserve Navy nurses on active duty but there are 550 'inactive' Reserve Navy nurses. By the end of November, however, the Nurse Corps has the first 7 Active Duty Reserve nurses on duty. At the end of the year there are 14 active duty Reserves and a total active duty force of 504 with 923 Inactive Navy Reserve nurses on the roster.[23] This Inactive Reserve roster is made up of nurses who have filled in all application forms for the Nurse Corps, who have taken their physical examination, who have taken an oath of acceptance and received their official appointment to the Navy Nurse Corps Inactive Reserve; they are the Navy Nurses immediately available for mobilization if needed. The Red Cross Nursing Service is still actively involved in this process; the recruiting of nurses. To explain: all nurses, upon graduating from nurses' training, are urged to register with the Red Cross. When nurses register with the Red Cross, they are asked their preference for military service. "As soon as the Navy receives a nurse's card from the Red Cross, the routine application and information forms are forwarded to her. . . . If a nurse cannot comply with Navy regulations for appointment in the Naval Reserve Nurse Corps, the Navy would like a statement of her intentions so that in this progressive state of organization, it can know definitely the number of appointments it can depend on."[24]

One of the Regular Navy Nurses, Ann Bernatitis, is stationed at Annapolis, Maryland in 1940 when she receives orders to the Philippines. She reports to Norfolk, Virginia where she boards a Navy transport ship. This ship is assigned the task of carrying U.S. Marines from Charleston to Honolulu and then returning to the States before heading out to the Philippines. Ann and another Navy Nurse are temporarily assigned to this ship for the trip to Honolulu and back. Ann says, "I went to Norfolk to get aboard this ship and I was joined by Mary Chapman who was the other nurse assigned for this trip and we went to Charleston. The Marines came from Parris Island; it was a whole detachment of marines embarking. . . . [In traveling through the Canal] it was interesting to see how, you know, the ship was way down low and then they close off the locks . . . and then the ship would gradually rise to another level and then the same thing would happen there. Then the ship would rise some more. They'd close the locks, the water would enter it, the ship would be elevated up to the next level and over you'd go. . . . From Panama we went to San Diego and again picked up some more Marines, then on to Honolulu. These Marines were headed for Wake Island. They were disembarked at Pearl Harbor. . . . We stayed on in Honolulu for about a week, as I recall, and of course . . . [in Honolulu] there was much sightseeing to be done."[25] The reason the transport returns to the States is to participate in landing exercises being held by Marines at San Clemente Island off the California coast. After the exercises, the ship prepares for the trip to the Philippines. As Ann tells us, "[It] was at this time that the third nurse joined us. That was Martha Smith from the hospital at Mare Island. . . . So we set sail for the Philippines. . . . We had dependents this time and . . . the nurses were assigned the duty of taking care of the dependents' children during the meal hours while the parents went out for their meals. . . . We were really in a passenger status with the extra duty of babysitting. That's what it amounted to really. . . . [But] being that the Captain [of the ship] is boss and he says 'you will be babysitters,' we were babysitters. . . . We got to Guam. We stopped over for the day and again went ashore. . . . [We had a small Navy hospital and] I imagine about maybe six nurses on duty. And the nurses that were assigned to Guam, as a rule, spent one year in Guam and then came to the Philippines for the other year. Now if you went [directly] to the Philippines, you spent your two years in the Philippines"[26] They finally arrive in Manila where they are met by some of the Navy Nurses from the Naval Hospital. They have lunch at the elegant Army/Navy Club that overlooks picturesque Manila Bay. Then they proceed to the other side of the Bay and the Canacao Naval Hospital. Ann relates that the hospital is of "about 250 to 300 beds. We had a main building . . . then they had a small dependents' unit. They had sick officers' quarters which was a separate building. Then they had the contagious unit, again a separate building."[27] According to Ann, "duty was very, very pleasant out there. [There were 12 Navy nurses there.] We worked roughly, I guess, from maybe eight o'clock until noon. Went over for lunch to the nurses quarters, only one nurse returned to stay on duty until the afternoon nurse came on. So she would come back from one until three o'clock or three thirty when another nurse would relieve her and then, of course, another nurse, the night nurse would have to relieve her."[28] "We had lovely quarters . . . and it was interesting, and we weren't accustomed to this, in that for something like five pesos (which would amount to about $2.50) a month, you had two women who came in and did your personal laundry. . . . There was really no need to take a lot of clothes out there because most of [the] people out there, say the Filipinos or the Chinese . . . all you have to do is show them a pattern and they'll make anything for you. So most of the girls had their clothes made."[29]

Miss Bernatitis says, "In November of 1940, I think people were beginning to suspect that war was going to come and the Chief Nurse suggested that we pack and send home some of our things that we had bought. I packed my trunk to send home. . . . I packed my belongings to send home with Mary Chapman [who] had put in her resignation because she was to be married and she was sending her things home. So I packed my belongings and sent them along with hers. And everybody else's belongings that they wanted to send home were sent home. So we definitely knew that something was in the air. . . . And well, all the wives had been sent home, so you knew they weren't doing that for no good reason. . . . Just the feeling in the air, really."[30]

In 1940 the Navy has only one hospital ship, the USS *Relief* and she is assigned to accompany the U.S. Navy's Pacific fleet on its maneuvers and exercises in the Pacific. Along with the rest of the crew and medical personnel are 12 Navy nurses. However, a passenger ship (the *Iroquois*) is currently being refitted as another hospital ship (the USS *Solace*) in light of the world tensions.

As for 1940 legislation pertaining to the Nurse Corps, on 17 October Congress authorizes "retirement benefits for certain nurses who had served in WWI and were discharged before 20 June 1930 with physical disability."[31] This is welcome news to the several nurses that fall into this category and for nurses contemplating the Navy in a world looking at war: it reassures them that they will be taken care of in case of service connected injury.

1941. The "British beat off German air attacks. . . . Germany conquers Yugoslavia and Greece."[32] The turmoil being created by Germany's Hitler increases. "At four o'clock in the morning of June 22nd . . . the German armies [charge] into the territory of the Soviet Union."[33] (So much for the 1939 German non-aggression pact with the Russians.) "The German army [stomps] forward . . . the Russians [burn] or [blow] up all they [can] as they [go], to leave nothing for the conqueror. Savage brutality [marks] the German advance."[34] By October the Germans are within 20 miles of Moscow[35] when the onset of the bitter Russian winter suddenly slows them down.

Leaving the war for now; back in the U.S., the Secretary of the Navy approves the 'Uniform Regulations, U.S. Navy,' on 31 May 1941. This is "the first publication to include the dress of the Navy Nurse Corps. From the creation of the Nurse Corps in 1908 until 1941, the uniforms to be worn by nurses had been prescribed by the Chief of the Bureau of Medicine and Surgery, subject to the approval of the Secretary of the Navy. These instructions were directed solely to the Nurse Corps, and were distinct from any regulation which covered the dress of men of the Navy. . . . Chapter XVII of the 1941 uniform instructions [specifies] the uniform for nurses and [includes] only the ward uniform and outer protective clothing. No provision [is] made for an outdoor uniform. The order [states] that the prescribed uniforms [are] to be worn at all times when on duty. Civilian clothes [are] to be worn when off duty or on leave. For wear out of doors, a hat similar to that of 1929, a blue sweater, a cape and a blue rain coat [are] provided."[36] On the 18th of June 1941, the "Bureau of Navigation [approves] the wearing of an outdoor uniform by Navy Nurse Corps members `in distant ports and in foreign countries under severe climatic conditions; but not otherwise unless approved by the Chief of the Bureau of Navigation.' No money allowance or provision for gratuitous issue [is] authorized for [said] outdoor uniform."[37]

In the meantime, the strength of the Navy Nurse Corps has been on the rise. On 31 May there are 643 nurses on active duty: 522 are regular and 121 are Reserve with 1010 nurses in the Inactive Reserve. On 31 July there are 694 on active duty with 1037 in the Inactive Reserve. On 30 November 1941 there are 621 regular Navy nurses on active duty with 166 Reserves on active duty for a total of 787 and 966 nurses are in the Inactive

Reserve.[38] It is through the efforts of the Red Cross that most of the Reserve and inactive Reserve Navy Nurses are obtained. (The Red Cross tries to reach every graduating nurse in the country, to request that they register with the Red Cross and to indicate on their registration which branch of the service they would be interested in, if needed in time of emergency.) In 1939 the Secretary of the Navy "had requested the aid of Red Cross in obtaining a sufficient number of nurses to meet the Navy mobilization requirements quickly. . . . The Chairman of Red Cross promised `whole-hearted cooperation.' . . . Conferences are held [with the Superintendent of the Nurse Corps and her staff] . . . [and] the following arrangements [are] made:

1. We [the Red Cross] will send to the Navy the names of all nurses who have indicated the Navy as their preference, and to send all cards in duplicate.

2. We will send a note to every nurse whose name is given to the Navy, telling them that they will hear from the Navy. [2,000 at first, then individually as new enrollments are sent over.]

3. The Navy will get in touch with the nurse -
    a. asking her if she is willing to serve, and telling her it will be required that the nurses take an oath to serve, and the understanding is that they would be ready in 24 hours.
    b. requiring them to report for a physical examination."[39]

But, the Navy also sends applications to nurses who write directly to the Navy Department or to the Superintendent of the Navy Nurse Corps asking how to join. Additionally, applications are given to nurses who ask for them at the local recruiting offices. This causes some dissention with the Red Cross. The Red Cross wants the Navy to have the Red Cross Nursing Service as the only way for the nurse to come into the Navy Reserve (which is the way the Red Cross has it set up with the Army Nurse Corps.) The Navy Nurse Corps does not wish to make such a commitment. The Red Cross continues to have "cordial relations with the Navy Nurse Corps, however, and an arrangement for procurement of nurses that [according to the author of `The History of The American National Red Cross'] was only slightly less satisfactory than that with the Army."[40]

June 1941 and the first five nurses report to their new duty station in Kodiak, Alaska. The Chief Nurse is Ruth Abrams, USN. 15 August 1941 and nurses report aboard the hospital ship, USS *Solace* with Chief Nurse Grace B. Lally, USN. Then on 25 November Navy Nurses report aboard Bourne Field, St. Thomas, Virgin Islands along with Chief Nurse Jane Mary Lynch, USN.[41]

December 7, 1941 and in the far east Japan makes "a strange miscalculation. At a time when at least half the United States [is] strongly isolationist, the Japanese [do] the one thing that [can unite] the American people and [motivate] the whole nation for war."[42] The Japanese bomb Pearl Harbor and declare war on the United States. "Japan seems never to have considered that the effect of an attack on Pearl Harbor might be not to crush morale, but to unite the nation for combat. This curious vacuum of understanding [comes] from what might be called cultural ignorance, a frequent component of folly. . . . Japan [gives] her opponent the one blow necessary to bring [the U.S.] to purposeful and determined belligerency."[43]

"[Early] December 7 [my roommate and I were in the nurses' quarters at Pearl Harbor Naval Hospital and] were getting ready to go on a double date picnic and then around [Oahu] island. Navy planes from Ford Island Naval Station often flew overhead, but this morning I told [my roommate], `The boys are sure getting low this morning, aren't they?' A few minutes later, loud explosions started and we were told, `This is no drill. This is no drill. Get to the Hospital.' I was sent to Ward A where patients were being received. . . . I was especially trying to save two badly shot up men. The Chaplain came by and said, `Keep track of their names and next of kin so that you can later write to their families.' . . . Later that December 7th, I and another nurse, Ann Tucker Newton, went to a 40 bed outlying ward and began receiving complete-body-burn patients. Burns constituted a great majority of the Navy's casualties [because] the [water] channel [near the Hospital] had been coated with oil when the *Arizona* was bombed [and] the entire channel caught fire. Thus, Navy men who were trying to leap from their ships to safety, were badly burned. I recall looking up and seeing a graying man standing in the doorway and thinking, `Why is he gray?' It turned out he was nude and burnt gray and still [he walked] into the Hospital."[44]

"December 7, 1941, I was on duty that day, before 0800, and was trying to collect the morning reports from the outlying buildings when I saw the planes coming over with the painted red [circles on them]. I could even see the faces of the Japanese in these low flying bombers [as they] headed for [Ford] Island and the anchored ships [of the Navy's Pacific Fleet]. But coming back they were strafing the hospital laboratory [where staff members were] hit and most of them were killed. Later, when we were already taking in casualties, the high flying bombers came over and from the dressing room where we were busy with the injured, you could hear the bombs being dropped and hurling down to their targets."[45]

Ruth Erickson (destined to become a Director of the Navy Nurse Corps) speaks of the 7th of December at Pearl Harbor, "It was my Sunday off. We didn't have a five day week. I had been on duty until 10 o'clock Saturday night, so Sunday was my day off. We had vacated our permanent [nurses'] quarters. There was a dry dock being built in there, so we [all the nurses from the quarters] had moved over to our temporary quarters which was a one-story structure shaped like an E.... I was preparing to go out the next day; I was going to the beach the next day for a full day. But, I went to have breakfast in the dining room about 7:30 that morning; sitting there and chatting with some of the other girls [Navy Nurses] who were off duty and then here's this drastic, terrible noise overhead. We said, `Ford Island is really busy today, they must have all [their] airplanes up in the air.' Then all of a sudden we started talking and I had an eerie feeling as I dashed out the door [since] the telephone was ringing at the far end and [it was] the Chief Nurse.... She said, `Girls, get into your uniforms, this is the real thing!' ... [We] go look out the window and see those planes flying so low. You could just see the rising sun on their wings, they were that low.... I hurried up and got dressed... We were right across the street from the hospital so I dashed in there and as soon as I got on the lanai, I felt kind of safe, but yet you weren't. So I dashed out the orthopedic section to the orthopedic dressing room and it was locked. I said to the corpsman `get to the OD's office as quickly as you can.' I thought he would **never** return. But it was just a split second and he was back there again.... So the first casualty came into the orthopedic dressing room at 8:25 and it was a wound in the abdomen. Well, I can still see the Chief of Medicine, who was on his way to go play golf that morning, but was making rounds before he left, and he came by our place.... [He] started intravenouses and transfusions and his hand was shaking as he inserted the needle in the vein. And then, of course, [getting] the patients out of bed; those that were convalescing in the orthopedic ward. If you could breathe, get up, because we needed the beds. The burn cases were just streaming in from the [ship] *Nevada*, because the *Nevada* was beached just opposite the hospital.... Here were patients with charred legs and arms, walking to the hospital three blocks away. So we would get them as pain-free as possible and quickly and then we had big fly sprays filled with tannic acid that we sprayed the burn areas with. This was almost a continuous thing until around four o'clock that afternoon [when] Miss Arnest [the Chief Nurse] came along and said, `We don't know how long this is going to be, so let's get some people off here, [as] the situation allows, because we're going to have to go on night duty real early. So I went off at four o'clock and then at eight o'clock I went back."[46]

On Sunday morning, 7 December, the USS *Solace* is sitting at anchor in Pearl Harbor near the *Arizona* and the *Nevada*. Shortly before 8 a.m., the Chief Nurse, Grace Lally, is on deck waiting for Mass.[47] "She [leans] on the rail.... A group of sailors [are] fishing from a small boat nearby.... [Suddenly, seemingly out of nowhere, comes] plane after plane, wings decorated with the sign of the rising sun, Japan's emblem. Bullets [trace] their way across the water.... [Miss Lally sees] men fall before the guns, she [sees] the bombs fall and the big ships - some of the world's great fighting ships - explode, burst into flames and capsize as desperate men [swarm] over the sides to plunge into the oil-covered waters of the harbor.... Miss Lally [has] to convince herself that it [is] happening. Adding to the air of unreality ... [is] the fact that the hospital ship [does] not fall under attack"[48] even though nearby ships are all but destroyed. "Miss Lally quickly [organizes] the 12 other nurses on the *Solace*. Wounded sailors [are] being brought aboard even before the bombs [stop] falling. Anchored next to the badly bombed battleship USS *Arizona*, the *Solace* [remains] constantly in danger throughout the attack. The hospital ship [is] moved, however, before the old battlewagon [explodes]. The nursing staff of the *Solace* [treats] 327 burn cases from that first day of the war, working three full days without sleep. `We could hear the fighting raging outside and wondered what was happening,' [says] Miss Lally. `But our job was inside the ship, and there we stayed for 10 days.'"[49]

("The smoothly-working medical organization placed at Pearl Harbor to serve the Fleet went into this unexpected action so efficiently that Admiral Nimitz gave a field citation to each of these three medical units:

The U.S. Naval Hospital, Pearl Harbor, T.H.

Mobile Hospital No. 2, Pearl Harbor, T.H.

The hospital ship *Solace*.

The citation, issued to the [hospital ship] under date of 29 October 1942, which became a part of the official record of every officer and man on board on 7 December 1941, reads as follows:

Citation

For meritorious achievement and distinguished service during and subsequent to the Japanese air attack on the United States Fleet at Pearl Harbor, Territory of Hawaii, on 7 December 1941. At the time of the attack and afterwards, this unit displayed conspicuous devotion in line of duty. Its ability to cope with this disaster was responsible for the successful care of all casualties and the saving of many lives. The professional skill displayed and distinguished service rendered by this hospital ship were in keeping with the highest traditions of the naval service."[50])

The *Solace* had been newly commissioned as a hospital ship in August of 1941; formerly, she had been a luxury liner named *Iroquois*. "Sending a four hundred and thirty-two-bed hospital to sea was no easy task. The big ship, . . . had six hospital wards, each with its own pantry; two main operating rooms, three auxiliary operating rooms, three main medical storerooms, an X-ray department, an eye, ear, nose and throat operating room, a urological operating room, a physiotherapeutic department, a pharmacy, and a clinical laboratory. . . . The [staff of twelve] young nurses were proud to serve under the woman [Chief Nurse Grace Lally] who, with twenty years of service, held the Navy Nurse Corps' record for sea duty, and who was one of only four women in the corps entitled to wear the China ribbon. This distinction commemorated [Miss] Lally's baptism of fire at the time of the Japanese invasion of China in 1938, when she had helped to evacuate American women and children."[51]

Back on shore at the Pearl Harbor Naval Hospital after the initial attack period, Navy Nurse Phyllis Dana tells us, "We worked eight hours on and four hours off around the clock everyday for many weeks. The blackout meant that all windows were covered with oilcloth and soon the stench of dying men and of complete body burns etched itself into our minds and hearts. [Another Navy nurse] and I and four Corpsmen made continuous rounds keeping over-bed cradles with the lights in them, to try and warm the [patients]. Limbs and torsos were wrapped in gauze and then mineral oil and sulfa powder saturated these dressings. . . . [Intravenouses] were attempted, but very difficult [to do] in burnt limbs. It was bad, bad, bad. Many died. But a wonderful redeeming point was the help received from other servicemen who came over to our ward to help feed the patients. I recall one man in an airplane splint with arms extended at right angles to his body, but he could hold a spoon in that [one] hand at the end of the splint. And he would come over and help feed his buddy who was badly burned."[52]

Also, at the Hospital, Navy Nurse Ruth Erickson says that on "the morning of the 17th of December, the Chief Nurse [Miss Arnest] came around and said, `I want you to go off duty, pack a bag and you're going to be leaving.' I said, `Where am I going?' She said, `I don't know, but you're going back with some patients.' So I carried out the orders. I went to the quarters and then found out that there were two others beside myself [to go] . . . . [We were driven] down to a pier in Honolulu and there we met up with the SS *President Coolidge*. [The ship had] zig-zagged its way in from the south Pacific filled with missionaries and many civilian passengers." Miss Erickson goes on to tell us that they were assigned to care for the patients to go back to the States aboard the ship. Another ship, the Army Transport *Scott*, is also filled with patients and is to accompany the *President Coolidge*. The Army Transport is staffed with volunteers from the Queens Hospital in Honolulu along with eight volunteer nurses. They return to the States with several destroyers as escorts, reaching San Francisco on Christmas Day. They go with their patients to the Naval Hospital at Mare Island, California. She tells us that they make sure their patients are `squared away' and by then they, all the nurses, are starved and longing for some Christmas dinner. Miss Erickson had been at Mare Island before, for a short time, so she knows where the galley is located. "We went in there and scrounged around and found some cold turkey and things like that." They have their Christmas Dinner. Then on December 27th they are sent aboard the Navy ship *Henderson*. She states that this ship is going to Hawaii with about 10,000 troops aboard. Navy Nurse Erickson says, "We could hardly wait to get back. We had a bond that was so strong between those of us who had gone through this thing out there."[53]

As far as hospital ships are concerned, the only other one besides the *Solace* is the Navy's USS *Relief*. "In 1941 *Relief* [is] reassigned to the Atlantic Fleet, serving as a base hospital in the waters from Charleston, SC, to Argentia, Newfoundland. When the Japanese [attack] Pearl Harbor, *Relief* immediately [sails] from Argentia to Casco Bay, ME, to provide for the needs of the victims of the war in the Atlantic."[54]

Overseas, there are twelve Navy Nurses at the U.S. Naval Hospital, Canacao, Philippine Islands, when the attack on Pearl Harbor occurs. They are:

1. Laura M. Cobb, Chief Nurse at Canacao, graduated from nurses' training at Wesley Hospital, Wichita, Kansas in 1917. She was appointed a Navy Nurse in the U.S. Naval Reserve in 1918 with orders to the U.S. Naval Hospital, Fort Lyon, Colorado. In 1919 she reported for duty at the U.S. Naval Hospital, Canacao, Philippine Islands until January 1921. She was honorably discharged in July 1921. Miss Cobb applied for and received reappointment to the Navy Nurse Corps in 1924. She was promoted to Chief Nurse in September 1938. In 1940 she received orders to the U.S. Naval Hospital, Guam, Marianas Islands. In January of 1941 she received a Letter of Commendation from the Medical Officer in Command.[55] The letter reads as follows:

"To: Chief of the Bureau of Medicine and Surgery
Subject: Commendation, case of Laura M. Cobb, Chief Nurse, U.S. Navy

1. I wish to commend Miss Laura M. Cobb, Chief Nurse, U.S. Navy, Guam, for the excellent manner in which she   performed her duties during the typhoon of November 3, 1940. Miss Cobb was on continuous duty for forty-eight (48) hours, and during this time she repeatedly risked life and limb in her efforts to insure the safety and comfort of the patients and to prevent undue risks to be taken by the nurses of this Command.

2. A copy of this letter will be attached to the next Fitness Report submitted in the case of Miss Cobb."[56]

From Guam, Miss Cobb is ordered, once again, to the U.S. Naval Hospital, Canacao, Philippine Islands in February 1941.

2. Ann A. Bernatitus. (Background provided in Chapter 4.)

3. Mary F. Chapman (Hays) was appointed a Navy Nurse on July 3, 1936. Her first duty station was the Naval Hospital, Portsmouth, Virginia. From there she went to Philadelphia then she had two TAD (Temporary Additional Duty) assignments aboard the *Chaumont* before reporting to Mare Island in June of 1940. She was there for a little over a month when she received orders to the Naval Hospital, Canacao, Philippine Islands in July of 1940.[57]

4. Bertha R. Evans (St. Pierre) had her nurses' training at the Good Samaritan Hospital, Portland, Oregon and graduated in 1928. She joined the Navy in 1931. (She is mentioned in Chapter 3.)

5. Helen C. Gorzelanski (Hunter) took her oath as Navy Nurse on 31 May 1935. She then reported to the Naval Hospital in Philadelphia. In 1937 she was transferred to Annapolis followed by orders to San Diego in March of 1940. She left there in April of 1941 with orders to Canacao where she reported aboard on 13 May 1941.[58]

6. Mary Harrington (Nelson) graduated in 1934 from nurses' training at St. Joseph's Hospital, Sioux City, Iowa. She joined the Navy Nurse Corps in 1937. Her first duty station was the Naval Hospital, San Diego, California for two and a-half years, then she received orders to Mare Island, California. In January of 1941 she left the States for duty at Canacao, Philippine Islands.[59]

7. Margaret A. Nash. (Background provided in Chapter 4.)

8. Goldia O'Haver (Merrill) had been a Navy Nurse for eleven years and was stationed at the Naval Hospital at Guam when she received her orders to Canacao in 1940. She had entered the Navy in mid December 1929. Her duty stations were Naval Hospitals at Great Lakes, Illinois, Portsmouth, Virginia, Washington, D.C., USS *Relief*, Puget Sound, Washington, and then Guam. She reported aboard at Canacao on 5 November 1940.[60]

9. Eldene E. Paige graduated from the Orange County Hospital School of Nursing, Orange, California, in 1936. She went into the Navy Nurse Corps on 1 August 1938.[61] She received orders to the Naval Hospital at Canacao and is stationed there as WWII begins.

10. Susie Pitcher received her nurses' training at Roseland Community Hospital School of Nursing, Chicago, Illinois, graduating in 1927. In September of 1929 she entered the Navy Nurse Corps. In 1939 she took a post-graduate course in anesthesia at the Jewish Hospital, Philadelphia, Pennsylvania. She received orders to the Naval Hospital, Canacao, Philippine Islands in 1941 and arrived there for duty on 16 September 1941.[62]

11. Dorothy Still (Danner) attended the Los Angeles General County School of Nursing, Los Angeles, California and graduated in 1935. In December 1939 she becomes a member of the Navy Nurse Corps.[63] She too, is aboard the Naval Hospital at Canacao as the war begins.

12. C. Edwina Todd was appointed a Navy Nurse on 20 July 1936. Her first duty station was at Mare Island, California followed by Puget Sound, Washington in 1938. She left Puget Sound on 19 February 1940 and reported in to the Naval Hospital, Canacao, Philippines on 24 April 1940.[64]

Being located well to the west of the International Date Line, it is one day later in the Philippines than it is at Pearl Harbor. Navy Nurse Ann Bernatitis says that "we heard the news about six o'clock in the morning [Monday morning]. . . . [Bertha Evans] popped into my room yelling at me, 'Ann, Pearl Harbor's been bombed! Pearl Harbor's been bombed!' Well gosh, I guess I got out of that bed in a flying leap. . . . All heck broke loose in the nurses' quarters. Everybody got up. But, you know, just before that Monday, on Sunday afternoon, Mary Chapman and I had gone to Manila to see a movie. The title of the picture we went to see was 'Hold Back The Dawn.'"[65] Many people would have willed that dawn to be held back.

Navy Nurse Mary R. Harrington tells us that she was on night duty at the Canacao hospital "and we knew that things [meaning the possibility of enemy actions] were getting tight because we had been blacked out for some long while. The main hospital building was set back from Manila Bay a little bit, and the officers' houses were all along the water front. After the families left, people who had been living out (off the compound) moved in together. Three or four doctors occupied a house . . . and the sick officers' quarters was also in that row of cottages. I had just made rounds down there; it was a beautiful moonlight night. I thought, well, I'm not going into the administration building and walk through, I'll just walk outside and go on into the building then. . . . [The] Commanding Officer and the Exec [Executive Officer] had the next house, and I heard voices in there. [I wondered] what in the world were they doing up at that hour of the night; it was 12:30 or so. . . . I looked down the street and I saw an overhead light on . . . [in] the war plans officers' room. They lived right across from the nurses' quarters. I wondered what in the world was going on, but, made my rounds anyway. We had two stories of general wards and I was just talking with the corpsman downstairs when the Assistant Master-at-Arms came in and he said, `We just got word that Honolulu has been bombed!'"[66]

According to Navy Nurse Edwina Todd, "At 0730 [December 8th, Philippine time] we gathered to hear the news officially [re Pearl Harbor] and were issued helmets, gas masks and a pamphlet dealing with the detection of various poisonous gasses and the treatment of gassed patients. A decontamination chamber was set up in the General Ward. By evening we were in dungarees, our uniform for many weeks."[67] "On Tuesday [December 9th, Philippine time] was our first bombing and that was at Clark Air Base [Army]. I remember that they [the Japanese planes] came over in squadrons, in fact we could look up and see them and hear the bombs drop. Although at that time, we didn't know where they were dropping, but we knew it was close by to us."[68]

Chief Nurse Laura Cobb keeps some written notes during this time and her entry for December 9th reads, "12:30 PM   Transfer of all patients (255) from Canacao Naval Hospital. Some to duty - ships and stations, remainder to Sternberg Army Hospital [in Manila] and Civilian Hospitals. Detached for temporary duty at Sternberg: Lt.(jg) E.F. Ritter (MC) [Medical Corps]; Ann Bernatitus, nurse; Mary Chapman, nurse; 20 Corpsmen."[69] The doctor, two nurses and corpsmen are given TAD (temporary additional duty) in order to care for those Navy patients being sent to the Army Hospital. Ann Bernatitus says, "it was that day that the Commanding Officer [of the Canacao Naval Hospital] received word to evacuate the hospital and those patients who were ambulatory and could return to duty were discharged from the Hospital. The Filipino patients that we had were sent home. The ones [patients] that couldn't be discharged were to be evacuated to the Army Hospital in Manila: the Sternburg. The Commanding Officer said that two [Navy] nurses had to accompany those patients being evacuated to Manila and [Chief Nurse Laura Cobb] asked for volunteers. Mary Chapman volunteered, but nobody else. Finally, [Miss Cobb] had us congregate in the living room and she asked for volunteers again. Nobody responded. It was getting a little tense that nobody wanted to go. Of course, you couldn't blame them, you know. They would go to Manila; they didn't know anybody over there; some place they'd never been before. They wanted to stay with their own unit. So anyway, I remember that we were in a semi-circle; Goldie O'Haver was the first person, I was the second and then I don't recall how the others were arranged, but I spoke up and I said, `Miss Cobb, why don't you make us draw straws?' I said, 'You know, if anything in the future comes up, no one will ever be able to say [that] this wouldn't have happened if you hadn't made me do that.' And she thought that was a good idea so she went out and she got applicator sticks. She came back holding them in her two hands: one hand above the other. She went to Goldie and Goldie pulled and she got a long straw. Well, she knew she was safe. She came to me and what happened? I drew the short straw! The second volunteer. So off Mary and I go to the Army Hospital where [our] patients had been evacuated; they took us over by car. We arrived at their [the Army's] nurses' quarters just about three or four o'clock. I always remember that the Army nurses were all gathered in the living room for their daily tea that they had when they got off duty. I said I guess it still hadn't really sunk in yet that war was declared. . . . I took night duty right then and there for our Navy patients and Mary went on day duty. Well, during the day I slept. Of course, if the bombers came over, I was up and out in the grounds where all the fox holes were dug. Then I'd go back to bed."[70]

December 10, 1941 (Philippine time) and Chief Nurse Laura Cobb at Canacao records, "12:35 PM - Air raid Alarm. Cavite [close-by town] bombed also Sangley Point Area and surrounding military objectives. 1330 [1:30 PM] - Casualties from bombed area began arriving at hospital. During next two hours between 400-500 [patients] were received consisting of both service [personnel] and civilians. Staff personnel were distributed in various wards and in addition 3 operating teams worked continuously in O.R. until time of evacuation of casualties to Sternberg [General Hospital] that night. There were [approximately] 35 deaths among those received at [the hospital], 10 of whom were naval personnel, the others being Filipinos, most of them [Cavite] Navy Yard employees."[71] Navy Nurse Margaret Nash tells us, "that was a day I'll never forget; never! And I think all the girls felt the same way. Patients were coming in helping other patients. Some were dead. They were on the roofs of the cars, on running boards. Maybe they'd be about 10 in one car, just sitting wherever there was space available. And they would help each other. The ones that were not too injured would help the seriously injured to get them into the wards. They continued to come until late that night, I remember. The ward that Bertha [Evans] and I were assigned to, ordinarily it had 78 beds but we must have had about 400 patients in that ward. . . . It seemed endless. You had to be careful when you were stepping around because there [might] be some that were even on the floor. . . . The only doctor that was available said the first thing we must do is try to help the ones that were suffering; that were just screaming with pain. . . . [We] had to have a routine and also to give tetanus [shots] to all the patients: tetanus toxoid. One did not have time to ask when [the patient] had [his] last injection. . . . So one [nurse] would fill up a 20 cc syringe with tetanus toxoid and the other [nurse] would follow her with the morphine and we went from patient to patient. Some beds you'd find a dead body, but you didn't have time to do anything, you just moved on to the next bed. . . . It went on until far into the night when our Captain [CO] evidently had a message from the Japanese commandant and evidently he told us that we had to evacuate the hospital because they were going to bomb it. The Red Cross was on the top [of the hospital] . . . [and] our Captain also reminded him of the Geneva Treaty, but he [the Japanese] said they knew nothing about the Geneva Treaty. They did not sign it so they did not have to live up to any Geneva Treaty. So the only thing we could do was to take the patients that were possible to transfer . . . across Manila Bay [to the Army Hospital]. I remember, believe it or not, I had my letter of appointment [as nurse in the Navy] in my pocket. I don't think I had a toothbrush. . . . So we started evacuating patients at midnight across Manila Bay in the small PT boats with whatever protection we could receive. But at this time I don't think we thought of protection, just getting out of there and trying to get as many patients as possible out before [the Japanese] arrived to do their bombing."[72]

Miss Cobb writes about these events, "1800 [6 PM] - The C.O. [Commanding Officer] ordered evacuation of all [patients] to Sternberg [Hospital], Manila. 1900 [7 PM] - Evacuation of [patients] began on Yacht `Mary Ann' and barges. Three trips to Manila were necessary. The last load leaving [hospital] dock at 0800 11 December 1941. December 11th: - Finished evacuation of [patients]. Evacuating hospital to Sternberg [and] Philippine Union College, Balintawak, P.I.. All medical officers, nurses [and] hospital staff [except for a small medical contingent] . . . leaving hospital for duty at Sternberg.

"December 12th: Naval Medical Unit established at Balintawak. Within next few days 6 Navy nurses reported for duty at this station. Six remained in Manila with the Army assigned with different Medical Units throughout the city, namely, [Santa] Scholastica, Jai Alai, Holy Ghost."[73] As Navy Nurse Margaret Nash says, "[We] went out to the Philippine Union College [Balintawak]. I don't know how many kilometers outside of Manila that was [but] we took as many patients as we possibly could. Some of the [nurses] went to Jai Alai and patients were transferred there. Jai Alai was a night club that many of us had visited in peace times. I do not know [but] there were at least two [nurses at Jai Alai] but we were taking a larger amount of patients and that's why there were [more] of us that were going out to the Philippine Union College. It was run by the Seventh Day Adventists. . . . [But] we had to put up tents for the patients. The Seventh Day Adventists . . . were filled and they were really very nice to us and they would do anything to accommodate us, but they couldn't accommodate us with any of their buildings. So we had to put up tents and put the patients in them. We slept on cots out in the open. I remember the mosquitos were crawling all over us. . . . We all looked as though we had the measles with all the mosquito bites. Of course we never slept all night. But the Corpsmen that we had with us (it's amazing how you improvise) they decided to put vaseline strips around the legs of the cots so the ants weren't able to crawl up and so that way the second night we were able to get some sleep. . . . [It] was quite a long time that we were out there. The Seventh Day Adventists would allow us to go in and take a shower occasionally, which was a real treat. We didn't have any clothes, so we were putting the same clothes back on. On Christmas Day, I remember; I don't know who had the radio, in fact, we never asked. That was one thing we would never do, was [ask] where they got or how; you just [accepted] it. They loaned us the radio and we heard President Roosevelt from the States, stating that Manila had been declared an open city. . . . [Whoever] was in charge (I can't remember, we were all so scattered) said the only thing for us to do was to take our patients and transfer them back into Manila. . . . [With] several of our wonderful Corpsmen [we] put our patients in the ambulances and we started evacuating once again into Manila. . . . We finally arrived into Manila and where we were going was Santa Scholastica. It was a College of Music, It was a huge building and it was run by the German Fathers. It was a German order. We arrived . . . about lunch time, I guess, because I remember hearing something ring, and we started unloading the ambulance when the sirens went off. That was alerting us [about] a bombing and the Japanese planes came over and start dropping their load of bombs. The patients that were unable to get out of the ambulance, the rest of them that we had on stretchers, we just lined them up alongside the fence at Santa Scholastica and we just [lay] down on the ground alongside them until the bombing was over. . . . [As] soon as that was over, we immediately jumped up and started transferring our patients into Santa Scholastica. And it seemed as though . . . someone [had] set up the wards and we were able to transfer our patients right into the beds for the first time."[74]

Meantime, Mary Chapman and Ann Bernatitis, who had been sent to Sternberg Army Hospital earlier on December 9th, had met briefly with their Navy Nurse colleagues when they came to Sternberg on December 11th. All of them were together just a few days when their commanding officer divided up the Navy Medical personnel to care for the Navy patients placed in sites other than Sternberg. Ann Bernatitis tells us, "Chief Nurse Laura Cobb, O'Haver, Page, Evans, Gorzelanski, and Nash [were sent] to take care of [the] patients at Union College. . . . Todd and Pitcher were assigned to Jai Alai. . . . Mary Chapman and Mary Rose Harrington [were sent] to Holy Ghost. Dorothy Still and I were to go to Santa Scholastica. We were on the bus to go to Santa Scholastica with two Navy corpsmen when someone came on board and told Dorothy Still that she would not be going with me; she was to go to Jai Alai. I was told the reason this happened was that Susie Pitcher . . . [was] being assigned as an anesthetist rather than as a staff nurse [at Jai Alai]. So I was left to go with two Navy corpsmen, the surgeon . . . [and] a dentist . . . who would compose the team that went to Santa Scholastica and that's how we [the Navy nurses] all got separated. Santa Scholastica was a girls' music school, I believe. The nuns were still there, but, of course, the school had disbanded. Our [the Surgical team with Ann Bernatitis] job was to set up the operating room and the first aid station. . . . I was there, by myself [no other Navy Nurses], with the two corpsmen, the doctor [surgeon] and the dentist. . . . [On] the 23rd of December . . . [the surgeon] told me . . . 'we're going to Bataan. We're leaving on Christmas Eve; on the 24th.' The reason for this departure to Bataan was that the Army was going to declare Manila an open city and they were sending the medical personnel, especially surgical teams, out to Bataan."[75] Chief Nurse Laura Cobb records in her handwritten notes for December 24th, "Army moving out to Bataan (Miss Bernatitus left with Army [Medical] Unit.)"

"A few days before Christmas, the bulk of the Japanese 14th Army had landed on Luzon, largest and northernmost of the Philippine Islands. . . . [The] well-trained, veteran troops poured ashore with only slight resistance and immediately launched a drive on the capital city of Manila. The defenders-hastily organized, poorly equipped, and ill prepared-were no match for the invaders. . . . [General Douglas] MacArthur declared Manila an open city and pulled his troops back to the shelter of Bataan, a small, mountainous jungle peninsula that juts out into the mouth of Manila Bay. He made his headquarters at Corregidor, the fortified island guarding the entrance to Manila Bay."[76]

On the 24th of December, Ann Bernatitis leaves Santa Scholastica on a bus to form up with the caravan going to Bataan. The caravan is forming at Jai Alai. She says, "[Being] alone, I didn't know what to do with myself, so I got off the bus [at Jai Alai] while they were getting everything organized and I sat on the curb in front of Jai Alai. And lo and behold, who comes out of Jai Alai, but Dorothy Still and she said, 'What are you doing here?' I said, `I'm going to Bataan.' She said, 'Well, where is Bataan?' I said, 'I don't know. I never heard of it before yesterday!' . . . [We] went into Jai Alai to see how they had set up their court [area] as a hospital. They had a hundred beds on the Jai Alai court. . . . [Then] she went back to her duty station . . . and I sat there until it was time to . . . get back on the [bus] and we [the caravan] started for Bataan. . . . [We] drove through all the villages. The Filipino people would greet us and wave to us giving us the victory sign. It was really very, very touching and at the same time it was scary as the devil because periodically the [Japanese] bombers would come overhead and everything [in the caravan] stopped dead. . . . [We would] jump off the bus and just dive into any where and everything . . . then get back on the bus."[77] Late that afternoon, the 24th of December, the caravan arrives at Army Hospital No. 1 at Limay, Bataan peninsula. (Ann tells us that Army nurses were on the caravan, but none were on the bus she was in.) From another source we learn that, "On Christmas Eve, 24 Army nurses, 25 [Filipino] nurses and . . . Ann Bernatitis, Navy Nurse Corps, were sent by motor convoy to the town of Limay on the Bataan peninsula. They were tasked to prepare a field hospital in a collection of rundown barracks. Their Christmas celebration consisted of cleaning floors, washing windows, assembling cots, and setting up a hospital facility from stored supplies."[78] Miss Bernatitis says, "[We had] to go over to this warehouse to get the equipment for the operating room. And I recall that nothing was marked. It wasn't packaged or crated according to a certain unit. It was just a crate. So you had to pull down crate after crate to find what you were looking for. I distinctly remember pulling down one crate, the two corpsmen [of her surgical team] and I; we pulled it down and we found surgical gowns in it wrapped in newspaper dated 1917! . . . The operating room was just a long narrow building with about eight operating tables through the center. Each table had a surgical team assigned to it and regardless of what type [of injury a] patient was placed on that table. That patient was to be taken care of by the physician whether he was a specialist in it [in that injury surgery] or not. And the ones that were brought in that looked like they were beyond hope, you gave them a hypodermic and eased their pain."[79]

Back in Manila, Chief Nurse Laura Cobb records this for the 26th of December: "Naval Medical Unit transferred to Manila [from Union College] by order of [Admiral] Hart. Stationed at Santa Scholastica. Census [approximately] 450 [patients]."[80] Then for the 27th she writes, "Army transferred several hundred [patients] from Sternberg to [Santa] Scholastica to await sailing of Red Cross Ship bound for Australia. Navy wounded were not included."[81] Navy Nurse Mary Harrington says, "We did not have any orders to leave the city as the Army nurses did. They went to Bataan. We had no orders to leave town. So we stayed in town and gathered up the rest of the wounded from the hospitals around. There was a Red Cross ship, inter-island boat, [that] went down to one of the southern islands for transferring patients on to Australia. And our corpsmen picked up patients from all over town and put them aboard the ship, but they didn't make any provisions for Navy patients, so we had to let our patients stay in, and that hurt."[82]

On the island of Guam in the Marianas Islands, five Navy Nurses are stationed at the U.S. Naval Hospital on the day Pearl Harbor is struck. They are:

1. Chief Nurse Marion Olds who has fifteen years' service in the Navy Nurse Corps. She graduated from George Washington University Hospital in 1919 and entered the Navy Nurse Corps in 1926. She had duty in Washington, D.C., St. Croix, Virgin Islands, New York, Boston, Annapolis, Maryland and San Diego, California. She arrived in Guam in February of 1941. Guam is her first assignment as a Chief Nurse of a Naval Hospital.

2. Navy Nurse Lorraine Christiansen (Halliday) graduated from the Holy Cross Hospital School of Nursing, Salt Lake City, Utah in 1934. She joined the Navy Nurse Corps in 1940. Her first duty station was the Naval Hospital at San Diego, California where she was assigned to operating room duty. From San Diego she received orders to Guam in 1941, reporting aboard on 6 September 1941.[83]

3. Navy Nurse Virginia Fogarty (Mann) went to City Hospital School of Nursing in Akron, Ohio in 1929; she graduated in 1932. She joined the Navy Nurse Corps in 1938. In 1941 she was stationed at the Naval Hospital in Great Lakes, Illinois when she received her orders to Guam. (Another Navy Nurse named Sylvia Lavache [Barnes] tells us that she had received orders for Guam, but she asked to be excused from the assignment. Then Miss Fogarty was given the orders in her place.[84]) Miss Fogarty sailed for Guam on the Navy troopship *Henderson*. She says, "[We] boarded the *Henderson* and set sail for Honolulu. We spent three days there and after that we set sail with the cruiser *St. Louis* guarding us. So it was that dangerous a period of time [this was in September 1941]. . . . [We] began to feel a little bit more of the tension that was undercurrent. And every day they would have target practice and so we would observe all this going on. We used to joke about eating fish and rice, in case our little brown brothers got too close to us."[85] Navy Nurse Fogarty reported for duty at Guam in September of 1941.

4. Navy Nurse Leona Jackson (destined to become a Director of the Navy Nurse Corps) graduated from nurses training at Miami Valley Hospital, Dayton, Ohio in 1930. She joined the Navy Nurse Corps in 1939. In January 1941 she boarded a ship for duty at Guam. On board the same ship she met her new Chief Nurse, Marion Olds. They arrived in Guam on 5 February 1941.

5. Navy Nurse Doris M. Yetter graduated from nurses training at Temple University Hospital, Philadelphia, Pennsylvania. She joined the Navy Nurse Corps on 14 March 1938 and reported to the Naval Hospital, Portsmouth, Virginia for her first active duty. She left there in 1941 for duty at San Diego, California. In mid-1941 she received orders to Guam and reported for duty at the Guam Naval Medical facility on 6 September 1941.[86]

"In October [1941] the women and children were evacuated [from Guam], leaving the five of us [Navy Nurses] and one expectant mother as the only American women on the Island. We missed them, but the men who remained looked after us and kept us entertained as best they could so that it was not too lonesome. . . . We had not been particularly worried about war with the Japanese, a number of whom lived on the Island. When we heard about the bombing of Hawaii on the morning of December 8 we did not believe it at first. As we were discussing it nine planes flew over us and started dropping bombs and we knew the war had started."[87]

Navy Nurse Leona Jackson writes that "I wasn't surprised at the Japanese attack, and I think for many of the people there it didn't come as a surprise. . . . In about an hour, I should say, the casualties had come in. The first objectives of the Japanese raid had been the *Penguin*, which was one of the station ships there [at Guam], and the Marine barracks, and the Marine post at Sumay [Guam]. The report came to us that the *Penguin* had been attacked and that the Skipper had scuttled her. A little while later the Skipper himself . . . was brought in and we knew then that the reports were true; we got the information straight from him. . . . The Japanese raided twice the first day. . . . I had gone on duty after lunch and was making rounds in the hospital when we heard them come over again [for the second time]. They came low over the hospital attempting to get the communications building, which was not awfully far from our ward. The clatter was terrific, but there really wasn't anything to get excited about because there was no place to go. The island was completely and entirely unfortified and so I think most of us just went on with our routine things as they would be done in ordinary circumstances. When we left and took our turns at sleep that night I think each of us wondered if the Japanese would attempt a landing,, but dawn came and no Japanese on the island, at least as far as we knew, and the day began again and the Japanese began again. This time there were three raids. The last raid of the day the Japanese were strafing as they came over, we never did know whether they were just trying to get the communications or whether they were just plain strafing. There weren't a lot of bullets [that] came into the hospital, I think just two or three; something of that sort landed in the various wards as they [the Japanese] came over. There weren't a whole lot of casualties from the second day. The roads were filled during the two days with natives who were making their way from Agana to their ranches in the interior of the island. They had been warned that in event of hostile aircraft action they should leave the settled areas and go into the cover of the palm jungles in the interior.

The actual landing on the island came about 3:30 [a.m.]; I think we heard the first shots on the third morning [10 December] of war. I was awakened from sleep by the sound of shots and walked out of my room onto the Lanai and everything looked so peaceful it seemed very difficult to realize that war had broken out in the Pacific. I listened and things were quiet. I noticed a curtain in the room next door to me move and said to Miss Fogarty - 'I wonder if that is a landing party.' And she said - 'Well, it might be a landing party, or perhaps it is just the sentries firing at looters.' So, both of us waited and in about half an hour we heard shots again. This time I said - 'Joe [Miss Fogarty], I am quite sure that it's a landing party, and I am going to make rounds in the hospital and see what's going on over there.' And she said - 'I'll go with you.' So, all of us went over to the hospital. The shots came closer and increased in volume as the Japs proceeded toward Agana. We had made our rounds and had come down to the library which was just off the emergency room and which we thought would be the most logical place to get any news or information. The Captain at the hospital had sent a messenger over to the government house asking if he knew anything about a Japanese landing on the island, and the only word was that they had received no word. Evidently, they had received no word because the sentries had been killed by the Japanese as they landed. However, it was quite evident that there was something more than usual afoot. They, that is the Japanese, came into Agana about six o'clock that morning. The first actual word of their landing on the island was brought to us by . . . one of the Public Works foremen. He and his native wife and brother-in-law had been coming in toward Agana from their ranch and they ran into an ambush of Japanese soldiers. At first they had thought that it was a Marine patrol, because of the darkness all uniforms look much alike, but as the Japanese jumped onto the running-board of the car they realized that it was Japanese and not our own Marines, and he had thrown the car into gear and thrown the Japanese off as he accellerated [sic] it and had left them shooting at him, but before he got away from them they had bayoneted his native wife and brother-in-law. He himself had been bayoneted, but he had brought them into the hospital for treatment. Then we knew that the Japanese were on the island. The firing ceased about dawn, about six o'clock. I think the most bitter moment in my life came at sunrise when standing in the library door I saw the Rising Sun on the flag pole where the day before the Stars and Stripes had proudly flown."[88]

Navy Nurse Virginia Fogarty also feels strongly about the flag, saying, "I think the hardest thing was to see our American flag come down and the Japanese flag go up in its place. . . . And when I saw that flag go down and another one go up I was so incensed. But there was nothing I could do about it. . . . No, they didn't desecrate it. Just a sense of joy that they [the Japanese] were able to do that to us. And [with a] 'look what we're doing to you' attitude."[89]

Leona Jackson writes that "The Japanese appeared in the hospital compound about 8:30 [a.m.], I think, a few of them had been in during the actual landing, but they appeared in force about 8:30. They used the hospital as a headquarters at first . . . the American officers and men who were stationed on the island, were captured or required to surrender and as they did they were brought into the hospital compound. The officers were lodged in the upper section of SOQ [Sick Officers Quarters] and the men downstairs. Conditions were extremely crowded, of course. . . . The prisoners were moved from the hospital after several days. . . . At the hospital the American nurses remained, the native nurses remained, the Commanding Officer was allowed to designate two doctors and a warrant officer as Administrative Staff."[90]

Navy Nurse Fogarty states, "Well, one day (this was after they [the Japanese] had been there about a week or so) . . . I was over on duty at the hospital, checking on the wards there and doing the best I could. And I was talking to . . . one of our corpsmen and one of the senior corpsmen. . . . [Passing by us] was one of the Chamorro [native] men who had [had] a stroke; he was on his way to the head [bathroom]. I was watching him and thinking how well he was doing; how well he was walking these days. We had urged him to do that and to walk by himself as much as possible. . . . This Japanese came over to me and he muttered something to me in

Japanese and pointed to that man. . . . I just ignored the man [the Japanese]. I just went on talking to the [corpsman] I was talking with and just ignored him. He yelled at me again and I still didn't pay any attention. And he hit me on the arm and I said `don't you do that!' With that he raised his bayonet in front of my nose so I felt, well, I can't hit him back and I had better watch and do what he's telling me or I'll have a bayonet stuck in me. So I walked over to the patient and said to him, `Be careful the next time you go to the head [and] try to see there aren't any Japanese around so they won't interfere with you.' And he nodded yes. But, this Japanese [soldier] thought that I was neglecting my duty and wanted me to go over and look after that man and he was giving me a very bad time because of misinformation. I just tried to ignore him and I knew how I felt toward him so I tried not to do what he wanted me to do, but I had to."[91]

Mrs. Jackson continues the Guam chronicle, "The Japanese had taken over by this time all of the hospital except for one ward. Part of the hospital they used as barracks, one ward of it, I think, they used as a ward. But we had nothing to do with those patients, the Japanese did not want us to know the extent of their casualties. . . . The hospital ward which was left to us housed all sorts of patients. It was probably the most amazing ward I'll ever see. . . . We had war casualties there, and natives, and men and women and children, we even had a Cassearian [sic] section for variety. We were able to take excellent care of these people because the Japanese had confined the native nurses to the compound too, and inasmuch as there were about 30 of them, some of them had gone to their homes before the Japanese landing and didn't return, but we still had an adequate force. Several hospital corpsmen had been retained on the compound and [they] operated the laundry and the galley. The rest of them had been sent . . . with the other prisoners. Life went on this way, and it was extremely uncomfortable. We remained in our [nurses'] quarters, but we had no privacy in those quarters. We never knew when or how many people would be stalking through looking things over, picking up what they wanted."[92] Navy Nurse Fogarty also mentions the lack of privacy when she says, "we were allowed to stay in our quarters for about a month with the Japanese wandering around all the time. They'd go into the Supply Room where we kept the light on all the time because of the humidity. We didn't want mold to get into our trunks and that sort of thing. And they would turn the light off and we would turn it on and they would turn it off. So we'd have a go around about the light. They were always interfering with whatever we were doing in our quarters."[93] Then Leona Jackson continues, "The island was full, of course, of Japanese propaganda, Japanese version of the news. However, one rumor became current and seemed to have some foundation, that we were being moved from the island. This rumor was proven true when on Christmas day we were told to inventory all of our personal possessions, pack them. To pack a bag containing only the things that we ourselves could carry. The rest of our things it seems were to be stored for us, so the Japanese said, would be sent to us later if we needed them. We asked what sort of things we should put in this bag, if we needed heavy clothes. Oh! No, we were going south, we wouldn't need any. Just the same each of us took a heavy coat. . . . The men were very much more unfortunate than we were. None of them, I think, with the exception of one . . . had been allowed to return to their quarters to get anything, and the first few days after the Japanese landing their house girls had been able to bring in something in the way of clothing to them. The Japanese had looked things over and anything that they thought might be used in the future they refused to allow the officers and men to have. A few articles of their clothing they did allow them to have, however. But most of them had only the things which they wore on their backs."[94]

(Shortly before the Navy Nurses on Guam were captured by the Japanese, they were "given hastily made dogtags and identification cards to identify them as non-combatant military members."[95] This becomes significant later on when these nurses are released as prisoners-of-war.) And that is how 1941 ends for the Navy Nurses, now POW's, on Guam.

Back in the U.S., Navy Nurse Dorothy McKinley (Filip) is at her first duty station: the U.S. Naval Hospital at Bremerton, Washington. She tells us that the "red brick hospital building stood majestically on a hill with wards . . . jutting out at right angles from a main corridor. A few yards away stood our pretty white nurses' quarters where we ate all of our meals. . . . From my room in winter I could see the snow covered Olympic [mountain] range in the distance; it was truly a beautiful sight. . . . [On] December 7th, the peaceful picture of

Bremerton changed. Almost overnight huge barrage balloons were raised over the [nearby] Navy Yard for protection. I was told later that [a] war-damaged . . . English warship, in dock for repairs, was the only ship which had anti-aircraft guns available to ward off any air attack. [Also], within hours the Army had set up camp on the golf course just out front of the nurses' quarters and across the street. Now all leaves were cancelled and all personnel were restricted to Bremerton. And I admit that I was one of those who walked to the dock just to watch the ferries [to Seattle] come and go, wishing I could spend that hour it took to ride over to Seattle, but now our nation was at war."[96]

Over on the East Coast, Navy Nurse Mary Benner is at the old Naval Hospital in Brooklyn, New York. There, a Hospital Corps School had recently been set up with Chief Nurse Mary Benner and her two assistants. She says "then Pearl Harbor broke while I was there and I remember yet watching them mount the machine guns on top of the buildings in the Navy Yard. We had been teaching the corpsmen a sixteen week course [in nursing]. You know we cut that down to six weeks? It [first] went down to twelve [weeks], then nine, on down to six. And it was really pathetic, later on, when we began hearing of the [corpsmen] that [we] had taught that had lost their lives [in the war]."[97]

Navy Nurse Ethel Batton (Quadrini) is stationed at the Naval Hospital in Philadelphia, Pennsylvania on December 7th. This is her first duty station. She tells us of the Navy Nurses' environment at Philadelphia and her impressions of her new vocation, "This was an exciting time in my life. A new type of nursing, making new friends, and becoming acquainted with the Navy. . . . Newly appointed nurses were on probation for six months, in which time attitude for the Naval Nursing Service was closely observed. Base pay for nurses was $70.00 per month, and paid monthly. . . . Nurses quarters in Philadelphia was relatively new, [with] single rooms, comfortable and pleasant. All meals were served in the dining room. Seating was arranged with eight nurses at each table, and a senior nurse to serve. Tables were set with white table cloths and napkins, navy china, and silver. Each nurse provided her own napkin ring. If a nurse was absent from dinner, she received a reimbursement of 25 [cents]. Guests were permitted for dinner on Wednesday and Sunday Noon. During the indoctrination period, I was assigned to duty with a senior nurse for a period of several weeks, and met with Ms. Bunte [Chief Nurse] for a series of [conferences] on rules and regulations covering the Navy in general, and the Nurse Corps. . . . Duty was arranged in eight hour shifts, changing AM and PM duty weekly, with every other week-end off. Week-ends began at 1200 on Saturday and night duty every four months. My first challenge occurred the day I went on duty and walked into a 35 bed ward all filled with men, and to see the nurse's desk in the middle of the ward. I had come from a hospital where the largest ward held 12 beds, and the nurse's desk was behind a glass window. . . . Supplies for the ward were closely guarded and quite limited. Equipment tended to be quite old. At the completion of the probationary period, nurses were supplied with the Navy Nurse Corps uniform, white duty uniforms and caps, a blue sweater, full length blue cape with a red lining, and a small blue felt hat. These came from the uniform shop Naval Supply Depot, Brooklyn, New York.

"December 7, 1941 brought news of the bombing of Pearl Harbor, which spread through the hospital rapidly. Many changes occurred overnight. Greater security, a great urgency to return all patients to duty rapidly, bed capacities on wards were increased, new equipment arrived, and doctors, nurses and corpsmen of the Reserve forces began to report for active duty."[98]

The Navy Nurse Corps is going to war for the second time and 31 December 1941 finds the Nurses of the Navy deployed as follows:

Canacao:	12	Pearl Harbor:	29	USS *Relief*:	12
Cuba:	8	Kaneohe, T.H.	2	USS *Solace*:	13
Guam:	5	Kodiak:	5	Coco Solo,	
St. Thomas, V.I. 5				Panama Canal Zone	4
Total overseas and at sea:		95			
In United States:		733			
Total active duty:		828[99]	Total inactive Reserve:	940[100]	

In Washington, D.C. on 7 December 1941, it is "an unusual Sunday morning for officers in the War and Navy Departments . . . where the clock was five and a half hours ahead of Pearl Harbor. [It had been] more than a year since [an Army Colonel had broken] the Japanese diplomatic Purple Code [and] American intelligence [was] figuratively . . . reading over the shoulders of Japanese diplomats as they received their instructions from Tokyo. This morning there was a fresh radio intercept to study. The Japanese diplomatic corps in Washington was being instructed to break off diplomatic negotiations with the United States. . . . [What] was unusual was that the diplomats were to tell their American counterparts this news at exactly 1 P.M. Washington time [7:30 A.M. Hawaiian time]. . . . General George C. Marshall, army chief of staff, drafted a dispatch to Hawaiian Headquarters, noting the deadline and adding, `Just what significance the hour set may have we do not know, but be on the alert accordingly.' . . . It was 6:30 A.M. Hawaiian time when he filed the dispatch at the army's Washington message center, and he later checked to see that it was sent. It had been sent, but the message center had neglected to tell him how. Army radio was having problems that morning, so Marshall's warning was sent through commercial channels - via Western Union. Not until mid-afternoon did a telegraph messenger pedal his bicycle up to Pearl Harbor headquarters with the dispatch."[101] Too late. Immediately after the attack on Pearl Harbor, the Japanese declare "war on the United States and Great Britain. The following day, President Roosevelt [asks] Congress for a Declaration of War against Japan. He [calls] December 7 `a date which will live in infamy.'. . . On December 11, Germany and Italy [declare] war on the United States, and Congress then [declares] war on Germany and Italy."[102]

1942 begins with more Japanese activities. On 2 January they invade and take over Manila in the Philippines. On 11 January they land in the East Indies where, in February, they capture the British fortress in Singapore. At the end of February, the Allies lose the battle of Java Sea (between the island of Borneo and the East Indies.) In March, the Japanese capture Burma (country between India and Thailand.) In early April the Japanese take Bataan in the Philippines. Mid-April and U.S. planes from a Navy aircraft carrier bomb Tokyo followed by an early May Allied victory at the Coral Sea battle (between Australia and the Solomon Islands.) Then in June, the Battle of Midway halts Japan's advancement to the east. (Also, in June just before the Battle of Midway, the Japanese bomb "Dutch Harbor in the Aleutian Islands, and [occupy] Agattu, Attu, and Kiska islands."[103]) Over in the European War Theater, the British stop the German Army at El Alamein in Egypt in early July. Back in the Pacific, at the beginning of August, U.S. Marines land on Guadalcanal in the Solomon Islands. Mid-September in Russia and the Germans enter Stalingrad. Then at the beginning of November, Allied forces land in North Africa, but French resistance ends in this area just a few days later. Back in Russia, in mid-November, the Russians attack the Germans at Stalingrad as the notorious Russian winter takes hold of the countryside and a German Army ill prepared for it.[104]

After Pearl Harbor and the U.S. declared war, President Roosevelt "had to decide where to strike first. . . . Roosevelt conferred with Churchill . . . [and the] two leaders realized that the United States could not strike an effective blow against Japan until the navy had recovered from its losses at Pearl Harbor. In addition, German scientists were developing new weapons that could mean defeat for the Allies. Both the British and the Russians wanted to see Germany defeated as soon as possible. For these reasons, Roosevelt and Churchill decided that Germany, the most powerful enemy nation, must be defeated first. . . . On Nov. 7, 1942, the Allies invaded North Africa. It was the greatest landing operation in history up to that time. After the landings began, Roosevelt spoke by radio to the French people in their own language. He explained that the Allies had to drive the Germans out of French territory in North Africa. Roosevelt was the first President to give a radio address in a foreign language.

"Many changes in White House routine were made after the United States entered World War II. The Roosevelts reduced their entertaining. Wartime security regulations went into effect. Machine guns were set up on the White House roof, and Secret Service agents took over a special office in the East Wing. Engineers built a bomb shelter in the White House basement."[105] Many more changes began to take place in the homes, workplaces, and lives of the rest of the American people. "The U.S. government set up agencies to handle such wartime problems as communications, economic stabilization, housing, labor, manpower, mobilization, price controls, rationing, and transportation."[106]   "As men went into the armed forces, women took their places in war plants . . . . In shipyards and aircraft plants, 'Rosie the riveter' became a common sight. . . . [Ration stamps were used for items including] meats, butter, sugar, fats, oils, coffee, canned foods, shoes, and gasoline. . . . [and the government warned people] not to give away information that might be of value to the enemy. Well-known slogans . . . included 'Loose talk costs lives' and 'A slip of the lip may sink a ship.'"[107] The government sold more than fifteen billion dollars in "savings bonds, certificates, notes and stamps to individuals and firms."[108] Children could (and were encouraged to) buy savings stamps at school and set records for amounts purchased. Many family men held two jobs in order to help the war effort. The government "set up a civil-defense system to protect the country from attack. . . . Many cities practiced 'blackouts.' Cities on the Atlantic and Pacific coasts dimmed their lights."[109] Local air-raid wardens patrolled the streets during black-outs and notified those in homes where lights were visible. Children and teenagers were made part of the defense effort and went door-to-door collecting tin cans and metal of any kind for the war effort. Everyone felt the fervor of country, flag, and patriotism, creating an unparalleled, country-wide 'togetherness.'

It is not only the men that are joining the Armed Forces in the fervor of patriotism. Many women, other than nurses, are entering one of five military organizations:

1. WAAC - Women's Army Auxiliary Corps, in 1942, which a year later on becomes the WAC (Women's Army Corps.) "Most enlisted women serve in clerical, medical, and Communications fields. . . . Officers receive assignments in personnel, intelligence, training, supply and administration."[110]

2. WASP - Women's Airforce Service Pilots. These are women pilots who ferry military planes overseas, do some flight instruction and tow targets for fighter pilots.

(In 1943 another women's military organization will become an entity; the Women in the Air Force or WAF. Until the U.S. Air Force becomes separate from the U.S. Army, in 1947, these women are "known as *Air WAC's* . . . and [perform] a variety of jobs during World War II at air bases in all parts of the world."[111])

3. SPAR - This is the U.S. Coast Guard Women's Reserve. "The name *SPAR* is taken from the first letters of the Coast Guard motto and its English translation, *Semper Paratus* (Always Ready). [All] SPARS are in the military Reserve . . . [and] come under the command of the Coast Guard. . . . The organization [is] created in November, 1942, to release Coast Guardsmen from office jobs for sea duty."[112]

4. WAVES - Women Accepted for Volunteer Emergency Service. This is the Navy women's organization that is signed into law in July of 1942. The WAVES are assigned to technical or clerical positions after a period of basic (recruit) training. One of the technical positions is that of replacing Medical Corpsmen in the Naval Medical facilities, to free the Corpsmen for sea duty and battlefield duty with the Navy and Marine Corps.

5. Marine Corps Women's Reserve. Again, the women are utilized to release men for combat duty.

To turn now to the general field of medicine, the lives of many soldiers are being saved by "the effectiveness of blood plasma which could be transported to the battle field and administered by a trained medical corpsman. The use of penicillin and the sulfonamides in relation to infection . . . [is] responsible for recovery of many of the wounded. When overseas sources of quinine [are] cut off by enemy action, synthetic preparations [are] perfected. . . . [A new insecticide called 'DDT' is] evolved and [works] miracles in the elimination of insect-borne and rodent-borne diseases, notably malaria and typhus. Also among effective prophylactic measures introduced in World War II [is] the administration of tetanus toxoid and yellow fever vaccine to all members of the fighting forces."[113]

The nursing profession is critical to all aspects of WWII medical care and the National Nursing Council for War Service is "a coordinating link between organized nursing and the Federal program for supplying an adequate number of nurses to the armed forces. . . . By magazine, poster, letter, and radio, the Nursing Council [spreads] its message of need and opportunity. In addition, it [serves] as a consultant to the *Procurement and Assignment Service for Physicians, Dentists, Veterinarians, Sanitary Engineers, and Nurses*, a Federal agency [which is] delegated responsibility for equable distribution of professional personnel in accordance with military and civilian needs. . . . Working side by side with [the National Nursing Council is] the American Red Cross Nursing Service as it [campaigns] to enlarge the roll of Reserve nurses . . . [for] the Army Nurse Corps and the Navy Nurse Corps. . . . Also, a *Red Cross Student Reserve* [is] set up in which senior student nurses [are] enrolled with the pledge to become active in war service upon graduation. . . . In a determined effort to meet the desperate need of hospitals, first-aid stations, and similar organizations for trained assistants to professional nurses, the *Red Cross Volunteer Nurses' Aide Corps* [is] organized. . . . Composed of women between the ages of eighteen and fifty, many of them with homes and families, the Corps [is] trained by qualified nurse instructors in an eighty hour course, thirty-five hours of which [are] in the classroom, and forty-five in hospital wards. . . . They [prove] dependable and invaluable additions to professional staffs wherever they [are] asked to serve. Additional help [comes] from the American Red Cross in the employment of great numbers of nurse instructors to teach courses in *Red Cross Home Nursing* to housewives and mothers in order that they might take intelligent care of their families during minor illnesses, or periods of convalescence."[114]

Also helping is the United States Public Health Service which by carrying out "the National Survey of Registered Nurses, first promoted by the National Nursing Council for War Service, it [is] able to determine not only the total number of nurses throughout the nation, but also their preparation, experience, and availability. With its sanction and cooperation, Federal funds [are] granted to established schools of nursing of good standing, enabling them to increase their dormitory space and teaching facilities."[115] It is a congresswoman, Frances Payne Bolton, from Ohio who sponsors the congressional legislation (the Bolton Bill) that provides the funds for these and other nursing needs in 1942. But, there is still a great demand for more nurses both in the civilian and military sectors. Out of this demand is born a creative and innovative nursing program whose time could not be better. Again, it is Mrs. Bolton who puts this Bill before Congress in 1942. It is a Bill that will establish the 'United States Cadet Nurse Corps.' (The Bill and its ramifications will be discussed when it is passed in 1943.) Another advance in 1942 is the formation of the National Association for Practical Nurse Education to meet "the need for means of supplying great numbers of well-prepared auxiliary workers."[116] Further, with the increasing demand for nurses in the war factories and work-places, 1942 sees the organization of the American Association of Industrial Nurses.[117] Meantime, the National Association of Colored Graduate Nurses is struggling "both to prevent the exclusion of black nurses and simultaneously to encourage them to apply for service through the American Red Cross. Once the war began . . . [they struggle] to abolish the quotas established by the army. They [continue] to protest even when, in July 1942, the Army Nurse Corps [accepts] sixty new black nurses, assigning them to the recently opened large black station hospital at Fort Huachuca in Arizona. . . . However, in spite of continuous NACGN pressure, the Navy Nurse Corps [proves] unalterably opposed to the induction of black women nurses."[118] But meantime, the Mills Training School for Male Nurses at Bellevue Hospital in New York City is still graduating men nurses and in 1942 the first black man is graduated there. His name is Lawrence A. Sumler. Neither the Bellevue Training School for female nurses nor the Mills School for men nurses make any "distinction of race, creed, or color."[119]

As for men graduate nurses, in general, in early 1941 the Men Nurses' Section of the ANA requested that the ANA approach the Surgeons General of the Army and Navy about providing opportunities "equal to those for women nurses in the medical departments of the armed forces. . . . [The] offices of the Surgeons General . . . indicated that no changes in military procedures in relation to men nurses could be made. The [American Red Cross] was already well aware of the problem of men nurses and of the several types of medical technologists whose skills were also badly needed by the medical departments of the Army and the Navy. It [the ARC] arranged to enroll qualified men nurses as medical technologists. The Medical Department of the Army agreed that men nurses holding the registration card of the Red Cross should, after the initial four-months' service as trainees, be promoted to the grade of technical sergeant providing a vacancy in that grade was available. This was far from satisfactory to the men."[120] At the 1942 ANA convention a resolution is passed "that registered professional men nurses who [are] members of the ANA be given opportunity to serve as professional nurses as soon as possible after enlistment or induction into the armed forces."[121] The resolution is sent to the Armed Forces and again it is stated that no changes will be made.[122] In relation to this, an article in the American Journal of Nursing published in May of 1942 states, "for the first time, because of the expansion of the [Navy's] Hospital Corps made necessary by war-time conditions, registered men nurses may enlist in their correct professional status. This is the only branch of the armed service which has made this provision for men nurses. Registered men nurses may enlist for the duration [of WW II] and six months in the Hospital Corps of the U.S. Naval Reserve, Class V-6, as pharmacist's mates, second class, at a monthly salary of $72. . . . For comparison, the beginning salary of the Navy nurse is $70 per month."[123] (The disparity in pay is not a mistake.) This article is written by a male R.N. who is a Chief Pharmacist's Mate on duty at a Stateside Naval Hospital.

On the front cover of the Life magazine of 5 January 1942 appears a close-up photograph of a young Navy Nurse in her white ward uniform and cap with the thin black band and one stripe of gold across it. (Her name is Navy Nurse Alberta Rose Krape and she is stationed at the Naval Hospital, Brooklyn, New York.) She stands in front of a typical medicine cabinet and in the lower left hand corner of the portrait in small black letters is 'Wanted: 50,000 nurses.' The article inside the Life magazine tells of the severe nurse shortage in the Army and Navy, the U.S. Public Health Service, and the civilian sector of the country and what is being done about it. This is but one example of the all-out publicity efforts being made for professional nursing needs in war time.

In March of 1942, Navy Nurse Mary Benner reports in to the Bureau of Medicine and Surgery in Washington, D.C. for duty on the staff of the Superintendant of the Navy Nurse Corps. She tells us, "my job was to help bring in Reserve nurses through the Reserve Nurse Plan. And we really did expand. . . . We brought them in just as fast as we could."[124] To show the expansion, on 31 January 1942 there were 976 total active duty Navy nurses (668 regular and 308 active Reserve) then at the end of March 1942 there are 1315 total active duty (732 regular and 583 active Reserve.) At the end of 1942 there are 2907 Navy nurses on active duty (1144 regular and 1763 active Reserve.) Mary Benner goes on to state that the office of the Superintendent "was down on Constitution Avenue in the Navy Department; one of those old wooden buildings along Constitution Avenue. And later on we were moved to 23rd and E [streets]. When they moved the [Naval] hospital out to Bethesda, Maryland, we moved into the old hospital area."[125] This move of the Naval Hospital actually began back in 1937 when the Navy Surgeon General told a Congressional House Committee that the then Washington, D.C. Naval Hospital (at Observatory Hill) was too small with no room for expansion in case of need. Eventually, a large plat of ground was obtained in Bethesda "and the construction of the Naval Medical Center became Franklin D. Roosevelt's personal crusade. . . . On 31 [August] 1942 President Roosevelt dedicated the new Naval Medical Center in Bethesda and the hilltop in Foggy Bottom [a.k.a. Observatory Hill at 23rd and E streets] received yet another tenant - the 100-year-old Bureau of Medicine and Surgery."[126]

In June of 1942 Congress passes a law providing "new Permanent pay scale for Army and Navy nurses. [Base pay is] increased from $70.00 to $90.00 per month with an increase of [five percent] every three years."[127] (At least now they receive more pay than the corpsmen that they are teaching.) Then on the 3rd of July 1942, the 77th Congress finally authorizes Permanent Relative Rank for the Navy Nurse Corps. (Relative rank had been given the Army Nurse Corps back in 1920. Army "nurses were given officer status ranging from second lieutenant through major, but pay and allowances were not the same as for men."[128]) The new law authorizes the relative rank from Ensign to Lt. Commander for the Navy nurses. (At this time Superintendent Sue Dauser is given the rank of Lieutenant Commander.) The law also says, "As regards medical and sanitary matters, and all other work within the line of their professional duties, the members of the Navy Nurse Corps shall have authority in and about naval hospitals and other medical activities next after the commissioned officers of the Medical Corps and Dental Corps of the Navy."[129] There is no provision for a further increase in pay, but the new law does authorize the

Secretary of the Navy to assign a money value to the nurses' initial indoor uniform and to then either pay a money allowance for that uniform or to direct the issue of that uniform to newly appointed nurses. In September a money allowance for uniforms is authorized. When November comes, an order is issued for the mandatory wearing of the street uniform. Now that the nurses are officers, several changes must take place in the Nurse Corps' uniforms. In March of 1942, a letter from the Chief of the Bureau of Navigation to the Chief of the Bureau of Medicine and Surgery had authorized "new uniform items for the Nurse Corps: both blue and white service dress, a blue overcoat, and both blue and white caps. Then a uniform instruction issued to members of the Nurse Corps on December 1, 1942 [describes] their new uniforms in detail. . . . The instructions for the white indoor uniform and cap, the cape, and the raincoat [are] unchanged. The new blue service coat [is] double-breasted, with two rows of three gilt buttons each. The rolling [sic] collar, lapelled coat [is] to be worn buttoned, on the left-a concession to the feminine sex.

"Grade [is] shown by means of gold or yellow silk sleeve lace: two strips of half-inch lace with a quarter-inch strip between them for the Superintendent; two strips for the Assistant Superintendent; a strip and a half for chief nurses; and a single half-inch lace for all others. No corps device [is] to be worn above the sleeve lace, but a metal corps device-the oak leaf and acorn superimposed on a gold foul anchor, with the letters *N.N.C.* raised above the oak leaf-[is] to be worn on either side of the collar. The white service coat [is] single-breasted, with three gilt buttons, a rolling [sic] collar, and notched lapels. No sleeve insignia [is] worn. Grade [is] indicated by shoulder marks which [have] the same stripe arrangement as the blue coat-sleeves, but no corps device. The metal corps device [is] worn on the left side of the collar of the white shirt, and a rank device on the right side, in the same manner as the devices worn on khaki shirts by male officers. The Superintendent of the Nurse Corps [wears] the gold oak leaf of a lieutenant commander; the assistant superintendent, the two silver bars of a lieutenant; chief nurses, the silver bar of a lieutenant (junior grade); and all others, the gold bar of an ensign. The outdoor cap, either blue or white to match the uniform, [has] a vague resemblance to that of male officers. The band of the cap [is] an inch and a quarter wide in front and three-quarters of an inch wide in back, and [is] covered with a band of black mohair. The crown of the cap [flares] up into a circular shape, the slant in front being about half an inch longer than in back. This visorless cap [is] worn with gold lace chin strap half an inch wide, fastened at either side with small gilt buttons. In lieu of the male officer's cap device, the Nurse Corps device [is] fastened to the front of the cap, above the chin strap."[130]

Then on the 22nd of December 1942 Congress passes the law authorizing "temporary relative rank from Captain to Ensign and [a] higher temporary pay scale for Nurse Corps personnel for [the] war period plus six months."[131] (All of these changes in rank mean further changes in the uniforms that will be promulgated in 1944.) The pay of an ensign is raised from $90.00 a month to $150.00 per month. Margaret Lou Covington says, "I went in the Navy in 1942 . . . as a Reserve Nurse U.S. Navy with the relative rank of Ensign. I remember my first month's pay was ninety dollars. In December 1942, legislation changed things. . . . I remember my first month's pay then was one hundred fifty dollars and I believe that's the richest I've ever been."[132]

Also, on the 22nd of December 1942, Captain Sue Dauser, Superintendent of the Navy Nurse Corps, takes the oath of office as the first Captain in the Nurse Corps and the first woman to be a Captain in the Navy.[133] A short item appears in the American Journal of Nursing saying that "Captain Sue S. Dauser, Superintendent of the Navy Nurse Corps, is the first woman authorized to wear the captain's four gold stripes on the sleeve of her Navy uniform. . . . The Navy Nurse Corps is now authorized to have two assistant superintendents, Commander Loretta Lambert and Commander Mary D. Towse, and four directors to serve in the grade of lieutenant commander. Additional officers of these grades may be named, if further expansion of the Corps makes it necessary. . . . Captain Dauser, who has been in the Navy Nurse Corps since November 1917, has been superintendent of the Corps since January 1939."[134]

There are other events that take place in Washington, D.C. area in 1942. For instance, in October, the Naval Medical Research Institute at Bethesda is commissioned with a complement of thirteen officers and fifty enlisted personnel.[135] Then in early November 1942, the Surgeon General of the Army authorizes the Army

Nurse Corps to appoint married nurses under the age of forty, to the Army Nurse Corps.[136] Undoubtedly, this is done in order to meet the increasing and unrelenting need for nurses. But, the Navy does not follow suit. Also, in November, Ensign Jean Byers (NC) USNR is assigned as the first nurse "consultant to [the] Bureau of Medicine and Surgery Audio-Visual Training Aide program"[137] to help develop films for corpmen's instruction.

As for new Navy nurse assignments, the Naval Dispensary, San Juan, Puerto Rico receives Navy nurses in February of 1942. In October Chief Nurse Lieutenant(jg) Beulah Duxbury (NC) USN and four nurses are assigned to the Naval Dispensary at Trinidad, British West Indies. And, on the 11th of November 1942, the Aiea Heights Naval Hospital on Oahu in the Hawaiian Islands, is commissioned and the Chief Nurse is Lieutenant(jg) Gertrude B. Arnest (NC) USN.[138]

Now, to return to the War. In the February 1942 issue of the American Journal of Nursing, an article states that the "first American wounded of the armed forces have arrived in San Francisco from Pearl Harbor by ship. . . . The convoyed ships, wearing war paint, slipped unheralded into port; disembarkation of the wounded began immediately. Naval medical officers, Naval hospital corpsmen, Navy nurses, and Red Cross nurses took charge of the service wounded. Ambulances moved swiftly, bearing the Army wounded to Letterman Hospital at the Presidio of Sam Francisco, those of the Navy to Mare Island."[139] One of the Navy Nurses at Mare Island, California, is Rachel B. Todd. She tells us, "in 1940 I signed up for the Red Cross and stated a preference for Navy over Army. [I] received orders to report for my physical [examination] on January 6, 1942, and then received orders to report to Mare Island, which I did, on March 24, 1942 as a U.S. [Naval Reserve]. I switched to USN [regular navy] in June or July . . . I just knew I liked the Navy and wanted to continue serving my country after the war would be over. I was assigned to Ward 13 [at Naval Hospital Mare Island]. There were forty-seven patients on the ward, and all were victims of the Pearl Harbor attack. They had [been] burned in the escape from the *U.S.S. Arizona, Pennsylvania* and *Nevada* and other stations in [Pearl Harbor]. The men on this ward, and ward 15 also, were being treated by [LCdr. Ralph C. Pendleton Medical Corps USNR]. . . . He had been working in Salt Lake City for twenty years on his treatment that he was going to use on the boys [the wounded]. It consisted of a wax which was sprayed on the burned areas. The sailors were still in great pain, regardless of what treatment they had been receiving. With this wax treatment, they were sprayed and they immediately felt the pain drift away; it was really amazing how it worked on them. At first, the wax coated sailors felt naked without any bandages over their arms, but the wax, of course, covered it to a certain extent. When they realized that [the] painful changing of dressings [was] stopped and that they could bathe themselves and get around, they liked it very well and [some] were released back to duty. Some of them took the wax with them so that they could keep the [burn] area soft so as not to form keloid. [Keloid is hard, raised, scar tissue.] The wax was kept ready for use on an electric burner in the nurses' station at all times. Patients would stop and knock at the door whenever spraying was necessary. Corpsmen and nurses would end up with wax in their hair and in their nostrils, the spray was so fine. The boys recovered very well with this treatment. However, some were so badly burned that they required skin grafting at a later date. . . .

"Most of the sailors were just kids; 19, 20, and 21 years of age."[140] Margaret Jackson is another Navy Nurse at Mare Island also assigned to a burn ward. She states, "We used paraffin wax as medication in a fly sprayer to cover the severe burn area. We would do this every day to make it air free around the burned area. Then a tent was put on the bed to keep the covers off the person. The results were wonderful and with very little scarring."[141] Rachel Todd helps us understand this wax treatment when she donates, to the NNCA, a copy of the 'Open Air Paraffin Wax Treatment For All Types Of Burns' as written by Dr. Pendleton at the Naval Hospital, Mare Island in 1942. The items used to make the wax are noted as; paraffin wax, petrolatum, liquid petrolatum (heavy), cod liver oil, sulfanilamide powder, menthol, camphor, and oil of eucalyptus. "The wax and petrolatum are melted on a water bath then the other materials are stirred in. While still melted pour the Rx [items noted above - in the quantities listed in the prescription] into insecticide spray 'guns' and allow to cool (melting point 117 [degrees Fahrenheit].) The Rx will keep indefinitely, although it will turn brown if heated excessively. Reheat on a water bath and then spray it. Keep the mixture well agitated to keep the sulfanilamide in suspension. . . .

Spray the melted wax Rx directly onto all freshly burned surfaces. Do not traumatize by scrubbing the burned skin or removing the protecting blisters before spraying. NEVER APPLY GAUZE OR ANY OTHER MATERIAL DIRECTLY ON THE WAX. The coalescing mixture of the wax Rx, burned materials, dirt, perspiration, serum and any previously applied medications will slide off the burn into towels or any easily removed material, thus performing a slow gentle cleansing. Respray uncovered painful areas as often as discovered, or whenever requested by the patient. . . . The spray gun may be used from 20 to 3 inches away from the skin. Confidence is gained by spraying some normal skin before covering the burned area. . . . When the patient cannot be moved, flush the area with warm tap water by a flower spray [gun], fountain syringe, etc. When possible, set the patient on a chair in a tub and flush the burned areas with tap water from a dish rinsing or hand bath spray. As early as possible permit a shower bath, which accomplishers wonders. (A tub bath contaminates clean areas.) All wax need not be removed each day. . . . If the patient should be burned fore and aft, a sheet of waxed paper prevents adhesions to the bed sheet. A cradle with ONE electric globe may be used to protect the patient from sun, cold, wind or the oversensitive easily offended aesthetic sense of attendants."[142] Listed among the many advantages of this method are:

> "Stops pain instantly, thus preventing early shock from pain, and providing comfort throughout healing."
> "It is inexpensive, easily mixed and may be used in isolated battle stations with little equipment and no trained personnel."
> "Dressing time is reduced 90 [percent] over most methods. This is of vital importance in mass burns, whether civilian or military."[143]

Rachel Todd remembers another day in 1942 at the Mare Island Hospital and says, "[one] day, if I remember correctly, it was in the morning and . . . all the nurses in the nurses' quarters were advised to come down in their ward uniforms and stand at attention along the driveway that went up to the administration building and around the administration building. Our special guest was Eleanor Roosevelt [the President's wife] and she stopped and shook hands with each one of us, and thanked each one of us personally, as she was going along, for serving our country. It really was very impressive. It was something I will never forget."[144]

As an insight to one side of the routines of Navy Medicine, Rachel Todd describes the 'Captain's Inspection' that is carried out in Naval Medical facilities everywhere. "Every Friday was field day, in preparation for inspection on Saturday morning. All patients, unless bed ridden, turned to and helped [the nurses and corpsmen]. The beds were moved from Port to Starboard [left to right], and Starboard to Port while floors were scrubbed, waxed and squeegeed. Utility rooms were turned inside out and upside down to get everything clean. Windows were cleaned, beds were lined up, and I do mean lined up. The wards were spotless and ready for inspection. On Saturday morning at [ten a.m.], the [inspection] parties started their rounds. If you didn't pass inspection, you didn't rate liberty [freedom for those patients the doctors permit to leave the hospital for a specified period of time]. [The patients] would stand at attention along-side their bunks [beds] dressed in the appropriate uniform-of-the-day, ready to go on liberty at [twelve noon]. I was lucky enough to always be on a ward that passed inspection, so everyone was happy. Liberty was from [twelve noon] Saturday to [eight a.m.] Monday morning."[145]

In April of 1942, Madonna M. Timm is a 'new' Navy Nurse at the Naval Hospital, Corona, California. She states that she had been a private duty nurse at St. Mary's Hospital (her nurses training school) when, after "the Pearl Harbor attack, Eleanor Roosevelt arrived in Rochester, Minnesota to visit her son James Roosevelt who was a patient at St. Mary's Hospital and across the hall from my patient. She met and spoke with all the nurses encouraging us to join the Army or Navy Nurse Corps; otherwise we could be drafted. Waltman Walters, M.D. USNR and Charles Mayo II, M.D. USAR of the Mayo Clinic decided to form units which we could join up with and stay together as a Unit during the duration of WWII. I decided to join the Navy Nurse Corps Reserve Unit of the Mayo Clinics [on] Feb. 27, 1942 because I had two brothers in the Marines in the Southwest Pacific. Our Unit was organized at the . . . [Naval Hospital at Corona, California]. . . . [The Hospital] had been a Country Club and Hotel for the Hollywood movie stars. It was a large, beautiful Spanish structure overlooking a small lake outside of Corona. I arrived April 14, 1942. . . . Nellie Jane DeWitt was our Chief Nurse and Ruth Houghton [was] her Assistant. . . . We had not been issued hospital beds and other Navy supplies so all enjoyed the gorgeous Hollywood furniture, beds, china, linens, and silverware left for us - as well [as] their Filipino cooks and waiters. . . . Five regular Navy Nurses from San Diego were assigned to help teach us Navy Nursing procedures. . . . We were busy admitting patients weekly from the Pacific war zone."[146]

Navy Nurse Katherine M. Loughman is assigned a different type of Nurse Corps duty in 1942. "[It] was early in my career. In 1942 I was sent to Buffalo, New York to recruit females for the service. That included Navy Nurses, women for the WAVES, for the SPARS [of] the Coast Guard, for the Marine Corps, and that was very interesting. I had 18 months of that duty. We [there were two nurses] covered all upper New York [state]; that was Buffalo, Rochester and that area."[147] It is also early in another Navy Nurse's career over in the state of Massachusetts. Her name is Virginia Holt and she writes that, "[in] 1942, while at Chelsea Naval Hospital in Boston, I was on call for Emergency duty after my day shift ended. I received a call to report at once to the operating room. A foreign seaman had been plucked from the icy waters off the coast of Boston after his ship had been torpedoed by a German submarine. We were sworn to secrecy as the public must not be informed about an enemy submarine lurking off the [Massachusetts] coast. The wounded sailor was brought into the operating room. His legs had both been blown off during the explosion,but the cold salt water had stopped the flow of blood from his stumps. We treated him for shock and exposure and the Navy Doctors were ready to sew up his stumps. The patient's heart stopped beating and his blood pressure dropped. I was told to start artificial respirations. I had to get on the [operating] table to administer them [artificial respiration]. He started to improve and his condition stabilized. He opened his eyes and stared at me working on him. I smiled at him and told him he was in a U.S. Naval Hospital and we would take care of him. He then said in broken English, `Would [you] yost `old my `and [just hold my hand?]' I held both his hands and soothed him as the Surgeon told him he would take some stitches in his legs. He was only 15 [years] old and had lied to get into [the] Norwegian Navy. Afterwards, he would wheel his wheelchair around the wards and thank me profusely for caring for him that night. He was the pet of the wards and later was fitted for artificial legs."[148]

Down in Pennsylvania, Sue Smoker is another Navy nurse who reports to her first duty station, the Philadelphia Naval Hospital, on 6 January 1942. Sue says, "[as] it turned out, twenty-five nurses, mostly from Pennsylvania, reported with me, and we were the first group to live out of [nurses] quarters. We were housed at the Sylvania Hotel [at] Broad and Logan Streets in Philadelphia. Our [trip] to the hospital for duty was a new experience for me. First, [we took] the subway, then a bus met us at Snyder Avenue [the end of the subway]. Later, that summer, another hotel, the Ben Franklin, was needed for the large number of nurses reporting to the Naval Hospital for duty. Navy buses were soon used for service [to take the nurses back and forth to the hospital] which was much more convenient. . . . On reporting for duty, the large open wards were new to me. They were much different from private and semi-private civilian [hospital] wards. I was not familiar with the Corpsmen setup or any of the routines, but, because I had six years graduate [nurse] experience . . . I soon learned the routine. There were usually two nurses assigned to the wards plus four corpsmen for a.m. duty. The afternoon shift had one nurse that took care of two wards and [had] the same number of corpsmen. The ward medical officer made rounds every morning at eight [a.m.] before going to surgery. . . . Our patients were young sailors and veterans because this [hospital] originally was a VA [Veterans Administration] hospital."[149]

On 20 July 1942, Ensign Janina Smiertka is stationed at the Dispensary at the Navy Yard, Washington, D.C.. Nearby is a Naval Magazine [making ammunition] at Bellevue, D.C. where a First-Aid-Station is located. Miss Smiertka tells us that the Navy had been advertising for civilian nurses to work there, but "no civilian nurses were attracted to the position, even if the salary was good, because of prior explosions."[150] Therefore, Navy Nurses from the Navy Yard are sent to the Naval Magazine for the eight a.m. to three p.m. shift and for the three p.m. to eleven p.m. shift. On 20 July Miss Smiertka is working the three to eleven shift. At nine-twelve p.m. an explosion occurs. "One of the men workers was careless"[151] with one of the explosive ingredients. Another worker, a woman, is injured and dies the next day. "The explosion was like a low roaring boom and I knew what it was."[152] "Everybody was running out of the building and I was running in - feeling that somebody needed attention. When I got there, I couldn't do anything anyway. The ladies [women defense workers] that were hurt, we put them in the ambulance and took them up to the [Navy] Dispensary at the Navy Yard and from there the Naval doctors put these patients in private hospitals."[153] "The next day [the Officer-in-Charge of the Naval Magazine] interviewed me about the explosion and I . . . [asked] `who saw me?' . . . and he answered, `it was the Marine on the scaffold [above the building housing the First-Aid-Station] that saw you because you stuck out like a sore thumb in your white uniform and [he] saw your activities."[154] One week later, the Officer-in-Charge of the Naval Magazine forwards a Letter of Commendation to the Commandant of the Navy Yard. The letter says:

"1. On the occasion of the explosion at 9:12 p.m., Monday, 20 July 1942, at this activity, the Medical Department of the Yard arrived at Bellevue with doctors and ambulances within ten minutes after their receipt of a telephone call informing them of the explosion.

2. Immediately after the explosion, Ensign J. Smiertka, (NNC) U.S. Navy, and Blain, B.H. PhM2/c, U.S. Navy [Pharmacists Mate], then on duty at Bellevue, went calmly and efficiently about their duties of administering aid to the injured and calming the hysteria of employees until aid arrived from the Yard.

3. The immediate response of the Medical Department Personnel from the Yard and the effective manner in which Ensign Smiertka and PhM. Bain discharged their duties is worthy of high praise and commendation."[155]

The Commandant of the Navy Yard also presents Ensign Smiertka and PhM Bain with a Letter of Commendation. And yet, as you may have noticed, Miss Smiertka says in her narration, that she 'couldn't do anything.' It seems that this is how many Navy nurses feel about what they do; it is not anything special, it is what they are expected to do - it is their 'duty.'

Meantime, in January of 1942 at the Naval Hospital, Bremerton, Washington, Navy Nurse Norma Bartleson and three others receive "orders to go to the Naval Hospital in Pearl Harbor. Another nurse . . . received orders to the hospital ship, the USS *Solace*, docked in Pearl Harbor. The five of us left for San Francisco and sailed from there aboard [a] transport ship . . . and four of us experienced our first sea voyage while enroute to our first overseas duty station. There were many troops aboard the ship and about twenty-five newly graduated Annapolis midshipmen of the class of `42 who had graduated early. We spent eight days on a constantly changing course, zig-zagging to avoid enemy submarines. We traveled in a convoy of ships and I remember well the destroyer ships as they bobbed over the waves. They were smaller ships and the bobbing was more noticeable than with the other ships. There were general alerts day and night and we were instructed to get to our stations and life boat as quickly as possible when the alert was sounded. We arrived safely at Pearl Harbor, and looking around, a different view met our eyes. In Bremerton we had felt safe looking at ships, but in this harbor we saw nothing but devastation . . . . The waters were covered with oil and remained that way for many, many months. We were the first Navy Nurses to arrive in Pearl Harbor after the war had been declared. Soon after, more nurses were arriving from the East and West coasts and all sectors of the States. . . . I was assigned to the surgical ward and cared for the casualties of Pearl Harbor as well as battles of Midway [Island], Coral Sea, Guadalcanal and others. . . . I will always remember the battle of Midway [June 5-6, 1942] and the wounded who were brought to the hospital, many with [perforated] and distended abdomens as a result of being thrown into the waters with great impact resulting from the depth bombs that had been discharged. Although the sights and men in our eyes were heartbreaking, the knowledge that we were helping a world at war offered consolation."[156]

A few months after her arrival at Pearl, Miss Bartleson is given TAD orders to help evacuate women and children to the mainland aboard the transport USS *Republic*. She tells us that during the trip "another nurse from our ship was sent to another transport in our convoy to assist with a delivery [birth]. She was taken by boat across the water and we watched intently as she sailed across and then climbed up the Jacobs Ladder to get aboard the ship. All went well."[157] (Climbing a Jacobs Ladder of heavy rope with wooden rungs on the side of a moving ship in the middle of the ocean, is no mean feat!) When Norma Bartleson returns to Pearl Harbor, she returns to the "frequent alerts that sent us to the air raid shelters. We carried our gas masks and even tucked in a candybar in case we had to stay awhile. One afternoon the alert sounded and as we were walking hurriedly down the corridor, my friend said 'I have to go back to my room.' `What for?' I said. `I forgot my eyelash curler.' There was always some humor along the way. . . . We were allowed four uniforms [white wards] a week in the laundry [and] in a warm climate, this was more than sufficient [even though] our white uniform served both as duty and dress uniform. We did not wear civilian clothes except around the nurses quarters. We received our white dress uniforms later in 1942. Until then the dress uniform consisted of the white duty uniform, blue cap and anchor on it and gas masks carried over the shoulder. This was the uniform of the day and was to be worn during daylight hours away from the hospital compound. We often had to press our uniform in order to look our best for social occasions such as dances at the Officers Club which were held in the afternoon hours. After sundown we were always either on duty or at the nurses quarters."[158]

In April of 1942 at the Philadelphia Naval Hospital, Navy Nurse Ethel Battin receives orders to Pearl Harbor after only one year of active duty. "Jacob Reed and Sons [Company] in Philadelphia worked in great haste to make dress white uniforms for me and two other nurses who had received the same orders. [The Superintendent of the Nurse Corps, Sue Dauser] had requested that we wear these uniforms to shore upon arrival in Honolulu. [By the time they arrive in Honolulu the new legislation will be passed, they will be officers, and thus the uniform will be in order.] . . . For this trip we traveled the United States by train, taking four days; tickets supplied by the Navy. We were directed to keep an accurate statement of expenses during our travels, in order to submit a claim, [with] included receipts, so that we could be reimbursed after we reached our destination. Expenses were to be kept within Navy instructions; an example of this was [an] allowance for dinner [of] $1.25. We had a few days to explore San Francisco and then departed for Honolulu aboard a transport; sailing under the Golden Gate Bridge at sunset. There are few comforts, if any, aboard a military transport, but we manage to survive, forty nurses in all, as the convoy zig-zagged across the Pacific. Pearl Harbor was an awesome sight; so many sunken ships in the harbor and so many young men lost. The Navy Yard was very active repairing ships that had limped back to the Yard from the battle zone. . . . Gas masks were a constant companion. Marshall law and 'black-outs' were enforced. Patients coming from the battle areas had injuries and wounds of the type rarely seen, except in time of war, and new to many doctors and nurses. These patients came [in] on any ship that was returning to Pearl Harbor. Even an ocean liner that had been converted to a transport brought in a full load of patients. The slogan of the day was 'don't talk, the enemy is listening,' therefore, we had no idea what was happening, or how the war was progressing."[159]

"On December 7, 1942," Rachel Todd says, "twenty-four of us [Navy Nurses] sailed for Pearl on the USS *Henderson.* . . . We, along with three other ships, zigged and zagged across the Pacific for six days. One night at 0400 [4 a.m.], the alarm sounded and we all reported in robes to our assigned stations. We stood and stood, getting colder every minute, and we never saw a thing. Finally, the all clear sounded . . . whatever it was, we never saw anything.

"On arriving at Pearl we were met by LCdr. Gertrude Arnest, Chief Nurse [of] the U.S. Naval Hospital at Aiea Heights. With a cigarette hanging out of the corner of her mouth, she came to me and said, `I understand your family lives in Honolulu, do you suppose there's room for you to live at home?' [Rachel Todd was born and lived in Honolulu until going to the Mainland, the States, for her nurses training.] 'I'm sure there is,' I replied, 'my room is still available.' 'Fine,' she said, 'you can have Dispensary duty. Have your family come and pick you up.' It seems that apartments were very hard to come by and the nurses couldn't find anything, so, as long as I had a place to go, that relieved her of having to find quarters. . . . Anyway, I lived at home [and worked at the Dispensary] for the next two years and got overseas pay for this."[160]

Over on the Island of Guam, Marianas Islands, at the end of 1941 the captive Navy Nurses were packing for a forced removal from the island. On 8 January 1942, the Navy Nurses are all moved to the quarters of the native Guamanian nurses. On 10 January the five Navy Nurses, the wife of a Chief Petty Officer and her young baby, and their luggage are put on a pick-up truck and driven about five miles to the Navy Yard on Guam. All the men (Doctors, corpsmen, other officers and enlisted) are required to march to the Navy Yard. They are loaded aboard a Japanese ship, the *Argentina Maru*, along with all but two of the patients from the Naval Hospital. Of the two patients left behind, one is paralyzed from a bomb fragment and the other is a Chief Yeoman who had bullet and bayonet wounds. "He had been wounded by a machine gun at the taking of the island [and] when a Japanese commanded him to get up and he said he couldn't, the Japanese had stuck a bayonet in his chest."[161] (Navy Nurse Jackson also says that earlier, "I, myself, saw the bodies of the American Marines being brought in. I said to the corpsman later who was in the morgue at the time they came in following the invasion - 'What wounds were on those bodies?' and he said - 'Bayonet wounds.' I said - 'I thought so.' They were bayonet wounds in the back. The men who had surrendered had been required to strip off all of their clothing except shorts, had been searched, evidently had been required to kneel at the feet of the Japanese and had been bayoneted in the back."[162])

The men were sent to the cargo hold of the ship, below the water line. The patients and some corpsmen were put into a twelve-berth steward's cabin. The Navy Nurses, the CPO's wife and baby are placed in a four-berth stewardess' cabin in the hold of the ship. The nurses took turns in sleeping on the cabin's deck each night "but the deck being Japanese Tatami [woven mat] was just about as soft as [the] Japanese [mattresses] on the bunks so nobody . . . thought much about it."[163]

It takes five days at sea to reach their destination in Japan. During that time, they are given two meals a day consisting mainly of rice with weevils in it and a few times they receive fish or macaroni. The women are allowed on deck, most days, for half-an-hour and usually for twice a day, but always under guard. The morning of 15 January, the ship drops anchor in Japanese waters. The women are given two slices of bread for breakfast then around noon-time the crew left the ship, the heat was off and all is very quiet. "After nightfall we were taken up on deck and from there were put aboard a barge, which nearly upset in the process of loading."[164] Navy Nurse Jackson indicates that it is bitterly cold and the clothing of all the prisoners is inappropriate for the conditions. Further, some of the prisoner patients have only a sheet to cover them. She records that the ferry or barge is open and exposed to the elements except for the wheel-house and that the wheel-house is where the Japanese send the six women and the baby. They are taken to shore then driven to a Prisoner-of-War Camp in Zentsuji, Japan.[165] "The night that we arrived there, it was a cold wintry night . . . it was blowing and snowing."[166]

The Navy Nurses are taken to the second floor of a dimly lit, unheated, old Army barracks building where they are led into a large room with rows of mats placed on straw. There they find the prisoner patients that had been brought to Japan on the same ship with them. A Japanese officer indicates that the nurses are to occupy this room and sleep on the mats along with the patients. (The patients are not seriously ill and no longer require skilled nursing care; they are convalescing patients.)[167] Navy Nurse Fogarty says, "This very officious Japanese said, 'Patients sleep here, nurses sleep here.'. . . And I thought, 'Well, I'm not going to let that go by.' And so I said, `No. Patients sleep here, corpsmen sleep here.' He said, 'No. Patients sleep here, nurses sleep here.' I still said 'no.'"[168] Navy Nurse Jackson continues, "After considerable argument the [Japanese] Colonel came in and he said - 'Patients here and nurses here.' and we said - 'No.' He stamped his foot and walked out. . . . He came back eventually and directed us to another room . . . where we could have a little amount of privacy and [meantime] the hospital corpsmen shared the [room] with the patients."[169] About ten that night, the nurses finally receive some food; bread and what is supposed to be hot cabbage soup, but they decide is hot water. During the following days and weeks, the nurses have no nursing duties so they go about the business of keeping clothing in order for those in the camp. Miss Fogarty says that everyone tried to keep a good attitude and that some of the Navy officers and the corpsmen, also prisoners, came in to see them and talk with them from time to time. Mrs. Jackson notes that she did not see any brutality; there may have been some, but she never saw any. Then the question of their status as non-combatants comes up. The Japanese tell them that even as non-combatants, the doctors, nurses and corpsmen, if they are released, could be of service to the war effort. Therefore, they are not to be released. So they try to settle down for the duration even though "We are continually annoyed by Japanese soldiers, mostly the guards, who would come in and out of [the] dormitories anytime day or night, curiously examining all articles of clothing and possessions. Some guards are belligerent in attitude, others friendly, all are curious."[170]

On 10 March 1942, the five Navy Nurses are surprised to learn that they are to be moved to Kobe, Japan. They leave Zentsuji on 12 March, board a ship (under guard) and sail to Kobe, arriving the 13th of March. They are taken to what had been an old hotel and is called the 'eastern lodge' and where they are now interned. After some time, some missionary priests and an American missionary arrive, soon followed by other 'Allied nationals.' "The conditions of life at the detention house were considerably better than they had been at the camp. We had beds to sleep on and there was hot water . . . [for] about two or three hours during the morning." They are even allowed to go shopping, under guard, "on a couple of occasions. The Swiss [consul] had come and we were able to get a very limited amount of funds but, at least, we could buy some hose of which we were in desperate need. . . . . Then [in June] the Swiss consul came and notified us officially that we were all on the list to go home [including the woman from Guam and her baby]."[171]

Under guard they go by rail from Kobe to Yokohama and then aboard the *Asama Maru* in Yokohama Bay. The ship did not get under way and the next day the Naval Attache from Tokyo, Commander Smith-Hutton comes aboard to speak with the Navy Nurses. They give him their report of all they had endured "and he was extremely thoughtful to us and many of the things that needed straightening out were straightened out for us by the Naval Attache and the State Department."[172] (On June 25, 1942 The New York Times, in an article entitled 'Scheduled for Repatriation by the Japanese,' lists the names of the five Navy Nurses along with the other 624 Americans due to return from incarceration. The Times does not indicate that they are Navy Nurses, only their names are published.) They leave Yokohama on 25 June at night. Mrs. Jackson speaks of looking out the porthole, as they get under way, and seeing reflected in the water the large cross marked on the side of the ship; marking the ship as diplomatic. They go south to Hong Kong where they pick up another group of American internees. From there they go to French Indo-China where they pick up some diplomats and others before heading to Singapore. From Singapore they go through the Straits between Java and Sumatra. Miss Fogarty states, "when we were going through the Straits, we were later told that we were almost hit by an American submarine. They saw the Japanese ship and they were . . . aimed, ready to fire and all of a sudden they caught the red cross on the side and they held their fire."[173] They go across the Indian Ocean and up the east coast of Africa to Lourenco Marques in Portuguese East Africa (Mozambique.) It is here that they leave the *Asama Maru* and become 'free' once more. Better yet, there in the harbor awaits the white hulled diplomatic ship *Gripsholm*, flying the Swedish flag and waiting to take them home. The nurses and others who had been aboard the *Asama Maru*, are exchanged for Japanese prisoners. The Japanese go aboard the Japanese ship and the ones who had previously been aboard, now go aboard the neutral Swedish ship, the *Gripsholm*, in this 'diplomatic exchange of prisoners-of-war.'[174]

Meantime, Navy Nurse Fogarty tells us, "this young foreign service officer had seen my picture along with the other four nurses in the Osaka [newspaper] and he decided that he wanted to meet me. So after three days aboard [the *Asama Maru*] he found someone to introduce us and from that time . . . all during the day and in the evening he was my companion. It was two days before we got to port that we became engaged. . . . We expected to get married after we got back to New York, but when we arrived at Lourenco Marques there were orders for him from the State Department to proceed to Brazzaville in French Equatorial Africa. . . . So we decided maybe we could get married [in Lourenco Marques]. . . . We had to get permission from the diocese at Lourenco Marques to have the marriage there so two of our [Maryknoll] priests [from aboard the ship] went with my husband-to-be and myself over to the Archbishop's residence. . . . The Archbishop could speak in French and Portuguese and our [priests] could speak in English and maybe one of the oriental languages so Latin was the [language used] to discuss it. He gave permission and in the meantime my husband [to-be] had to consult a lawyer to get civil exoneration for a quick marriage [and he did]. . . . [As for the Navy,] we had two Naval Charge d'Affaires aboard [the ship]. One of them said, 'Don't do it, you'll be AWOL [Absent WithOut Leave].' The other said, 'It's quite all right. I'll cable the State Department and the Navy Department.' So he did and it came back with permission. . . . So we had permission from the church and civilian authorities and my Navy authorities. . . . So by Saturday noon it was all accomplished and one of the [Maryknoll] priests married us. The second [Maryknoll] priest was my husband's best man. . . . At that time when you were married, you were automatically out of the Navy. That was your resignation. . . . I did write a letter to Miss Dauser [Navy Nurse Corps Superintendent] after we arrived in Brazzaville and I apologized to her for my abrupt departure from the Navy. . . . She wrote back the nicest letter."[175] This is what the 2 October 1942 letter from the Superintendent says:

"My dear Mrs. Mann:
    Your letter of September 11, was indeed a welcome piece of mail. We are all so happy for you and never for a moment must you think that we had any harsh thoughts, for that was furthest from our minds. It was with comfort and satisfaction that we learned of your happy marriage, and we are inclined to agree with you that the choice you made is a wise choice.
    I am forwarding the information about your pay accounts to the department that was carrying your pay and also asking them to contact you if there is need for further correspondence regarding the matter.
    Needless to say how happy we were to welcome the four nurses who did arrive [home], and they all were so eager to tell us about your fortunate marriage, and they all spoke so highly of your husband. I am sure that you are hearing from some of these nurses and they are telling you whatever news might interest you. Naturally there will be a great deal that will have to wait for your return, but they will know what news will be of most interest to you.
    If at any time I can be of any service to you do not hesitate to let me hear from you.
    Wishing you all the success and happiness possible in your new life, I am,

                    Sincerely yours,

                    SUE S. DAUSER, R.N.
                    Supt., Navy Nurse Corps"

Chief Nurse Marion Olds, and Navy Nurses Leona Jackson, Lorraine Christiansen, and Doris Yetter leave Africa on the diplomatic ship *Gripsholm* which sails down the coast of Africa, around the Cape of Good Hope and across the southern Atlantic Ocean to Rio De Janeiro, Brazil. Mrs. Jackson tells us that "Rio is truly a beautiful city, many people have said that it is one of the three most beautiful ports in the world, and I will certainly never argue with them. It is one of the most beautiful places I have ever seen, but I assure you that nothing has ever looked so good to me as the Statue of Liberty in New York Harbor."[176] The *Gripsholm* arrives in New York harbor on Tuesday, the 24th of August 1942. Mrs. Jackson says, "After we docked we had a little session with the FBI and the ONI and the Army Intelligence and a few other people."[177] From there they report to the Bethesda Naval Hospital, Maryland for medical exams[178] and reports for the Navy Department in Washington, D.C.. In the following days they are given some official leave before returning to Navy nursing duties.[179] Chief Nurse Marion Olds receives orders to the Naval Hospital at Charleston, South Carolina. Navy Nurses Lorraine Christiansen and Doris Yetter are sent to the Naval Dispensary at Long Beach, California.[180] In December 1942, an item in the AJN notes that "almost one hundred Navy nurses [are] assigned to assist with physical examination of WAVES applicants. . . . They are assigned all over the United States in offices and universities. . . . Mrs. Leona Close Jackson . . . has been assigned to the Naval Officer Procurement Office in Washington. She will assist in physical examinations of the WAVES."[181]
    In September 1942, the American Journal of Nursing reports that "Some Army and Navy nurses are proudly wearing service ribbons on their uniforms. The American Defense Service Medal is authorized for issue to all military personnel including nurses, for honorable service of twelve months or longer, at any time between September 8, 1939 and December 7, 1942. Since the medal has not been and will not be issued for the present, the ribbon only is worn. It is gold color, about 3/8 inches by 1 3/8 inches with vertical red, white, and blue stripes 1/4 inch from each end. . . . There will be another service medal some time in the near future for Navy personnel,

including Navy nurses, who were engaged in the evacuation of civilians at the time Shanghai was being bombed by the Japanese."[182] Now that Navy Nurses are also Navy Officers, they are eligible for these richly deserved awards.

Back in January of 1942, when the Navy Nurses at the Bremerton, Washington Naval Hospital received their 'dispatch' (immediate) orders, one of those nurses had orders to the hospital ship *Solace*. Her name is Frances Quebbeman. She accompanied the others to Pearl Harbor where she finds and boards the ship. She writes that, "The *Solace* headed south the latter part of February and we arrived in Pago Pago, Samoa where we stayed for a month then went on to Tonga [The Tonga Islands are 'about 3,000 miles southwest of Honolulu.'[183]]. ... Then to New Caledonia to await the first casualties. ... Duty aboard the *Solace* was the most memorable of my Navy career. A wonderful and enthusiastic staff of nurses and doctors who all worked tirelessly whether sea sick or not. How many trips from the forward area to Mobile Hospitals in Auckland and Wellington, New Zealand and to Mobile Army Medical Units in Figi? We were soon adept in loading patients quickly, sometimes 500 in two hours and then names, rates, serial numbers, life boat stations, sight muster, x-rays done prior to clearing the harbor. Three nights and days when we traveled blacked out and reached debarkation points. Then ashore for a few brief hours, back North and do the same. The nurses in New Zealand greeted us each trip with a bouquet of flowers. The government of New Zealand sponsored our trip to Rotorua [a health resort in the Hot Springs District[184]] where the Maoris sang for us - that was while the ship was in dry dock."[185]

On the last day of September 1942, several Navy Nurses, stationed at San Diego Naval Hospital, received 'dispatch' orders. Ensign Ruth Moeller is one of the nurses and she says, "Very unexpectedly on September 30, 1942 I received my orders for the [hospital ship] *Solace*. I had been in the service for six months. I recall that there were many nurses who were disgruntled about the fact that I had only been in the service such a short time and received my orders to a hospital ship. Why I received them I have no idea, but I did. That was the plum assignment - to go to the South Pacific and be on a hospital ship where all the action was. So I received my orders with the stipulation that I was to report to the Commandant in San Francisco ... on October 1 which was the next day. I did not receive these orders until approximately nine o'clock in the morning when I was on duty in the clinic and was told, 'You are being detached.' I was not able to turn over the clinic to anybody. I just told them I was leaving. I ran all the way from the Naval Hospital [to the nurses quarters] because there was no transportation. Buses used to take us. A bus would pick us up and take us to Balboa Park [nurses quarters area] which was some little distance and bring us back again to the hospital. ... So I ran over all the way to tell my roommates and ask them to get my gear together (all my civilian gear, etcetera) and pack those things up and send them to my folks. In those few hours that I had, I threw whatever uniforms I had into my suitcases and the Red Cross picked me up. There were several other nurses involved in this. The Red Cross took us over to the paymaster to pick up our records there and we got our health records. The Red Cross called the [train] station and asked [that] the train be delayed a little bit so we could make the train from San Diego to San Francisco. We left about twelve or one o'clock. ... We had to travel all night into the morning of October 1 in order to report to the Commandant of the 12th Naval District [in San Francisco] according to our orders. After doing that, provisions had been made for us to stay at [a] hotel. ... Nothing in our orders stated a perdiem [per day pay while traveling on orders]. We were drawing ninety dollars per month. We were there a matter of weeks because there wasn't any transportation available. [No ship to take them to the hospital ship *Solace*, out in the Pacific.] Most of us ate two meals a day. I finally, as some of the other nurses did, contacted home and asked them to send some money because there was nothing in our orders except for drawing on subsistence [small amount allowed for living out of government quarters]. Ninety dollars a month is all we had to pay our hotel bill and our meals.

"The people of San Francisco were very nice. I think we were probably the first Navy nurses in uniform. We had just received our uniforms, so they would talk [to us] and we were invited out for meals and there were some social things that were planned for us. Some other [Navy] nurses came a little bit late and we were all housed in the [same hotel].

"After all the hurrying from September 30 and arriving on October 1, finally on November 24 we were all detached to go to the South Pacific to meet up with the USS *Solace*. The ship we were assigned to was the USS *Mount Vernon* which was a converted luxury liner; a huge ship. They were carrying enlisted personnel and officers on this ship. We were not able to get a ship prior to this time because there were so few ships, so much going on in the war zones and they needed all the ammunition and supplies and medical equipment they could get. . . . So we had to wait such a long time, but there was good reason for it. . . . We were on that ship for Thanksgiving and until December 12 when we were detached at Noumea, New Caledonia [an island about 800 miles east of Australia]. The interesting thing about Noumea was the fact that there were all these Marines and they had never seen a Navy nurse before. We were all in uniform. . . . [The song `White Christmas' had just come out when these nurses had left the States so, since it is so close to Christmas, these nurses introduced these Marines to the song; `I'm Dreaming of a White Christmas.'] That song always brings back so many memories. These were all fighting men, the troops, the Marines and the Navy people. This was when we were ashore for a little while before we got on [board another] ship and traveled down to New Zealand where we got the *Solace*. . . . Miss Lally was the Chief Nurse aboard the ship when we reported aboard. She was only in civilian clothes; she did not have a uniform at that time, nor did any of the nurses who were aboard the hospital ship. We were all Reserves who went out there and relieved [some of the] nurses who were aboard."[186]

It is in November of 1942 that the first "detachments of Navy nurses leave [the] West Coast for [the] South Pacific. LT(jg) Jessie B. Crump (NC) USN [leaves to become the] Chief Nurse for [the] USN Mobile Hospital #4, Auckland, New Zealand. LT(jg) Ida M. Ildstead (NC) USN [goes to the] USN Base Hospital #2 [at] Efate, New Hebrides [a South Pacific Island group]. Ensign Hazel B. Allison (NC) USN [leaves for] Base #4 [at] Wellington, New Zealand."[187]

Out in the Philippine Islands, in January 1942, Navy Nurse Ann Bernatitis is with the Army at a Bataan Field Hospital at Limay, called Hospital #1. She tells us, "things were getting pretty heavy. The front lines weren't holding and they were beginning to retreat so the hospital had to be moved further down the [Bataan] peninsula. On January twenty-third, the hospital moved to `Little Baggio.' [Named after `Baggio' a Philippine summer resort area.] There we found the wards set up. There was an operating room and there was a nurses quarters with a mess hall for the officers and there was a building for the doctors. . . . Things were generally better, but we worked very hard. . . . On March the thirtieth of `42, the hospital was bombed even though we had a red cross on top of it. The Japanese apologized saying it was a mistake, but on April the seventh, it was bombed again; one of the bombs hitting directly in a ward among the ward patients. It was really tragic to see. And at that time, two of the Army Nurses were injured by shrapnel."[188] "We were located right next to an ammunition dump . . . they were looking for the ammunition dump . . . instead they caught us."[189] "Things quieted down for a while, but we were overcome by medical patients, especially dysentery, malnutrition, beri-beri. . . . By this time, rations were really low. All the time we were on Bataan, it was two meals a day; about nine in the morning and four in the afternoon. . . . There wasn't much to eat. So anyway, [with] all the medical patients coming in, the operating room [nurses] were not busy helping the doctors in the operating room, but [we] were busy. We saved all the dressings, washed them, re-sterilized them and mended [surgical gloves,] patch after patch on the gloves. . . . Everybody did their best. We always claimed that help was going to come; that a convoy was going to steam in. In fact, there was a tree right outside the operating room and someone had built a platform up in it and every day somebody would climb that platform to scan the horizon to see if the convoy was coming.

"We had some Japanese patients in the prison section. In fact, I remember going down with [one of the doctors] one day to put a Kirschner wire in a Japanese's leg. I remember saying, 'He doesn't have a pillow case on his pillow.' And [the doctor] said, `Listen girl, you forget, he's your enemy. This is war. You don't have white sheets and white pillow cases.' It's funny how it all goes back [to your basic nurses' training]: 'he's a patient and he should have the best, regardless; war or not war, enemy or not enemy'. . . . Then April comes along when we receive word that the frontlines are falling back . . . and that they're going to evacuate the nurses."[190] "Everybody was coming down the [Bataan] peninsula and from the peninsula there was no place to go, but Corregidor and actually Corregidor wasn't big enough to hold all the forces from Bataan and . . . there was no way to get them over there . . . they didn't have that many small boats and they had no ships of any kind. . . . One evening about eight or nine . . . two days before Bataan fell . . . they were evacuating all the nurses to Corregidor. . . . They got us in buses and we started down to where the boat would come in to pick us up. A very treacherous road, it was steep and all down grade. . . . As we started it was dark, no lights on the bus, no headlights. As we were going down we would meet tanks that were coming up. . . . Some [tanks] were coming down . . . because the front lines had broken and everybody was retreating down. I remember some of the [troops] would try to hang on to the windows [of the bus] . . . so they could ride part of the way. They'd make us close the windows so they couldn't do that. The road was so dangerous they could hang on to [the bus] and all of a sudden just drop off and go down a gully. . . . Finally we get down there [and] there's no boat. . . . Then finally a boat came over and we got on it and all the time we were going . . . across, the Japs were shelling . . . over towards Corregidor so you never knew just quite what was going to happen to you. . . . [It's] getting close to midnight when all this is happening. But, you know, there you sit on that boat and everybody left somebody behind that they were especially friendly with, feeling bad, wondering what's going to happen and what have you. And we get over to Corregidor, finally. . . . They had, I think it was, ambulances waiting for us when we got off the boat and just pushed us in the back and took us up to the tunnels where the hospital was. . . . Corregidor is a rock with a lot of tunnels. It's all tunnels, nothing but tunnels."[191]

"They took us up to the tunnel where the hospital was. . . . They weren't expecting us apparently, because no provisions were made for where we were going to sleep. So, that night we slept two in the bed, you know, [the] head to toe thing. . . . While I was on Corregidor, I only worked one day in the operating room because I had amoebic dysentery. I wasn't very active, you know, staying close. I forget what kind of medicine they were giving me, copper something or another and coppery powder that you mixed in water and had to swallow. So you kind of stayed in the nurses section in the quarters . . . we couldn't go outside except only maybe at night. You would go just outside the tunnel, but not very far because every time you got out there they might start shelling. . . . Then on April the 29th was when [word was received] that two Navy PBY's [seaplanes] were coming in and they would be evacuating some people. No one knows how people were picked to be on that, but I wasn't one of [the ones] picked. . . . You know, everybody knew that there was that one lone Navy nurse there . . . on Corregidor. . . . They'd say, 'Hey, how come they didn't load you on the PBY?' I'd say, 'Haven't you heard? I'm waiting for the Army to come in and rescue me.' . . . So they [the PBY's and the evacuees] went out but, unfortunately, they went to, I think it was, Mindanao [another island in the Philippines] first and, I think, they [the PBY's] damaged their landing pontoons or something . . . they did repair one of [the PBY's] enough to take off, but all [the people left behind at Mindanao] were taken prisoner. . . .

"Life on Corregidor resumed, then] on May the third [1942], I remember being told to report to the mess hall in the afternoon. And we [Ann and eleven Army nurses] were told that we were going to be leaving that night. . . . We were to meet in the tunnel [twenty-six people] . . . early in the evening. . . . [We met and were] standing around when the Japanese started shelling `The Rock' so they had to postpone [leaving] until later that night. Then [when gathering together later that night, someone called] your name, you stood up [and] General Wainwright [who had replaced General MacArthur] shook your hand, wished you 'God speed' and said, 'Tell them how it is here.' Then [you] got in the car and off you went to the dock. It was pitch black."[192] "Nobody talking together - this is all silence. We get down to the docks and there's a small launch waiting for us. We get into that and it started off. It just seemed like we rode for ever so long. Everything pitch black. Nobody saying a word. Then, all of a sudden, we were going through the mine fields. You see, that's where the submarine had come in and was waiting for us. And finally, out of nowhere, this big, black shadow appears and it was the submarine. Just as we got up to the submarine, the Japanese, over on Bataan, started playing their searchlights on the water. . . . Well, no time was lost, I can assure you. You had to get over the rail [on the submarine]. Someone got hold of your hand as you were getting over the rail, and gave you a yank. You were on something solid; you'd hear this water sloshing against the side of the submarine and then suddenly you were going down a hole. You get to the bottom of the hole and it's all bright and lighted and everybody is looking at you."[193] The evacuees "consisted of *thirteen* women (eleven [Army] Nurses, one Navy Nurse, one civilian) six Army Colonels, and six Naval Officers; the ship U.S.S. *Spearfish*; the rendezvous point - a spot in the China sea four and one half miles S.W. of Corregidor P.I.."[194] Miss Bernatitis tells us there were also, "two stowaways. [The two stowaways were: `One Navy enlisted and one civilian that was with Army Transportation.'[195]] They [the stowaways] just walked aboard on the launch. . . . If you had the nerve to get on that launch, no one had the nerve to say you can't go."[196] Corregidor fell to the Japanese just two days after Ann and her companions left.

The submarine USS *Spearfish*, which had been on a successful patrol for several weeks, heads for its base in Australia. It takes seventeen days to travel the three thousand miles from Corregidor.[197] With the evacuees the submarine has "a [fifty percent] personnel overload"[198] so that sleeping arrangements, among other things, are critical. The women are assigned to the Chief's quarters which has just four bunks in it. "We were assigned shifts to sleep; eight hours to sleep. [This] meant one of the shifts had an extra girl so they'd take turns. They'd either double up in the bunk or one would sleep on the deck. . . . If you got tired of staying in the mess hall, and playing cards or listening to records, talking, you'd look for a place to sleep or lay down. Space was just not available for things like that. One of the favorite spots was the radio shack. The radioman had his bench right in front of the panel and there was enough space between the bulkhead and his bench where someone could lay flat if they put their feet up [on] the bulkhead. . . . You would find someone laying there all the time. Across the hall . . . was the yeoman's office. That was filled with mattress covers filled with paper. You know they never threw anything overboard, paper especially. They'd put it in [mattress covers] and save it until they hit port. So this room was filled with mattress covers filled with paper. . . . You'd find somebody [lying] on top of those. . . . We got into Freemantle, Australia on the 20th of May."[199]

They are met and welcomed; Navy Nurse Bernatitis by the Navy Admiral there as well as others. After a few days, Miss Bernatitis flies to Melbourne where she eventually boards a liner, taken over by the military, to return to the States. She arrives in New York then goes down to Washington, D.C. to give her reports. She speaks with Captain Dauser who takes her in to the Surgeon General and a press conference is held. Also, she is taken out to Bethesda to get her uniforms, since she is now a Naval Officer (Ensign) in the Nurse Corps. After a period of leave, she reports to the Bethesda Naval Hospital for duty where she not only has her nursing duties, she is also asked to do public relations work by going on Bond drives to help sell War Bonds, to speak at Chamber of Commerce meetings, various banquets, and other gatherings.[200] (Later on Ann Bernatitis is awarded the Legion of Merit Medal. It is the first Legion of Merit ever awarded to anyone.[201])

On 1 January of 1942, in the Philippine Islands, the city of Manila falls into the hands of the Japanese. There are eleven Navy nurses still in the city at their hospital at Santa Scholastica. Chief Nurse, of the small Navy Unit, writes, "Jan. 1st, 1942 - Capt. Rob't Davis, C.O. interned our [Medical] Staff and [patients]. Japanese troops on outskirts of City of Manila. Manila burning."[202] Another of the Navy Nurses writes, "New Year's Day ushered in a new life for us. Across the street where Japanese prisoners had been quartered we saw them released, they all shouted `Banzai' and waved miniature Rising Sun Flags at us as the Japanese Army marched in. The next day we were prisoners. Our men were immediately set to work stringing barbed wire to fence us in. At night Jap sentries moved through our sleeping quarters every half-hour stamping their feet as they walked to insure that you didn't sleep. Sometimes you would awaken to find a bayonet stuck through your mosquito netting and a Jap sentry leering over [you]. Providentially none of us were harmed."[203] For 6 January, Miss Cobb writes, "Our Unit was officially taken over by the [Japanese] Army. During [the] next 8 weeks, as our wounded recuperated, groups were transferred to prison camps located in Manila. One or two M.D's were transferred with them."[204] Navy Nurse Margaret Nash tells us that she remembers "the day when the Japanese Commandant came in . . . and told us we were under the Imperial Japanese Army and gave our Captain the instructions [of] what they expected. . . . So, as usual, we lived day by day and night by night. In the ward, some of our Filipino patients escaped . . . they would just ride out with their people. I don't know how [the Japanese] found out about it, but anyway they did . . . and a few days after, the higher command of the Japanese Imperial Army came by and told our Captain that if any more patients escaped, the Captain, the doctor on the ward, the corpsmen on the ward and the nurse on the ward, which, of course, happened to be me, would be shot. . . . But then the Filipinos were more cooperative with us and they realized what they were putting us through."[205]

Then on 8 March the Navy Nurses are interned at the Santo Tomas civilian internment camp in Manila. The camp's "population was approximately 3540. This heterogenous collection of people included every character imaginable from the highest to the lowest - Society people, businessmen, professional people - the prostitute and beachcomber. . . . Seventy percent were Americans, most of them Manila residents. The British totaled [twenty-eight percent] and the other remaining nationalities - such as - 30 Polish, 28 Netherlanders, one each Belgian, Mexican, Nicaraguan and Cuban. Approximately [thirty-eight percent] of this group were women. There were about 300 children under 12 years of age. The camp was predominately middle aged, this included several hundred married couples - who were required to live separately."[206] Navy Nurse Edwina Todd recalls that, "On arrival in Santo Tomas hundreds of men, women, and children gathered to see who we were and what our entry was about. They watched while we were searched by both Japanese and Civilian Internee Guards. After three or four hours had elapsed they realized they had no room for us so that night we all slept on the floor in the small dispensary in the main building. The next day an unused classroom was opened."[207] "We were in [a] room with sixty-nine other people. . . . [Our] beds were lined up along side the windows. . . . The bed was there and whatever you had accumulated you stowed under the bed. In order to get out in the morning, you'd have to go over the bottom because the beds were all so close together. Then surrounding us were all the civilians and some of the mothers that were in there. . . . We also had some youngsters [under five or six years old] in there with their mothers. . . . And all the rooms . . . were about the same size . . . because they were the class rooms of [the] Santo Thomas College . . . [a] big University run by the Dominican Fathers . . . [and] turned into an internment camp. . . . Then we started working in the [camp] hospital."[208]

"Two Rockefeller Foundation men [Doctors] with the help of [another Doctor] opened the [beginning] camp hospital. An old Mineralogy building was cleaned out and with a few donated beds and medicines brought into camp by these doctors, the hospital [had] started functioning. As [the] weeks went by this institution increased to a 60 bed hospital. . . . [And its Out Patient] Clinic was a very busy place treating over 50 percent of the camp. There were 2 isolation tents where TB's [tubercular patients] and venereal cases were isolated. . . . Professional medical people donated their services to the running of the Hospital. Several Filipino doctors and Filipino Red Cross nurses volunteered their services to the Camp to help Civilian Nurses and Doctors. The Navy nurses volunteered their services immediately upon arrival (March 1942) in Camp which helped the situation. By July 15, 1942, the Japanese issued an order prohibiting most of the Filipino Red Cross Nurses entering the Camp. This created a situation which was relieved by 6 Maryknoll Sisters, from St. Paul's Hospital in Manila, being permitted to enter Camp and give their services to the Hospital."[209] Meanwhile, on 2 July, the Japanese brought the Army Nurses, captured during the fall of Corregidor, to Santo Tomas, but placed them in isolation from the rest of the camp's internees. They were placed in a school across the street from Santa Tomas until August when they joined the rest of the camp. Also, at that time, the Japanese agree to the transfer of the Camp Hospital over to the larger quarters of the school where the Army nurses had been.[210] The Army Nurses, after resting from their ordeals at Bataan and Corregidor, then join with the Navy Nurses to provide professional services at the Camp Hospital and to the rest of the internees.

Back in the States, in Philadelphia, on Tuesday morning the 14th of July, 1942, a morning newspaper (the Philadelphia Inquirer) carries a news item entitled "11 NURSES MISSING IN MANILA SECTOR." The subtitle is, "Some or All May Be Jap Captives, Navy Announces." Parts of the article state, "Eleven Navy nurses were officially reported missing today in the Navy's seventh casualty list of the war. The young women were last heard from in the Manila Bay area prior to the conquest of that section by the Japanese early in the war. . . . The only Navy nurse now known to have escaped from the Manila area was Miss Ann Agnes Bernatitus native of Exeter, PA. She went from Manila to Bataan Peninsula with an Army medical group when American forces retreated into that wilderness stronghold, later was assigned to the island of Corregidor and eventually was removed from there to Australia by submarine." The Navy Nurses may be missing, but they are not forgotten and they carry on, as best they can, as Navy Nurse Nash has said, "day by day and night by night," as prisoners of war throughout the rest of 1942.

[1]   Goble, CDR Dorothy Jones, NC USN (Ret.), information from her unpublished history research notes.

[2]   Information prepared by the Navy Nurse Corps Officers on the staff of the Director of the Navy Nurse Corps, prior to 1972.

[3]   Goble, op. cit..

[4]   Information prepared by the Navy Nurse Corps Officers on the staff of the Director, op. cit..

[5]   Laird, LCDR Thelma NC USNR, Jones, LCDR Dorothy NC USN, Feeney, LCDR Elizabeth NC USN, Seidl, CDR Elizabeth NC USN (Ret.), Blaska, CDR Burdette NC USN, *Chronological History NAVY NURSE CORPS*, Prepared by: Nursing Division, Bureau of Medicine and Surgery, 1 August 1962, p. 21.

[6]   "Navy Nurse Corps," *NWMM News (National Womens Military Museum)*, Researched by Isabel Van Lom, NWM Museum, P.O. Box 68687, Portland, Oregon 97268, December 1990, p. 4.

[7]   Laird, et al, op. cit., pp. 21, 22.

[8]   Hickey, Dermott Vincent, *The First Ladies In The Navy - A History of the Navy Nurse Corps, 1908-1939*, June 1963, P. 143.

[9]   Goodnow, Minnie, R.N., *Nursing History*, W.B. Saunders Company, Philadelphia and London, 1948, p. 270.

[10]   Jamieson, Elizabeth M., B.A., R.N., Sewall, Mary F., B.S., R.N., *Trends In Nursing History*, W.B. Saunders Company, Philadelphia, 1944, p. 551.

[11]   Wells, H.G., *The Outline of History*, Revised and brought up to date by Raymond Postgate, Garden City Books, Garden City, New York, Volume II, 1961, pp. 924-926.

[12]   *The World Book Encyclopedia*, Field Enterprises Educational Corporation, Chicago, Volume 16, 1966 edition, p. 419.

[13]   *Great Events of the 20th Century*, Editor: Richard Marshall, The Readers' Digest Association, Inc., 1977, p. 297.

[14]   Wells, H.G., op. cit., pp. 926-928.

[15]   Ibid., p. 928.

[16]   Ibid., p. 929.

[17]   Ibid..

[18]   *The World Book Encyclopedia*, Field Enterprises Educational Corporation, Chicago, Volume 20, 1966 edition, p. 385.

[19]   Roberts, Mary M., R.N., *American Nursing History and Interpretation*, The MacMillan Company, New York, 1963, p. 665.

[20]   *The World Book Encyclopedia*, op. cit., Volume 16, p. 419.

[21]   Jamieson and Sewall, op. cit., p. 513.

[22]   Ibid..

[23]   *Nurse Corps, U.S. Navy Monthly Census*, Xerox copy, figures from Monthly Reports of Superintendent, Nurse Corps, to Bureau of Naval Personnel (Planning & Control Div.)

[24]   "The Naval Reserve Nurse Corps," *The American Journal of Nursing*, Volume 41, No. 4, April 1941, pp. 385, 386.

[25]   Bernatitis, Ann Capt. NC USN (Ret.), *Oral History Interview Tape Transcript*, Interviewer Irene Smith Matthews Lt(jg) Navy Nurse Corps, taped 19 May 1971.

[26]   Ibid..

[27]   Ibid..

[28]   Bernatitis, Ann Capt. NC USN (Ret.), *Oral History Interview Tape Transcript*, Interviewer Capt. Doris M. Sterner NC USN (Ret), taped 7 May 1990.

[29]   Bernatitis, Interviewer Irene Matthews, op. cit..

[30]   Bernatitis, Interviewer Doris M. Sterner, op. cit..

[31]   Laird, et al, op. cit., p. 22.

[32]   Wells, H.G., op. cit., p. 978.

[33]   Ibid., p. 931.

[34]   Ibid., p. 933.

[35]   Ibid..

[36]   Tily, James C., *The Uniforms of the United States Navy*, Thomas Yoseloff, Publisher, 8 East 36th Street, New York 16, New York, 1964, pp. 250 and 256.

[37]   Laird, et al, op. cit., p. 22.

[38]   *Nurse Corps, U.S. Navy Monthly Census*, op. cit., pp. 2 and 3.

[39]   "Red Cross Nursing Service In World War II," *The History of the American National Red Cross*, by: Portia B. Kernodle, Administrative Unit, The American National Red Cross, Washington, D.C., 1950, Volume XVI, pp. 261, 262.

[40]   Ibid., p. 262.

[41]   Laird, et al, op. cit., p. 22.

[42]   Tuchman, Barbara W., *The March of Folly from Troy to Vietnam*, Ballantine Books Edition by arrangement with Alfred A. Knopf, Inc., New York, March 1985, p. 31.

[43]   Ibid., pp. 31, 32.

[44]   Dana, Phyllis M., former Navy Nurse, *Oral History Interview Tape Transcript*, self interview, 28 February 1991.

[45]   Entrikin, Helen, retired Navy Nurse Corps Officer, *Oral History Interview Tape Transcript*, self interview, 12 August 1990.

[46]   Erickson, Ruth Capt. NC USN (Ret.), *Oral History Interview Tape Transcript*, Interviewer LCdr. Alice Laning NC USN (Ret.), 9 January 1990.

[47]   Matthews, Irene Lt(jg) Navy Nurse Corps, *Oral History Tape with Grace Lally, Transcript*, unpublished transcription.

[48]   Van Atta, Burr, "Grace B. Lally; nurse on Pearl Harbor ship," *Philadelphia Inquirer*, 23 June 1983.

[49]   "Succor Aboard the Solace," *Army and Navy Nurses in World War II*, Edited and designed by Wallace and Anne Clark, Military Nurse Publishing Company, 230 W. 41st Street, New York 18, New York.

[50]   Dixon HC USN, Lt. Ben F., "The `White Lily,'" *Hospital Corps QUARTERLY*, Hospital Ships Number, July 1945, p. 3.

[51]   Newcomb, Ellsworth, "The Solace:Mercy Ship," *Great Adventures in Nursing*, Helen Wright and Samuel Rapport, editors, Harper and Brothers, New York, 1960, pp. 264, 265.

[52]   Dana, op. cit..

[53]   Erickson, op. cit..

[54]   Curto, LCdr Christine NC USN, "Nurse Pioneers and the Hospital Ship *Relief*," *Navy Medicine*, Jan Kenneth Herman, editor, Department of the Navy, Bureau of Medicine and Surgery, Washington, DC, Vol. 82, No. 3, May-June 1991, p. 24.

[55]   "LT. (jg) LAURA M. COBB, (NC) USN, NOW A PRISONER OF WAR IN THE PHILIPPINES," *Biographical Sketch*, reproduced at National Archives, from Navy Nurse Corps Historical Documents, Box #2, National Archives, Washington, D.C..

[56]   Ibid., page 2.

[57]   Information obtained from the file card of Mary F. Hay's assignments, Bureau of Medicine and Surgery, Washington, D.C., provided by Captain Joan Engel Nurse Corps USN, Deputy Director, Navy Nurse Corps, 1993.

[58]   Information obtained from the file card of Helen C. Hunter's assignments, Bureau of Medicine and Surgery, Washington, D.C., provided by Captain Joan Engel Nurse Corps USN, Deputy Director, Navy Nurse Corps, 1993.

[59]   Nelson, Lt. Mary Rose Harrington, former Navy Nurse, *Oral History Interview Tape Transcript*, Interviewer LCdr. Alice Lanning NC USN (Ret.), 12 August 1989.

[60]   Information obtained from the file card of Goldia A. Merrill's assignments, Bureau of Medicine and Surgery, Washington, D.C., provided by Captain Joan Engel Nurse Corps USN, Deputy Director, Navy Nurse Corps, 1993.

[61]   "Lieutenant Eldene Elinor Paige, (NC) USN," *Biographical Sketch*, reproduced at National Archives, from Navy Nurse Corps Historical Documents, Box #2, National Archives, Washington, D.C..

[62]   "LCDR SUSIE JOSEPHINE PITCHER, (NC) USN, RET. (Deceased)," *Biographical Sketch*, reproduced at National Archives, from Navy Nurse Corps Historical Documents, Box #2, National Archives, Washington, D.C..

[63]   "LIEUTENANT DOROTHY STILL, (NC) USN," *Biographical Sketch*, reproduced at National Archives, from Navy Nurse Corps Historical Documents, Box #2, National Archives, Washington, D.C..

[64]   Information obtained from the file card of Edwina C. Todd's assignments, Bureau of Medicine and Surgery, Washington, D.C., provided by Captain Joan Engel Nurse Corps USN, Deputy Director, Navy Nurse Corps, 1993.

[65]   Bernatitis, Ann Capt. NC USN (Ret.), *Oral History Interview Tape Transcript*, Interviewer Doris M. Sterner, op. cit..

[66]   Nelson, Lt. Mary Rose Harrington, former Navy Nurse, op. cit..

[67]   Todd, CDR. C. Edwina (NC) USN, "NURSING UNDER FIRE," speech presented at the annual convention of the Association of Military Surgeons, Detroit, Michigan, October 9-11, 1946, then printed in *The Military Surgeon*, Vol. 100, No. 4, April 1947, p. 74.

[68]   Nash, CDR Margaret A. NC USN (Ret.), *Oral History Interview Tape Transcript*, Interviewer Florence Alwyn Twyman NC USN (Ret.), 28 September 1990.

[69]   Cobb, LCdr. Laura NC USN, Handwritten notes on notebook paper, reproduced at National Archives, from Navy Nurse Corps Historical Documents, Box #2, National Archives, Washington, D.C..

[70]   Bernatitis, Ann Capt. NC USN (Ret.), *Oral History Interview Tape Transcript*, Interviewer Doris M. Sterner, op. cit..

[71]   Cobb, LCdr. Laura NC USN, Handwritten notes on notebook paper, op. cit..

[72]   Nash, CDR Margaret A. NC USN (Ret.), *Oral History Interview Tape Transcript*, op. cit..

[73]   Cobb, LCdr. Laura NC USN, Handwritten notes on notebook paper, op. cit..

[74]   Nash, CDR Margaret A. NC USN (Ret.), *Oral History Interview Tape Transcript*, op. cit..

[75]   Bernatitis, Ann Capt. NC USN (Ret.), *Oral History Interview Tape Transcript*, Interviewer Doris M. Sterner, op. cit..

[76]   Kallsch, Philip A., Kallsch, Beatrice J., "Nurses Under Fire:The World War II Experience of Nurses on Bataan and Corregidor," *Nursing Research*, Vol. 25, No. 6, November-December 1976, pp. 410,411.

[77]   Bernatitis, Ann Capt. NC USN (Ret.), *Oral History Interview Tape Transcript*, Interviewer Doris M. Sterner, op. cit..

[78]   Manning, Michele Major USMC, "Angels of Mercy and Life Amid Scenes of Conflict and Death: The Combat Experience and Imprisonment of American Military Nurses in the Philippines 1941-1945," *STUDENT RESEARCH AND WRITING AY: 1984-85*, Marine Corps Command and Staff College Education Center, Marine Corps Development and Education Command, Quantico, Virginia 22134, 1 April 1985, pp. 12, 14.

[79]   Bernatitis, Ann Capt. NC USN (Ret.), *Oral History Interview Tape Transcript*, Interviewer Doris M. Sterner, op. cit..

[80]   Cobb, LCdr. Laura NC USN, Handwritten notes on notebook paper, op. cit..

[81]   Ibid..

[82]   Nelson, Lt. Mary Rose Harrington, former Navy Nurse, op. cit..

[83]   Information obtained from the file card of Lorraine Halliday's assignments, Bureau of Medicine and Surgery, Washington, D.C., provided by Captain Joan Engel Nurse Corps USN, Deputy Director, Navy Nurse Corps, 1993.

[84]   Barnes, Sylvia Lavache Navy Nurse, *Written Personal History*, May 1991, p. 5.

[85]   Mann, Virginia Fogarty Navy Nurse, *Oral History Interview Tape Transcript*, Interviewers Capt. Doris M. Sterner NC USN (Ret.) and CDR. Patricia Warner NC USN (Ret.), 13 December 1989.

[86]   Information obtained from the file card of Doris M. Yetter's assignments, Bureau of Medicine and Surgery, Washington, D.C., provided by Captain Joan Engel Nurse Corps USN, Deputy Director, Navy Nurse Corps, 1993.

[87]   Olds, Marion Chief Nurse U.S. Navy, *I Was A Prisoner At Guam*, an article reproduced at National Archives, from Navy Nurse Corps Historical Documents, Box #2, National Archives, Washington, D.C..

[88]   Jackson, Leona Lieutenant (jg), U.S. Navy Nurse, *Capture Of Guam By The Japanese, 9 December 1941*, Secret Document declassified by Law of 3 May 1972, Recordgraph narrative made at the Office of Naval records and library on 31 March 1943, with notes concerning the capture of Guam made by Mrs. Jackson aboard M/S *Gripsholm*, while returning from Japan, reproduced at the Navy Department Library, Naval Historical Center, Washington Navy Yard, Washington, D.C., pp. 1, 2.

[89]   Mann, Virginia Fogarty Navy Nurse, *Oral History Interview Tape Transcript*, op. cit..

[90]   Jackson, Leona Lieutenant (jg), U.S. Navy Nurse, *Capture Of Guam By The Japanese, 9 December 1941*, op. cit., p. 2.

[91]   Mann, Virginia Fogarty Navy Nurse, *Oral History Interview Tape Transcript*, op. cit..

[92]   Jackson, Leona Lieutenant (jg), U.S. Navy Nurse, *Capture Of Guam By The Japanese, 9 December 1941*, op. cit., p. 3.

[93]   Mann, Virginia Fogarty Navy Nurse, *Oral History Interview Tape Transcript*, op. cit..

[94]   Jackson, Leona Lieutenant (jg), U.S. Navy Nurse, *Capture Of Guam By The Japanese, 9 December 1941*, op. cit., pp. 3,4.

[95]   Frank, Mary E.V. Major, Army Nurse Corps, *Army And Navy Nurses Held As Prisoners Of War During World War II*, from the Department of Defense, Office of the Assistant Secretary of Defense (Manpower, Installations and Logistics, April 1985,) p. 2.

[96]   Filip, Dorothy McKinley Lt. Navy Nurse Corps, *Self-interview*, 27 April 1991.

[97]   Benner, Mary CDR Navy Nurse Corps, *Oral History Interview Tape Transcript*, Interviewer Irene Matthews, 6 February 1970.

[98]   Quadrini, Ethel Batten LCdr. Navy Nurse Corps, *Oral History Interview Tape Transcript*, self-interview, 15 August 1990.

[99]   Laird, LCDR Thelma NC USNR, et.al., *Chronological History NAVY NURSE CORPS*, op. cit., p. 23.

[100]   *Nurse Corps, U.S. Navy Monthly Census*, Xerox copy, op. cit..

[101]   *200 Years, A Bicentennial Illustrated History of the United States*, Joseph Newman, Directing Editor, Books by U.S. News & World Report, Inc., 2300 N Street, N.W., Washington, D.C. 20037, 1973, book 2, p. 159.

[102]   *The World Book Encyclopedia*, op. cit., Volume 20, p. 393.

[103]   Ibid., Volume 1, p. 288c.

[104]   Ibid., Volume 20, p. 385 and p. 402.

[105]   Ibid., Volume 16, pp. 419, 420.

[106]   Ibid., Volume 20, p. 409.   122 Matthews, Irene Lt(jg) Navy Nurse Corps, *Oral History Tape with Grace Lally, Transcript*, unpublished transcription.

[107]   Ibid..

[108]   Ibid., p. 410.

[109]   Ibid..

[110]   Ibid., p. 2.

[111]   Ibid., p. 3.

[112]   Ibid., Volume 17, p. 595.

[113]   Jamieson, Elizabeth M., B.A., R.N., Sewall, Mary F., B.S., R.N., op. cit., pp. 512, 513.

[114]   Ibid., pp. 513-516.

[115]   Ibid., p. 516.

[116]   Ibid., p. 535.

[117]   Roberts, Mary M., R.N., op. cit., p. 666.

[118]   Hine, Darlene Clark, *Black Women In White: Racial Conflict and Cooperation in the Nursing Profession 1890-1950*, Indiana University Press, Bloomington & Indianapolis, 1989, p. 171.

[119]   Ibid., p. 316.

[120]   Roberts, Mary M., R.N., op. cit., pp. 319, 320.

[121]   Ibid., p. 320.

[122]   Ibid..

[123]   Brown, Daniel M., R.N., Chief Pharmacist's Mate, Mare Island Hospital, Mare Island, California, "Men Nurses and the U. S. Navy," *The American Journal of Nursing*, May 1942, p. 501.

[124]   Benner, Mary CDR Navy Nurse Corps, *Oral History Interview Tape Transcript*, op. cit..

[125]   Ibid..

[126]   Herman, Jan K., Historian at the Naval Medical Command, Department of the Navy, *A Hilltop in Foggy Bottom (Home of the Old Naval Observatory and the Navy Medical Department)*, Reprinted from U.S. Navy Medicine, 1991, pp. 81, 82.

[127]   Laird, LCDR Thelma NC USNR, et.al., *Chronological History NAVY NURSE CORPS*, op. cit., p. 24.

[128]   Donahue, M. P., *Nursing: The Finest Art. An Illustrated History*, C.V. Mosby Company, St. Louis, Missouri, 1985, p. 408.

[129]   Laird, LCDR Thelma NC USNR, et.al., *Chronological History NAVY NURSE CORPS*, op. cit., p. 24.

[130]   Tily, James C., *The Uniforms of the United States Navy*, op. cit., pp. 260, 263.

[131]   Laird, LCDR Thelma NC USNR, et.al., *Chronological History NAVY NURSE CORPS*, op. cit., p. 25.

[132]   Covington, Margaret Lou CDR Navy Nurse Corps, *Oral History Interview Tape Transcript*, Self-Interview, 22 July 1990.

[133]   Laird, LCDR Thelma NC USNR, et.al., *Chronological History NAVY NURSE CORPS*, op. cit., p. 25.

[134]   "With Army And Navy Nurses," *American Journal of Nursing*, March 1943, pp. 305, 306.

[135]   Laird, LCDR Thelma NC USNR, et.al., *Chronological History NAVY NURSE CORPS*, op. cit., p. 24.

[136]   Ibid., p. 25.

[137]   Ibid..

[138]   Ibid., pp. 23-25.

[139]   "Indispensable!," *American Journal of Nursing*, February 1942, p. 137.

[140]   Todd, Rachel B. LCDR Navy Nurse Corps, *Oral History Interview Tape Transcript*, Self-Interview, April 1989.

[141]   Blair, Margaret Jackson LCDR Navy Nurse Corps, *Oral History Interview Tape Transcript*, Self-Interview, May 27, 1991.

[142]   Pendleton, Ralph C. LCdr MC-V(S) USNR, "Open Air Paraffin Wax Spray Treatment For All Types Of Burns," circa. 1942. Donated by Rachel Todd.

[143]   Ibid..

[144]   Todd, *Oral History Interview Tape Transcript*, op. cit..

[145]   Ibid..

[146]   Hanf, Madonna M. Timm LCDR Navy Nurse Corps, *Written Self-Interview*, August 1990.

[147]   Loughman, Katherine LCDR Navy Nurse Corps, *Oral History Interview Tape Transcript*, Interviewer Dorothea Tracy LCDR Navy Nurse Corps, 11 May 1990.

[148]   Cavanaugh, Virginia Holt Ensign Navy Nurse Corps, *NNCA Autobiographical Survey Addendum*, 6 July 1989.

[149]   Hummel, Sue Smoker Captain Navy Nurse Corps, *Oral History Interview Tape Transcript*, Interviewer Helen Barry Siragusa LT Navy Nurse Corps, 29 January 1991.

[150]   Davenport, Janina Smiertka Lt(jg) Navy Nurse Corps, *Oral History Interview Tape Transcript*, Interviewer Helen Barry Siragusa LT Navy Nurse Corps, 27 March 1988.

[151]   Davenport, Janina Smiertka Lt(jg) Navy Nurse Corps, "Most Memorable Duty in The Navy," one page typewritten account, 1988.

[152]   Ibid..

[153]   Davenport, *Oral History Interview Tape Transcript*, op. cit..

[154]   Davenport, "Most Memorable Duty in The Navy," one page typewritten account, op. cit..

[155]   O'Donnell, J.J. Officer-in-Charge, "Commendation of the Medical Department Personnel," 27 July 1942. Copy of letter donated by Janina Smiertka Davenport.

[156]   Bartleson, Norma CDR Navy Nurse Corps, *Oral History Interview Tape Transcript*, Interviewer Patty Hoff, 22 August 1990.

[157]   Ibid..

[158]   Ibid..

[159]   Quadrini, *Oral History Interview Tape Transcript*, op. cit..

[160]   Todd, *Oral History Interview Tape Transcript*, op. cit..

[161]   Jackson, Leona Lieutenant (jg), U.S. Navy Nurse, *Capture Of Guam By The Japanese, 9 December 1941*, Secret Document declassified by Law of 3 May 1972, op. cit., p. 6.

[162]   Ibid..

[163]   Ibid..

[164]   Ibid..

[165]   Ibid..

[166]   Mann, Virginia Fogarty Navy Nurse, *Oral History Interview Tape Transcript*, op. cit..

[167]   Jackson, Leona Lieutenant (jg), U.S. Navy Nurse, *Capture Of Guam By The Japanese, 9 December 1941*, Secret Document declassified by Law of 3 May 1972, op. cit..

[168]   Mann, Virginia Fogarty Navy Nurse, *Oral History Interview Tape Transcript*, op. cit..

[169]   Jackson, Leona Lieutenant (jg), U.S. Navy Nurse, *Capture Of Guam By The Japanese, 9 December 1941*, Secret Document declassified by Law of 3 May 1972, op. cit..

[170]   Ibid..

[171]   Ibid., p. 11.

[172]   Ibid..

[173]   Mann, Virginia Fogarty Navy Nurse, *Oral History Interview Tape Transcript*, op. cit..

[174]   Halliday, Lorraine Christiansen LCdr Navy Nurse Corps, *Oral History Interview Tape Transcript*, Interviewer Dorothea M. Shore Tracy, 13 June 1990.

[175]   Mann, Virginia Fogarty Navy Nurse, *Oral History Interview Tape Transcript*, op. cit..

[176]   Jackson, *Capture Of Guam By The Japanese, 9 December 1941*, Secret Document declassified by Law of 3 May 1972, op. cit., p. 12.

[177]   Ibid..

[178]   Information obtained from the file cards of Marion B. Olds', Doris M. Yetter's, and Lorraine Christiansen's assignments, Bureau of Medicine and Surgery, Washington, D.C., provided by Captain Joan Engel Nurse Corps USN, Deputy Director, Navy Nurse Corps, 1993.

[179]   Halliday, *Oral History Interview Tape Transcript*, Interviewer Dorothea M. Shore Tracy, op. cit..

[180]   Information obtained from the file cards of Marion B. Olds', Doris M. Yetter's, and Lorraine Christiansen's assignments, op.cit..

[181]   "Navy Nurses Help Induct WAVES," *The American Journal of Nursing*, December 1942, p. 1452.

[182]   "Army and Navy Nurses Have Told Us," *The American Journal of Nursing*, September 1942, p. 1081.

[183]   *The World Book Encyclopedia*, Field Enterprises Educational Corporation, Chicago, Volume 18, 1966 edition, p. 254.

[184]   *The Columbia-Viking Desk Encyclopedia*, by staff of the Columbia Encyclopedia, William Bridgwater, Editor-in-chief, The Viking Press, New York, 1933, p. 854.

[185]   Quebbeman, Frances, CDR Navy Nurse Corps, *Written Personal History*, 13 May 1991, pp. 4-5.

[186]   Moeller, Ruth Captain Navy Medical Service Corps, *Oral History Interview Tape Transcript*, Interviewer Doris M. Sterner Captain Navy Nurse Corps, 17 October 1988. (Captain Moeller was Head, Medical Specialists Section, Navy Medical Service Corps at BUMED prior to her retirement. A DOD directive dated 27 August 1963 authorized Director status for her position.)

[187]   Laird, LCDR Thelma NC USNR, et.al., *Chronological History NAVY NURSE CORPS*, op. cit., p. 24.

[188]   Bernatitis, Ann Capt. NC USN (Ret.), *Oral History Interview Tape Transcript*, Interviewer Doris M. Sterner, op. cit..

[189]   Bernatitis, *Oral History Interview Tape Transcript*, Interviewer Irene Matthews, op.cit..

[190]   Bernatitis, Ann Capt. NC USN (Ret.), *Oral History Interview Tape Transcript*, Interviewer Doris M. Sterner, op. cit..

[191]   Bernatitis, *Oral History Interview Tape Transcript*, Interviewer Irene Matthews, op.cit..

[192]   Bernatitis, Ann Capt. NC USN (Ret.), *Oral History Interview Tape Transcript*, Interviewer Doris M. Sterner, op. cit..

[193]   Bernatitis, *Oral History Interview Tape Transcript*, Interviewer Irene Matthews, op.cit..

[194]   Parker, Captain T.C. U.S. Navy (Retired), "Thirteen Women In A Submarine," *United States Naval Institute Proceedings*, The Institute, Annapolis, Maryland, July 1950, p. 717.

[195]   Bernatitis, Ann Capt. NC USN (Ret.), *Oral History Interview Tape Transcript*, Interviewer Doris M. Sterner, op. cit..

[196]   Bernatitis, *Oral History Interview Tape Transcript*, Interviewer Irene Matthews, op.cit..

[197]   "Thirteen Women In A Submarine," Parker, Captain, op.cit..

[198]   Ibid., p. 718.

[199]   Bernatitis, *Oral History Interview Tape Transcript*, Interviewer Irene Matthews, <u>op. cit.</u>.

[200]   <u>Ibid.</u>.

[201]   Bernatitis, Ann Capt. NC USN (Ret.), *Oral History Interview Tape Transcript*, Interviewer Doris M. Sterner, <u>op. cit.</u>.

[202]   Cobb, LCdr. Laura NC USN, Handwritten notes on notebook paper, <u>op. cit.</u>.

[203]   Todd, CDR. C. Edwina (NC) USN, "NURSING UNDER FIRE," <u>op. cit.</u>, p. 76.

[204]   Cobb, LCdr. Laura NC USN, Handwritten notes on notebook paper, <u>op. cit.</u>.

[205]   Nash, CDR Margaret A. NC USN (Ret.), *Oral History Interview Tape Transcript*, <u>op. cit.</u>.

[206]   Cobb, LCdr. Laura NC USN, Handwritten notes on notebook paper, <u>op. cit.</u>.

[207]   Todd, CDR. C. Edwina (NC) USN, "NURSING UNDER FIRE," <u>op. cit.</u>, p. 77.

[208]   Nash, CDR Margaret A. NC USN (Ret.), *Oral History Interview Tape Transcript*, <u>op. cit.</u>.

[209]   Cobb, LCdr. Laura NC USN, Handwritten notes on notebook paper, <u>op. cit.</u>.

[210]   <u>Ibid.</u>.

CHAPTER 6

Superintendent - Captain Sue S. Dauser
(1943 - 1946)

☆ ☆ ☆

Captain Sue Dauser has been offered and accepts another term as Superintendent of the U.S. Navy Nurse Corps. She assumes her second term in January of 1943. With the Nurse Corps expanding rapidly to meet the war-time nursing care needs of the Navy and the all too hectic pace related to these activities, this is not the time to have a change in the Head of the Nurse Corps. The explosive growth of the Nurse Corps reaches 3293 at the end of January; 1255 are Regular Navy and 2038 are Reserves.[1] There are Navy nurses deployed outside the United States at fourteen duty stations and one Prisoner-of-War camp as follows:

1. Puerto Rico, in the West Indies
2. Trinidad, in the West Indies
3. Cuba, in the West Indies
4. Samoa, in the South Pacific
5. Kodiak, Alaska
6. Dutch Harbor, Alaska
7. Newfoundland
8. Oahu, Hawaiian Islands
9. USS *Relief*
10. USS *Solace*
11. New Hebrides, in the South Pacific
12. New Zealand
13. Panama Canal Zone
14. Virgin Islands
15. Santo Tomas Prisoner-of-War camp, Philippine Islands[2]

At the POW camp in 1943, life goes on, but is becoming even more strenuous and difficult. The Japanese captors add more and more prisoners to the camp. Illnesses and hardships increase with the population. "In May of 1943, the Japanese Military decided to open a new Internment Camp at Los Banos for military age men (Civilians.) There were a large [number] of businessmen and English seamen. [The] greater portion were Civil Service employees of [the] Navy and Army. Dr. C.N. Leach offered his services as Medical Director for the Camp. The Navy Nurses, one British nurse and a Filipino nurse volunteered their services to care for [the] health of [the] Camp."[3] The Japanese choose the site for the new camp at an agricultural branch of a Philippine University where the Filipinos already have a small hospital. The Japanese force the Filipinos out and the Filipinos leave taking all their medical supplies and equipment.

Navy Nurse Mary Harrington says that she heard about the new camp and "I went in and sat on my haunches outside the Chief Nurse's [Laura Cobb] mosquito net that night and I said, `Laura, why don't you volunteer for our group to go up and set up this Camp?' So she went down and volunteered and we had a British nurse with us and a Filipino nurse whose husband was a Naval Officer. . . . [The day they leave] Laura wanted to be sure she had everybody's service record [so] she stuck them inside her blouse. She wasn't very full, kind of skinny, so they made her some leis [to hang around her neck to hide the fullness of the service records from the Japanese]. The girls got some leaves and some . . . hibiscus and stuff, [and] made some leis, and here was Laura wearing all the records on the inside of her shirt. She was going to get those through. . . . They put all the nurses in one truck and they put a little Japanese guard on it and you never saw a man who looked so much like he had been whipped or something. The poor soul, I'm sure, had lost face being put up to guard a bunch of women. . . . We were the last truck out of the Camp. When they [some of the Camp's internees] played [over the Camp's PA system] 'Anchors Aweigh,' I cried all the way down the driveway out to the [railroad] station."[4]

"800 men [internees for the new camp] and [the] nurses entrained for the new camp. . . . We were placed in Steel Box Cars, 65 to a car (where normally 30 men would have been a load) one to [two] nurses placed in a box car with [the] men (we were thought to be held as hostages provided any men tried to escape.) One Jap guard in each car. Both doors closed when [the] train got under way. After some persuasion, the doors were opened. Some of the men almost suffocated."[5] "This trip took 7 hours by box car to cover the distance of 45 miles. It was the hottest time of the year. The average person lost 7 to 10 lbs. on this trip."[6] "When we [had] left Santo Tomas at five o'clock that morning, they gave us a hard boiled duck egg and a piece of bread and that was our ration for the day."[7] "Naturally we were thirsty upon arrival [at Los Banos]. After we were counted we went up to a bungalow where 50 men were assigned to a water detail as all water had to be boiled. However, before we were allowed to drink, Jap photographers came up and had us sit on the grass with a few of the men. We were photographed as if pouring with our empty bottles 'just like a tea party.' It would make good propaganda for Tokyo."[8]

"They put us in a cottage . . . and we didn't have anything to eat. I remember we looked outside the barbed wire fence and we could see chickens and banana trees surrounding us. . . . I don't know how, but one of the chickens came close to the fence and we grabbed the chicken and we killed it. We made chicken stew."[9] They had practically no supplies or equipment for the hospital but with the help of some ingenious men internees and a great deal of improvising, eventually they had a hospital, of sorts.

Navy Nurse Margaret Nash speaks especially of an Australian man who helped them. He had been on his way to Australia from Singapore with a stopover in Manila where he had been captured and sent to Santa Tomas and then to Los Banos. Miss Nash says, "Everyone in the camp called him 'Chum.' . . . He'd come to the quarters because I was walking down [to the dispensary] in the dark at five-thirty in the morning and he did not want me to be walking down with only the sentries and the guards . . . around. Chum would come up to the cottage [where the nurses were quartered] and walk with me down to the dispensary. One day he came in and said to me, 'Why do you have to go so early?' And I said, 'To boil the instruments.' He said, 'Well, the clinic doesn't open until eight o'clock. Does it take that long?' And I said, 'Yes, because I only have a little hot plate. I have to boil all these instruments that the doctors use.' (The instruments came from the doctors that were in the camp.) . . . So Chum said, 'What did you use in America?' . . . Then I drew him a picture of a sterilizer and in about a week after that, Chum came into the clinic and brought in a sterilizer and I asked him, 'How did you get the material to make this?' He said, 'Never ask questions, just accept.'"[10]

"We lacked trained personnel so Miss Harrington and Miss Still [both Navy Nurses] conducted classes to volunteer candidates. Many of the men in camp had worked in the Cavite Navy Yard. They proved handy with tools and did for us what the Seabees did for the Navy."[11] "So they got corrugated tin and they beat the ripples out of that and made basins and other things for us. When they got some iron pipe, they made bed frames. . . . Sometimes you got some things. We got some unbleached muslin and made some sheets out of it. . . . We got a bolt of denim and . . . [Navy Nurse Goldie O'Haver] made us denim uniforms. They were very practical. . . . Well, they might have been heavy but denim is a strange fabric. It's heavy but it isn't as hot as a lot of other things. It breathes more. So we weren't that uncomfortable. . . . We took old mosquito nets and boiled them up [for dressings]. No adhesive? One of the men tapped a rubber tree and made a . . . sort of a pasty mess and you can put that on a patient and stick a little dressing on top of it.

"There was a Polish doctor [in the camp] . . . [and] he knew some home remedies. We made cough medicine out of onions and brown sugar; made a cough syrup out of that. And in a little while they began sending some things up from Santo Tomas; they were sharing a little."[12] "Our first emergency operation was a ruptured appendix (6 weeks after arrival.) This was the beginning of a general hospital. Daily we had from 170 to 200 cases at the Clinic; infection from bamboo. They were clearing the Camp to make it livable, also digging post holes (forced by Japs to do so) for boundary of our Camp and helped stretch barb-wire fence around our enclosure."[13] The ten Navy Nurses and their Chief Nurse struggled on, doing what they could with what they had. Then in December, Miss Cobb notes that, "Following the arrival of [a] Red Cross Ship, [in] December 1943, we then had a fair supply of linen and drugs of all kinds."[14]

Out in the South Pacific Ocean, the hospital ship *Solace* is shuttling "back and forth between [the] New Hebrides [Islands], New Caledonia and New Zealand. We would pick up the patients . . . sometimes they would be brought from ashore and sometimes directly from ships. . . . We would usually be out a ways [from shore] when the barges brought all the patients in. . . . The medical officers were there and it was a triage sort of thing. . . . They would put a tag on them [with] where they were to go to, what was wrong with them [and] if any treatment was to be started immediately. Of course, we [the Navy Nurses] were right on the wards awaiting these patients as were the corpsmen. . . . Sometimes we would load 400 patients in a matter of two or three hours' time and we would be under way again heading south to New Zealand"[15] where they unload the patients at the hospital. The patients came from "Guadalcanal [and] from ships that were hit so you had burn cases, a large number of malaria cases, [and] combat fatigue.

"My ward was part medical and we had one locked area adjacent to it which had the psychiatric patients in it. Those [patients] who were more disturbed were kept on the top deck. There was a locked word up there because they could not be controlled very well. We had orthopedic cases. . . . You couldn't put [any of] them in traction because they had to be in a condition [so] that they could be moved readily in the event that we had to abandon ship. Every night, an hour before sunset, we would go through the wards and put all our patients in life jackets and we did that every morning, one hour before sunrise. Those were, apparently, the times that the Japanese submarines would come out and hit the ships. Our ship was not hit.

"On our runs back up [from New Zealand back to the islands to get more patients], there were no patients so we had to get the wards in order. All the supplies had to be gotten ready. . . . In those days there were no such things as 4 by 4's that you could take out of a package. You folded all [the] 4 by 4's; all our dressings were folded. There were no disposable things. Everything was reused, the needles, syringes, etc., all these things.

"[Chief Nurse] Edna Morrow [came aboard] to relieve Grace Lally as Chief Nurse. Not too long after she came aboard, they discovered a lump in Edna's breast so she had to be sent back to the States."[16] Lieutenant Morrow goes by plane to the States. On the 21st of January 1943 that plane is reported missing. On the 31st of January, an Associated Press article from Ukiah, California reports the missing Navy transport plane "on a flight from Pearl Harbor to San Francisco, had been found wrecked and burned in the mountains ten miles southwest of here [Ukiah]. All aboard were dead. . . . The sheriff's report said the plane, flying through one of the heaviest rainstorms in years in this area, hit a vertical cliff." Another Associated Press report datelined Washington, January 23, gives the names of all those aboard. It lists Rear Admiral Robert H. English, commander of the Pacific fleet submarine force, three Navy Captains, three Commanders, two Lieutenant Commanders, Lt. Edna Owella Morrow (Nurse Corps), and the crew of the plane. This news report says, "That the loss of so many high-ranking officers was a severe blow was easy to discern through the terse statements by Navy headquarters." And the Nurse Corps lost one of its own.

In 1943 the *Solace* traveled over 37,000 miles. "On Thanksgiving Day she put into a port of the Gilberts, and took aboard 238 Tarawa casualties. December 17 of that year was a gala day - for Admiral Nimitz came aboard and presented 289 Purple Hearts to wounded veterans of the Pacific War."[17] Speaking of decorations, thirteen Navy nurses who were aboard the *Solace* during the attack on Pearl Harbor, are cited for outstanding performance of duty under fire at that time. They are: Lieutenants Dorothy Bogdon, Loraine Ceaglske, Ruth Cohen, Hilda Combes, Teresa Duggan, Margaret Haley, Genevieve Hickey, Chief Nurse Grace Lally, Agnes Shurr, Ida Thompson, Marjorie Von Stein, and Ensigns Anna Danyo, and Irene Galiley. After continuous duty in many locations in the war zone, these nurses were recently relieved from sea duty and returned to [naval] hospitals within the continental limits of the United States. "The roster [complement] of nurses on the 'Solace' has been increased to twenty-one."[18]   Also, "During the first twenty months of the war 7,500 casualties were treated aboard the U.S.S. *Solace*. Only sixteen were lost."[19]

The other Naval Hospital ship, USS *Relief*, left Casco Bay, Maine in early February 1943, to "put into a Boston yard to prepare for Pacific duty. By 23 [February], she was on her way to the South Pacific Advanced Fleet Base at Noumea, New Caledonia, via the Panama Canal."[20]

The July 1943 edition of the American Journal of Nursing contains an article entitled, "Nurses Christen Two Navy Hospital Ships." The two ships referred to are the *Mercy* and the *Comfort*. Navy Nurses Lt(jg) Doris M. Yetter and Lt(jg) Lorraine Christensen (former POW's from Guam) christen the USS *Mercy*. Two First Lieutenants from the Army Nurse Corps christen the USS *Comfort*.[21] The reason for the Army nurses christening a Navy ship is because the Army have their own hospital ships during World War II. Three of them are staffed with Navy personnel for the running and maintenance of the ships while the Army staffs the medical side of the ships. The USS *Comfort*, the USS *Mercy*, and, eventually, the USS *Hope* are "designated as hospital [ships] by the Navy for the Army; operated by the Navy for the Army." All three ships will go into service in 1944 and all three will serve in the Southwest Pacific with one other all-Army hospital ship. The rest of the Army's hospital ships will serve the European and Mediterranean war areas.[22]

Navy Nurse Florence Wisneski tells us about traveling across the Pacific on a ship transporting "I would say close to two hundred [nurses]. Very crowded conditions. If you wanted any space out on deck during the day, someone had to give up breakfast . . . and hold the corner otherwise there was no place for you to stand up. We dropped part of the nurses off at Guadalcanal and another [place of call in the Solomon Islands]. Guadalcanal had a hospital and, I think, the other place was also a base hospital. . . . My destination was . . . in the Solomons group at Mobile Hospital #10. We cared for the First Marine Division primarily. . . . Arrived one day and [the patients] arrived the next day.

"The Navy had this very well planned. . . . [The patients] arrived on hospital ships and most of the injuries were at least three days old and sometimes as high as six. You could tell what kind of a [battle] landing [they had been in] and where the mines were place and how they [the troops had] approached. You would receive some that had all leg injuries and you knew they were walking into the beach. Then you'd [have some] where they were all face and head injuries and you knew they had had to crawl. . . . We had about 50 [Navy Nurses at the Mobile Hospital]. . . . It was a different kind of treatment for the fractured wounds. The fractures were held in place by . . . [metal] pins and the wounds were left open. Patients were put out into the sunshine and the air for circulation and they had no coverings on their wounds. The dampness in the islands and dressings did not go together. And the sunshine and the fresh air would help. It had a drying effect that enhanced the healing."[23]

Navy Nurse Charlotte Sprague writes about her 28 day trip aboard the USS Henderson to New Caledonia, "We had no idea where we were going. We arrived at our destination just as the sun was setting. It was too late for the French Pilot to [navigate] us through the mined coral reefs that evening; we were to wait until daylight to go through the safety route with the pilot. For the first time, we were allowed to keep the lights [of the ship] on and the port holes uncovered. Little did we realize that a two-man Japanese submarine had followed us and was now nestled directly under our ship. The sub slid in with us the next morning as we were guided in. It was captured the next day. . . . The two Japanese men were taken to the Prisoner-of-War camp on the island. The sub was put on display in the town of Noumea's central square."[24]

Another Navy Nurse to go to New Caledonia, is Sue Smoker and she tells us of her duty there, "It was a new hospital; we were situated right on the Bay. Our next door neighbor was the Army Camp on the left and on our right was a recreational facility for the whole island. Admiral Halsey invited the nursing staff to a reception. We arrived wearing our dress blues and our high collars and our blue ties, and going through the receiving line, he removed our ties and hung them over the picture in the hallway and said there would be no dress uniforms worn on this island and no long ties. . . . After the Battle of Bougainville [one of the Solomon Islands], we received a shipload of patients to await transportation to the United States. Among them was a young boy from Brooklyn, who [was an] amputee. He was very upset that at each transfer, they would take his crutches away and make him a non-ambulatory patient. He became friends with a Seabee and asked [him] if he could make arrangements to have a peg leg made for him. Several weeks went by and this young man would be absent from the ward. He would sign out to various spots on the station, but when you went to check on him, he wasn't there. Several days later, after questioning him at great length, I found out he was getting rides out to the Seabee station and . . . they had crafted him a peg leg. It was beautifully done. They had leather tools, they had special nails in there, it was really a masterpiece.

"The doctors did not want him to wear it because his stump was not healed properly, so he promised us if we gave him a pair of crutches, he would not wear it. But, our Executive Officer found out that Bob Hope was on the island and thought that perhaps he would like to see what had been done. He made arrangements for the young man to put the peg leg on and go down to see Bob Hope. Bob signed [the peg leg] with his pen and promised he would write a letter informing the Seabees of their wonderful work. My Brooklyn patient came back to the ward and showed me . . . [where Bob Hope] had signed it . . . and he promised he wouldn't wear it again until the stump was healed."[25]

Yet another Navy Nurse in New Caledonia, Grace L. Smith, tells us that she is the second senior of the twenty-five nurses stationed there and goes to New Zealand to be Chief Nurse. "My orders came to proceed to USN Base Hospital #5, Wellington, New Zealand. I went aboard the USS *Argonne* [on] 15 June '43 [and we] departed 16 June '43. And being the only female aboard ship - I . . . occupied the vacant quarters of [Admiral] Halsey. While on board I was given the job of sewing on buttons, insignias, and rips in the uniforms of Officers and enlisted men which kept me busy during the day. This was my duty until we disembarked 21 June 1943 in Auckland, New Zealand. . . . Oh, yes, the men stood 4 hour watch at the foot of stairway . . . leading to my quarters. (Adm. Halsey's [quarters].) He was not on board."[26]

East of New Caledonia lie the islands of Samoa and there at the Navy medical facility, a new Chief Nurse arrives in 1943. She says she traveled by ship to Honolulu from San Francisco then by plane to Wallis Island in the South Pacific where there was a contingent of Marines. She and five other nurses had to wait there on Wallis Island for five days before they could get transportation to American Samoa. Chief Nurse Mary Lindner says, "We didn't have any service personnel, [it] was mostly Samoans that we were caring for. We also had patients who had leprosy but they were isolated by themselves.

"The Samoan people . . . would come in [to the hospital] and help take care of their [relative] that was ill and they would sleep under the bed at night. While I was there I had a school room built right there by the nurses quarters and had a bed set up so [that] they were all taught how to give baths and everything like that, before they went on the wards to help the people. I was the Chief Nurse in charge and six [Navy nurses] were mostly there for instructing the Samoan nurses. . . . Some of them were student nurses; they had to go to school for two years before they were on their own and all of them worked at the hospital. . . . The Marines had been on that island before we came; the island had been fired upon but apparently [they] had moved out very quickly. There were graves of deceased Marines on that island. Maybe once a month a ship would come in and bring us supplies."[27]

Also, in 1943, Navy Nurse Helen Gavin receives orders, as Chief Nurse, to Mobile Hospital #9 at Brisbane, Australia.[28] On 22 November, Chief Nurse Gavin and a large number of other Navy Nurses board the USS *West Point* for deployment to the South Pacific. "We didn't know where we were going. At that time you never knew where you were going. . . . So we got on the *West Point*. It was a troop ship. All these soldiers and sailors and so many; three thousand."[29] Navy Nurse Madonna Timm notes that they boarded the ship on 22 November 1943, "it was crowded. They served two meals a day as by the time they finished . . . breakfast, it was time to start serving dinner. . . .

"We were given Japanese [words] to study and remember in case we would become their prisoners. So we decided to each learn only one word as we most likely would be taken together anyway. I'll always remember mine as it was `Hung Chow' (meaning `Constipation') and thank the good Lord I never had the chance to use it. After 2 weeks zig-zagging in the Pacific, [in a Bay in New Guinea] the Navy Nurses disembarked the USS *West Point* by rope ladders [Jacobs ladders] in our dress blues [uniforms] (as we were not issued slacks as the Army nurses had) into a landing craft and onto the Australian TSS 'Katoomba.' It was a very old ship carrying their casualties from the New Guinea battle zone. It had an Australian doctor with a peg leg wearing khaki shorts and two older nurses who they call 'Sisters.' Leaving the Coral Sea area we landed in Townsville, Australia. Helen Gavin . . . our chief nurse went ashore and found a Red Cross house that we could all stay [in] overnight and [then we] could leave via plane in the A.M. to our destination. No one [knew] exactly where we were going for sure as all . . . of our orders read differently. . . .

"[We] left early the next morning for Brisbane, Queensland, Australia."[30] "We went down to Brisbane and the Navy met us. When we saw our beautiful little Navy Corpsmen, they were all there to meet us, we felt like we were at home because we'd been with the Australians now all this time and we were with the Army, also. So we got into Brisbane and . . . MOB 9 [Fleet Hospital 109]. . . like a MASH unit. . . . It was a mobile unit but it was a [complete] hospital unit," says Navy Nurse Swanson.[31] Miss Timm continues, "Some of the Navy Nurses from Sidney had been there and organized the wards as great numbers of Navy and Marine Casualties were arriving daily. The 1st Marine Division arrived from Guadalcanal for rest. Seventy percent of them had malaria and other tropical diseases that were new to us. Soon we were daily admitting 500 to 700 to the new wards. They came by ship, planes, and ambulances. Many of them just stared at us in our white dress ward uniforms and caps.

"The boys in the laundry seemed to enjoy starching our uniforms STIFF - in fact we were able to stand them in a corner of our room and jump into them when necessary. We called them 'Bustle Butts' as they ballooned out in back under the wide belt. . . . Brisbane MOB 9 Hospital was south of the equator so our first Christmas was spent enjoying their summer weather . . . [and time] off could be spent down at . . . a beach house reserved for the Navy Nurses. We made many life time friends with the people in Australia who were very good to us all. . . . Their kindness to us will never be forgotten."[32] Miss Swanson mentions the Nurses Quarters Fleet Hospital 109 or, as she calls it, MOB 9, "our quarters were very nice. We were in little cabins. There were five in a cabin. We had five rooms and then the center was a living room. . . . They had our bathrooms or the latrine, at they called it, was naturally a little distance away. That was an adventure in itself because when you went out to go to the bathroom, it was pouring down rain. We had rain gear and it was these old leather raincoats that they had in the Army and our hats. We had to get all dressed up with boots to go to the bathroom."[33]

Navy Nurses are spread all over the South Pacific during WWII and each one of them has a sea story or more to relate; a whole book could be written on each of them. However, almost every Navy Nurse we've met and spoken with (whether from WWII or not) says the same thing, "But I didn't do anything special to write or talk about; I only did what had to be done; I did my duty."

Besides Navy Nurses, in November 1943 an amazing and new medication makes its appearance in the South Pacific; 'penicillin.' At New Caledonia it is used to treat osteomyelitis in a wounded patient. And over in New Hebrides, "41 cases [are treated] with penicillin. Medical personnel administered the drug by I.V. and intramuscular injection. In six of the cases, the patient's conditions did not respond to the drug. Nonetheless, penicillin proved effective in treating gonorrhea and blood stream infections. With penicillin now available in increasing amounts, Allied medical personnel would no longer have to depend solely on the less effective 'sulfa' drugs."[34]

Back in the 'States' in 1943, Navy Nurses are doing their war-work in other medical facilities besides Naval Hospitals. For instance, there are many Naval Dispensaries staffed with Navy Nurses and one of these is at the Naval Air Station, Deland, Florida. Lt(jg) Sarah O'Toole is Chief Nurse at this dispensary and, in an American Journal of Nursing article she writes, "Having served three weeks as assistant to the chief nurse [at a naval hospital], I received orders detaching me from all duties at the naval hospital and was transferred to a small naval air station dispensary as chief nurse. This dispensary has an outpatient department, treatment and examination rooms, a 'sick officers' quarters' of ten rooms, a 30-bed ward for enlisted men, two quiet rooms for very ill patients, a 'sick WAVES' quarters' with five beds and three isolation rooms. There are also a dental clinic, operating room, laboratory, pharmacy, x-ray department, and a well-equipped physiotherapy department.

"We take care of all crash and accident cases occurring at the Base and do minor surgery. Major surgery and very ill patients are generally transferred to naval hospitals. . . . We have on our staff five doctors, four nurses, approximately twenty-five corpsmen, an ensign (HC), and chief pharmacist's mate. . . . Both naval hospital and naval dispensary duty are pleasant, but my personal desire is to be on the fighting front. I want to be actually of assistance to our boys out there where they need it most and I hope to have duty on one of our grand, big, beautiful hospital ships before the war is over."[35]

Also in Florida is Navy Nurse Jeanne Grushinski, originally from New Jersey. She tells us that getting her orders to the Naval Hospital at Pensacola is her introduction to the state of Florida. She says, "The Chief Nurse was Miss Morris and she was from New Hampshire and was a very warm person . . . very interested in her nurses and we really got very good [professional] experience. It didn't matter that we worked 28 nights straight without a night off. We still seemed to have time to go horseback riding, go to the beach and, of course, the Officers' Club which was a beautiful spot right on the beach. . . . [One] of the requirements for night duty was to turn the 'Obstacle Lights' on or off. . . . Those [the obstacle lights] were the lights on the top of the tallest buildings; there was a smoke stack there [and] a chimney stack. [The buildings] had to have that light because [they] were quite tall and with the airplanes flying [around] in the air for flight training, why, that was something that was [designated] the [night] nurse's duty."[36]

As Navy Nurse Grushinski points out, her Chief Nurse, Lt. Margaret Morris NC USN, is indeed interested in her nurses and their welfare. An example of this concern is a letter Lt. Morris writes to the Superintendent of the Navy Nurse Corps, Capt. Sue Dauser, on 29 August 1943. She begins the letter by noting that even though the nurses quarters are full and the overflow has doubled up in other areas, there is still a need for more nurses. She justifies this with, "I know my report of the number of future [obstetrical] deliveries sounded rather fantastic but I had to relieve the nurses, who had the watch [on-call after regular working hours], three times last week. They had six deliveries each night for two nights and seven the next night. . . . They [obstetrics] have 540 cases to be delivered before Xmas. I also need nurses for afternoon duty when I take the P.M. nurse for relief it means that one nurse takes four wards and the wards are too heavy for one nurse."[37]

Then Chief Nurse Morris goes on to describe another problem involving attempts to wrongfully pressure for the nursing services of the Navy nurses. A nursery was established on the Naval Base for the care of the children of mothers (dependent wives) who wanted to volunteer for Red Cross work or for other tasks to help out the war effort. The wife of one of the officers on the base had her husband call the Naval Hospital's Executive Officer and request the services of two Navy Nurses on a volunteer basis from 5 p.m. to 11 p.m. every day. The two volunteers would each be paid four dollars a day. "I told [the Executive Officer] it would not work out for it would have to be the A.M. nurses [who would have] to volunteer. The nurses are tired at 3 P.M. [when they get off duty], and working from 8 A.M. to 11 P.M. with only two hours off would be too much in this heat. But he wanted me to try it out and it did not work just as I thought."[38] (Some of the details given the Navy Nurse volunteers at the nursery were, "Wash cribs when the babies left, sweep deck, count linen and clean cupboards and of course change the babies and heat the bottles and feed the babies."[39])

Miss Morris then consults with the Commanding Officer of the Naval Hospital and tells him the situation and that she "went over to the nursery myself to see the situation and what they need is nurse's aids. The object of the nursery is to relieve the mothers so they can do Red Cross Work and vital things of that sort but from what I see and hear the mothers are at the movies, parties and dinners. . . . The Commanding Officer does not approve of it and we are not sending any more nurses. . . . My attitude is if we are going to be officers we should have the duties of the officers and not maids."[40] The officer's wife that originally made the request and gave the volunteer nurses their volunteer 'duties' informed the Navy Nurses that she would go to the Admiral of the Naval Base and "have him write to Washington to have nurses detailed there [at the nursery]."[41] That is why Chief Nurse Morris relays the incident to Captain Dauser; in case the matter is forwarded to Washington. A few days after receiving Miss Morris' letter, Captain Dauser writes back, "Your letter of August 29, has been read with real interest. You have had the experience that I hoped was behind us in this war. How many times we have had to be on the alert for just such infringements on the rights of the nurse corps. I wonder if the time will ever come when the public will be educated to the exact status of our nurse and not scheme for all the extras they might have. I feel certain now that you have stopped all nurses going over to help with the nursery situation and that this matter of extra duty will soon be forgotten."[42]

Up at the Naval Hospital in Charleston, South Carolina, Ensign Margaret Covington tells us, "My background was pretty typical of the majority of the nurses who arrived in Charleston those first months of 1943. [She is a native of North Carolina.] We were small town girls who had led a somewhat sheltered life. We were young and eager and inexperienced. This was an entirely new way of life for most of us. We were a close-knit group. Most of the doctors and nurses and the corpsmen came from North and South Carolina and Georgia. . . . The Army had several bases in and around Charleston . . . there were French and British ships in the harbor and the French and British Officers were often guests on our Guest Night at the nurses quarters [at dinner/mess]. . . . Wednesday night was a very special night at the nurses quarters because it was our guest night and we had the opportunity to invite our male guests. And we really 'put on the dog' that night; our silver service, our silver, our white tablecloths, our Navy china, and each table had its own hostess, which was traditional at the Navy dining rooms at that time. . . . Since Charleston was very crowded at that time, and many establishments were 'out of bounds' for Navy Nurses, most of the time we entertained our guests either in the nurses quarters or at the Officers Club. Occasionally we were invited aboard a British ship or a French ship for dinner. . . .

"The first months [at Charleston] were an indoctrination period for us. We received classes in Navy protocol, Navy policy, and procedure; [we] were taught primarily by Lt(jg) Marian Olds who was our Chief Nurse. . . . I remember her well as quite a lady; firm but understanding. We all respected her very much. She had been on Guam when it was captured by the Japs. . . . In addition to those classes [already mentioned], we had classes in [marching] and drilling which were conducted by a Marine Sergeant [and] also, swimming classes

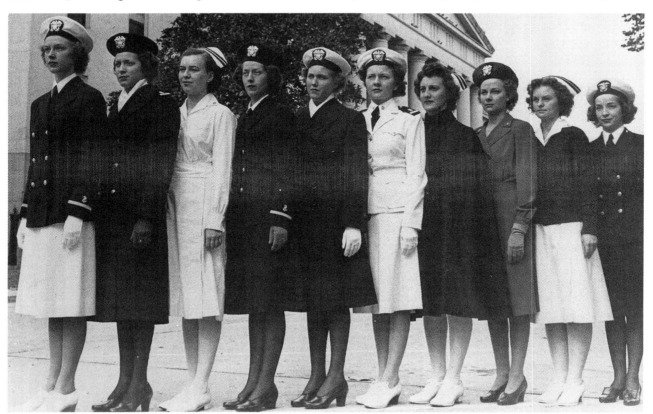

Uniforms worn by Navy Nurses in the 1940's. (Photo courtesy of Navy Bureau of Medicine and Surgery.)

. . . . At the end of my six months in Charleston, I was given a written examination and after passing was given the opportunity to join the Regular Navy [versus the Reserve], which I did. This lasted for twenty-two years.

"During these early months we were also fitted for our Navy uniforms. Our Navy uniform wardrobe consisted of the white traditional ward uniform. . . . The navy insignia at that time was the large anchor with the oak leaf with the acorn on the side. Our Navy dress blue [uniform] was the two piece double-breasted suit . . . with the gold buttons down the front. We wore our Navy insignia on our lapels. . . . Our Navy hat was the round, flat top, tam-type hat . . . [and] we had the white flat top [and] we also had the navy-blue flat top. In Charleston, because it was considered a tropical station, a white flat top was worn year around. . . . In addition . . . we wore black hose and black shoes. . . . The dress white uniform was the traditional white uniform . . . with the shoulder boards. I failed to mention that at this time we were wearing the man-type shirt and the man-type tie. I thought I would never learn to tie that tie. We also had a bridge coat [overcoat] with which we wore a white scarf and gray gloves. In addition to that, we were issued a Navy cape which was dark navy with a maroon lining."[43]

Up in North Carolina, Ensign Nancy Aulenbach says, "I helped set up the hospital at Camp LeJuene. Camp LeJuene [Naval] Hospital had just been built and we outfitted it and supplied it. The hospital was dedicated at 10 A.M. on May 1, 1943 and at 12 o'clock the patients started rolling in from Cherry Point [Marine Corps Air Station Medical Facility about 30 to 40 miles Northeast of Camp LeJuene] and I found myself on P.M. duty that day. Camp LeJuene was a large hospital. They were preparing to take care of the wounded from the war, so there were 40 patients in every ward. Then it was so built that the corridor outside the ward could also hold many beds. There was one nurse to a ward; a doctor, a nurse and corpsmen. For night duty there was one nurse on the upper deck [floor] and one nurse on the lower deck."[44]

Further north at the Norfolk Naval Hospital in Portsmouth, Virginia, a 35 year old nurse, Evelyn Hope George, reports aboard for indoctrination and duty as a new Ensign in the Nurse Corps. She had graduated from nurses training in 1930 and had been doing industrial nursing as well as studying physical therapy prior to joining the Navy. She says, "There were 14 or 15 of us in one room [in the nurses quarters at Portsmouth]. They converted a pool room for us. We had double bunks and had a good time together. . . . While we were there, the Cadet nurses [a program to be discussed later on in this chapter] were starting to come in. I think they got us mixed up with the Cadet nurses. Most of us were older. Our picture was in the paper marching with the Marines, one time, and they called us Cadet nurses [when] we were 'boots' [individuals new to the Navy]. . . . [The] Marines taught us to march. . . .

"[While at Portsmouth] I had an interesting experience. I believe I helped pick up a spy on the staff. It was a doctor. . . . He had the therapy department and I had been assigned to the therapy department - because I was the only nurse there who had had any training in that field. . . . [We] had a 'fever' therapy department and we would run patients with venereal disease in these fever cabinets and they would become delirious. This doctor would question the boys that were delirious and ask them questions about boats and ship movement and things. I thought it was irregular. . . . So I felt it was out of ordinary and I asked another doctor that was a friend of mine, who I could trust, and I asked him if he thought that that was proper procedure. He said he didn't think so but that I had better not discuss it with anyone. The following day two men came in the department and questioned me about the machine . . . they were in civilian clothes and they went into the main office and got [the 'therapy'] doctor and then I was called in to say good-bye to him. He apparently had orders but they ushered him out and he left his cap with his scrambled eggs on it [Male Officer's hat with gold embroidery on the visor]. It was left on the desk and he was taken. We didn't see him again.

"Then [Chief Nurse] Bunty called me [to] her office and commended me. . . . She said, 'Sometimes we can't say why we're commending somebody,' but she commended me for my work I had been doing and didn't say specifically why."[45] Miss George also tells us about Norfolk having 'blackouts' at night. She mentions that the nurses had to move to Norfolk to a barracks as a nurses quarters for a short period of time. She says, "We were transported by bus back and forth and, of course, [at] six o'clock in the morning we'd be getting dressed without lights on, due to the blackout, and one morning I had one black stocking on and one white on"[46] with her white ward uniform. She didn't notice it until she was on the bus and on the way to the Naval Hospital for duty.

The American Journal of Nursing carries a 1943 article by Lt(jg) Edna Scheips about a special recreational facility for the Navy Nurses in the Fifth Naval District (the area including Norfolk and Portsmouth.) It is the Navy Nurse Officers' Club at Virginia Beach. "The club was conceived and organized by Commander Helen M. Bunty, Nurse Corps, U.S. Navy, ranking officer of the Corps in the Fifth Naval District."[47] Miss Scheips notes that the club is started in the summer of 1943 and the property was leased. It is "just off the ocean front . . . [and] the club includes among its facilities twenty-five rooms, eighteen baths, living-room, dining-room, kitchen, third-floor dormatory, and spacious terraces. . . . One of the rooms on the main floor has been converted into a small chapel, and here, on Sunday mornings, mass is read by a priest from Virginia Beach, and a Navy chaplain from the Chaplain's School at Williamsburg conducts Protestant services. The majority of the members are stationed either at the Norfolk Naval Hospital in Portsmouth or at the naval hospital at the operating base in Norfolk. . . . Week-ends find the already crowded buses from Norfolk to Virginia Beach carrying many Navy nurses, for with the ban on pleasure driving in this area, this is the only transportation to their club. They do not find the hour and a half trip too much of an inconvenience. . . . The club is run on a co-operative basis and every member upon registering is assigned a small detail."[48] Even though the Club is so close to the beach, activities on the beach are limited to daylight hours. "Because of war time security, everyone had to be off the beach by dark and the beaches were patrolled by service men with dogs."[49]

Back in March of 1943, another 'first' event takes place: the first members of the Women's Reserve (WAVES) report to the "Hospital Corps Schools at USNH San Diego and NNMC [National Naval Medical Center], Bethesda for orientation courses."[50] In addition, as Lt(jg) Esther Schmidt writes in the American Journal of Nursing, "WAVES of specified qualifications are daily being recruited for actual [naval] hospital duty within the continental limits of the United States, and are being trained as adequately as limited time allows. . . . [As] the outline of courses [for such training] has been made and presented by the Bureau of Medicine and Surgery, uniformity can be maintained throughout all schools which are to be organized. . . .

Classes for WAVES in [the naval hospital at] Corpus Christi began April 19, 1943. A group of forty-five is being sent to us every four weeks. At the present time these girls attend classes four hours a day, have one hour of drill weekly, and at the end of the first week are assigned to two hours of ward duty daily."[51] Miss Schmidt then outlines the courses and course contents as set-up by BuMed. The Major categories are: eight hours of Anatomy and Physiology, forty-five hours of Nursing, six hours of Hygiene and Sanitation, ten hours of First Aid and Minor Surgery, four hours of Materia Medica, and two hours of Metrology. (The latter has to do with weights and measures, percentages and solutions.) "All WAVES who take this training come to us with a rating of hospital apprentice, second class. Upon completion of the above course, they are rated up to and including pharmacist mate, second class, depending upon previous experience, education, age, professional qualifications, and corps school grades. Recommendations for these ratings are made to the Bureau of Medicine and Surgery by the commanding officer of the hospital. . . . If the future classes continue to measure up to the standards the first two have set, I would say the hospital WAVES are an excellent group from which to draw student nurses."[52]

The WAVES are not the only ones going to school, even in war-time, the Navy Nurse Corps continues the professional improvement and education of its members. "Fourteen members of the Navy Nurse Corps serving in various U.S. Naval Stations, are enrolled in a special course in dietetics given at George Washington University, Washington, D.C."[53] And, in December 1943, the first two Navy nurses report to the Army Air Force School of Air Evacuation at Bowman Field, Kentucky. These are the first of the Navy Flight nurses. They are Lt(jg) "Stephany J. Kozak (NC) USNR and Lt(jg) Dymphna M. Van Gorp (NC) USNR."[54]

Dymphna Van Gorp had graduated from Marquette University in Wisconsin with a BS in nursing in 1940. At the beginning of the war she was working for the Milwaukee Visiting Nurse Association. She had joined the Red Cross and "regularly received double post cards from the Red Cross in Washington asking my preference [for the Army or Navy Nurse Corps]. The return card was addressed to their local office. I returned the cards each time with my Navy choice marked but was never contacted. A year later I learned that it was local policy to keep nurses working in public health as long as possible. Meantime, I received orders from the Army's Sixth Service Command to report to . . . Oklahoma prepared for overseas deployment. I had had no official contact with the Army and most certainly had not taken their oath of office. . . . I also received some very strong letters later from the Army representative when I didn't respond to the orders. In the fall of 1942, I wrote to Captain Sue Dauser, Director of the Navy Nurse Corps, and as a result, . . . I became an Ensign. . . .

"It was at the US Navy Hospital on the base at Sampson, New York, that I reported on the 9th of March 1943. A new base, not yet completed, six miles of barracks and mud, was in the lovely 'finger lakes' area seventeen miles from Geneva, New York. Although there were wings of empty wards, the hospital was working. . . . There was need for a school for hospital corpsmen and I was assigned to this project with another nurse, but she was soon transferred. There was a war-time sense of urgency. No guidelines for the organization of the school were available nor were there any educational materials; no books, charts, equipment or instructors. [The Chief Nurse] said that . . . Manuals would arrive some time but I never saw one. Interviews with doctors reporting in from sea duty gave an idea of what a corpsman needed to know aboard ship. A curriculum evolved. Class room space and supplies had to be negotiated. All this gave me a chance to draw on past experience . . . where I had learned to improvise equipment, and we needed to improvise here.

"I wrote a small procedure manual with simple diagrams and looked for a way to duplicate it other than the blurred, blue ditto sheets used by the hospital. I was in luck when someone called 'the roving Chief,' who was really the night security watch, investigated the light under my office door. The fellow wore thin tennis shoes and rode a bicycle over what seemed miles of ramps. The entire hospital, all on ground level, . . . was spread over acres of land and, of course, there [were] war-time blackouts. The Chief told me of a store room of equipment no one yet knew how to use. To my joy I found a new . . . Mimeograph, far superior to the one I had learned to use at the age of sixteen. It never occurred to me to ask permission to use it. . . . So I produced my little manual. Nurses interested in teaching were assigned to the school. Students arrived at intervals of two or three days in various sized groups. . . . Procedures were at first learned in the wards. . . .

"We worked under the supervision of a medical officer, but for the most part I was left alone to do my job with minimal interference. Corpsmen were shipped out immediately on completion of final exams and we had, at one time in the beginning, 150 corpsmen and 50 WAVES. We put a good deal of effort in projects to help motivate learning even if that meant unorthodox methods of teaching. The idea was to make this learning experience unforgettable. Many students had had little choice - [they] had requested torpedo squadron or some other [field]. Their ages varied as did backgrounds, from the helper at a grocery store to the optometrist who was used to being called 'doctor,' now he was called by his last name only [as all other enlisted personnel below Chief Petty Officer]. . . . At the end of nine months I left nurses who were a joy to work with and a sense of a job well done. You don't always end this way."[55] From Sampson, Lt(jg) Van Gorp is ordered to flight school.

In 1942, a chain of islands off the Alaska Peninsula, the Aleutian Islands, had been attacked and two of the islands, Attu and Kiska, invaded by Japanese forces. Attu is the Aleutian Island farthest from the U.S. mainland and closest to Russia and Japan. Then, about two hundred miles east of Attu and about one thousand miles from the tip of Alaska Peninsula in the chain of the Aleutians, is the Island of Kiska. In May 1943, Allied forces attack the Japanese on Attu and, after several brutal battles, reclaim Attu. Then, in August, the Allies reclaim Kiska without a battle and without finding any enemy forces left on that Island. Navy Nurses are stationed at Naval Facilities on two of the Aleutian Islands; both of these Islands are closer to the Mainland but still near to 'harm's way.' They are stationed at the naval medical facility at Adak Island (about two hundred fifty miles east of Kiska) and at Dutch Harbor on Unalaska Island (about four hundred fifty miles east of Adak and about two hundred miles west of Alaska Peninsula.) Navy Nurses are also stationed at the Naval Facility on Kodiak Island but that is southeast of the Aleutians;directly south of Alaska Peninsula.

This, then, is the background for the narrative of Ensign Bettie Fuller Navy Nurse Corps. She is stationed at the Oakland Naval Hospital, California, in April 1943, when she receives orders to Sitka, Alaska. She is detached and travels to Seattle where she has to wait for further transportation. "I was there with five other nurses for about five days when we were given orders to board the USS *North Sea*, which had been a cruise ship before the war. The Navy had taken it over, but had retained the Captain and crew. . . .

"[The ship's] Captain Williams was delightful and gave us a wonderful cruise up the inland waterway. At night we would stop . . . and he and his officers would take us ashore and show us the sights. One day while we were waiting for the tide to change . . . Captain Williams lowered a life boat over the side and took us ashore and we dug clams, which were then taken back to the ship and cooked for our dinner. I arrived in Sitka about the 29th of April, 1943. Sitka was a Naval Air Station and had a small dispensary which we six nurses enlarged somewhat to form more of a hospital. In July . . . four of us received orders to Adak and were scheduled to leave . . . [on a ship] with a battalion of [Navy] SeaBees [C.B. which means Construction Battalion] who were headed for Adak. Our orders were to proceed to Dutch Harbor to await transportation. The SeaBees went on to Adak and, among other things, [they] built our nurses quarters [at Adak].

"We were at Dutch Harbor for about six weeks and then, with several other nurses, we boarded a plane and flew to Adak on August 13, 1943. Adak was a very austere, cold, foggy, muddy place. We were delighted to find our quarters in Adak unbelievably well built. The SeaBees had done a tremendous job of setting up five Quonset huts. Three of the Quonset huts were divided by a bath into two bedrooms accommodating four nurses. The fourth Quonset hut was the chief nurse's with bedroom, bath and living room. The fifth Quonset hut was a living room and kitchen, complete with all electric appliances. Eventually, the SeaBees added a sixth Quonset hut which was our recreation room complete with ping-pong tables, juke box, [and] suntanning equipment. A wonderful area for getting away from the miserable Aleutian weather."[56]

"In Adak the nurses' duties were difficult in many ways because the hospital was scattered over quite a bit of terrain. The hospital had been planned in this way because if there was a bombing the whole hospital wouldn't be destroyed. So that inspite of the mud and wind we had to walk from one end to the other between these various buildings. Also, to get to the hospital from the nurses quarters we had a long, deep, wooden stairway. During one of the famous Aleutian 'williwaws' [wind storms], the stairway was blown down and the only way we could get to the hospital was to have an ambulance come up the road and pick us up and drive us back down. . . . As we walked between our various [hospital] buildings, we would be ankle deep in mud, in our full button galoshes, and the dust would be blowing in our faces. This is because the wind never stops blowing in the Aleutians and while it was muddy under foot the wind dried the top off enough to produce dust.

"Not many people knew about the war in the Aleutians, although some very tough battles were fought [there]. . . . The battle [of Attu] had already taken place when I arrived in Adak but, now we were getting ready to invade Kiska and recapture that island. The [Navy] fleet built up in the harbor until the harbor was almost covered with ships (battleships, destroyers, etc.) and we were making plans to take care of casualties. August 15 was the date set for the invasion of Kiska. When our ships and men arrived and went ashore they found nothing. They searched the island and were amazed to find nothing but a few dogs on the island. Apparently under cover of the heavy Aleutian fog, the Japanese had evacuated all of their personnel from Kiska. During this period of time, one of the ships backed onto a mine and the stern was blown off. Those casualties were brought to us at Adak. But, those were the only casualties of the Kiska invasion."[57]

The Chief Nurse at Adak, at this time, is Lt(jg) Mildred Terrill. Miss Terrill tells us that while there in the Aleutians, all the nurses were given a copy of a diary purportedly written by a Japanese soldier on the island of Attu when it was invaded by Allied forces in May of 1943. She notes that, "We were given the diary so we would understand the Japanese better. They wanted us to know what the Japanese were doing."[58] Portions of entries at the very end of the diary are,

> "Life Facts:
>   March 6, . . . Graduated from . . . Medical School [in Japan]. . . .
>   Sept. 15, . . . to May 22, . . . [three years] Pacific Union College Medical Dept. Agwin, Cal. . .
>   Jan. 10, 1941 Transferred to 1st. Imperial Guard Inf.   Reg. . . . .

Sept. 1, [1941] Entered Army Medical School. Graduated Oct. 24. Acting Officer since December."[59]

The diary covers each day from May 12th through May 29th of 1943 and describes the fierce battles from the viewpoint of a Japanese medic. For May 21 the entry is, "Was strafed when amputating a patient's arm. It is my first time since moving over to . . . Harbor [on Attu] that I went in an air raid shelter. Enemy plane is a Martin. Nervousness of . . ., Commanding Officer is severe and he has said his last words to his N.C.O.'s and Officers that he will die tomorrow, gave all his articles away. Hasty chap, this fellow. The Officers of the front are doing a fine job. Everyone who heard this became desperate and things became disorderly."[60] On May 26 he writes, "The last line of . . . was broken through. No hope for reinforcements. Will die for the cause of Imperial Edict."[61] Then the last dated entry is for May 29th, "Today at 2000 we assembled in front of Headquarters. The Field Hospital took part too. The last assault is to be carried out. All patients in the hospital were made to commit sucide [sic]. Only 33 years of living and I am to die. I have no regrets. Banzai to the Emperor. I am grateful I have kept the peace in my soul, which Edict bestowed upon me. At 1800 took care of all the patients with grenades. Good-bye . . ., my beloved wife who has loved me to the last. Until we meed [sic] again, grant you God-speed. . . . The number participating in the attack is little over 1000, to take enemy Artillery positions. It seems the enemy is expecting an all out attack tomorrow."[62] On 29 May, Allied forces secured Attu.

In 1943 the need for professional nurses is critical. Many more are desperately needed in the military as well as on the homefront. "The vigorous recruitment by the armed forces created serious shortages in the civilian sector, and the manner in which this problem was solved had several long-range consequences. The movement to stratify nursing started before the war, but the wartime experience in both military and civilian hospitals was the deciding factor in changing nursing from a single entity to a multi-level system."[63] As mentioned previously, nurse's aides are being trained and used at this time to help in the WWII national shortage of professional nurses. "The second approach to the shortage was governmentally sponsored refresher courses to bring inactive nurses back into the work force. Since many of these women were married and had significant family responsibilities, they were available only part time. They were accepted on these terms, and employers found they could make significant contributions. As a consequence some of the old prejudices against married and part-time nurses crumpled. The third strategy was to bring massive numbers of students into nursing schools, not only to prepare them for nursing after graduation, but also to use their services while they were in training."[64] This third approach leads to the creation of the **U.S. Cadet Nurse Corps**.

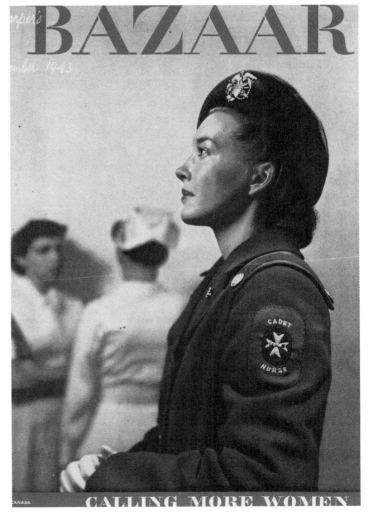

Cadet Nurse uniform WWII. (Photo courtesy of [Nursing Section] U.S. Public Health Service, Rockville, MD)

"In consultation with nursing and defense agency leadership, in 1943, the PHS [Public Health Service] determined that 65,000 women, 10 percent of all high school graduates that year, would need to be recruited into nursing and that a new approach . . . should be tried."[65] "These deliberations resulted in an administration bill creating the U.S. Cadet Nurse Corps. It was introduced in the House of Representatives by Francis Payne Bolton, congresswoman from Ohio and became law on June 15, 1943."[66] The bill was signed into law by President Roosevelt and becomes known as the Bolton Act placing responsibility for the program under the U.S. Public Health Service. Within the PHS, "A new Division of Nurse Education was created to administer the Bolton Act appropriations, which soon amounted to more that 50 percent of the entire USPHS annual budget. . . .

"This operation was headed by Lucile Petry (now Lucile Petry Leone). . . . To recruit 65,000 new student nurses in FY 1944 and another 60,000 in FY 1945 - about twice the number of students admitted to schools of nursing in peace time - a massive recruitment and publicity campaign was launched. All available media were used to spread the Cadet Nurse Corps message across the nation."[67] "The Cadet Nurse Corps was rapidly adopted by the Nation, receiving $13 million of donated publicity and technical assistance in its first year. Cadet nurses appeared on bill boards and radio spots, newsreels and magazine covers. A fashion show to [choose] the uniform was held at the Waldorf-Astoria and celebrities, such as Eleanor Roosevelt and Mrs. Winston Churchill, made regular appearances with Cadet nurses."[68]

(When WWII ends, "admission into the Cadet Nurse Corps was terminated and by 1949 the last student had graduated. Of the 170,000 students enrolled, 124,000 had graduated and 1,125 of the Nation's 1,300 nursing schools had participated. During 1945, 85 percent of nursing students in the country were Cadet nurses."[69]) It "was widely advertised that students entering schools of nursing would be provided with books, indoor uniforms, all entrance and tuition fees, and paid a generous monthly allowance for personal expenses. In addition, an attractive gray outdoor uniform was designed featuring crimson epaulets, insignia of the United States Public Health Service, and a distinctive sleeve emblem patterned after the Maltese Cross, emblem of the Knights of St. John of Jerusalem, organized during the Crusades. In return, students pledged themselves to remain in some type of active nursing for the duration of the war."[70] The 'monthly allowance' referred to above begins at "not less than $15 and [increases] to not less than $30 per month."[71] The Schools of Nursing training the Cadet nurses are "compensated from federal funds for:

1. Reasonable tuition and fees.
2. Maintenance for first nine months.
3. Uniforms and insignia. [The Cadet nurses wear the same indoor uniforms as the other student nurses.]
4. Stipends for all but the Senior Cadet period."[72]

This 'Senior Period' is the last six months of the Cadet nurse's training. The Senior Cadet Period can "be spent:

1. In the home hospital doing 8 hour duty with few or no classes.
2. In some other approved institution where the time would count toward graduation.
3. If requested by the student and a Federal hospital, in an approved Federal hospital.
4. The stipend of not less than $30 per month [is] to be paid by the institution using the services of the Senior Cadet nurse.

"Five Federal Agencies [plan] to use the services of the Senior Cadet nurses in their hospitals to augment the services of graduate nurses and sub-professional workers. These [are] the Army, Navy, U.S. Public Health Service in Marine hospitals, Veterans Administration and the Indian Service. All of these agencies except the Navy [are] permitted by law to employ under-graduate nurses under Civil Service."[73] The Law has to be changed to allow the Navy to utilize the Senior Cadet nurses. (Public Law 74 is amended in early 1944 and allows the Cadets in Navy hospitals. "Programs for the training of Senior Cadet nurses and the utilization of their services [are] first set up in the U.S. naval hospitals at Seattle, Oakland, San Diego, Chelsea, St. Albans and Portsmouth. Later Great Lakes, Sampson and Pensacola [are] added. . . . The program for Senior Cadet nurses in naval hospitals [is] in operation from April 1, 1944 to June 30, 1946. A total of 1150 Cadets"[74] are utilized in the Navy during that period.)

By 7 October 1943, about 860 schools of nursing receive Federal funds for the Cadet Nurse Corps.[75] ("The Cadet Nurse Corps enrolled 132,000 students to 1,125 nursing schools between July 1943 and October 1945."[76]) The program is very popular and, in fact, changes the face of nursing forever. Young women who would never have been able to afford higher education or the tuition fees for nurses training, find the Cadet Nurse Program to be their 'scholarship' to a bright future. As a result, the numbers of graduate nurses increase substantially and the profession grows in ways heretofore unsuspected.

The National Nursing Council for War Service, in its efforts to find further sources of nurses, has been looking not only at the practical nurses but also Black nurses and men nurses. "The NACGN (National Association of Colored Graduate Nurses) worked closely with the Council, and in the early days of the war, inquiries about Black nurses and opportunities for Blacks in schools of nursing were referred by the Council to the NACGN. Its small staff and limited budget, however, could not carry this increased load. With financial aid from . . . the Rockefeller Foundation, the Council elected to set up a Black unit on an experimental basis and appointed a Black nurse, Estelle Massey Riddle (Osborne) to direct it with the title of consultant. The preliminary work was so promising that . . . a second black consultant, Alma Vessells John, was added in 1943 and the work of the unit was integrated with the general program."[77] When Lucile Petry (Leone) is appointed to her position in the Public Health Service, she includes "on her staff . . . a Black nurse, Rita Miller (Dargan. . .), as a consultant on a part-time basis, on leave from Dillard University in New Orleans where she chaired the Division of Nursing. Miss Miller's responsibilities were to assist Black schools in applying for participation in the Cadet Nurse Corps program, to help Black schools qualify for the corps, and to facilitate inclusion of more Black students in the program."[78] "Her efforts combined with the generous grants awarded, allowed the stronger all-black schools dramatically to increase their student enrollment."[79]

In addition to this, in "order to qualify for a share of the Bolton Bill windfall, some white schools abandoned their discriminatory policies and extended equitable consideration to black applicants."[80] ("By 1945 approximately 2,600 black students were enrolled in schools of nursing, a 135 percent increase over the 1939 figure. By the end of World War II, `49 schools of nursing with black and mixed enrollments had admitted black students, as compared with 29 in 1941.' Furthermore, in addition to the outbreak of World War II, as Riddle and others observed, one of the indirect benefits of the Bolton Bill to black nurses was an enhancement of their chances to secure employment in institutions previously closed to them."[81]) In 1942 the Army Nurse Corps did accept some black nurses but, "in spite of continuous NACGN pressure, the Navy Nurse Corps proved unalterably opposed to the induction of black women nurses."[82]

"In 1943 there [are] four schools of nursing for men only: the Mills School, New York; the Pennsylvania Hospital School of Nursing for Men; and the two Alexian brothers', in Chicago and St. Louis. Seventy-five schools accepted men along with women, of which three were for [black] nurses, the students totalling about 900."[83] In 1943 the ANA does a survey of men nurses and "received more that 1000 returns. . . . The number of replies received from men already in military service was small but significant. . . . The men in the Navy who answered the ANA's questionnaire had all been assigned to the Hospital Corps with ratings from Pharmacist's Mate, third class, to Chief Pharmacist's Mate (permanent). Base pay in this group ranged from $78.00 to $138.00 per month."[84]

("In 1944 a member of the House of Representatives introduced a bill to give men nurses the temporary commissioned rank of second lieutenant in the Army and of ensign in the Navy which had been granted to members of the Nurse Corps. This bill had the active support of the ANA but was never brought out of committee."[85])

In Washington, DC, in 1943, 'The Manual of the Medical Department of the United States Navy' is published by the Bureau of Medicine and Surgery; printed by the U.S. Government Printing Office. In Chapter I, the main objective of the Bureau is succinctly stated under "Establishment, Organization, And Duties of the Bureau[:] . . .

> 6. Duties. - (a) General -
> The Bureau, under the direction of the Secretary of the Navy, is charged with and responsible for the maintainance of the health of the Navy, for the care of the sick and injured, for the custody and preservation of the records, accounts, and properties under its cognizance and pertaining to its duties, and for the professional education and training of officers, nurses, and enlisted men of the Medical Department of the Navy."[86]

The Medical Department is one of the 'support' entities for the Navy as a whole and the Bureau of Medicine and Surgery (BuMed) is the organizational and managerial center of that Medical Department. The Surgeon General of the Navy is the Head of BuMed which, at this time, is made up of the following sections; the "Medical Corps, Dental Corps, Nurse Corps, Hospital Corps, WAVES, and Civilian."[87]

Also published by BuMed in 1943, is a twenty-two page pamphlet on the Navy Nurse Corps. It shows black and white photos of Navy Nurses on duty, in dress blues and dress whites, a hospital ship, and an applicant for the Nurse Corps being sworn into the Corps, etc.. Along with the photos is a brief history of the Corps, and brief explanations of various aspects of the Corps. For instance, the requirements for entering the Corps are listed as:

> "1. Minimum preliminary education: High-school graduate.
> 2. Registered nurse; graduate from a school of nursing approved by the Surgeon General.
> 3. Age 22 to 28.
> 4. Citizen of the United States or naturalization of 10 years.
> 5. Single, widowed, or legally separated.
> 6. Physically qualified.
> 7. Satisfactory credentials from training schools and other sources."[88]

Additionally, the pamphlet states that the entering Navy Nurse's salary and uniform allowance are, "$150 per month with full maintenance for the first 3 years. 5 percent increase every 3 years. . . . There is a money allowance for complete initial outfits of the regulation ward and street uniforms."[89] On page 17 the pamphlet notes that, "Every Navy nurse and naval Reserve nurse serves a 6-month probationary period for observation of her adaptability, endurance, and professional qualifications for the Navy service. At the end of 6 months she is recommended for acceptance or rejection by the commanding officer of the station to which she is assigned." Even though there is a war and nurses are needed, the Navy Nurse Corps keeps its standards intact, just as the `Sacred Twenty' and especially the first Superintendent of the Corps, had intended.

Speaking of needing nurses, the American Journal of Nursing publishes the 'Quotas' needed from each State in the U.S. for the Army and Navy Nurse Corps for the year of 1943. The total number needed is given as 36,000. The highest quota of 4,164 nurses belongs to New York while Pennsylvania has the second highest at 3,960. The lowest is Nevada with a quota of 36 while Wyoming is next to last with 72.[90] But, Captain Dauser is worried about recruitment and the Red Cross. "During 1942-43, the Superintendent of the Navy Nurse Corps, Sue S. Dauser, indicated several times that she thought the Red Cross was overemphasizing the needs of the Army Nurse Corps at the expense of the Navy. In February, 1943, shortly after the public recognition of Red Cross Nursing Service as the recruitment agent for the army, . . . [it was] suggested to her that, if the two corps could be placed on the same basis, there would be less chance of discrimination.

But the trend in the opposite direction continued and by the end of 1943 the Navy Nurse Corps had taken over the processing of applications. The ostensible reason was that it was necessary to have complete data on all Navy Nurses. The Navy was always included in Red Cross publicity plans, however, and any recruitment or enrollment information gave facts about both branches of the military. Of the nurses who joined the Navy Nurse Corps after the Red Cross no longer processed the papers, more than half were referred by the Red Cross."[91] Meanwhile, the Army Nurse Corps announces that, "The marriage of an Army nurse to a member of the armed forces will no longer affect her assignment to duty. A married nurse will not be transferred to another station because her husband is serving at the same station."[92] The Navy Nurse Corps does not follow suit.

On December 31, 1943, the total active duty strength of the Navy Nurse Corps is 2907; 1104 are regular Navy and 1763 are reserve Navy.[93] And in 1943, "a convalescent hospital was commissioned at Santa Cruz on 8 March and the USNH Memphis, TN, officially opened on 17 March."[94]

In 1943, U.S. and Allied troops and naval forces begin to turn the tide of the war in the Pacific. "The American plan was to reach the Phillippines by two routes, one beginning at Guadalcanal and the other at the Gilbert and Marshall Islands. En route, islands would be either conquered or bypassed if possible."[95] General MacArthur leads his troops against the Japanese in New Guinea and New Britain to begin his island-hopping campaign back to the Philippines while Admiral Nimitz is preparing his carrier forces to support troops at the island battles necessary to carry out the American plan. Admiral Halsey leads the naval forces through the Solomon Islands battles then on to support MacArthur at New Britain. In late 1943, Admiral Spruance leads naval forces into the Gilbert Islands for the bloody battle at Tarawa.[96]

In the North African campaign of WWII, the "Axis desert fighters held the Allies to a stalemate during the winter of 1942-1943, but by mid-May, 1943, the Allied forces had conquered North African and were on schedule for the summer invasion of Sicily and Italy."[97] Meantime, out in the Atlantic Ocean, in "March, 1943, U-boat wolfpacks [German submarines] sank 108 ships. . . . But that was the peak. Slowly, month by month, the toll of German submarines went up."[98] And in Europe, on:

"July 10   Allied forces invaded Sicily.
Sept. 3   The Allies landed in Italy.
Sept. 3   Italy signed a secret armistice with the Allies.
Oct. 13   Italy declared war on Germany."[99]

All during the turmoil of war, there is, for the American people, the steadfast encouragement and pronouncements of the charismatic President; Franklin Delano Roosevelt. His 'fireside chats' make the radio a gathering place for families all over the nation. (Also, he is the first President to appear on television.) He leaves the "United States many times during the war for conferences with Allied leaders. He [is] the first President to leave the country in wartime. Early in 1943, he [meets] with Churchill in Casablanca, Morocco. The two leaders [announce] that they [will] accept only unconditional surrender by the Axis nations. In other conferences, Roosevelt [discusses] problems of war and peace with both Churchill and Premier Joseph Stalin of Russia. . . . Roosevelt also [confers] with Generalissimo Chiang Kai-shek of China in 1943. . . .

"In November, 1943, the Big Three [Roosevelt, Churchill, and Stalin, meet] at Tehran, Iran. During and after this conference, Roosevelt [works] to get Churchill and Stalin to agree on major war aims."[100] Then in 1944, President Roosevelt faces another election campaign, in addition to everything else. His Republican opponent is New York Governor Thomas E. Dewey. The "Republicans [argue] that no man should be President for 16 years. The Democrats [answer] by saying that America should not 'change horses in mid-stream.' Republicans [charge] that Roosevelt [is] in poor health. The President [replies] by driving around New York City in an open car for four hours during a rainstorm - and then making a major speech. Roosevelt [wins] an easy victory. He [carries] 36 of the 48 states."[101] But, the campaign and the war are taking their toll on the President's health.

As to the war in Europe, the "American high command had promoted a cross-Channel attack [from Great Britain] as early as 1942. The British, experienced in fighting the tough German war machine, counseled caution until the Nazis were considerably thinned and stretched, especially by their struggle with Russia. As it happened, a frustrating shortage of one essential, landing craft, meant postponement until 1944. 'The destinies of two great empires,' British Prime Minister Winston Churchill grumbled, 'seem to be tied up in some God-damned things called LSTs.' So England became, from 1942 on, a great armed camp. . . . So by the spring of 1944 the men and the weapons [are] massed in sufficient numbers."[102] "Long prepared, often adjourned (one actual false start was made), the gigantic expedition [takes] place in a short lull in the worst storms June [has] seen in the Channel for twenty years."[103] 6 June 1944; D-Day. The invasion of Normandy by British, American, French and Canadian forces. On 13 June the "first V-1 rocket fell on London."[104] Hitler is using the rockets his scientists have developed. But, by the end of 1944, the Allies are beginning to turn the tide on Germany.

Over in the Pacific, U.S. troops, Naval Forces, Marines and Allied forces are attacking, invading and raiding various islands in the island-hopping campaign begun in 1943. Then, on the 15th of June 1944, U.S. B-29 bombers raid Japan and:

"June 19-20 U.S. forces won the Battle of the Philippine Sea.
July 21 U.S. troops landed on Guam Island. . . .
Oct. 20 U.S. Army forces landed on Leyte. [Leyte is a Philippine island southeast of the main island of Luzon where Manila is located.]
Oct. 23-26 The U.S. Pacific Fleet crushed the Japanese Fleet in the Battle for Leyte Gulf."[105]

Away from the war itself and back in Washington, DC, on the 26th of February 1944, legislation is finally approved giving actual military rank (versus the 'relative' rank) to Army and Navy Nurses. But, it is approved only for the duration of the war plus six months and does not include pay or retirement or leave, etc.. These items remain the same as previously written in the laws governing the Nurse Corps specifically. According to a Navy JAG (Judge Advocate General) opinion, "Had such been the intent of Congress a specific provision to that effect would have been included in the [new] law. The only effect apparently contemplated by the legislation in question was to grant actual rank in lieu of relative rank to members of the Navy Nurse Corps."[106] Navy Nurses are now commissioned Naval Officers, albeit only temporarily. Temporary or not, in August, procedures are "established with [the] office of Naval Intelligence and [the] Civil Service Commission for [the] checking of applicants for commission in [the] Nurse Corps in [the] same manner as that followed for other candidates for naval commissions."[107] Then in September, the "Secretary of the Navy [authorizes] Nurse Corps selection in [the] ranks of Commander, Lieutenant Commander and Lieutenant (senior grade), on [the] basis of billet requirements."[108]

In May 1944, the Navy Nurses are authorized a slate-gray uniform, in addition to their other uniforms. "It was a one-piece double-breasted dress with notched lapels and a rolling collar. . . . The gray uniform was to be worn with black shoes, beige stockings and gray gloves. The purse was black corde without a handle. With the gray working uniform, either the standard, circular, visorless cap of the Corps with a commissioned officer's device, authorized in May 1944, or a garrison cap could be worn. The gray garrison cap had a miniature cap device on the left side and the . . . [rank insignia] on the right."[109] Then in August, a BuMed Memorandum signed by Captain Dauser, goes out addressed to 'All Officers of the Nurse Corps, United States Navy.' The subject is changes in the Nurse Corps' uniform regulations. First, there are the changes in the Nurse Corps insignia:

"(a) Elimination of the letters `NNC' from the present corps insignia.
(b) Elimination of large metal pin-on corps devices.
(c) A corps device made of gold embroidery or of yellow silk of approved shade will be worn on the sleeves of the blue uniform . . . above the gold stripe. . . .
(d) A corps device made of gold embroidery of yellow silk will be worn on the shoulder marks [shoulder boards]. . . .
(e) The miniature metal pin-on insignia of rank will be worn on the right collar tip of the indoor duty

uniform and miniature pin-on corps device on the left collar tip in the same position as the present large pin-on device."

The same memorandum then states, "The regulation for hose with the Service Dress, White, is changed from white to beige hose." Then at the end of the memorandum, the `Overseas duty uniform' is noted, "At overseas hospitals where laundry facilities are limited the officers of the Nurse Corps, subject to approval of the commanding officer, may wear the basic seersucker gray and white striped dress of the Women's Reserve. This will be worn without tie, and open at the neck, with the same miniature devices as with the white duty uniform, and with beige hose and black shoes."[110] "The instructions for the dress of members of the Nurse Corps were brought up to date by a Bureau of Naval Personnel letter of December 15, 1944. . . . For the first time, nurses were designated by their rank, not as Superintendent, Assistant Superintendent, and so on. Provision was made for ranks up to and including that of captain, and the same sleeve lace and metal rank devices were employed as for men."[111] "Although the [changes] of December 15, 1944 . . . specified a beige stocking for use with the blue uniforms, nurses were permitted to wear the formerly authorized black hose during the transition period."[112]

Back in April of 1944, the Cadet Nurses began reporting into Naval Hospitals to start six months of practice for the end of their senior year of nurses' training.[113] For the education and utilization of the Cadet Nurses, the "Bureau of Medicine and Surgery of the Navy set up policies, [and] selected six hospitals, and assigned two instructors to each [hospital]. The program was to be an integral part of the nursing service and under the direction of the Chief Nurse. . . . The U.S. Naval Hospital, Chelsea, Massachusetts, was one in which the program was to be instituted and it was here that we were assigned. [Lt(jg) Esther Schmidt NC USN and Lt(jg) Catherine Meredith NC USNR.] . . .

"In order to understand the position of the cadet nurse in the naval hospital, it is necessary to outline the organization briefly and to identify and state the duties of the ward personnel. A physician is designated as medical officer and in that capacity is ultimately responsible for all of the ward activity. The Navy nurse assists him to carry out the purposes of the ward and is essentially an administrator, supervisor, and teacher and not a bedside nurse. Her position corresponds to that of the head nurse in a civilian hospital. On a division there are never more than three nurses on day duty - this is the exception and the majority of divisions have only one. She is responsible for the management of the ward, the direction of the nursing care, the housekeeping, and clerical work. Two fundamental situations in this organization which have had bearing on our planning are that patients are kept in the hospital during the entire period of illness, that is until discharged from the service or able to return to duty; and that the nursing care is given by the corpsmen whose preparation at present is limited. . . .

"Corpsmen and WAVES carry out all the duties that in a civilian hospital would be assigned to staff nurses, student nurses, nurse's aides, orderlies and housekeeping personnel. Six weeks in a corps school affords the basic preparation they receive for carrying on their hospital duties. . . . The convalescent patients, whose duties are assigned on the direction of the medical officer, must be included in the working personnel as they assist in keeping the word clean and in good order. The above situation was the one into which the senior cadet was introduced. Our problem was to define her responsibilities and functions and make the best use of what she had to offer. . . . With this in mind, the cadet nurse was assigned to the nursing care of patients with the understanding that she was to teach the corpsmen and the WAVES. This was to be accomplished by setting an example of excellent bedside care and by supervising these workers in their nursing practice. . . . It was absolutely necessary to work through the charge nurse. We discussed with her the making of a plan for the specific work of the student, and her responsibilities and the student's need for guidance. She was designated as the assistant to the cadet instructor."[114] The program at Chelsea is planned on an average of fifty cadet students but in actuality, the number varies when the program goes into action.[115] In July of 1944, the first two Senior Cadet nurses complete their training at naval hospitals; Amy A. Reichert at Chelsea, Massachusetts and Georgette Marie Bayless at Seattle, Washington.[116]

On 1 January 1944, Navy Nurses are stationed at:

"Outside Continental Limits:

Adak [Alaska]	Kodiak [Alaska]
Argentia, Newfoundland	New Caledonia
Attu [Alaska]	New Hebrides Islands
Australia	New Zealand
Bermuda	Puerto Rico
Canal Zone [Panama]	Samoa
Cuba	Trinidad, B.W.I.
Curacao, N.W.I.	Virgin Islands
Dutch Harbor [Alaska]	USS *Solace*
Hawaiian Islands	USS *Relief*

Within [the] Continental Limits at 40 Naval Hospitals, 176 Naval Dispensaries, [and] 6 Hospital Corps Schools."[117]

One of the Continental Naval Hospitals is St. Albans on Long Island in New York. Navy Nurse Edith Colton reports there in July, 1944. "As I recall, there were close to five hundred nurses stationed there. It was at St. Albans Hospital that the Cadet Nurse Program was started. I was stationed there for only four months and had less than one month's ward duty. For my night duty, I was assigned the nurses' quarters. My main duty was to man the phone for emergencies. I also had to make sure that each nurse signed in and out of the log book when she left or returned to quarters. This log was scrutinized each morning by the Chief Nurse. The rest of my duty at St. Albans was [an assignment] in the dining room and kitchen where I was to oversee the help and make seating charts for the dining room. Once again we had very lovely service."[118]

By that Miss Colton means that the dining is similar to what she experienced when she first entered the Navy in 1942 at the new Naval Hospital in Seattle, Washington. She tells us that the nurses quarters there in Seattle were such that there "were two nurses in each room with a community bath down the hall. Our main meal was at noon. All the nurses gathered in the living room of the quarters in anticipation of the arrival of the Chief Nurse and her assistant. When they arrived, they led the way into the dining room. We were assigned tables with eight to a table. One nurse had the responsibility of being the hostess. When the main dish was brought to the head of the table . . . she proceeded to serve it. The nurse to the left or the nurse at the end of the table would serve the other dishes. The service was all silver. The entire meal was quite elegant, with all the dinnerware being silver and the service very posh. It was typical Navy tradition, even in wartime."[119]

Also, Navy Nurse Colton describes the ward routine that she learned at Seattle in 1942. Her description could be of almost any open ward in almost any Naval Hospital in the States. (In general, it could be of any open ward in almost any Naval Hospital throughout the 1940's, 1950's and early 1960's.) "In organizing a ward, I discovered that books were a very important part of ward management. We had a log that took care of the census of the patients. Every patient and his diagnosis was entered daily in the book, beginning with the more seriously ill listed first. We also had a linen book, a drug book, and no doubt others that I have forgotten! Each morning, after the Ward Medical Officer arrived, there was Sick Call. Each patient who was able to be out of bed was standing at attention at his bedside. If a patient was unable to get out of bed he was at attention in his bed. There were 30-35 beds with [about] 18 beds to a row. [From one end of the ward, the beds on the left were in the 'port row' and the beds on the right were in the 'starboard row.'] At the entrance to the ward was the doctor's office, the treatment room, the kitchen ['galley'] and quiet rooms. The quiet rooms were for the more seriously ill. The doctor and a nurse stopped at each bed with a corpsman who carried the chart rack and, when necessary, another who manned the dressing cart. The nurse recorded all the [doctor's] new orders, cancellations, and changes in the Sick Call book.

"The food was brought [to the ward] from the main kitchen in a food cart. The food cart was brought by a corpsman who was assigned that duty as well as by a patient who was assigned to help. It was a metal cart with bumpers on the sides. It plugged into the wall and had wells for soup, vegetables, etc. There were salads and desserts kept underneath. The patients would line up and be served on divided metal trays. Those who were unable to come to the chow cart had their tray carried to them by another patient. They all looked out for each other. . . .

"The patients, according to their physical condition, were assigned cleaning duties. As their physical ability progressed, so did their cleaning duties. There were never any civilians working for us; we completely depended on corpsmen and patients. There was also no such thing as limited duty for the patients. When a patient was hospitalized, he remained so until he was fully recovered and fit for duty; therefore we had many who were capable of being assigned more strenuous duties. Much to our consternation, the outside '[master-at-arms]' was ever on the look-out for these patients and would recruit the men for [his work details]. Since the liberty [permission to leave the compound for a specified time period] was always better, we would get a good man trained and lose him [to the master-at-arms]."[120]

In early 1944, Ensign Ruth Gouge reports into the Naval Hospital in Long Beach, California. She had her nurses training in Dayton, Ohio and obtained her Bachelor of Science degree in Denver, Colorado. She joined the Navy in 1943 and was stationed at the Brooklyn Naval Hospital in New York prior to her new orders. She states, "I proceeded to the Naval Hospital in Long Beach, California. I was awe-struck by the tropical [climate], never having experienced this. . . . On [one] occasion, while covering the evening emergency room, the Shore Patrol brought in a very tall and very young Marine. He obviously had over imbibed. As was the custom, I asked him to say 'around the rugged rock the ragged rascal ran.' Teetering unsteadily but without hesitation, he replied, 'lady, I can't say that but I've sure been there.' His injuries were minor but he had made me smile. All injuries in the ER were not minor nor with levity. On Christmas day of 1944, a devastating experience occurred. An ambulance arrived and a stretcher rushed into the department. A young sailor lay on the stretcher drained of all color and life. Beneath his head was a small wash basin to catch the seeping blood from a self-inflicted bullet wound from temple to temple. The tragedy was reflected [in the faces] of the two Navy uniformed ambulance drivers. It was no less apparent in mine. Needless to say, that Christmas remains indelible in my mind."[121]

Also, in California, at the new Naval Hospital on Camp Pendleton near Oceanside, is Ensign Freddie Tucker of the Navy Nurse Corps. She writes, "The hospital was built to care for servicemen returning from the Pacific battles as well as those in training. Camp Pendleton was the training center for the Third, Fourth and Fifth Marine Divisions which would fight in the final battles of WWII. The hospital was in such a remote area that we could hear coyotes howling at night. Many patients were veterans of the First Marine Division who had served in the South Pacific battles of Guadalcanal and [the] Solomon Islands. They suffered from malaria and other tropical diseases. Malaria cases were isolated which I thought strange having grown up in Alabama where malaria was common. There were cases of mumps, scarlet fever and spinal meningitis. Penicillin was the new wonder drug but was not in plentiful supply. . . . I [also worked] on a medical ward where young sailors from the Farragut, [North Dakota] training station, had contracted rheumatic fever and were sent to sunny California to recuperate. These young men were only 17-18 years old and had not finished boot camp. They were not disciplined in any way - quite a contrast to the Marines we usually had as patients. These sailors refused to obey the doctor's orders for bed rest and only a 'Captain's Mast' brought order. [The Commanding Officer, usually a Captain, is authorized to convene, for judgement, minor offense cases and, where deemed guilty, the Captain can assign certain punishments to the guilty service-persons. This is a Captain's Mast.] . . . Sometime in late 1944 . . . we were given a gray dress uniform which was more comfortable in the warm climate though not more attractive. We never wore the white uniform in California."[122]

In October 1944, Navy Nurse Rachel Todd and another Navy nurse stationed at Pearl Harbor, receive "orders to sail back to San Francisco with a dependent who had been shot by her husband. . . . It wasn't hard when the patient was not ill, but she was bedridden."[123] Once they turned the patient over to the Naval Hospital, they were given leave then reported into the Oakland Naval Hospital for duty. "Among other duties while at Oak Knoll, I was assigned to central supply. Those were the days when we had 2,000 patients aboard. We also, in those days, had to sharpen each needle, regardless of shape or length, wash out all the [IV] tubings and then set-up new IV trays, cut the gauze (the Red Cross ladies would make the 4x4's), and supply oxygen to oxygen tents on the wards. The corpsmen . . . [from the wards] came twice a day, at 9:00 in the morning and 3:00 in the afternoon to get the necessary supplies. 'I need 30 IV trays', 'I need 5 canisters of 4x4's', 'I need 8 canisters of fluffs', 'I need 14 IV's of 5%/10% Glucose', whatever it was, they came in and asked by the bunches. I finally ordered enamel buckets to use instead of the canisters because [the corpsmen] couldn't carry all the canisters they needed . . . and, of course, they couldn't wheel [any carts or guerneys] around with all the ramps [the hospital] had. . . . The nurses today have no idea what it is like to sharpen each needle, wash out each piece of tubing, make 2x2's, 4x4's, set-up each tray, [and do all the autoclaving/sterilizing necessary]. . . . You name it and we were responsible to have what was requested at any time."[124]

On the other side of the country, a young Navy Nurse, by the name of Ednoa Pauls, performs her active duty at the Naval Hospital, Bethesda, Maryland. She had joined the Navy in 1942 and was sent to the Naval Hospital at the Naval Air Station in Corpus Christi, Texas. After seventeen months, she received orders to the Naval Hospital at Bethesda, Maryland where she is assigned duty on SOQ [Sick Officers Quarters] in the 'Towers' of Bethesda. She writes that, "SOQ at 'Bethesda' . . . is in the tower of the main building. Eighteen floors from the eighth floor up were medical patients. There were two or more nurses on each floor, but my duty assignment was to all of the floors. The assignment required a lot of walking and many more responsibilities than at Corpus. The officers as patients were from all areas of the War and, for many of them, Bethesda was their last hope for treatment or recovery. There were also V.I.P. patients at Bethesda, as we served the Washington area politicians. As a nurse, I am reluctant to reveal all the important people who passed through or to share any gossip, but I will say that President Franklin D. Roosevelt, Senator Tom Connelly, Harry Hopkins as well as others were our patients. There was also a 'Mr. X', a German submarine Captain. He had a guard posted at his door 24-hours a day and since he was in traction and couldn't possibly run away, we wondered about the guard; was he there to keep intruders out?"[125]

Up in the Northeast part of the country, Ensign Claire Walsh is stationed at the Naval Hospital, Portsmouth, New Hampshire. The Navy's main 'Brig' (prison) is also there in Portsmouth. Miss Walsh is assigned to one of the military wards at the hospital. She says it was "my first experience in a military ward. While we were there, three German submarines were brought in and they came right into the Navy Yard [at Portsmouth] to the dock. The Germans were taken up to the prison, which we called the 'castle'; the large naval prison there in the Navy Yard. One of the men from the German submarine was taken to the hospital by ambulance and brought to our ward which was the prison ward [often this ward in the Naval Hospitals was also called 'the brig']. Marines guarded the ward at all times and the ward was very secure. . . . Anyway, the young man had [to have] an appendectomy and he was quite apprehensive until someone found someone in the hospital who had [a] smattering of German and he went to the operating room with the patient so he could help the anesthesiologist in all the communication."[126] So, Navy Nurses did not have to go to the war area to meet with Axis troops, but even the enemy patient is still a patient until proven otherwise.

In December 1943, two Navy Nurses were the first to attend 'flight' school; Lt(jg) Kozak and Lt(jg) Van Gorp. (As mentioned earlier in this chapter.) They finish their course in Air Evacuation Training in early 1944 and they are ordered to Rio de Janeiro, Brazil where they are to assist "in setting up an air evacuation training program for the Brazilian Air Force nurses."[127] Miss Van Gorp tells us that in early 1944, "we were on our way to Brazil in a small two-engine, propeller plane of a commercial air line. We boarded at Miami [and] had two overnight stops; the first at Trinidad . . . and the other . . . [in] Brazil at the mouth of the Amazon River. [After] landing at . . . [the latter stop], a large man came aboard announcing that he was from the Minister of Health and it was his duty to make sure travelers did not bring diseases into his country. From his shirt pocket he drew six mouth thermometers which he quickly thrust into the mouths of the first six passengers. When he retrieved them, he put them back into his pocket for the minute it took to speak to [his] assistant who was taking notes, then he continued to the next passengers.

"The two of us . . . arrived in Rio de Janeiro on the 30th of January 1944. It was still summer there where the seasons were reversed from ours [in the States]. We were members of the Navy delegation of the Joint Brazil-United States Military Commission. . . . Our immediate task was to introduce to Brazilian nurses methods of transporting patients by air. This was to be done while the Brazilian Air Force started the preliminary process for the organization of their nurse corps. We met the Director of the . . . School of Nursing . . . and [the] nurses from the school who were to be our students. We particularly sought out one of the senior nurse instructors . . . who had been in the United States and spoke . . . [English]. She was . . . a part-time instructor who would assist us in setting up our program. We also had access to the class rooms at the school, although our first group was to be small in number. The Brazilian Air Force base . . . (some 50 miles from the city) was the site of our training activities. We were provided with a physical education instructor and a swim coach and used an olympic-size pool to teach swimming and to practice ditching drills with life rafts. We were also provided with a mock-up of the cabin of a plane, in the beginning. Later on . . . we used a cargo plane which we had outfitted with straps and brackets for holding litters and equipment. . . .

"Nurses learned the fundamentals preparatory to getting patients aboard a plane, such as triage and smooth ambulance travel and positioning of patients on the plane according to need for specialized nursing care. . . . Later Brazilian corpsmen were added to the practice sessions with the cargo plane. Classes began at six in the morning and on days when they were scheduled at the air field, we had to leave the apartment at four or earlier to get to the commercial airport in the city. There we would catch the miserable bus for a bumpy ride to the base. Pilots and instructors were also passengers. Once or twice we were all lucky and went by small plane that had to be at the base too. . . . With modification, we taught what we had learned at the Army school in Kentucky, including desert, jungle and sea survival for patients and crew. Later, after . . . [Miss Kozak, the other Navy Nurse] had married and left the area, another Navy Nurse and I directed a training film of air transportation of wounded featuring Brazilian nurses and corpsmen. At the same time, at the Brazilian Air Force hospital, the two of us covered 24 hours of hospital duty with American patients when it was required.

"At the air field we had formed a routine where we simulated the process of patients arriving by ambulance to the plane where a loading crew was standing ready. From a balcony running the length of the two-story communications building, pilots observed our every move. One day we had a new ambulance driver and his driving was erratic enough to scare the rest of us. Small planes were parked near by and at one time it looked like he would shear the tail off one of them. By that time I had had some lessons in the language, but he was from the Amazon region and I spoke . . . [a different dialect] so I couldn't make him understand. . . . So I got in and drove the ambulance to show him how. . . . Then I saw that all activity had stopped. Corpsmen were holding patients on litters in mid-air, for [example]. They had never seen a woman drive before and certainly not a bulky machine like that [ambulance]. . . .

"Our uniforms and insignia were of special interest everywhere . . . and for two years we were never out of uniform. Ceremonies and official functions seemed numerous and we were expected to attend. We learned that an invitation from a high-ranking official was an order. . . . One day, in the morning, we were notified by phone that we were invited by Admiral Halsey to a reception that afternoon. We were finishing three grueling weeks at the hospital and were in no mood for a party. Our last patients were to be discharged the next morning. We were both expected at the reception and assumed we would be back in about two hours. As a guest of the Brazilian government, the Admiral was staying in the only house on a small island in the bay. With other guests we went by Captain's gig and on arrival were welcomed by the Admiral who was wearing an aloha shirt. We were the only ones in uniform until later when the Admiral made a broadcast and wore his for the cameras. . . . After a very late dinner and more talks, we were finally on our way back. We came ashore at two in the morning. That same evening I attended an embassy function. . . .

"Every Friday I submitted the report on our activities of the previous seven days. One Friday morning, after night duty, I went to the Naval Operating base to write the report. The spacious room was empty except for a large desk directly opposite the door [plus] a chair and a typewriter. I was barely started when the ragged shoeshine boy came in. I was in blue uniform. [I] kicked off my [black] pumps and continued to type. The boy, as usual, sat in the middle of the room . . . with his legs spread out and started his work. Suddenly, the door blew open [and] at the same time I heard a loud 'ATTENTION!' By habit I jumped up, acutely aware that the big opening in the desk revealed my stocking feet. In the doorway stood General Eisenhower. He quickly took in the scene, smiled broadly and said, 'Carry on.'

"Oh yes, our living conditions. On arrival we stayed at the . . . Hotel until an apartment became available in an area approved by the military. Other Americans told us that we had to hire servants or suffer finding a dead chicken on the door step as a sign that we refused to help the economy. However, our apartment was furnished complete with a combination maid/cook selected by the landlady who occupied the flat below [us]. All our food was purchased at small stores in the neighborhood and variety was limited. We also had a laundress who did the laundry at her place. Everything was so expensive that we counted sheets and towels closely and when things weren't returned for a month, discovered that the laundress was renting them out. Also, the maid did a job of babysitting in the place when we were not there. The second maid was much better but there were always little things for us to learn. At times, we went to Uruguay to hold clinic for the large diplomatic staff at Montevideo and once I returned to Rio with a large beef tenderloin, as meat was like groceries; limited in variety. We invited friends in for filet mignon and were all much in anticipation. When [the cook] set a platter of meatloaf on the table! She explained that meat with no bone in it was always ground-up."[128] Lt(jg) Dymphna Van Gorp, Lt(jg) Stephany Kozak and the Navy nurse in charge of the nursing service at the Central Aeronautical Hospital in Rio de Janeiro, LT Catherine M. Kain, all receive the Navy Commendation Ribbon for their service in Brazil.[129]

Speaking of flight nurses, in November 1944 Ensign Mary Ellen O'Connor (NC) USNR receives TAD orders to Washington, D.C.. She is a former flight stewardess for United Air Lines and she is called to BuMed to discuss and help make plans for training Flight nurses for the Navy.[130] Miss O'Connor had more that 8800 hours in the air with UAL and had been a flight instructress for them.[131] As a result, the first course in 'Navy Flight Nursing' is prepared for opening at the NAS (Naval Air Station) Alameda, California on 11 December 1944.[132] (Classes for the first corpsmen are held at the same time.) Ensign O'Connor is promoted to Lt(jg) and is designated as the flight nurse in charge at the Naval School of Air Evacuation for Casualties at Alameda. Twenty-four Navy Nurse Corps officers are selected for the first course of instruction.[133] The Navy Nurses are:

"Kathryn Burke	Mary Leahy Hudnall
Mattie Dillard Hill	Stella Makar Smith
Dorothy Doll Dolan	Gladys Markell Teefy
Irene Freeburger Oddo	Lydia Masserine
Lucile Gemme Findley	Gweneth Nolan
Myrtle Hanna Boring	Emily Purvis Dace
Mae Hanson Ankeney	Kathleen Redmond
Norma Harrison Crotty	Evelyn Schretenthaler Wisner
Gwendolyn Jensen Murray	Miriam Serrick McAllister
Winnie Jennings	Emma Urgitis Barbiero
Jane Kendeigh Cheverton	Kathryn Van Wagner Pribram
Rachel Larue Nichols	Dorothy Wood Murphy"[134]

The course instructors are "flight surgeons whose responsibility it [is] to teach everything they [can] regarding the care of patients in flight. The two-month course [includes] training films, lectures and demonstrations. At this time, the Army [has] been evacuating patients for several years and their flight surgeons and nurses [are] very helpful to us."[135]

Back in Brooklyn, New York, Ensign Eveline Kittilson is stationed at the Naval Hospital. She says, "It was a very old hospital located by the Navy shipyard so it was noisy and dirty. We didn't have any air conditioning in those days so we left our windows open. Every day when I came off duty my bedspread would be covered with dirt. There was so much to see and do there when we got liberty. Manhattan was only 15 - 20 minutes away on the subway and it was perfectly safe to ride the subway then, night or day. . . . While at Brooklyn, hospital ships were being built in the shipyard and I kept hoping to be assigned to one of them when completed but instead I received orders to San Juan, Puerto Rico [in the latter part of 1944]. We referred to it as the 'fur lined foxhole' as we didn't get any war casualties. The hospital was a single story frame building with outlying wards. Our patients were active duty men in the San Juan area. Occasionally a merchant ship would be sunk in the area and we would receive casualties. Here we lived in two and three bedroom houses near the hospital and a native Puerto Rican maid did our cleaning and washing. We had our own mess in another house. All of the corpsmen were conscientious objectors. There were only about a dozen nurses here and the work was very routine."[136]

Ensign Rita F. Reed has been in the Navy for just six months when she receives her orders for overseas duty. "The Chief Nurse called me to her office one afternoon; [the] subject [is] overseas orders. [The Chief Nurse says,] 'Pack all your gear. Be sure to take your small scrubbing board to wash head covers and gloves.' She issued me orders to report to the Commandant of the Third Naval District for transportation. In Norfolk, Virginia I met our [new] Chief Nurse, Lt(jg) Clyde Pennington. Our group consisted of two Lt(jg)s and twenty-two Ensigns [and the Chief Nurse]. We reported, as ordered, to our ship. . . . Employing rank, we rode the Captain's gig to our ship, climbed the ladder, requested and received permission to come aboard the . . . [ship] which was the Admiral's flag ship. We occupied his staff's quarters for the next two weeks.

"At sea, from the 4th of March until the 18th of March 1944, our convoy consisted of our ship and two destroyer escorts. Aboard ship we first had life boat and survival drill. We certainly surprised the male officers aboard when they saw 25 Navy Nurses. Soon we were all friends [and] under war-time conditions, we zig-zagged our way across [the ocean]. Enroute Miss Pennington discussed hospital routines and our assignments. I was to be the anesthetist. We had strict blackout conditions, kept life jackets nearby or on, constantly sang songs, played games and enjoyed sunshine on deck. [The ship] anchored 24 hours off shore at Gibraltar, then proceeded to the harbor in Oran, North Africa, arriving on March 18, 1944. We learned our hospital was about seven miles from the port. Once that area had large homes, formal gardens, vineyards, palm trees and farming. Much of this had been damaged during the German occupation. [Navy] Base Hospital No. 9, which had been built by the SeaBees, was already staffed with doctors and corpsmen. We were the first group of Navy Nurses.

"We soon learned to find our way around the large compound. We had medical, isolation, surgical wards, operating rooms, central supply and special treatment rooms. We were a city of quonset huts. Our quarters consisted of three buildings plus a recreation hut. All officers shared another recreation hut and the mess hall. We wore our starched white uniforms and white shoes and stockings. Fortunately, there were native people to do our laundry. We rotated shifts and carried on all the routines that we'd done at the Naval Hospitals in the States. The night nurse had one additional duty, it was to go into the three huts around 4 a.m. to turn the oil heater up because the nights were cold as well as the early mornings. We had some busy times. Our patients were coming from Sicily and Italy at that time.

"Periodically the hospital ships would come into the harbor, mostly the USS *Refuge*, and take the patients who required long-term care and specialized treatment back to the States. Our other patients were treated and returned to duty. There were times when we were on call [and] we worked long hours and then [there were times when] we had short days. Depending upon the hospital conditions, we could request a Jeep and driver to take us to the very lovely beach near the harbor or into the city of Oran for some errands. We were allowed to shop in a few of the stores, although there was very little to buy and very little that we wanted to buy. . . . In early June 1944, we all became aware of much unusual and secret activity. Our hospital was put on stand-by alert. Later we learned that this was due to the D-Day, June 6, 1944 invasion. We were part of it without being aware of it. . . . This [tour of duty in Africa] is probably my most challenging duty due to the fact that I was very new to the Navy and also [it was] my first time out of the United States, or actually, out of New England."[137]

Three young Nurse Corps Ensigns at Bethesda, receive overseas orders and join a large group of Navy Nurses at Lido Beach, New York where, in January 1944, they board the British ship, HMS *Aquitania*. "All of us were teary eyed when the Army band played 'I can't give you anything but love, baby' and 'Lady, be good to me.' Jean [Jean Reichard] and I [Sara Marcum] shared a stateroom with four other nurses from various hospitals, there [were] 3 tiered bunks on either side. Only two of us could get dressed at one time, then we would go to the library or topside so the others could get dressed. . . . About 1 day from Scotland some enemy planes were observed overhead and the gunnery crew fired at them. We had to stand by with abandon ship gear on. I heard one of the English sailors say 'I bloody hope this doesn't ruin our tea time!'"[138] They land safely and then proceed to London. "When we arrived in London we had fog and air raids, which were additional experiences."[139] After a short time in London, the Navy Nurses travel, by train, to the Royal Victoria Hospital in Netley, England, arriving on 30 January 1944. The hospital is about five miles south of the port of Southampton. It is an elderly, historic facility, whose foundation stone was laid by Queen Victoria in 1856 and finally completed in 1863. "Queen Victoria and Florence Nightingale are both known to have worshiped in the Royal Chapel."[140]

"Ensign Helen Converse Kusenberg . . . spoke reverently of their privilege in walking through the wards where Florence Nightingale had made her rounds. They met and visited with an English matron who had known Miss Nightingale, and they saw the lamp . . . which she [Florence Nightingale] had used on her nightly rounds through the wards at Scutari as she tended the wounded heroes of another war [Crimean War]."[141] "Formerly a British hospital, this institution is a quarter of a mile long, is three stories high with more than a hundred wards, operation rooms, and laboratories, and is maintained in a state of constant readiness. Sixty outbuildings can be utilized in emergencies, almost doubling the normal capacity. The hospital maintains a staff of 50 doctors, 12 hospital corps officers serving as technicians, 98 trained navy nurses and 400 skilled hospital corpsmen."[142] Ensign Desmarais (NC) USNR writes, in an article in the AJN, "We received our first casualties on D [D-Day] plus 4 (June 10, 1944) in England. They were fresh battle casualties that had been given only first aid and the sulfonamide routine in France and aboard the LST's which brought them into Southampton, England. . . . My station was in the upper third deck operating room, but I was also senior nurse on a medical ward and stayed there to direct the admission of casualties until it became necessary to start serving as an anesthetist. . . . I was called to the operating room about 11:00 A.M. on that day and began immediately to give anesthesia. There was no time for meals or rest. The line of casualties was endless, it seemed. . . . I worked that day, as did all the staff, until 3:00 A.M., then had a sandwich and coffee and three hours of sleep. . . . Everyone worked for four consecutive days under these circumstances, then the casualties came in sporadically for a few days in small groups of 250 to 300 patients. We had an opportunity to rest and get supplies ready for the next large group of admissions four days later."[143] Not only do they have the influx of battle casualties, there are the air raids and bombs to contend with. "Air raid alerts, A.A. [anti-aircraft] fire, and explosions had become commonplace during the 'baby blitz' of February to April and the news on June 13th of the robot bombs (V-1) was not received at first with the seriousness it merited. The stereotyped announcement that flying bombs had fallen on 'Southern England, including the London area' and that 'damage and casualties were caused' become real for us on June 24 when the first one fell in our vicinity. During July, the Portsmouth-Southampton area, a strip of about 18 miles in length and five in breadth, was a target and it is believed some five hundred bombs were launched. On two nights within a period of several hours, 25 fell within a radius of about four miles from the hospital. . . . The bombs seemed to pass directly over the reservation and the motor to cut out directly over wherever one was. The knowledge and sound not only of A.A. rocket fire but also cannon fire from pursuing night fighters made one realize the gunners had to be good not to bring the bomb down on us. They were good and the nearest miss was about a quarter mile distant in Southampton Water. Despite the massive construction of some of our buildings they shook and trembled and one could feel the blast and see it in the movement of blackout curtains. . . . Example is a potent force and to see the nurses proceeding calmly and to know that on the exposed third deck, medical officers, nurses, and corpsmen were circulating among the N.P. patients reassuring them, was a behavior guide for all of us."[144]

"Almost 10,000 [invasion casualties] were treated up to 30 September 1944 with [the] death rate among combat casualties of only 33 hundredths of one percent."[145] In October of 1944, Lieutenant Commander Mary Martha Heck NC USN is awarded the Bronze Star Medal for "meritorious service as [the] chief nurse at a US Naval Base Hospital established in England [Base Hospital No. 12, the above mentioned Hospital], prior to, during and after the assault on the coast of France in June 1944."[146] The Bronze Star Medal is "presented her by Admiral Harold R. Stark, U.S. Navy Commander, Naval Forces in Europe, for 'meritorious service' and 'untiring effort.' Miss Heck insists, however, that the meritorious services and untiring efforts were evenly distributed among the 99 nurses in her charge."[147]

On 16 February, the USS *Bountiful* is boarded by its complement of Navy Nurses. The Chief Nurse is Lt(jg) Ethel P. Himes NC USN. This is a newly commissioned hospital ship. Then on 1 March the USS *Samaritan* receives its Navy Nurses and joins the rest of the hospital ships on active duty. Lt(jg) Elizabeth Schaak NC USN is the Chief Nurse. On 2 March, the hospital ship, USS *Refuge*, is commissioned. Navy Nurses go aboard with Lt(jg) Mildred Marean NC USN as the Chief Nurse.[148] One of her young nurses is Ensign Elizabeth Torrance NC USNR. Miss Torrance tells us, "we cruised around the Chesapeake Bay for degaussing [similar to removing static electricity] and after . . . [the shakedown,] our first trip was over to Oran, North Africa where we got casualties from North Africa and also the Italian campaign. We returned to the United States and our first port of call was Norfolk. We debarked all the patients there and then we went back again to the Mediterranean area to Naples. . . . We had quite a bit of free time in Naples. . . . One of the Chaplains arranged for us to go up to Rome. . . . Then we had an audience with the Pope with many, many other people, but then something extraordinary happened; he asked for an interview with us. He said he had never seen American Marine sisters before and he wanted to meet us. So they took us into a chamber behind the audience hall and he spent a good half-hour with us. . . . We were in uniforms but in our fatigues; those horrible gray dresses. He was very charming. He came along the line, there were only 14 of us, and he asked where we were from. . . . It was really an experience. . . . The other half of the nurses [from the ship] went later in the week but they didn't get to see the Pope like we did. . . . Then [the ship] made several trips from Naples over to . . . [the] south of France [but] we did not go ashore there. . . . We got many, many [German patients] in horrible condition. They had been left in a field hospital, absolutely alone, because they knew the Allies would be getting there very shortly. Their dressings were, if they had any at all, of newspapers and bags and things like that. They had obviously run out of most of their supplies. [The German patients] created quite a sensation on the ship."[149] Ensign Torrance says that the German patients are placed on the ship's wards just as any other patients are and the other patients did not like it at all. She also notes that one of the corpsmen heard one of the Germans on the ward say, "You've got 16 live Frenchmen here today; you're going to have 16 dead ones in the morning."[150] To top things off, Miss Torrance says that a corpsman finds, but manages to obtain without a struggle, a loaded gun from one of the Germans. They take these patients back to Naples without too many additional incidents. Then she tells us that at the time of D-Day, they were headed into Normandy but are diverted to Liverpool, England for the safety of the hospital ship and its personnel. "At Liverpool they brought us patients from Normandy by all sorts of boats."[151]

Meanwhile, back in Alaska, there are seven Navy Nurses stationed at the 75-bed Naval Dispensary at Dutch Harbor. Navy Nurse Margaret Jackson reports that one day in 1944, a Russian ship sinks some distance away from Dutch Harbor. Eight survivors manage to get into a lifeboat where they remain for seven days before being found. Miss Jackson goes on to say that the Russians have some frostbitten toes and some have to be amputated. The patients do not understand English but an interpreter is finally found and when a Russian ship docks close by, the patients are sent aboard. Navy Nurse Jackson also tells us, "One Sunday [morning] in May of '44, some of us [nurses] saw LT J.D. Lucille Hendricks [the Chief Nurse; who had been Chief Nurse, previously, at Sitka] and [two Ensigns] . . . take off for a visit at . . . Bay. . . . [After] they took off, the tower only heard from them once. They never arrived at their destination. A few days later they were spotted on the side of a volcano. The theory was that they wanted to see a volcano and a down draft took them. There was much grief on our island as they were so well liked. They were buried on that island; a sad day that was."[152]

A change of pace here, for just a moment, to discuss a curious phenomenon that takes place after being stationed overseas. On coming back to the States/mainland after a year or two, there is a strangeness, a feeling of something lost or missing and even a taste of fear. Strange new things have occurred since leaving the mainland. New laws have been passed, new cars have appeared, clothes have changed, things of importance have happened that people discuss but the newly returned has no knowledge of these things. If one has been overseas where driving on the left hand side is a way of life, the fear of driving again on the right brings fear you wouldn't believe. Everything is new again; familiar but with a disconcerting difference. It takes a while to readjust. Even so, there remains, a niggling feeling of a few blank spots in your life.

A Navy Nurse leaving Adak, Alaska after her tour of duty there, says, "I received orders to report to [the Naval Hospital] Seattle. I flew out of Adak and landed in Seattle. . . . My first reaction in Seattle was absolute fright at having to cross the street because I hadn't seen traffic or a crowded street in so long that I didn't quite know how to approach it. That and the fact that in the Aleutians we had to wear our rank on everything, including our raincoats and, as I walked down the street in Seattle, I was approached by a Warrant Officer who brusquely came up to me and said, 'What are you doing with that on your shoulder?' I was so taken aback I had to stop and wonder why or whether or not I was supposed to have that [insignia] on my shoulder."[153]

Moving out to the South Pacific, Navy Nurse Charlotte Sprague comments on the twenty months she spends at Mobile Hospital #7 and Fleet Hospital #107 in New Caledonia. "The area where our Naval Base was located was on a Frenchman's Ranch. It was loaned to the US Navy via the Lend Lease Agreement. The understanding was the Navy could build and put up tents, a commissary, etc. but the Frenchman's animals had the run of the land. There were cows, chickens, goats, etc. roaming like free spirits. They were #1 priority. The compound was built on the side of a very large hill or very small mountain. A frequent [sight] while going down into the town of Noumea was a native farmer following his wife who carried a huge basket on her head, while nursing an infant on one breast and a baby goat on the other and a child by her side clinging to her hand. . . .

"The Lepers were allowed to roam the streets although there was a leper colony in the hills for the white French and another for the natives. . . . [The] nurses and the Dermatologist would visit the colony and carry medical supplies and clothing to the lepers, prn [as indicated/as necessary]. . . . I recall the send off of Admiral Halsey. It was a real occasion. He was being sent to Hawaii (as the fighting had moved so far North.) The send off party was being held in our Officers Club. I remember this 'Giant Among Men' with the huge grizzly eyebrows walking toward me with his hand extended, and saying 'Halsey's my name and what is yours?' I am never at a loss for words but when I finally answered in a tiny squeak of a voice, I said, 'Sprague, is mine sir!!' He was a bull of a man with the kindest eyes and the firmest handshake!

"I recall the first patient to receive penicillin. There was a board of doctors. It was decided to use it on a young Marine whose leg was shattered [and] badly infected. The ward doctor had to get up every 3 hours at night as that is how it was dispensed; [every] 3 hours by the ward medical officer. It was considered the miracle medication. Before that we only had sulfa to fight the wounds with and of course a lot of prayers."[154]

Up on the island of New Guinea, Navy Nurse Claire Vecchione and twenty other nurses arrive at the Navy Facility at Hollandia in West New Guinea. "It was a lovely base. . . . It was all set up. We had our wards set up; they were quonsets. . . . Our [the nurses quarters] quonset huts were built sort of like on a hill. . . . We had little cots and we all had mosquito netting. Every night we had to put our mosquito netting down. . . . It was the end of `43 going into `44 and we were kind of in a lot of danger. That's when Tokyo Rose would get on the . . . radio and say, 'If the nurses on Hollandia will wear their best clothes at the Easter Service, they'd better because this is their last service they will see.' She would say different things like that. . . . We were always kind of in fear. . . . You always had to go out with another date. . . . They had to carry 45's because of the fear of trouble. And one day we did [have trouble]. . . . I was coming in off a date; from a date. I came on into my quarters. Now, we had four [nurses] on one side, four on the other. Of course we had our little mosquito nets. Our quonset butted up against the mountain . . . and they did tell us that there were caves up there. That the Japs were up in there but we never believed it. . . .

"As I [said], I was coming in; it was 12 o'clock and that's what time we had to [be] in. I was just lying down on my bed and I heard this [nurse] scream; one of the [nurses] in our quonset. I jumped up and turned on all the lights and just as I did, I saw this man running out. The [nurse] in the last bunk near the door to the back, was just hysterical. This guy had gotten in . . . first, he closed her mouth then he hit her on the shoulder. . . . I put on the lights then she started screaming and he ran. . . . We [all] screamed. . . . We kept yelling, all eight of us. . . . All the lights start going on. The Commanding Officer came. . . . [We say], `We're not going any place unless you put locks on our doors and you give us guards. We can't take this kind of thing!' So he said, `Don't worry, we'll take care of it.' Well, they did. They put the guards on and we did get locks on."[155]

Miss Vecchione relates another incident that helps describe one of the other difficulties in the life of a Navy Nurse. "I was night supervisor of the wards. . . . I was a Lt(jg) at the time. I went on the wards and I was making the rounds. . . . I could see some light underneath [one of the rooms]. I said to the nurse, 'Are they awake?' She said, 'I think they are.' So, I went in and they were gambling around this big table; the officers [patients]. I said, `Sir, I'm real sorry. You're not allowed to gamble.' They said, 'Well, we're officers.' I said, 'I know, but it's just a rule, you can't gamble.' So they took up their money, mad and all, and we [turned off] the lights and I went. . . . So, the next night I make my rounds and they are there again. So I went in and I said, 'Sir, I'm real sorry. I told you we are not allowed to gamble. I'm afraid I'm going to have to take all that money.' There was a bunch of money in the pot, so I just took all that money. I said I'd give it to Navy Relief and this guy who was quite young, a Commander, said, 'I'm Commander . . . Doesn't that mean anything to you?' I said, 'Sir, I'm very sorry, but I understand once you're a patient, you're in pajamas and your rank doesn't count here.' He said, 'Miss, I'm going to put you on report. I'm reporting you to the Commanding Officer tomorrow.' I said, 'Well, I'm sorry, sir. Those are my orders.' I was shivering in my boots! . . . When morning came, the first thing I said, 'Where's Miss Gavin [the Chief Nurse], I have to tell her.' So, I told her what happened last night. She said, 'Don't worry, you were right..' She went to the Commanding Officer. [The Commander] did go to the Commanding Officer, but the [CO told him], 'She did her duty and that was what she was supposed to do. There's nothing I'm going to do about it.' "[156]

Also, in the South Pacific at this time is LT Faye Elmo White of the Navy Nurse Corps. (She served with the Army in WWI and joined the Navy Nurse Corps in 1921. She was promoted to Chief Nurse in 1936, commissioned a Lieutenant in April 1943, appointed Assistant Superintendent in September 1943 and promoted to Lieutenant Commander in October 1944.) In September 1944 she is returning to the States after 20 months as Chief Nurse of two different hospitals in the Pacific. Just before returning, she makes "a 12,000-mile tour of inspection of all the hospitals in the South Pacific Area."[157] She is awarded the Bronze Star Medal just prior to her return to the mainland. The citation reads, "For meritorious service to the Government of the United States while serving as chief nurse of a Fleet Hospital in the South Pacific Area from June 29, 1943, to August 30, 1944. During this period, Lieutenant White displayed exceptional ability and worked tirelessly in the indoctrination and training of nurses and hospital corpsmen under her supervision. Through her professional skill and thorough knowledge of the personnel problems involved in hospital administration, she rendered invaluable assistance to the Force Medical Officer in assignment of nurses to other hospitals in the South Pacific. Her initiative and skillful leadership were an inspiration to the officers and men with whom she came in contact, and were in keeping with the highest traditions of the United States Naval Service."[158]

During 1944, Navy Nurses arrive at the Fleet Hospital in the Russell Islands (near the Solomons), the Fleet Hospital on Guadalcanal in the Solomon Islands and at the Base Hospital at Tulagi, also in the Solomons. Over in New Guinea, in addition to the naval facilities already mentioned, Navy Nurses arrive at Base Hospital 14 at Finschafen in eastern New Guinea and at Base Hospital 13 at Milne Bay on the very tip of eastern New Guinea. The Chief Nurse at this latter hospital is Lt(jg) Ruth Houghton NC USN. (She will rise to become a Director of the Nurse Corps.) Another facility, Base Hospital 8, on Oahu, Hawaii, is opened and staffed with twenty-nine Navy Nurses in 1944. The Chief Nurse is Lt(jg) Veronica Bulshefski. (She, too, is destined to be Director of the Corps.) Then, on the 24th of December 1944, Lt. W. Leona Jackson NC USN returns to Guam which has now been recaptured by the American forces. (She, too, will eventually head the Nurse Corps.) She reports to Fleet Hospital 103 as the "first Navy Nurse to return since Japanese occupation. [And isn't that most appropriate, after having been a POW there?] On 19 January 1945, Mrs. Jackson [reports] to the Island Command, Guam, as Senior Nurse Corps Officer"[159] of the newly opened Base Hospital, Guam.

In November 1944, the "Destroyer USS *Higbee*, first combatant ship to be named after a woman in the service, [is] launched at Bath, Maine, christened by Mrs. A.M. Wheaton in honor of her sister, the late Mrs. Lenah Sutcliffe Higbee, second Superintendent of the Nurse Corps, USN. [The] vessel [is] commissioned 27 January 1945."[160]

On 31 December 1944, there are 8,893 Navy Nurses on active duty in the Corps; 1,895 are regular Navy and 6,998 are active duty reserves.[161] And, at the end of 1944, Navy Nurses are deployed outside the Continental Limits of the U.S. as follows:

"Alaska & Aleutians	New Guinea
Argentia, Newfoundland	New Hebrides Islands
Australia	Oran, Algiers
Bermuda	Palermo, Sicily
Brazil	Puerto Rico
Canal Zone [Panama]	Russell Islands
Cuba	Samoa
Guam, M.I.	Solomon Islands
Hawaiian Island	Trinidad, B.W.I
Naples, Italy	Tunisia, Bizerte
New Caledonia	

Hospital ships: *Bountiful, Refuge, Relief, Samaritan, Solace.*"[162]
Los Banos prisoner of war camp, Philippine Islands.

With the POW Navy Nurses at Los Banos in 1944, life "went along day after day and the clinic was always filled up. We had jungle rot as we called it. You, know, athlete's foot.... By this time there were a lot of deficiencies.... They were coming in with all kinds of diseases and scurvy."[163] Navy Nurse Edwina Todd notes that "In 1944 we had several cases of malaria.... Although treated with atabrine and intravenous quinine, one young man died.... The lack of urinary antiseptics was tragic, chronic kidney conditions were common, caused by many months of standing in line waiting to go to the bath-room, improper diet, especially certain vegetable substitutes ... which contained oxalic acid crystals and other kidney irritants. We had sulfa drugs with which to treat acute urinary infections, but nothing for the chronic cases."[164]

Navy Nurse Mary Harrington says, "A few people got shot trying to go through the wires, but on the whole we kept our distance and they [the Japs] kept theirs. Mostly we worked.... Supplies kept going down and we tried to make it on what we had."[165] POW Margaret Nash indicates that she is fairly healthy "until September of 1944, when I started running this high temperature. My legs and arms were all swollen and I had great big welts all over my arms. They would just raise. They looked like boils.... So when my temperature got so high, they put me in the hospital. Dr. ... said he never saw anything like it before and neither did Laura Cobb [Chief Nurse] or anyone else. And so by this time I wasn't caring very much so Dr. ... told Laura the only thing they could do for me, they had some typhoid ... vaccine and they could give me an injection and ... you know, the fever therapy, and raise my temperature up to 106. It was very difficult for me. Then they gave me the second shot and that one almost killed me. Dr. ... wanted to give me three but Laura said 'no way, she could never tolerate any more.' So I stayed in the hospital for at least five or six weeks. But finally, I guess with the rest I was getting, it seemed to subside to the point that I was able to return back to duty."[166] And the year 1944 ends on that note for the eleven imprisoned Navy Nurses.

1945. The Navy Nurses at Los Banos face the new year with trepidation as the food situation becomes worse in the POW camp. Chief Nurse Laura Cobb writes, "No dogs or cats were safe in the camp the last few months. Our Camp had one to two deaths per day from starvation. Santa Tomas had 6 to 7 similar deaths per day. Over 80% of [the] Camp had beriberi and all were suffering from malnutrition."[167] "The last two months of internment we were without laxatives or cathartics of any type. While we had cathartics they were frequently administered as the constantly deficient diet lacked bulk and beriberi produced an atony of the intestinal tract. Patients were so starved for fat they would beg for a dose of castor oil, drink an ounce and smack their lips. Even rancid cocoanut oil seemed palatable. Internees would go as long as eleven days without a bowel movement before coming to the hospital — then an enema would be administered. Our tubing was very worn by the time we were liberated. . . . Throughout the existence of the Los Banos camp, Miss Evans [Navy Nurse Bertha Evans] served as dietician. Patients always ate three meals a day to the rest of the internees two. During the last three months lunch was prepared merely by dividing breakfast in half. . . . When the Japs slaughtered, they sometimes let us have the bone to use for soup, and blood when congealed was fried and fortunately passed as liver to the patients."[168]

An article in a 1945 issue of the American Journal of Nursing states that, "The only food eventually issued to them was 'lugas,' an inferior rice cooked with so much water that it took on a mucilage-like consistency. . . . `We got so we didn't especially mind the weevils,' says Commander Cobb, 'but the cockroaches and worms made eating tough going much of the time.' . . . Systematically, brigades of internees dug pig grass, banana tree roots, and slugs to supplement the meager prison fare."[169] Miss Cobb notes that, "The last 3 days we were given only palay (unhusked rice) to eat."[170] "Almost all of the prisoners were plagued with edema - hands, feet and abdomens were swollen and as time went on the condition became worse."[171]

Navy Nurse Edwina Todd writes, "Our rubberkneed corpsmen were no longer able to push the 'Camp guerney' used as a stretcher for patients, the carpenters were no longer able to make coffins, the grave-diggers to dig graves, the nurses literally pulled themselves up the stairs. . . . You fell down a couple of times enroute to and from work. Your hand shook as you gave an injection as well as when you assisted in the OR or gave medications. The surgeon was in a similar state. Though loathe to admit it you were often incontinent. . . . We realized that it was no longer a question of our liberators coming but our survival until they arrived. Though we all thought this we did not admit it even to each other, and then one day after two days of going without food, while gazing out of the door of the barracks in which I lived, looking up, I saw a little white patch floating down, surely a parachute - a parachute dropping food. Soon there were many parachutes and nine planes flew in straight formation, the words RESCUE painted on their sides. Tears were trickling down my cheek. I'd thought I could no longer cry. . . . Before we could fully absorb this, tanks came crashing right through the camp walls."[172]

POW Margaret Nash tells us, "it was February 23rd, 1945 that I . . . was at the stage that if I saw there were steps there, I couldn't walk them. So it was better for me to go out on the level ground and then I just had a short incline to walk up, to go up for roll call because roll call was every morning at seven o'clock. Just as I was going to walk up the hill, I looked up and I could hear planes flying and something dropping out. . . . But the planes got low enough that we could see 'RESCUE.' They had written that on the planes. . . . Oh, dear! I'll never, never forget it regardless of how long I live. . . . So then the paratroopers landed and the amphibian tanks crashed through the gates. They got all the Japanese. . . . Someone told me at one time there were about 263 guards in the camp. So they got them all. . . . But everything happened so quickly. . . . I ran up to one of the paratroopers . . . and I said, 'Did you bring anything to eat?' And he just looked at me. He said, 'Here's half my (Hershey) bar.' . . . I said to him, 'How long will you be here?' And he said, 'Not very long. As soon as we can get all of you people out.' And I said, 'Our patients?' He said, 'Soon; we've got to leave here as soon as possible.' . . .

"We had two new born babies. One was nine days old and the other was only three days old. The mothers were quite ill and so Laura [Cobb] said to Edwina Todd and I, 'I want you two to take the babies and protect them with your life.' The mothers were on stretchers and Toddy and I were lucky enough to be put in one of the amphibian tanks with many of the patients. And each one of us carried a baby."[173] The other nine Navy nurses and the rest of the internees that are ambulatory, walk the one and a half miles to the beach area where transportation is available. As Laura Cobb writes in her notes, "McArthur's forces liberated our Camp on Feb. 23, 1945 in a daring rescue raid 25 miles inside enemy territory. The mission, said to be the most perfectly timed and coordinated of the Philippine campaign, was accomplished by a combined force of guerrillas, paratroopers and amphibious troops. The entire camp of 2,157 internees were saved."[174]

On the 3rd of February, American troops had entered Manila and freed all internees at the Santo Tomas site. "The Army was also under orders to attack, as soon as possible, the nearby Japanese internment camp at Los Banos and to free, if possible, the 2,147 prisoners of war and the 11 Navy nurses held there. This camp was some 24 miles within the enemy lines, so a rescue attempt involved considerable risk. But intelligence reports indicated that the plight of the internees was desperate and that their death rate was very high from lack of food and medicines, and so the risk was justified. A special force was directed to liberate them at the earliest practicable hour. . . . The assaulting troops annihilated the entire enemy garrison of 243 soldiers, liberated the internees and the Navy nurses, and brought them safely within American lines. The casualties were slight: two men were killed and three men wounded from the task force, and three internees were slightly wounded."[175] But to return to Miss Nash's recollection of the event; she tells us of reaching the beach area where transportation is assembled, "to the trucks and the jeeps - the first jeep I ever saw."

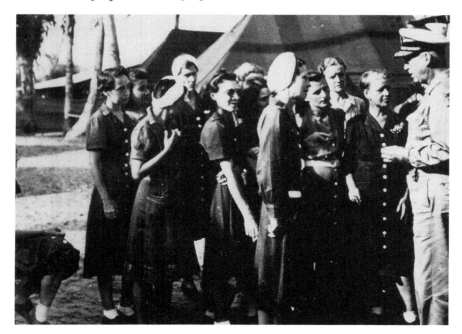

Navy Nurse Prisoners of War just released from Los Banos Prison Camp, Philippine Islands 1945. (Photo courtesy of Navy Bureau of Medicine and Surgery)

The Army is in the process of setting up a hospital in an area nearby and the internees are to be transported there. Miss Nash, with the baby assigned her, continues, "As soon as I got up there [to the hospital], I went to one of the Army doctors and I told him that the baby that I had was very ill. . . . He had someone take the temperature and it was 106 and he said to me, 'You'd better give her some penicillin.' And I just looked at him and said, 'Penicillin? What's that?' And it was only then that he recognized the anchors on my collar. And he said, 'My God! Are you one of the Navy Nurses?' And I said, 'Yes, we were just rescued from that camp.' He said, `Let us have the baby. Could you help us [set up the hospital]?' And I said, 'Sure, if we had something to eat.' I was always thinking of something to eat to get me through the next hour. So he sent Toddy and I down and we had army beans and graham crackers. Of course, I put some of the graham crackers in my pocket in case we didn't get any more food.

"So Toddy and I went up and we started setting up the wards. . . . What they wanted was to get the beds set up to open up a hospital there. We worked there for five days and then they brought in some Army nurses . . . . They wanted us to stay a few days longer because they [the Army nurses] were exhausted, but, as Laura

[Cobb, Chief Nurse] told their Chief Nurse, 'Your girls may be just in and exhausted, but my girls are starving to death and we're going back to the States as soon as our orders arrive.' "[176] Miss Todd continues the saga, "having been relieved by Army nurses we flew by C-47 to Leyte [Philippines] where Army nurses lent us uniforms and gave us silk stockings; from Leyte to Samar [still in the Philippines] in Adm. Kinkaid's plane."[177] Then they are flown to Guam where Miss Nash meets with Leona Jackson whom she had been stationed with, previously. They are there for only a short while and take off again for Kwajalein, then Johnston Island and finally to Pearl Harbor for two days. As Edwina Todd writes, "At the Navy Hospital [at] Aiea Hts., we were re-introduced to cosmetics, cologne, hot baths, and beauty parlors and other things delightful to the feminine heart. Best of all we met our fellow nurses and changed to Navy uniforms."[178]

Of this episode, Miss Nash says, "that was the first time that I saw the Navy uniform. And so many of our friends were out there. . . . There they tried to outfit us with our Navy uniforms and it's the first time that we knew that Navy Nurses had rank. We were so pleased at that. But everyone was so kind. Then we left there and went into Oak Knoll Naval Hospital . . . in Oakland. That is when they started our physical examinations."[179] Shortly thereafter, Ensign Margaret Nash is sent to St. Alban's Naval Hospital in New York where she is diagnosed with tuberculosis, beri-beri and pellagra. (She remains at St. Alban's, under treatment, for a year then she is medically surveyed out of the service in 1946. This heroic and valiant Navy Nurse, Commander Margaret A. Nash NC USN (Ret.), dies in November 1992.)

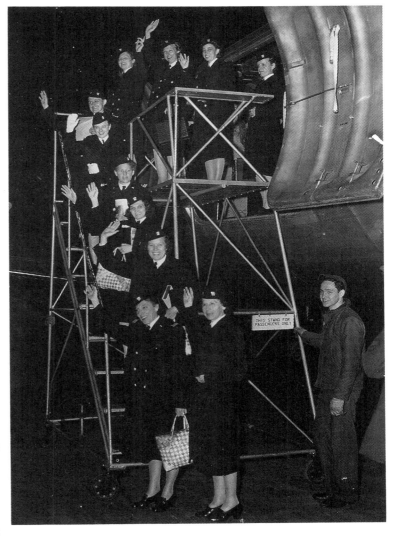

POWs welcomed home. Top to bottom: Goldia O'Haver, Eldene Paige, Dorothy Still Danner, Mary Rose Harrington Nelson, Mary Chapman, Edwina Todd, Susie Pitcher, Margaret Nash, Bertha Evans St. Pierre, Helen Gorzelanski, Laura Cobb. (Photo courtesy of Navy Bureau of Medicine and Surgery.)

As for the other POWs:

Laura Cobb is kept at the Oak Knoll Hospital until well enough to return to active duty. She is then assigned as Chief Nurse at Treasure Island, California. Miss Cobb retires in 1947. She is now deceased.
Mary Chapman resigns in October 1945 to get married; Mary Chapman Hays.
Bertha Evans remains on active duty until 1957 when she retires with the rank of Captain. Her married name becomes Bertha Evans St. Pierre.
Helen Gorzelanski returns to active duty and then receives a physical disability retirement in 1949. Her

married name becomes Helen Gorzelanski Hunter.

Mary R. Harrington marries in 1945 and leaves the Navy. Her married name becomes Mary Harrington Nelson.

Goldia O'Haver is given a physical disability retirement as a Commander in 1946. (She had entered the Navy in 1929.) Her married name, Goldia O'Haver Merrill.

Eldene Elinor Paige remains on active duty. She is sent to the Bethesda Naval Hospital Maryland. She resigns in February 1946, reappointed in February 1950, released to inactive duty in February 1952 and resigned in January 1955.

Susie Josephine Pitcher had developed cardiac problems while a POW (as noted in the interview of Mary Harrington Nelson) and is given a physical disability retirement in February 1946 as a Lieutenant Commander. She had been on active duty since 1929. She dies in 1950.

Dorothy Still stays on active duty and receives orders to Bethesda Maryland. She resigns as a Lieutenant in 1947. Her married name is Dorothy Still Danner.

C. Edwina Todd stays on active duty. She has a wide variety of duty stations ending as Chief Nurse at the Naval Hospital Portsmouth, Virginia. She retires (a permanent disability retirement) in 1966 with the rank of Captain and with thirty years of active duty service.

On the 4th of September 1945, the above eleven valiant and courageous Navy Nurses are awarded the Bronze Star Medal by the U.S. Army "'For meritorious achievement, while in the hands of the enemy, in caring for the sick and wounded.'"[180] The Navy awards the same eleven, on the same day, a Gold Star in lieu of a second Bronze Star Medal.[181] In addition to these two awards, the eleven Navy nurses (and Navy Nurse Ann Bernatitis) are given the Army Distinguished Unit Badge for the Unit of Nurses at the Canacao Hospital: " 'As public evidence of deserving honor and distinction is awarded to all units of both military and naval forcer of the United States and Philippine Governments engaged in the defense of the Philippines since Dec. 7, 1941.'"[182] The eleven Navy Nurse POWs are additionally given the American Defense Service Ribbon with star, the Pacific and Asiatic Service Ribbon with two stars, The Philippine Defense Ribbon with one star, and the Philippine Liberation Ribbon with one star. "The Navy also awards Bronze stars to 3 civilian nurses who served with the Navy Nurses."[183] All of these fourteen ladies were Prisoners-Of-War for thirty-seven long months; just imagine - over three years of hunger, fear and not knowing if you would ever be free again!

In early 1945, Navy Nurse Mary Benner tells us, "There were 125 nurses gathered in San Francisco. I was the senior, the Head Nurse, Chief Nurse, and we were there three weeks before our transports would take us out [overseas]. . . . My job was to get these girls to all learn how to swim. One of the women's clubs . . . lent us their pool and we had swimming instructions even with packs on their backs and helmets and so forth. I saw that everyone of those girls learned to swim, but the joke of it was - I never could swim myself and nobody knew that. I always said I would stay aboard ship and go down with the Captain when the band played 'Nearer My God To Thee.' Nobody checked on the Chief Nurse. . . We went out [to sea] with two transports with nurses and doctors and we had destroyers in front of us and beside us as far as Honolulu. I didn't know then where I was going until I got into Honolulu and I was just going to Honolulu; just five of us got off there. The rest all went out beyond Guam and various places. So as soon as I got into Honolulu, I was assigned to Pearl Harbor, the 14th Naval District, to assist . . . the District Medical Officer [an Admiral]. . . . While I was in the District, in the Admiral's office, there were about 22 Dispensaries I had to visit once a month. They were on the islands of Hawaii and Maui and I even visited the lepers on Molokai. I would fly in all kinds of craft to go over to these other islands once a month and drive around the island of Oahu and visit these various Dispensaries and keep them staffed. [Additionally] my job was to meet every transport that came in . . . [and] the big flying plane that would bring nurses in. When they came in, I was to assign them either . . . down under or keep them on the island there."[184]

(Commendable emergency planning; having an experienced senior Navy Nurse Corps Officer on hand to assign incoming nurses to medical facilities; medical facilities that she visits to acquaint herself with staffing needs, patient loads, and problems.) In September of 1946, Lieutenant Commander Benner is assigned to the Naval Hospital Aiea Heights as Principal Chief Nurse, in addition to her assignment at COM 14. "So when I went up to Aiea Heights, I really had both duties then, although things were . . . lessening a bit. But we were getting all these patients in from Iwo Jima and Guadalcanal; it was really pretty bad. . . . We had wards of blind and amputees and so forth and we would send them back on the transports; 2200 at a time, sometimes. They came in so fast; we just kept them long enough to straighten some of them out and then send them on back to the States."[185] Lieutenant Commander Mary Benner is a recipient of the Bronze Star Medal for her service at COM Fourteen from 26 December 1944 to 21 January 1946. (Commander Mary Benner retires as Chief Nurse at the Naval Hospital, Bainbridge, Maryland on 1 February 1956.)

There are about 200 Navy Nurses stationed at the Naval Hospital at Aiea Heights, so you can well imagine the size of the hospital and the patient loads they experience. To give us another insider's view of Aiea, Lieutenant(jg) Freddie Tucker reports, "In March 1945, a group of nurses from Camp Pendleton [California] were sent to Hawaii to replace nurses that had been transferred to a station in the Solomon Islands. We flew from Oakland. . . . I remember the flight as being long and cold. When we stepped out into the warm, humid night air in Honolulu, it felt nice. We were met by a Senior Nurse who gave us assignments. Most of us went to the Aiea Heights Hospital. Aiea was a large hospital with huge wards, each with about 100 beds. There were four rows of beds with the nurses' station in the center on one side. Patients needing the most care were in beds nearby. The center rows of beds had the headboards together. Each bed was equipped with headphones so the patient could listen to the radio. We arrived during the Iwo Jima invasion, followed by that of Okinawa. We were so busy that we did not have a day off for weeks. . . "Patients were admitted in large numbers, arriving by ship or plane. It was not unusual to admit twenty-five or more at a time. All had received emergency care and had tags attached to clothing telling when they last received medication. Though there were many fatalities in the field, the wounded who survived to reach a base hospital had a good chance of recovery. In the entire time that I was in service, not a patient died while I was on duty which says a lot about the care given and the stamina of the young Marines. After the rush of admitting and treating, perhaps days later, we filled out forms so that the wounded could receive `purple hearts' [military decoration for being wounded]. These were bestowed in mass ceremonies from time to time. Patients were entertained by USO groups and occasional sightseeing rides provided by the Red Cross. The hospital had provision for handicrafts and recreation. Religious services were conducted for every denomination.

"My longest duty was on a plastic surgery ward. Dr. . . . did a wonderful job reconstructing faces, ears, etc.. The corpsmen deserve much credit. They did magnificent jobs in difficult situations. I do not remember many individual patients but do think of the young man with most of his face missing and the one who helped make the plate to cover the hole in his skull. . . . Once I did private duty with a WAVE officer who had been attacked and beaten. Until the war was over the nurses did not go anywhere alone. Our dates signed out with the Officer of the Day so there was a record of when we left, returned and with whom. In Hawaii when leaving the hospital compound we wore the dress white uniform or the gray dress. Naturally because there were few women and many men, our social life was as busy as we wanted."[186] In her personal history account, Mrs. Freddie Tucker Wright also mentions the nurses who had been POWs. She notes that they stopped at Aiea on their way home and that "[their] ordeal was obvious in their faces and state of health."

Among a group of other Navy nurses arriving at Aiea just before Lt(jg) Tucker is Lt(jg) Ruth Gouge. She notes, "Due to the yet undetached 'Old Timers' the new arrivals were assigned to the basement of the nurses quarters which was dormitory style. We occupied this area with a degree of apprehension. We quickly dubbed it 'Lizard Lane' since indeed the little creatures flitted about over the concrete walls. We never failed to put on our shoes without their being shaken as there were also spiders exaggerated in our minds to tarantula magnitude. Mosquito netting was essential for protection during sleeping hours. This created a hazard when attempting to disentangle a head covered with bobby pins and arms searching for a gas mask and flashlight in response to [air-raid] alerts and the need to report to the duty station. We were finally liberated by the detachment of our predeces sors. . . . While awaiting assignment to the operating room, until others departed, my duty was on a burn ward. The odor of seared flesh conjured up flashbacks to my very young days when the inspired minister presented his version of 'Hell, Fire and Brimstone.' If such a place indeed exists, this ward was the gateway. Present were burns of many kinds and sources: ship explosions from kamikaze attack, flame throwers, shells and mortars into fox holes.

"On March 28, 1945 Keith Wheeler, a war correspondent who was shot through the jaw and recovering at Aiea Heights, reported in the Honolulu Star Bulletin this account relating to a young man on the ward and to whom I gave nursing care. These are his quotes: `White phosphorous is a combustible explosive, when it strikes flesh it burns and keeps on burning through skin, muscle and bone. There is a 21 year old in the burn ward who caught the burst of a white phosphorous mortar in the back three weeks ago. They doused his burns first with copper sulfate to extinguish the tiny fires that burned and burrowed deeper and consumed his flesh. They replaced the sulfate dressings with wet saline packs. Four days later they found he was still burning. They put the fires out again. A week later another spot was discovered where the flesh continued smoldering. His pain was such that morphine kept him under constantly. I talked to him this afternoon. His talk of the future did not include any knowledge that when grafts were started new places were still burning. He knew not that the greedy phosphorus is down in his bones now and still going. His pain is less now because the nerves are burning away.'

"This was Keith Wheeler's perception. Mine were even more vivid and distressing. Only we, as the health care team, who changed his dressings daily and attempted to remove the ever present flecks of white phosphorus, witnessed the pea sized beads of perspiration which ultimately drenched his tortured body along with his cries of agony. Skin from his buttocks had long ago succumbed to the invasion. The muscle mass was markedly reduced and when exposed appeared not unlike a raw beef steak. I do not know the ultimate fate of this young man, but it could not have been good. Prior to this experience I had been exposed to other atrocities visited upon our fighting men. This particular sight revulsed me. I was angered at the blatant disregard for human life and man's inhumanity to man. . . . Much time passed before I could reconcile in any way the enemy's acts. Introspection brought the realization that the 'other side' was fighting a cause which they were led to believe was a justified war for them and that they were indoctrinated into and to participate in. Their bodies and lives too were shattered."[187]

In mid December 1944, twenty-eight Navy Nurses leave San Francisco for a rough sea voyage to Honolulu. They only know that their ultimate destination is LIRP. When they arrive in Honolulu they find out that LIRP is the code name for a small island in the Marianas named Tinian; located North of Guam and just South of Saipan. After about five weeks or so, they arrive at their destination. Lt(jg) Sarah O'Toole writes in an article for the American Journal of Nursing, "Tinian is a very beautiful island, small and picturesque. We are pioneers, the first white women, as well as nurses, to come to this particular Pacific island. We were greeted royally at the docks . . . and quickly transported in a large truck to the hospital, amid the cheers of the men who had gathered to unofficially welcome us to Tinian."[188] They then take up their duties at the naval hospital there in this small island.

On another island, not as small as Tinian, Navy Nurses arrive in March of 1945. The island is Manus in the Admiralty Islands which are located northwest of the Solomon Islands and northeast of New Guinea. Lt. Elizabeth A. Walsh is the Chief Nurse of this group and of Base Hospital 15 at Manus.[189]

In January 1945, Base Hospital 18, Fleet Hospitals 103,111, and 115 at Guam in the Marianas, are staffed with Navy Nurses. The Chief Nurses are Lt(jg) Edythe M. Fielder NC USNR, Lt(jg) Ruth V. Wilhelm NC USNR, Lt(jg) Ruth M. Reed NC USN and Lt(jg) Jervace L. Crouse.[190] Then in June of 1945, Lt. Elizabeth Italia Sears NC USNR and seven other Navy Nurses arrive on Guam to re-establish the training school for native nurses. Also, north of Guam in the Mariana Islands, on the island of Saipan, another training school is started. The Senior Nurse Lt. Edna A. Hinnershitz writes, "August 11th we [eight Navy Nurses] arrived here on Saipan for temporary additional duty in connection with the inception of a native nurses training school. A program for teaching practical nursing and ward routine was started 20th August for the native girls working at the hospital and the two dispensaries. . . . The classes are conducted by a navy nurse with an interpreter. Since the classes are fairly large for this type of teaching, two nurses and two interpreters are often used. There is an enrollment of 80 pupils, with a usual attendance of about 76. There are 50 Japanese, 28 Chamorros, and 2 Koreans. Of these, 5 are males."[191]

On the 8th of July in 1945, LCdr. Ruth B. Dunbar NC USN, Chief Nurse, and her contingent of Navy Nurses arrive at Fleet Hospital 114 on Samar in the Philippine Islands.[192] (There are many other small and not so small islands where Navy Nurses serve with little known distinction amid the casualties and horrors of World War II. They cannot all be mentioned but these excerpts written herein are meant to describe the assignments and to pay a small tribute to the many who courageously served there.)

To turn now to the hospital ships in 1945. As one Navy Petty Officer writes, "with the commissioning of six new ships during April, May and June of this year, our mercy fleet is being swelled to a total of 15 hospital ships, including three manned by Navy crews but staffed by Army medical and surgical men. The six new ships are the USS *Tranquility*, the USS *Haven*, the USS *Benevolence*, the USS *Repose*, the USS *Consolation* and the USS *Sanctuary*. They are known as the `Haven class' - first time in history the Navy has had a class of hospital ships. They are designed to be of maximum service in forward assault areas and will function not only as floating hospitals but also as medical supply ships servicing advance base hospitals and warships."[193] Among other new specifics, these ships have, "Complete air-conditioning throughout both hospital and crew's quarters. . . . Increased recreational facilities. For the first time, two Red Cross workers will be aboard with Red Cross supplies to assist in recreational work."[194] These six hospital ships "were built as U.S. Maritime Commission C-4 hulls by the Sun Shipbuilding and Dry Dock Co. of Chester, Pa. They are full conversions. . . . Their speed is 17 1/2 knots with cruising radius of about 12,000 miles.

"Hospital beds are provided for 802 patients - 742 enlisted men and 60 officers. In an emergency, of course, the capacity can be increased by several hundred. In contrast, the older hospital ships accommodate from 450 to 760 patients each.

"For ship's company, there are accommodations for 58 officers, 30 nurses and two female Red Cross workers, 24 chief petty officers, 230 crewmen and 238 hospital corpsmen. The `nurses' country' is self-contained, with separate mess. For the corpsmen 181 berths are on the second deck and 57 on the main deck for night detail.

"The hospital consists of two main operating rooms, fracture operating rooms, plaster room, apparatus room, anesthesia room, clinical laboratory, dispensary, dental clinic, dental prosthetic laboratory, radiographic room, endoscopic room, eye-ear-nose-throat operating room.

"All medical rooms and wards are arranged so that there is access between them without going into the weather.

"The typical ward consists of two tiers of berths, which may also be used as single berths. Wider than usual ship berths, ward berths are detachable so that a patient may be handled if necessary without taking him from his berth. For further convenience of movement, the berths are accessible from both sides."[195]

Hospital ships "are always painted white with a wide green band painted around the hull and large Red Crosses marking them for easy identification. At night, they are fully lighted. All this was decided upon at the Hague Convention of 1907 when the immunity of hospital ships was agreed to by representatives of many nations."[196]

The U.S. Army also, "has a hospital fleet. By the end of summer it will total 29 vessels, including three manned by Navy crews but staffed with Army medical personnel under Army command. The others are manned by civilian crews of the U.S. merchant marine in the employ of the Army Transportation Corps.

"The Army uses hospital ships primarily for evacuation of wounded, although for limited periods they may become emergency hospitals. For instance, during the invasion of southern France 12 of them lay off the coast and served as emergency hospitals until orders sent them, laden with casualties, to hospitals in North Africa and England. . . . Many of the Army ships are also used in shuttle service. They lie at anchor off an invasion beach taking on casualties and, when loaded, debark for a port of safety where hospital facilities are available on land."[197]

The USS *Rescue* is commissioned in early 1945 after being converted from a "coastwise cruise ship. . . . [The] Medical staff aboard consists of 17 medical officers, 25 nurses, 8 chief pharmacist's mates and 156 hospital corpsmen."[198] Lt. Dorothy M. Davis NC USNR is the Chief Nurse and all nurses board the ship on 25 February 1945.[199]

The USS *Tranquility* is the first of the new class of Hospital Ships, the Haven class, to be commissioned and Lt. Sylvia M. Koller NC USN is assigned as Chief Nurse. The nurses board the ship on 24 April 1945.[200] The ship is sent to the South Pacific. On the 30th of July, the Navy's heavy cruiser, the *Indianapolis*, is sunk by Japanese torpedoes in the South Pacific. The ship is carrying the "first atomic bomb to Tinian [in the Mariana Islands]."[201] There are 316 survivors and 880 men lost. The survivors are in the water for 87 hours before they are spotted by a Navy PBY (plane.)[202] Navy Nurse Edna Park, who is aboard the USS *Tranquility*, tells us that the survivors were rescued and taken to an island "and we picked them up from . . . [that island] . . . their skins had been rubbed raw from the life-jackets. A lot of them had swallowed a lot of oil. They were dazed and a lot of them were burned. . . . There was just a whole feeling of; a different feeling from any other people that we picked up."[203] Miss Park goes on the say that not too long after that experience, some nurses are sitting at breakfast, on the ship, when someone tells them, "'Oh, they dropped an atom bomb!' And everybody looked at everybody else and said, 'What the hell's an atom bomb?' And a few days after that we found out. Then we had a real victory celebration at sea."[204]

The next hospital ship to join the fleet, is the USS *Haven*. The Chief Nurse is Lt. Ruth A. Erickson NC USN. (Destined to be a Director of the Corps.) She and her 28 nurses board the new ship on 5 May 1945. Only a week later on the 12th of May, Chief Nurse Lt. Helen M. Ernest NC USN and her nurses board the next hospital ship, the USS *Repose*. Also, on the 12th of May, Lt. Erma Richards NC USN, Chief Nurse and her staff of nurses board the USS *Benevolence*. The fifth and sixth of the fleet of new hospital ships are commissioned and staffed shortly thereafter: the USS *Consolation* with Chief Nurse Lt. Gertrude H. Nelson NC USN and nurses on 22 May and on 20 June the USS *Sanctuary* with Lt. Hazel Bullard NC USN, Chief Nurse with her nurses.[205]

Meantime, the USS *Relief* and the USS *Comfort* (one of the Navy ships staffed with Army Medical personnel) are in the South Pacific in preparation for the Okinawa invasion. The two hospital ships are gearing up to receive casualties and to transport casualties to medical facilities on nearby islands, as necessary. The Chief Nurse aboard the *Relief*, Lt. Ann Bernatitis, tells us that the invasion begins and "on Easter Monday the two hospital ships came in. The morning that we went in, about six o'clock in the morning, we were greeted with bombs falling on either side of us. The Jap ships were bombing. . . . We went in first to pick up casualties. When we would fill up, we'd pull out and go to one of the three places - Guam, Saipan or Tinian [Mariana Islands] - then the *Comfort* would come in and load . . . [and] we would retire at night and go out to sea. We would go out to sea all lighted up."[206]

During one of these trips to and from Okinawa, the *Comfort* is attacked and hit by a Japanese kamikaze plane. (The Japanese pilot commits suicide by deliberately flying his plane into his target, in this case, the hospital ship.) Another Navy Nurse on the *Relief*, Beatrice Rivers, provides us with a copy of the official Navy Communique which is posted on the bulletin board of the Ward Room on the *Relief*: "CINCPOA COMMUNIQUE NUMBER 347 RELEASED AS OF 2345 GCT 29 APRIL 1945 AS FOLLOWS X PARA ONE X A NAVY HOSPITAL SHIP USS COMFORT WAS ATTACKED AND HEAVILY DAMAGED BY A JAPANESE AIRCRAFT ABOUT 50 MILES SOUTH OF OKINAWA AT 2058 LOCAL TIME ON 28 APRIL . . . THE CRASHED JAPANESE PLANE WHICH MADE THE SUICIDE ATTACK IS STILL ON THE COMFORT X THE VESSEL WHICH WAS ENGAGED IN EVACUATING WOUNDED FROM OKINAWA SUFFERED 29 KILLED 33 SERIOUSLY WOUNDED AND MISSING INCLUDING PATIENTS PASSENGERS AND CREW [including Army Nurses and other medical personnel] X AT THE TIME OF THE ATTACK SHE WAS OPERATING UNDER FULL HOSPITAL PROCEDURE WAS CLEARLY MARKED AND WAS FULLY LIGHTED X SHE IS NOW PROCEEDING TO PORT UNDER HER OWN POWER X"[207]

Meantime, the Navy's first flight nurses are on the way to war. The first course for flight nurses opened at Alameda on Monday, 11 December 1944. The theoretical course is completed on 10 January 1945.[208] "Upon completion of the theoretical work, the nurses and corpsmen made practice flights from Oakland airport to the Floyd Bennett Airport in New York. Purposely, the convalescent patients [from Oakland Naval Hospital[209]] were chosen, to allow the medical attendants to become accustomed to the sensation of flying and acquainted with the situation in an evacuation flight.... [These] hospital express planes are comparable to a small 20-bed airborne hospital ward. Tiers of litters, four high, line one side of the plane while across the aisle are comfortable reclining chairs for ambulatory patients. Space is provided for 36 men - 12 litter and 24 ambulatory; if all are litter patients, 20 may be carried with the maximum of comfort.... On the left side of the cabin, toward the back of the plane, is a small complete galley set up. This is an electrically heated oven capable of heating six Maxson meals in 15 minutes. The Maxson platters are pre-cooked, frozen breakfasts, lunches, and dinners and are supplemented with bread and butter, a hot beverage, and dessert. A large electric hot-cup is put aboard for soup for those patients who are on a liquid diet and jugs of milk for those on a Sippy diet.

"At the extreme right side of the plane are adequate head (toilet) facilities for ambulatory patients. The medical kit which is put aboard for each flight, provides the equipment usually found in the ward's medicine cabinet and dressing room. There is a bedpan and urinal for the litter cases, first-aid articles, and sterile supplies such as needles, syringes, catheters, Levin tubes, and dressings, It also contains stimulants and narcotics, blood plasma and intravenous fluids. The flight nurse is responsible for the medical kit and the key is in her possession at all times. She keeps account of the narcotics, signs for the amount issued, and for each one she uses. A prescription form is filled out with the necessary data and turned in to the flight surgeon in charge, after each flight. Her kit is then replenished before her next flight."[210]

Navy Nurse Margaret L. Covington is in the third class for flight nursing, and she says, "There were 36 nurses in my class. The first two classes each had 24 nurses in them and in March of 1945, a fourth class joined us; that class also had 24 nurses, so we had a total of 108 nurses at that time in Alameda.... What we didn't know at the time was that plans had started in early 1944; we were being groomed to participate in what would be the first massive evacuation of casualties from a battle area and also the largest. The school lasted about six weeks. Many of our classes were with the corpsmen who were part of the unit. Each class was assigned a flight surgeon, its own corpsmen, and its own nurses. At first the classes were mostly in theory and adjusted to flying; later we concentrated on air evacuation such as setting up planes, loading patients, ditching procedures and so forth, and the care of different type casualties. Emphasis throughout the program was on team work and unity of purpose. I had my first practice flight, after I had been there about a month, from Alameda to Olathe, Kansas. I guess I was frightened over my first flight [she had never flown before] for I surely got air sick, but I kept it to myself because I was afraid it might boot me out of flight. I finally worked this air sickness out.

"While we were in school at Alameda, we were fitted for our flight uniforms. These were designed by some well-known designer in New York and I have always thought they were quite attractive. They were winter green, the same material as the pilot's winter uniform. They were slacks with side pockets, a wool shirt which was quite attractive. The zipper started at the bottom and ran transversely up to the neck, which made it a little different. On the collar of this shirt, we wore our rank and our insignia. The insignia was the anchor with the oak leaf with the acorn in it. In addition, we had an Eisenhower-type jacket that went with this outfit, black braid on the sleeves, as the pilots wore, designating rank. There was a baseball-type cap out of the same material. And, of course, our wings, which we received at Alameda and were quite proud of, we wore over our heart."[211] The 'wings' that Miss Covington refers to is the Naval Flight Nurse Aviation Insignia and is designated for and described in Naval correspondence as follows: "Nurses who have been designated as Naval Flight Nurses shall wear the following insignia:

Gold-plated metal pin, winged, with slightly convex oval crest with appropriate embossed rounded edge and scroll. The central device shall be surcharged with gold anchor, gold spread oak leaf and silver acorn, symbol of the Nurse Corps insignia. The metal pin shall be of dull finish. The insignia shall measure 2" from tip to tip of the wings. [The remainder of the description contains the precise measurements of the items appearing on the 'wings.']"[212]

The flight nurses also have "a working uniform [made] out of cotton and washable material and I will say that it wrinkled badly. It was slacks and shirt made very similar to the green uniform. That too had a baseball cap out of the same material. For our fatigues, we were issued a dark green nylon coverall which was like the pilots wore. Also, we were issued a fatigue dark green baseball cap. We wore our fatigues over our gray slacks with an open-neck white shirt. We only wore our flight clothes while flying. . . . [In January 1945, Flight Nurses are issued uniforms of gray cotton shirt and slacks with matching visored cap and `aviation' green wool shirt, slacks, battle jacket with matching visored cap and an overseas cap.[213]]

"The Battle of Iwo Jima was in February 1945 and nurses from the first two classes left for Honolulu some time shortly after that."[214]

"The first class of 24 flying Navy Nurses completed flight indoctrination January 22, 1945. They immediately started active flying service on 24 flying teams, consisting of a nurse and a pharmacist's mate. Each 12-plane squadron operated with the following medical personnel: 1 flight surgeon, 24 flight nurses, 1 hospital corps officer, and 24 pharmacists' mates."[215]

The Navy assigned "the task of air evacuation to the Naval Air Transport Service, commonly known as NATS. As the Iwo Jima campaign closed and the stage was set for the invasion of Okinawa, NATS organized its own special air evacuation squadron - VRE-1 (Air Transport Evacuation Squadron ONE) which did a two-fold job. The planes flew to the target area loaded with air mail, blood plasma, ammunition and other vital supplies. Transformed after arrival at the forward area by installation of removable litters into airborne hospital wards, they returned to rear hospitals with capacity loads of wounded fighting men. . . . It was Squadron VE-2, based on Guam, that first began this evacuation. . . . [They] went into Iwo Jima and evacuated the wounded to hospitals on Guam where the patients remained for a few days before continuing on their journey to points nearer the U.S..

"VRE-1 began operating on Okinawa just 6 days after fighting began on that Island. . . . Approximately 6 to 8 flights left Guam each night anytime after midnight and arrived on Yonton airfield at Okinawa sometime after 0730. Landings in the wee hours of the morning were not made for the Japs would bomb this area nightly at that time.

"The crew consisted of the plane commander, co-pilot, relief pilot, navigator, radioman, flight nurse and flight corpsman.

"The patients were Army lads, Marines, and Sailors. They were brought down to the revetment (a stone shelter [built] similar to a sea shell by the Japs) from the clearing hospitals via ambulance.

"Some of these patients had been injured just four hours previously while others had been injured four days ago.

"Patients with head wounds, chest wounds, extensive burns, fractures, amputations, malaria, combat fatigue, etc. were evacuated.

"Facilities on this island were [meager], crude, and temporary and so the patients presented a pitiful appearance. Their clothes were dirty and worn for days, their hair was mussed and they were badly in need of a shave. They were worn and haggard and in need of sleep let alone being hungry. Their food consisted mostly of canned and K rations.

"As the trip was long and no refrigeration was on board the plane, canned and dried foods and fruit juices were taken along. Canned boned turkey was the main staple and we usually made this into sandwiches. Served them with hot soup, hot chocolate, coffee, and fruit juices. Packages of candy, gum, and cigarettes were passed out later. And how the lads devoured this food!! The fresh baked bread from Guam was a God-send to them after going without it for so long.

"Besides preparing and serving food, the flight nurse and flight corpsman were kept busy administering medicines, giving blood plasma, [penicillin], whole blood, changing dressings and watching over the patients for signs of hemorrhage, shock and other complications. Should one be restless and in want of sleep, they would work over him, make him comfortable and give him a sleeping pill so he would relax and sleep. . . .

"Another strange thing about . . . [flying] is that the higher up you go, the less the air pressure is and more energy is needed in breathing and working. Working for 8 hours on a plane in air would be equivalent to 16 hours of work on the ground.

"We would leave on a trip around midnight and return to Guam about 8:00 P.M. that following evening. We average about eight hours in flight going to the target area and eight hours returning."[216] (As Navy Nurses well know, no one in the Service gets paid overtime. When there is an emergency or a need, everyone works until the job is done or until the adrenalin runs out and they can no longer function.)

"The actual Okinawa Campaign began on April 1 and ended June 21. The newly formed [VRE-1] evacuation squadron's first operation was the evacuation of the wounded from Okinawa. Air evacuation in itself was no new operation, but at the time [VRE-1] went into Okinawa, it was the most massive air evacuation of patients from a battle zone ever attempted. Within days after the battle of Okinawa began, the skipper of [VRE-1] . . . took the first . . . hospital plane for the air evacuation of patients into the island. The officers and men that made up the . . . ground crew were organized and waiting. In 45 minutes after the skipper's plane landed, it had been unloaded and 32 wounded men, many on stretchers, had been loaded and secured and was headed over the Pacific for Guam."[217] (The flight nurse on this first flight, as well as the previous pioneering flight into Iwo Jima, is Ensign Jane Kendeigh.[218] She is a graduate of Alameda's first class of flight nurses.) "In a six-week period of time, [VRE-1] evacuated 9600 casualties under extremely bad weather conditions. I remember so well the rain and the mud in both Guam and Okinawa that summer. . . . I know that my flight wings and the [Navy] Commendation Ribbon with the Battle Star of Okinawa [given to all members of VRE-1 in 1946] are two of my most prized possessions."[219]

Navy Flight Nurse Irene Freeburger tells of her experience just after the invasion of Okinawa began. She notes that when they begin their flights to Okinawa, the air-strip and the communications system are somewhat skimpy. She says that on 10 April 1945, the plane commander, a corpsman, the "co-pilot, a young pilot being checked out, a navigator and myself left Guam for Okinawa at 0640 hours. Eight hours later we reached the vicinity of Okinawa. Our mission was to pick up casualties and return them to the base hospital in Guam. The weather was foul in Okinawa and the island was closed in; zero visibility. Instructions via radio ordered us to come up so high at so many degrees, etc.. These directions lead us directly toward a mountain higher than our position. Through a miracle the clouds opened up and . . . [the plane commander] was able to turn the plane and miss the mountain by 30 seconds. It was declared that the Japanese had monitored our communication. The pilot tried in vain to land. In the meantime, our right inboard engine began to feather. Since there was no land around, we had to select an [alternate] route. The choice was between the Philippine Islands or Iwo Jima.

"Since our concern was fuel, the choice was Iwo which was about one-half to one hour shorter time than the Philippines. About one hour into the flight to Iwo, the left inboard engine began to feather. The pilot talked it over with his crew and it was their opinion that eventually we would have to ditch the plane, but we continued to fly on two strong-functioning engines so we kept going. . . . When the pilots decided that we [might] have to ditch the plane, the plane commander said someone would have to check me out in the `Mae West' (the survivor jacket) and tell me about ditching.  The crew drew straws to determine who would tell me and take care of the screaming woman.  The navigator drew the short straw.  He came to me, cautiously, and said, `The pilot wants me to check you out in the 'Mae West' because we may have to ditch the plane.' Until this time, the crew kept [the Corpsman] . . . and me informed of all happenings. My reply to the navigator was, `Let me get my ditty bag.'  This was a bag given to us by the Red Cross.  It contained cards, toothbrush, soap and my lipstick, of course.  The navigator could not believe what he heard.  He said, `I expected a screaming woman.'

"We flew over the Third Fleet which was under the command of Admiral William Frederick Halsey. [The pilot] . . . did not open up the radio for fear of giving away the position of the fleet. The fleet radio called . . . [the pilot], it said, `We see you big boy, come in.' When . . . [the pilot] gave his reason for not calling, he was told that the fleet was hunting the Japanese fleet and hoped to bait them. We learned later that the Japanese fleet was in home waters awaiting the invasion by the Americans. In the meantime, the Third Fleet radioed and said, `We understand your situation. If you have to ditch the plane, we will send out a Destroyer to pick you up.' I guess that could be a comforting feeling when you're all alone flying a four-engine plane operating on two engines over the Pacific in war-time.

"After flying steadily for 12 hours and 39 minutes, we arrived at the island of Iwo Jima and we were not allowed to land immediately. It was a . . . [Japanese] attack going on on the island. [This type of Japanese] . . . attack was when Japanese, holed up in caves, came out periodically and killed Americans. A fighter plane was sent up to verify that we were friends, not foe. (At that time Japanese planes with American markings would come into the air strip and strafe.) When the fighter pilot saw an American girl waving to him, he let us land. [The pilot] . . . and the second pilot, both armed, escorted me to the tent which was the Operations office. The Operations officer took one look at me and threw up his hands to his head and said, `My God, a woman!' The question was what to do with me. The Officer said, `We could put her in a tent with guards around her, but I wouldn't trust the guards.' He said I was the only woman on the island. It was decided to lock me in the food compartment of the plane and the crew would remain in the fuselage of the plane. [The pilot] . . . gave me his gun and said, `Shoot first and then say, `Who's there?'' I refused the gun but he hung close by me and ordered me to use it if necessary.

"Four engine planes were not permitted to remain over-night on the island at that time, because the enemy came out at night and bombed the big, shine jobs [planes]. Due to needed repairs for our malfunctioning plane, we had to stay over-night. Early in the evening the young marines and sailors gathered around the plane to receive fresh bread that was intended for the patients we were unable to pick up in Okinawa. These boys hadn't seen fresh bread in a long time. The plane commander finally announced that I was to retire to the forward part of the plane. He said, 'The reason that those boys are here is because they haven't seen an American girl in a long time.' . . . [And] I thought it was because of the fresh bread. That night there was a great deal of shooting outside the plane and I learned, the next morning, that the Japanese did see the plane and attempted to attack it. . . . The plane was repaired and we headed on to Guam. What we didn't know was that we had been reported missing in action and crews all along flights up to the target area were instructed to watch for flares and markers of the downed plane.

"When I returned to our Quonset hut in Guam, a be-draggled, tired individual, I was rejuvenated by hilarious whoops of, `She's back; she's back.' And I was glad to be back.

"During the 12 hour plus flight, I never lost faith. I knew we would make it safely. [The corpsman] . . . was down at one point. He showed me pictures of his wife and son who lived in California. With tears in his eyes, he expressed fear that he would never see them again. Before that flight, I was reading the book called `The Robe,' . . . which seemed to strengthen my faith as a Christian. And I knew, and I reassured [the corpsman] . . . that we would make it back."[220]

Another flight nurse tells us of one of her flights, "Must recall the flight from Guam to Kwajalein at the very end of World War II. My load consisted of battle-scarred Marines - ambulatory and litter. Also 3 Japanese prisoners - ambulatory and important military figures. They were to be interrogated at the headquarters on Kwajalein. It was most evident that those 3 officers were scared - and rightfully so. The Marines were very anti [Japanese] - and voiced their ideas of ridding the plane of the enemy! The 3 Japanese officers were placed in bucket seats in the rear of the plane. They were across from the hatchway and near the [plane's] `head.' The Marines' plan was obvious. It took hefty doses of sedatives to quiet everyone. The corpsman and I sat next to the hatchway and the prisoners, watching every move until we landed. The sedatives worked and the 3 officers were off-loaded at once."[221]

Meantime, back in the States, Navy Nurse Edith L. Colton tells us she arrives for duty at Fort Pierce, Florida on 4 January 1945. "We were assigned quarters in town which had been occupied by the Coast Guard women (S.P.A.R.S.). There were nineteen of us at Fort Pierce. Our quarters were [in] a flat building that housed four nurses in each flat, with the Chief Nurse occupying one apartment. One other nurse and myself were assigned to clean up this building before the nurses moved in.

"Every morning we were picked up in the station wagon and taken to the BOQ [Bachelor Officers Quarters] for breakfast. This BOQ must have once been a hotel, it was located right on the Indian River. . . . After breakfast we were driven across the river to our dispensary. All of this was done very secretly. After I had left, I learned that the men [at Fort Pierce] were being trained for the Bikini Project. Of course, none of us knew it.

"Fort Pierce was a very small base. I had the duties of the sick officers quarters [SOQ], galley duty, and teaching classes for the corpsmen. Laura Kamp was the Chief Nurse . . . Gertrude Merz was assigned the duty of opening a hospital for the dependents (located in town) and the other nurses were assigned to the wards [and one nurse to the operating room]. The C.O. [Commanding Officer] of the Base was Captain . . . (a line officer) [and he] was far from receptive [to] having nurses on the Base and he immediately put a guard around our quarters from sunset to sunrise."[222]

Navy Nurse Geraldine Houp speaks of another duty oddity; a Navy Hospital at an Army Base in Virginia. "I don't remember the dates that the Navy had the hospital, but the Navy had the hospital at Fort Eustis, Virginia, an Army Base, for a period of time and I was there in 1945. At that time they had a large contingent of the German Prisoners of War at Fort Eustis. They worked on the grounds. They served in the mess hall. They did a lot of the cleaning. . . . Of course we were not to communicate with them in any way. . . . I remember one day one of them came to the door of the nurses quarters . . . and asked if he could have a drink of water which I gave him and I felt kind of guilty because we weren't supposed to talk to them. But, they were plain, ordinary young men like our young men were."[223]

In Washington, DC, President Roosevelt begins his fourth term in office by traveling to Yalta, in the Crimea of southern Russia to meet with England's Prime Minister Churchill and the Russian leader, Stalin. The meeting takes place in February 1945 and the three "leaders mapped the final assault on Germany and the postwar occupation of that country. They also planned a meeting in San Francisco to lay the foundations for the peacetime United Nations organization. In a secret agreement, Russia promised to enter the war against Japan after the surrender of Germany. In return, Russia was to receive the Kuril Islands [islands lying north of Japan] and other concessions."[224] The President returned to DC, made a report on Yalta to the Congress, then on 29 March, "left for a rest at Warm Springs [Georgia]. He had prepared a speech for broadcast on April 13. Roosevelt had written: `The only limit to our realization of tomorrow will be our doubts of today. Let us move forward with strong and active faith.' April 12 began as usual. . . . He planned to attend a barbecue in the afternoon. Before the barbecue, Roosevelt was working at his desk while an artist . . . painted his portrait. Suddenly [the President] fell over in his chair. `I have a terrific headache,' he whispered. These were Roosevelt's last words. He died a few hours later of a cerebral hemorrhage."[225]

"Late in the afternoon of April 12, 1945, [Vice President] Truman was suddenly summoned to the White House by telephone. He was taken to Mrs. Eleanor Roosevelt's study, and she stepped forward to meet him. `Harry,' she said quietly, `the President is dead.' . . . At 7:09 P.M., Truman took the oath of office as President."[226]

As for the War, "The Russians entered Vienna on April 13th, and shortly afterwards surrounded Berlin with the Fuhrer [Hitler] within it; [General] Patton drove towards Czechoslovakia stopping short of Prague; the British reached the Elbe. On that river on April 25th the Russian 58th Guards met the 69th U.S. division; and the Reich was cut in half. . . . Crazier than ever in his last days, and feeding himself to the end with delusions about German armies advancing to rescue him, he [Hitler] decided on a more melodramatic end; as the Russians fought their way to his air-raid shelter in Berlin he committed suicide on the last day of April with Eva Braun, and their bodies were afterwards burnt by his order. Mussolini two days before had been shot, with his mistress, by Italian partisans, and hanged upside down in the street."[227]

"At last Admiral Karl Doenitz, Hitler's successor as head of state, agreed to surrender unconditionally. On May 7, at Eisenhower's headquarters . . . the instrument of surrender was signed. The Supreme Commander signaled V-E (Victory in Europe) Day to the Combined Chiefs of Staff: `The mission of this Allied force was fulfilled at 1241, local time, May 7, 1945. Eisenhower.'"[228]

Now all the war efforts of the U.S. and the Allies turn to the Japanese adversary. "On August 6, a B-29 [plane] called `Enola Gay' dropped the first atomic bomb used in warfare, destroying 4.7 square miles in Hiroshima. ... On August 9, another atomic bomb destroys 1.8 square miles in Nagasaki. ... On August 8, the Russians had declared war on Japan, and invaded Manchuria. ... On August 14 (in the United States), the Allies received a message from Japan accepting Surrender. The Allies appointed MacArthur supreme commander for the Allied Powers. On September 2 (Tokyo time), aboard the battleship *Missouri* in Tokyo Bay, the Allies and Japan signed the surrender agreement. MacArthur signed for the Allied Powers, Nimitz for the United States, and Foreign Minister ... for Japan. President Truman proclaimed September 2 as V-J (Victory Over Japan) Day."[229]

On August 17, three days after Japan surrenders, three U.S. Navy Hospital ships accompany the Third Fleet into the entrance of Tokyo Bay. The hospital ships are the USS *Rescue*, the USS *Tranquility*, and the USS *Benevolence*. Aboard the *Rescue* is Navy Nurse Dorothy M. Davis. The mission of the hospital ship and its personnel is to collect and process the prisoners of war interned by the Japanese. They begin to take the POWs aboard on the 4th of September and travel along the coast of Japan doing this work. "They [the POWs] were brought to us in small landing craft. Those who were too ill to walk came in stretchers and were admitted directly to the hospital wards for immediate treatment. The ambulant cases were taken to the decontamination ward where they discarded all their clothing, showered, and were thoroughly sprayed with DDT powder. New clothing was issued, and they were examined by a medical officer. This examination determined whether or not they were able to be transferred to waiting ships for passage home.

"Each one was carefully questioned by military investigators before leaving the `Rescue.' ... It was an interesting experience, though heartbreaking at times, to learn that an elderly-looking, emaciated gentleman before you was a boy in his twenties. ...

"All those who passed through our hands for transfer were given good, hot, nourishing meals before leaving. This was the highlight of their day aboard. We were impressed particularly with the little children's consideration for each other. Not one of those babies would drink a full glass of milk or fruit juice without waiting to make certain that all the others were receiving the same amount.

"The ex-prisoners suffered mainly from malnutrition and the vitamin deficiency diseases such as beriberi, both wet and dry; pellagra; night blindness; and scurvy. Tuberculosis was common as well as the various dysenteries. Some suffered from old fractures and wounds incurred through the enemy's disciplinary measures. ... On September 19, 1945, the USS `Rescue' was ordered to sail for San Francisco. This was wonderful news for all hands; for we were the first hospital ship to be ordered home with the prisoners-of-war patients. ...

"We were fortunate to have with us, from the first group in our new assignment, a Catholic priest who had been with those men throughout their imprisonment. He understood them and their problems and helped keep up their desire to live. He gladly accepted our invitation to the nurses' wardroom and, over a `feast' of homemade cookies and milk, he told us the true story of life in a typical Japanese prison camp. He made us proud of the opportunity to help these men. With the knowledge of their experiences, we were better able to care for them understandingly. His advice was both simple and effective. First: no obvious sympathy. Second: lots of `T.L.C.,' tender, loving care. This last had become so foreign to them that it had overwhelming results. ...

"On October 7, 1945, we sailed under Golden Gate bridge into San Francisco Harbor with 764 of the happiest men alive. Grateful tears were shed unashamedly as the ex-prisoners-of-war read the `Welcome Home' sign that glowed through the misty sunset from Marin's shore line."[230]

Navy Nurse Ethel Buler is aboard the *Benevolence* when it comes into Japanese waters. She notes that one of the "Highlights of my career was viewing the signing of the treaty with Japan. The *Benevolence* was docked to the port side of the *Missouri* and we were able to see the ceremony with the aid of binoculars. Peace at last!"[231] Another Navy Nurse on the *Benevolence*, Mary E. Price, tells us, "We were out in Tokyo Bay waiting for the prisoners [POWs] to come out to the ship. Many of them didn't even wait for the ship, they swam out because they were so glad to see us. We took care of civilians, British; we took care of everyone as they came out of the

POW camps. . . . We didn't keep everyone, we just processed them. The ones who were sick we kept. The ones who were well enough were sent on to Hawaii. [General] Jonathan Wainwright came through our ship and Pappy Boyington and many prominent people were processed through our ship. It was very interesting. Everybody worked all night. We sent some of the corpsmen to try and get some rest, next minute they'd be back. They couldn't sleep; they said they had to come back and help."[232]

Out in the South Pacific on VJ day is the hospital ship USS *Relief* with Chief Nurse Ann Bernatitis aboard. Ann says, "I remember we were out top side watching the movie or getting set, waiting for the movie to start when general quarters sounded and everybody thought we were getting bombed. And it was the VJ day; the Japanese had surrendered. . . . And of course everybody on the ship just went wild. . . . Everybody saying, 'Now we can turn around and go home.' . . . I said, standing out on deck talking to one of the officers, and I said, 'No, I don't think we ought to go home now. You know what I'd like to do? I'd like to go pick up those people that we left behind three and a half years ago. . . . Then I'd really feel like the war was over.' Of course we didn't know, but we were going. . . . Sure enough we get orders a day or so later that we're going to Manchuria [in China] to pick up the war prisoners."[233] "We started out to go to . . . [in Manchuria] to pick up the war prisoners and we were accompanied by the Destroyer. . . . There were two mine sweepers that went along with us and cleared the way of mines. They took us up to Manchuria, to . . . [where] we sat there at the dock. . . . Russian soldiers [the area had been taken over by the Russians] were on the dock and we [the nurses] weren't allowed ashore. . . . [It] took about four or five days for the prisoners that we were to pick up to arrive and every night the ship was all lighted up and music was always blaring. But anyway, they finally arrived."[234]

"[They'd] come aboard and some of them would actually bow down on their knees and kiss the deck. They were so happy to think they had survived all this and finally here were the Americans who were taking them home. . . . Roughly 700 some [POWs were taken] aboard."[235] "[In] the group were the two doctors that I had left behind, Dr. . . . the Navy Dentist on Bataan, and Dr. . . . the surgeon on Corregidor. After three and a half years in prison camp!"[236] "We brought them back to Okinawa Harbor [but] a typhoon comes up and we can't put them ashore. We had to go out to sea. We had to sit the typhoon out, so we go out there and mill around until the typhoon passes and then we put them ashore."[237] Another Navy Nurse on board the USS Relief, Beatrice Rivers, shares with us a 'thank you' sent to the staff of the ship, "The following communication was received on board, by the Captain and is quoted herewith:

September 15, 1945.

"We, group of 45 Dutch Officers and 7 other ranks taken aboard the U. S. hospital ship 'Relief' at Dairen Harbour [Manchuria, China] after our release from the Japanese P.O.W. Camp at Moukden, wish to express our deepest gratitude and admiration for the way in which you, Captain, and your crew received and welcomed us on board your ship. You have done everything that was humanly possible to make us feel at home, to help us forget the mental and physical sufferings we have gone through during our captivity and to give us the assurance that you welcomed us as wholeheartedly on board your ship as you did your own fellow-countrymen. We want to thank you out of the depth of our hearts for the memorable days we have passed aboard the 'Relief.'

"One more favour we ask. We all felt that your ship was not just a U. S. hospital ship, but indeed part - and however small a truly representative part - of the American nation and that your conduct towards us stands for American helpfulness, hospitality and generosity. We, therefore, would appreciate it very much if you would convey our thanks to the American people in general and give them the assurance that we shall never forget what America has done for us.

(signed) . . .

Colonel Royal
Netherlands Indian
Army, Senior Officer
of the Group."[238]

Navy Nurse Marion Caesar is aboard the hospital ship USS *Samaritan*, about three hours out of Honolulu, "when the Captain came over the loud speaker and said, 'The destination of this ship is Tokyo, Japan.' So we went into Tokyo Bay about three weeks after the Armistice. There were three hospital ships in there. While we were there, there was a terrible explosion in the harbor and we were the closest to it. So we had those patients aboard. There were about 21 Japanese and 14 Americans. And it was an American who caused the explosion. They were discarding ammunition. There was one powder that's used . . . and the other was dynamite. They just threw it over and one of the American sailors threw the dynamite and blew them all up. And they all came aboard our ship. Of course we operated for, oh probably 24 hours steady because many of them were in terrible shape. And I have a copy of a nice thank you letter we got from one of the Japanese survivors, but several of them died. Then we had orders to go down and be the hospital to the 7th Fleet. We went down to Sasebo [Japan] and we were down there until the following . . . [year.]"[239]

In September 1945, the USS *Repose* arrives in Okinawa but must go to sea again in order to ride out a typhoon in the area. The winds of this storm are so severe that the fire plugs on the main deck are sheared off at deck level and paint is literally blown off some of the ship's metal. The damage is repaired and the *Repose* is ordered to Shanghai, China for duty with Service Squadron 10 of the Seventh Fleet.[240]

The Chief Nurse of the USS *Haven*, Ruth Erickson, tells us, "the highlight of my career was [that] I was in Pearl Harbor when it [WWII] started and I was on a hospital ship, the *Haven*, in Honolulu when hostilities ceased. I was there when it started and I was there when it ended. . . . We had sealed orders for somewhere out in the Pacific but when hostilities ceased then [they were] cancelled out."[241] The Haven receives new orders and heads for Japan to arrive at Nagasaki on the 11th of September 1945 "and [a] medical mission goes ashore to receive liberated allied prisoners of war."[242]

Back in the States, VJ day is a day of joy and excitement excesses. "In July, 1945 I received orders to the U.S. Naval Hospital in Long Beach, California, arriving there one week before VJ Day. A couple of nurses and I went into Long Beach that night, VJ Day, to watch the celebration. The town went wild, the people were shouting, kissing, tooting horns, throwing paper around and so forth. It was dangerous to be on the streets, so we came home early. The hospital was busy all night with injuries, and five died before they could do anything for them. They admitted around 80 injured during the night. The celebrating lasted two days and all stores were closed. . . . There were over 230 nurses, as this was a very busy hospital with all the servicemen returning from the war. More wards had to be built to accommodate all the returning patients. Many were amputees who were sent there for rehabilitation."[243]

Navy Nurse Margaret L. Larson notes that her most memorable duty is at the end of WWII. "As WWII wound down in the Pacific, the prisoners of war were returned to hospitals on the West coast. I recall night duty at Oakland Naval Hospital with several wards that were opened just for these men. Many had spent nearly the entire war in prison camp(s). They had joined a peace time Navy or Marine Corps and now they were part of a service that had changed dramatically in response to the war.

"There were stacks of Life magazines from 1941 through 1944 and current issues available so they could review their missing years. Many had not seen any girls or women from the USA during the time of their captivity and they were eager to refurbish their social skills. One of the most frequent questions was who won the World Series.

"The galley was open on each of the units so they could have food at any hour to restore their malnourished bodies. Some were severe: edematous legs, pot bellies with sores on their bodies and with decaying teeth. These latter day Rip Van Winkles had the strange situation of months and years of incarceration then release with an accumulation of back pay and leave time. Many spent that money quickly with no concern for the future. Most hid their emotional scars and trauma under a front of bravado. Too many drowned the pain of the hardships they had experienced in alcohol. The war was over and the period of adjustment to peace had just begun."[244]

One of the Navy flight nurses tells us how their work continues after the war, "Early months after VJ Day continued to be busy months relaying AEROVAC flights and carrying patients and servicemen back to Honolulu and to the West Coast. Among these were many of the . . . POWs that had recently been liberated from Japanese prisons. They were brought to Guam and then on to Honolulu and the States."[245] "Hospital flights arrive regularly in Oakland, California from such points as Shanghai, Tokyo, Samar, Guam, and Honolulu. Once weekly, the [huge] MARS [plane] arrives in California with 100 patients. The war is over, but casualties still exist and illness and sickness take their toll of people. Some of the recently evacuated were war injured being moved to hospitals for specialized treatment, patients with fractures resulting from jeep and motorcycle accidents, rheumatic fever, skin infections, diabetes, cancer, tuberculosis, leukemia, and mental disorders."[246]

Navy Nurses of World War II distinguished themselves and their Nurse Corps with their many heroic actions and devotion to duty under wartime conditions. Not all of them receive recognition or awards but the following list notes some of the WWII awards:

Distinguished Service Medal
>   Captain Sue Dauser USN - for duty as Superintendent of the Navy Nurse Corps during the pre-war National Emergency period and during the war.

Legion of Merit and
Distinguished Unit Badge (Army)
>   LT Ann Bernatitus USN (mentioned previously herein)

Bronze Star Medal (Navy)
>   LCDR Mary L. Benner USN (mentioned previously)
>   CDR Mary Martha Heck USN (mentioned previously)
>   LCDR Faye Elmo White (mentioned previously)

Bronze Star Medal (Army) and
Gold Star (Navy) in lieu of Second Bronze Star Medal and
Distinguished Unit Badge (Army)
>   LCDR Laura May Cobb USN
>   LT Bertha Rae Evans USN
>   LT Helen Clara Gorzelanski USN
>   LT Mary Chapman Hays USN
>   LT Goldia Aimee Merrill USN
>   LT Margaret Alice Nash USN
>   LT Mary Harrington Nelson USN
>   LT Eldene Elinor Paige USN
>   LT Susie Josephine Pitcher USN
>   LT Dorothy Still USN
>   LT C. Edwina Todd USN
>   (all mentioned previously)

Commendation Ribbon with Metal Pendant
>   Arnest, Gertrude B. LTJG USN- USNH Pearl Harbor
>   Bateman, Vera J. LTJG USN- USS *Bountiful*
>   Belanger, Bernadette LT USNR- USS *Bountiful*
>   Boyd, Dorothy M. ENS USNR (duty not noted)
>   Brady, Patricia LTJG USNR- USS *Bountiful*
>   Condon, Jean M. LT USNR- USS *Bountiful*
>   Doll, Irma F. LT USNR- USS *Bountiful*
>   Felder, Mary E. LT USNR- USS *Bountiful*
>   George, Helen M.J. LT USNR- USS *Bountiful*
>   Goldthwait, Marjorie F. LTJG USNR- COMNAVEU, England

Hambright, Nora J. LT USNR- USS *Bountiful*
Hardman, Anita M. LT USNR- USS *Bountiful*
Henry, Mary L. ENS USN- Base Hospital, England
Hames, Ethel LT USN- USS *Bountiful*
Jackson, Wilma L. LT USN- Hdqtrs. Island Command, Marianas
Janca, Ablina C. LT USNR- USS *Bountiful*
Jungferman, Rhea A. LT USNR- USS *Bountiful*
Kain, Catherine M. LT USNR- Aeronaut Hospital, Brazil
Klesius, A. Gertrude LCDR USN- USNH San Diego
Kozak, Stephany J. LTJG USNR- Aeronaut Hospital,   Brazil
Kreider, Anna M. LT USN- Fleet Hospital, Guadalcanal
Large, Edythe I. LT USN- USS *Bountiful*
Lindner, Mary J. LTJG USN- Fleet Hospital No. 107,   New Caledonia
Linville, Delma U. LT USNR- USS *Bountiful*
Marinak, Margaret T. LTJG USNR- USS *Bountiful*
Monteville, Sophia G. LCDR USN- USS *Relief*
Netter, Ida A. LCDR USN- USNH Seattle
Ozmore, Mary L. LTJG USN- COMNAVEU, England
Pennington, Clyde LT USN- Base Hospital No. 9, North Africa
Povlovsky, Helen F. ENS USNR- COMNAVEU, England
Powell, Augusta M. LTJG USNR- Base Hospital, England
Reynolds, Georgia LT USNR- USS *Bountiful*
Richardson, Catherine LT USN- USS *Solace*
Smith, Mary I. ENS USNR- Base Hospital, England
Squires, Bertha O. LT USNR- COMNAVEU, England
Staben, Lois M. LT USNR- USS *Bountiful*
Szpakowski, Mary U. ENS USNR- COMNAVEU, England
Terrell, Lenora A. LTJG USN- Fleet Hospital, Pacific
VanGorp, Dymphna M. LTJG USNR- Aeronaut Hospital, Brazil
Vestal, Sallie L. LCDR USN- USNH Philadelphia
Weir, Primrose C. LT USNR- USS *Bountiful*
Wilder, Elizabeth A. LT USNR- USS *Bountiful*
Yarnall, Catherine E. LT USN- Base Hospital No. 7, Pacific
Zuber, Florence B. LT USNR- USS *Bountiful*[247]

One other award of note, is mentioned in a San Francisco Newspaper article on Sunday the 24th of February 1946. The article states, "One of the Navy's own - Lt. Cmdr. Laura M. Cobb, NC, with twenty years of United States Navy service behind her - will receive a top civilian award Monday to add to the medals represented by the ribbons on her trim uniform.

"At the Soroptimist Club luncheon at the St. Francis Hotel, Commander Cobb will be presented with the Avon Award for Achievement (Medallion of Honor and $1,000 Victory Bond) - for heroic and selfless work among sick and wounded internees in Japanese prison camps."[248] The award, given by Avon Cosmetics, is presented to selected women of achievement and it is called "the Avon Medallion of Honor for Women of Achievement."[249] The citation of this award states, "Avon Award for Distinguished Service to Lt. Comdr. Laura M. Cobb (NC) USN. In recognition of your courage and perseverance in your duties as a Lieutenant (jg) of the United States Navy Nurse Corps under dangerous and difficult conditions as a prisoner of war in a Japanese Internment Camp, we deem it a privilege to present to you The Avon Medallian of Honor for Women of Achievement. [Signed

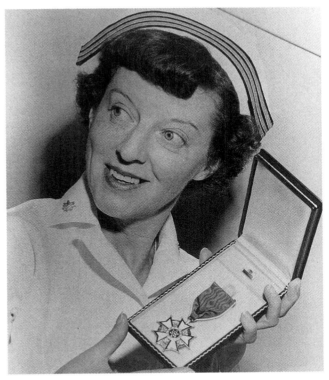

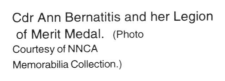

Cdr Ann Bernatitis and her Legion of Merit Medal. (Photo Courtesy of NNCA Memorabilia Collection.)

by the Committee of Award - Fannie Hurst, C. Mildred Thompson, Gladys Swarthout and for Avon Products Inc. - J.A. Ewald, President.]"[250]

As you will recall, Miss Cobb was Chief Nurse of the group of POW Navy Nurses in the Philippines. In December 1945, the Commanding Officer of the Naval Hospital at Canacao in the Philippines at the start of WWII, recommends Miss Cobb for the Legion of Merit Award. He sends his letter to the Secretary of the Navy via the chain of command for such actions. The following endorsement is placed on the request as it goes through the chain to the Secretary, "The records of the Navy Department Board of Decorations and Medals reveal that Chief Nurse Laura Maye Cobb Nurse Corps, U.S. Navy, has been awarded the Navy Bronze Star Medal and the Army Bronze Star Medal, which awards completely cover her services both during the campaign in defense of the Philippines and while a prisoner of the Japanese. The Board, therefore, recommends no further award in this case."[251] Laura Cobb did not receive the medal

During World War II, the build-up of the Navy Nurse Corps peaks on 30 June 1945 when the strength of the Corps reaches 11,086 Navy Nurses on active duty; 9,273 are Navy Reserve and 1,813 are Regular Navy.[252] Also, from the beginning to the end of the war, 37 Navy Nurses died in service but "none of these died as a result of enemy action."[253] As for WWII deployment of Navy Nurse Corps Officers, "within the continental limits [of the U.S., they] were assigned to 40 Naval Hospitals, 176 dispensaries and 6 hospital corps schools. They brought nursing care to the front lines aboard 12 hospital ships, in air evacuation of casualties, and to foreign lands where American women had never before been seen. At land based establishments overseas, they were assigned to"[254] these activities:

Admiralty Islands   Italy
Africa   Marianas Islands
Alaska   New Caledonia
Aleutian Islands   Newfoundland

Australia	New Hebrides
Bermuda	New Zealand
Brazil	Puerto Rico
Canal Zone	Russell Islands
Cuba	Solomon Islands
England	Trinidad
Hawaii	

By September of 1945, overseas deployment is rapidly being discontinued, leaving Navy Nurses stationed at:

"Alaska & Aleutians	Hawaiian Islands
Argentia, Newfoundland	Manus, Admiralty Islands
Australia	New Caledonia
Bermuda	New Guinea
Brazil	Puerto Rico
Canal Zone	Saipan, [Marianas]
Cuba	Samar, [Philippines]
Guam, [Marianas]	Trinidad, B.W.I."[255]
Hospital Ships: 12	

Now that the war is over, the Nurse Corps faces the huge task of demobilization. At the end of August, the Nurse Corps' demobilization officer at the Bureau of Medicine and Surgery, Washington, DC and six other Nurse Corps Officers receive temporary additional duty under instruction orders to the Demobilization School at Great Lakes, Illinois. (The BuMed Nurse Corps officer is Lt(jg) Charlotte C. Maas USN.) Then in early September, 5 Naval Personnel Separation Units are designated for releasing active duty Navy Nurses to inactive duty. The Navy Nurses who attended the Demobilization School are assigned to the Units as Assistant Civil Readjustment officers and Lt(jg) Maas is placed in charge. Then on the 15th of September a 'Point' "formula and score for demobilization of" USNR Nurse Corps Officers becomes effective.[256]

Navy Nurse Ednoa Pauls writes about 'points' in describing her active duty. Miss Pauls was appointed a Reserve in early 1941 and reported for active duty in January 1942. "August 11, 1944, I received orders to transfer [from USNH Bethesda] to the Advance Base Assembly and Training Unit at Lido Beach, Long Island, N.Y. (Called A.B.A.T.U.). The unit assignment was to organize a complete hospital to go to Guam. I stayed at A.B.A.T.U. and this time I didn't have to report to the Chief Nurse as it was me. There was a small dispensary to take care of short illnesses and 'short arm' examinations for Navy personnel unloaded off ships returning from Europe. 'Short Arm', I learned, was a spot check for venereal diseases, lice, and scabies. While at A.B.A.T.U., the War in Europe ended, May 7, 1945. The War in the Pacific ended August 15, 1945. At that time, I had enough 'points'—39-1/2— to be discharged from active duty in the Navy. I was released from the Active Navy at [US Naval Air Station], Corpus Christi, Texas, with some flyers who were being released.... All I wanted at the time was to get civilian clothes and find a place to live. Nurses were in demand so after Christmas [1945], I joined a group of ex-Navy doctors at the Texas Medical Center, Houston, Texas."[257]

A Charleston, South Carolina Naval Hospital Newsletter of October 1945, carries an article on points that states, "An important ALNAV (No. 345) relative to the reduction of points has just been released which gives the point scores up to 1 January 1946. . . . Medical Officers had their points reduced from 60 to 53 on 1 November, which remains constant until 1 January when they are again reduced to 51. The Navy Nurse Corps will have no change from their present scale until 1 January when the points go from 35 to 33."[258] But, the Nurse Corps 'demobilization' moves at such a rapid pace that the strength of the Nurse Corps goes from 10,968, at the end of September 1945, to 2,304 at the end of August 1946! Of that 2,304 in 1946, 1248 are Regular Navy and

1,056 are Reserve nurses.[259]

The government, meanwhile, is busy preparing for the huge influx of veterans into the civilian economy and is trying to help with the job market for returning service personnel. One Naval Hospital's newsletter carries information on this, "Personnel returning to civilian life, who wish to return to their former jobs (either with private concerns or the Federal Govt.) may rest assured that those jobs will be available to them. ALNAV No. 296 informs that special boards will aid in securing seniority and a return to the former wage scale. . . . Civil Service positions will be open and the Civil Service will offer other definite advantages for any veterans who wish to apply. . . . Veterans, unemployed, or partially employed (at less that $23.00 per week) as well as those who, self-employed, have a net earning of less than $100 the previous month are entitled to money allowances through the G.I. Bill of Rights. . . . For complete unemployment, there will be an allowance of twenty dollars per week. . . . For the self-employed, the difference between the monthly net and one hundred dollars will be paid."[260]

Meantime, during 1945, there are many policy and regulation changes that affect the Navy Nurses. On 10 January there is a change in the regulations concerning marriage. A Navy Department press and radio release says, "Vice Admiral Ross T. McIntire, Surgeon General, United States Navy, today announced a modification in Nurse Corps regulations which will permit Navy Nurses now in service to marry without being required to resign. In December, 1944, the Bureau of Medicine and Surgery received applications for resignation from 138 nurses who gave `marriage' as the reason for their action. Resignations for the same cause averaged more than 100 a month in 1944, reaching a high point in November — 160. . . . There is no change in present policy which disqualifies married nurses for entrance into the Nurse Corps."[261] Then on February 1945, the "Secretary of the Navy approved modification of appointment policies to permit temporarily the reappointment of former members of [the] Nurse Corps, USN or USNR, whose resignations were accepted between 1 Janurary 1944 and 10 January 1945, solely by reason of marriage."[262]

One of the marriages taking place due to the policy changes, happens in the Admiralty Islands, South Pacific, on 1 August, 1945. The Base Hospital's newspaper headlines the event and reports, "Amid a setting of tropical splendor, Lt. Margaret Keegan (NC) USN became the bride of Lt. Thomas V. Kiernan (D-S) USNR at the attractively decorated Chapel of Base Hospital FIFTEEN in what was described as a precedent-making event. This ceremony has the unique distinction of being the first wedding of its kind to take place in the long chain of Admiralty Islands. Father . . . staff Navy Chaplain, performed the double ring ceremony attended in the Chapel's sanctuary by Father . . . Navy Chaplain of the Ship Repair Unit. The lovely bride wore the traditional Navy white fitted dress uniform [dress whites]. Her flowers in the form of a corsage were a spray of multi-colred tropical beauties. . . . Guest soloist was Lt. Helen Sullivan (NC) USNR who . . . was accompanied at the piano by Lt. Mabelclaire Ralston (NC) USNR. . . . On leaving the Chapel the bride and groom were met with a hail of rice— at the hands of enthusiastic well-wishers. A wedding reception followed . . . at the Officer's Club, Naval Base Hospital No. 15. . . . Both Lt. Kiernan and Mrs. Kiernan have resumed their respective duties following a brief honeymoon at ————— Island-(A military secret)."[263]

It's fortunate the Kiernans married when they did because on the 17th of September, the "Temporary suspension . . . of [the] policy re marriage in [the] Nurse Corps [is] rescinded."[264] On the 17th of October, a Memorandum is sent by BuMed to the Editors of all Journals, "Announcement has been made that effective 1 November 1945 all married officers, Regular and Naval Reserve Nurse Corps, will be released. Prior to 10 January 1945, a member of the Nurse Corps who married became ineligible for retention in the Naval Service. Last January, this policy was suspended as a temporary measure during the period when a large Nurse Corps was urgently needed. The new announcement reinstates the former policy."[265]

Back in January 1945, the Nurse Corps and Navy Recruiting began to work more closely together when the "Chief of Naval Personnel directed active participation of Offices of Naval Officer Procurement in prospecting, processing, and delivery of commissions to candidates for [the] Nurse Corps."[266] Perhaps this is in response to a statement in President Franklin DeLano Roosevelt's message to Congress, on 6 January. The statement is, "Since volunteering has not produced the number of nurses required, I urge that the Selective Service Act be amended to provide for the induction of nurses into the armed forces. The need is too pressing to await the outcome of further efforts at recruiting."[267] "The effect of the President's request for a draft of nurses was electric.... [The] official appeal for a draft of nurses, followed in three days by the introduction into the House of Representatives of a draft bill, was sensational. The nurses' organizations at once took a stand in favor of a National Service Act for all men and women. The Red Cross, recognizing its responsibility as recruiting agent for the army and navy and following its policy of taking no stand on pending legislation, merely intensified efforts to meet the need by recruitment of volunteers."[268]

Hearings were held and many Nursing Organizations testified. A "revised draft bill was sent to the Senate, where hearings continued through March, but it was never brought to the floor.... On May 24, a little more than two weeks after VE Day, a letter from the Acting Secretary of War to the Chairman of the Senate Committee on Military Affairs suggested that further action on the bill be dropped."[269] However, back in the early part of the year, when the draft seemed a real possibility, questions about another source of nurses come to the surface. "Present threats of a nurse draft throw a dramatic spotlight on the shortage of nurses in the armed forces. ... Yet, in the midst of this dire need, numerous qualified nurses who are willing and able to serve their country are being ignored by both branches of the armed forces. The National Association of Colored Graduate Nurses estimates that there are some 9,000 registered Negro nurses in this country. But at this writing there are only 308 Negro nurses in the army and not one in the navy, though the navy has signified its intention of including Negroes in its Nurse Corps. This is no reflection on the patriotism of Negroes, for numerous nurses of this race who have tried to enter the services have been mysteriously classified as 'unavailable' for the army or have received letters that 'the navy does not accept Negro nurses.'"[270]

The Army and Navy Nurse Corps did finally open their ranks to black nurses when, in early 1945, "the War Department declared an end to quotas and exclusion."[271] Phyllis Mae Daley is said to be the first black nurse to come on active duty in the Navy Nurse Corps. She is a graduate of Lincoln School of Nursing in New York. Her oath as Ensign NC USNR is executed 8 March 1945 and she proceeds to active duty 11 April 1945. Ensign Daley reports to her first active duty station at the Naval Dispensary, Boston Navy Yard on 14 April 1945. (She is released on points the 9th of August 1946 for marriage.)

Another black graduate nurse, Edith M. DeVoe, executes her oath as Ensign NC USNR on 18 April 1945. She proceeds to her first active duty station 13 June 1945 and reports to her first active duty station the same day. (Miss Devoe has the distinction of being the first black nurse to transfer to the Regular Navy. In a Navy Department release for newspapers dated 22 January 1948, it is stated, "Ensign Edith DeVoe, U.S.N.R... . one of the four Negro nurses commissioned in the U.S. Navy during World War II, was sworn into the Regular Navy (Nurse Corps) January 6, 1948 at the Navy Department.... She is now on duty at the Navy Communication Annex Dispensary ... Washington, DC." Then on 1 April 1956 Miss DeVoe is placed on the temporary disability retired list.) From this time onward black graduate nurses have their opportunity to serve their country, too.

In March 1945, the "1st ALNAV ... promulgating enblock promotions for certain Ensigns and Lts. (jg) of [the] Nurse Corps, [came out] with new ranks to date from 1 March 1945."[272] (The important phrase here is 'enblock promotions.') As for uniform changes for Navy Nurses, in the beginning of this year, "Black hose of the Navy Nurse Corps has been replaced by beige, and the gray gloves have given way to black ones. During the necessary transition period, nurses may wear either color until such time as those in possession are worn out."[273] Then in April 1945, active recruiting of nurses for the Navy is discontinued (!) and "surplus applicants [are] referred to the Army Nurse Corps."[274] (This one step, halting active recruitment, is to have a tremendously detrimental impact on the recruitment of nurses for the Navy and the strength of the Navy Nurse Corps for the next two decades.)

In August 1945, a Bill for Congress appears, H.R. 3449, proposing that the 'Commanding Officer' of the WAC, Women's Army Corps, be given the temporary rank of Major General. The War Department submits the following comment and recommendation to this Bill:

"(a) That at present the highest ranking officer of the WAC is a colonel who is not commanding officer, but has the title `Director, Women's Army Corps';

(b) That it is considered that the duties and responsibilities of the Director, WAC, do not warrant the grade of major general but that there would be no objection to statutory authorization of the grade of brigadier general for the Director, who is believed, however, to be the only general officer required for the WAC;

(c) That if the Director, WAC, is to be a brigadier general then the Superintendent of the Army Nurse Corps also should be given the rank of brigadier general in the Army of the United States as her duties and responsibilities are as great as those of the Director, WAC."[275]

Once again, now that the war is over, the Navy Nurse Corps is not even mentioned in the above Bill. Both the Navy Surgeon General and the Superintendent of the Navy Nurse Corps, Captain Sue Dauser, write letters and comments about the omission and the Surgeon General recommends the inclusion of the Superintendent of the Navy Nurse Corps; that she be given the rank of Commodore, temporarily, for the duration of the emergency and six months thereafter.[276] Nothing ever results from all this.

In September of 1945 yet another Bill appears; HR 3923. This one is "introduced to provide for establishment of [a] USN training school for nurses" and this is turned down; not approved.[277] Also, in September the Secretary of the Navy approves a change of the upper age limit for appointment of nurses to the Regular Navy Nurse. Current members of the Reserve Nurse Corps who began active service prior to their 38th birthday, can now request transfer to the Regular Navy.[278] On 3 December 1945, Congress approves a law that provided Physical Disability retirement pay as 75% of active duty pay, if retired on or after 22 December 1942.[279] The law also provides, for the nurses, the "same pay in grade as for other naval officers . . . [and] increased rental and subsistence allowances for dependents."[280]

As for the U.S. Cadet Nurse Corps and the U.S. Navy in 1945, the first two graduate Cadet nurses to join the Navy Nurse Corps report for active duty on 3 January 1945. Marion Hogue reports to the Naval Hospital at Philadelphia and Joyce Marie Hudson reports to Naval Hospital at Oakland, California. (Miss Hogue remains in active service until 1948 when she resigns to get married. Miss Hudson stays on active duty until resigning in 1954.)[281] In October plans are made to close out the Cadet nurse student program in the Navy. Captain Dauser writes a letter to the Navy Finance Division saying, "The Surgeon General wishes the [Cadet nurse] program closed out at the end of the fiscal year, June 30, 1946. . . . There are 285 [senior Student] Cadet nurses now assigned to seven Naval Hospitals and 73 more will be reporting by January 1, 1946. These will all finish by June 30, 1946 and are included in the budget for this fiscal year."[282]

Then in November 1945, the Navy Surgeon General writes to the Surgeon General of the U.S. Public Health Service. He says, "It is with regret that we write the last set of orders for a Cadet nurse to proceed to a Naval Hospital for her Senior Cadet Period. . . . Since April 1, 1944, nearly 1100 Cadet Nurses from Schools of Nursing in forty states and the District of Columbia have been assigned to Naval Hospitals for their Senior Cadet Period. They have given expert nursing care to critically ill patients and assisted the members of the Nurse Corps in the administration of the wards and the instruction of the members of the Hospital Corps. . . . May we take this opportunity to thank the members of the United States Cadet Nurse Corps, those who served in Naval Hospitals and those who remained at home to release Senior Cadets and graduate nurses for service."[283] ("The last class of Cadet nurses left the Navy in June 1946. In all, from 1943-46, 1,155 nurses spent their last six months of training in the Navy. Of these 59 entered the Navy Nurse Corps after completion of training, that is, to this date [February 1947]. While the Cadet was spending her six months in the Navy she received from the Navy $60 per month in salary, and she was also furnished subsistence and quarters, in kind. Equivalent value of quarters was set at $45.00 per month regardless of number of days in the month. Equivalent value of subsistence was $0.75 per day, computed on a day to day basis. . . . The Cadet received, thus, $360 in actual cash for the six months."[284])

Now the Navy Nurse Corps is beginning to return to some of its peacetime activities which is evidenced

by some new orders. On 18 October 1945, "LT Elmora J. Merte (NC) USN and 5 nurses report [to the] U.S. Military Government Hospital 204, Tinian, M.I., to assist in training native women as nurse attendants."[285]
Then on the 14th of December 1945, the Secretary of the Navy, James Forrestal, presents Captain Sue S. Dauser with her Distinguished Service Medal. Part of the citation states, "For exceptionally meritorious service to the Government of the United States in a duty of great responsibility as Superintendent of the Navy Nurse Corps during the prewar period of the National Emergency and during World War II. . . . By her sound judgment and careful planning, she was directly responsible for expanding the Navy Nurse Corps from 600 in the prewar period to 11,500, the number essential to provide adequate nursing care for the Navy, Marine Corps, and Coast Guard personnel as the war progressed. Loyal to the ideals established as a standard for her profession, Captain Dauser maintained a high morale and splendid efficiency in the Navy Nurse Corps, and her constant devotion to duty throughout reflects the highest credit upon herself, her command, and the United States Naval Service."[286]

As for the civilian side of nursing in 1945, there are 1295 Schools of Nursing with 127,000 student nurses.[287] Though the war had interrupted the National League of Nursing Education's accrediting program, the work goes on now and there are 110 accredited schools of nursing in 1945.[288] Also, in 1945, there are about 140 schools with collegiate affiliations which give courses leading to a degree.[289] As a matter of interest, "In 1945 more than fifty Negro nurses received college degrees, half of them being M.A."[290] Now that the war is over, the profession must carry out its plans for the process of returning to a peacetime environment. "A National Nursing Planning Committee functioned . . . from 1944 to 1948. In preparation for the work of this committee, a study of nursing needs and resources was made by a committee . . . [and estimates] were projected to 1946. . . . By sheer coincidence, the comprehensive program developed . . . was published in the first issue of the AJN to appear after V-J Day."[291]

The plan is called the "Comprehensive Program for Nation Wide Action in the Field of Nursing."[292] However, "The close of World War II by no means put an end to the need for nurses. While they were no longer recruited for the armed forces, requests poured in from other sources, and the staffs of civilian hospitals and public health agencies remained critically depleted. Nurses returning from front-line duty took extended vacations, found means of securing advanced education, or even engaged in other occupations, while married and retired nurses who had given service left the field once more."[293] "Shortage of nurses! In that irritatingly recurrent phrase, which was to be replaced by the more accurate 'increased demand for nursing service,' may be found the motivation for sharp acceleration of processes in both nursing education and nursing services which were already in existence.

"The special characteristics of the evolving post war program were summarized as: (1) recognition of nursing as a service to be planned in relation to community needs, (2) the preparation and licensure of practical nurses, (3) critical evaluation and reconstruction of educational programs-basic and advanced-for professional nurses, (4) removal of nursing schools from the control of service agencies to an appropriate place in the educational system of the nation, (5) reorganization of the professional organizations to ensure unity of action within the profession and in interprofessional and community relationships in the development of nursing education and nursing service, and in promoting the welfare of the members of the profession."[294] The coming years would see many, and more, of these types of objectives attained.

Also, in 1946, the passage of a Public Law raises "the status of nurses and nursing service within the Veterans Administration. These professional nurses were removed from the General Schedule for Civil Service pay and a separate Nurse Schedule was developed, in their recognition as members of the Department of Medicine and Surgery of the Veterans Administration."[295]

In early 1946, the Navy Nurse Corps begins its own post-war program - for educational enrichment. "The Navy Nurse Corps has, throughout its history, attracted to its service women who were the products of the better educational systems of their times. But they were not to be allowed to settle into complacency. In 1923 the Superintendent of the Navy Nurse Corps was knocking on the door of one of the outstanding universities of the country, asking that a few of her nurses be admitted in order that they might be better prepared for the task of teaching basic nursing to the hospital corpsmen. Her efforts to develop the program failed at that time but that did not deter her or her successors. At the end of World War II, when Navy Nurses finally had time to take stock of the situation, we had lost several years out of our educational lives. Caring for battle casualties on Pacific Islands had left no time for formal programs in nursing, though our experiences added immeasurably to our professional background. In 1946, with the post-World War II emphasis on university preparation in nursing and the benefits of the G.I. Bill as a talking point, we won approval of a program of education benefits for regular officers [USN not the USN Reserve] in the Navy Nurse Corps."[296] On the 8th of January 1946, "New opportunities for assignment to postgraduate courses [are] announced to members of the Nurse Corps:

> [1] 12 months Physiotherapy at the Medical College of Virginia, Richmond . . . with openings for 18 students.
> [2] 12 months Anesthesia at the University of Utah School of Medicine, Salt Lake City and at the University Hospital, Cleveland, Ohio and 9 months anesthesia at Baylor University Hospital, Baylor, Texas, with openings for a total of 17 students. . . .
> [3] 4 months Neuropsychiatric nursing at Pennsylvania Hospital Department of Mental and Nervous Diseases, Philadelphia, with openings for 20 students. . . .
> [4] 18 months in Occupational Therapy at the Boston School of Occupation and at the Philadelphia School of Occupational Therapy, with openings for 36 students. . . .
> [5] 9 months of Teaching and Ward Administration at selected universities . . . with openings for 10 students.
> [6] Continuation of the 9 months Dietetics course at George Washington University, with openings for 20 students.
> [All of the above] programs to be continued in accordance with the need for personnel trained in these specialties."[297]

One of the 18 Navy Nurses accepted for the Navy sponsored Physiotherapy education, is Lt(jg) Ruth Moeller. She states, "At the beginning of 1946, I was stationed at Portsmouth, Virginia. I received a letter from Captain DeWitt stating that they had my letter that I was interested in [physiotherapy] and that the Navy would be sending Navy Nurses to the Medical College of Virginia and that I would be one of the pioneers in this field, because this was the first class that was being offered this opportunity. There were 18 Navy Nurses selected for that. . . . All 18 graduated [from what] was an accelerated program. We came after the first class that they offered was being given [at the Medical College.] The class had already started in the Fall, so they had to revise the curriculum for us. . . . I went there in February of 1946 for six months, then following that [was a] six month apprenticeship. . . . The apprenticeship was given in a Naval Hospital. Three Naval Hospitals were selected for the apprenticeship of the 18 nurses who graduated."[298] All 18 graduates had to take a Board Examination at the end of their apprenticeship to be qualified as physical therapists. (In addition, these 18 Navy Nurses had agreed to spend at least three years in the Navy in return for their education.)

"After I finished the apprenticeship, which was taken at the Philadelphia Naval Hospital, I was assigned to the St. Alban's Naval Hospital, Long Island, New York. The officer in charge [of physiotherapy] was a WAVE physical therapist."[299] The WAVE officer was being released to inactive duty due to demobilization. Further, due to the small number of physiotherapists in the civilian community, the Navy was unable to recruit any to fill its needs. "So the Navy decided it had to train its own people. . . . My orders [to St. Alban's] stated I was to be [assigned to] physical therapy and any such other duties as would be assigned me. When I reported for duty to the Chief Nurse's office, she said [I would] be going to [duty of] a ward. I asked, `What about my physical therapy?' She left me sitting on a bench outside of her office for approximately an hour while she went elsewhere. When she reappeared, she said, `You will report to physical therapy.'. . . Apparently, what happened [was that] she went to see the Commanding Officer and some things transpired during that time . . . and I was [assigned to] the hydro therapy room. So it was nothing but doing whirlpools [treatment for patients] and cleaning [the whirlpool] tanks; nothing very stimulating."[300]

Then, one of the Nurse Corps Officers from BuMed came to visit. She was the one who had started the Navy's Physiotherapy program and the one who was following the graduates of the program. Miss Moeller tells the BuMed representative of her duties "and asked that I be reassigned if a billet [for a physiotherapist] became available because I was only doing hydrotherapy and certainly was not using my training. In addition, every other weekend, I did ward duty . . . and supervising contagious wards. . . . In a matter of a few weeks, I received my orders to the Naval Hospital at Quantico, Virginia where I was in Physical Therapy with Corpsmen [to help.] . . . I had OR call, so there were some days I would work in the Physical Therapy Department and I was the Nurse Corps Officer on-call for the Operating Room [when surgery had to be performed.] There were times I worked all night in the Operating Room and then the following day I reported for my duty in the Physical Therapy Department. . . . On weekends I would do Supervisory duty, maybe even the Chief Nurse's Office or the Emergency Room but that was an every-other-weekend sort of thing. In other words, it was working 12 days and maybe some nights . . . to have two days off. . . . It never changed until I transferred to the Medical Service Corps in 1957."[301]

Another Navy Nurse (Edith Ferguson nee Colton) takes advantage of the educational chance and applies for the Navy sponsored 'Dietetics' course at George Washington University. She is accepted. She tells us, "At that time, a lone woman was not able to rent an apartment in Washington, DC, so I took up residence in Meridan Hall (a hotel for military women.) . . . I completed my schooling at George Washington University on May 26, 1947. I was assigned duty in the diet kitchen along with Louise Bueher Olsen and Kay Goggin (now deceased.) Myrtle Teisseire Warner was the Senior Dietician. . . . Even though we were in special departments [the diet kitchen], we each had to take our turn at night duty [on the wards]. We worked twenty-eight straight nights from 10:00 p.m. to 8:00 a.m.."[302] This type of practice continues for at least the next twenty years. Nurse Corps Officers trained in specialties could not depend on always being assigned duty in their specialties. And, even when assigned to their specialties they are often called upon to do rotational night duty on the wards and/or weekend ward duty.

Operating Room nurses often do double duty without recompense. They do their day shift then take call at night. If called out for surgery, they can work all night then still be expected to work the next day (and in rare cases, even longer) unless an understanding Supervisor allows them some compensatory time off - if the operation schedule allows it. Nurse Anesthetists have an exceptionally hard and rigorous duty situation. This is, in part, due to the fact that all Navy Nurses are assigned to the Nursing Service, no matter what their specialty and the Nursing Service has a quota limit. Chief Nurses have to have nurses for round-the-clock coverage of all wards and special patient areas. Because Nurse Anesthetists are on the Nursing Service, some Chief Nurses require them to work on the wards on the weekends or on holidays, and in some cases, even when the Anesthetist is on call she has to work on the ward. If she is called to surgery, then there is a mad scramble among the supervisors to find a replacement or combine duties for another Navy Nurse.

In addition, when a lone Nurse Anesthetist is ordered into a small stateside or overseas Navy medical facility, she is many times the ONLY anesthetist; there is no anesthesiologist with her. In these cases, the Navy Surgeon at the facility is supposed to take the responsibility for helping the anesthetist if problems arise. Also, at these small stations, the anesthetist is, again, utilized on the wards if the Chief Nurse so orders it. Although, it should be noted that not too much surgery, especially not complex surgery, is usually performed at these smaller stations. It must be noted, however, that Chief Nurses and Senior Nurses (at smaller duty stations the Chief Nurse is called Senior Nurse) are responsible for having adequate nursing coverage and this can mean that the specialty nurses must be utilized. Another fact is that by working on the various wards and units, the specialty nurses become especially adept at all types of nursing and not just their special field. Understand that in case of emergencies, war or battle it is entirely another matter. No Navy Nurse or any other Naval Officer cares or thinks of how long or where they work under those circumstances.

In February 1946, the "School of Nursing on Guam [is] opened to native girls from ex-Japanese mandated islands, now called [the] Trust Territory."[303]   Then on the first of April, 1946, Captain Sue S. Dauser retires having served on active duty for 28 years, 5 months and 15 days. She has gallantly and courageously led the Navy Nurse Corps through the most demanding and lengthy emergency/war period that the Corps has ever faced. (Captain Dauser retires to La Mesa, California. She enters a retirement home that she helped to start. In early 1972 she suffers a heart attack and dies a few hours later.)

[1]   *Nurse Corps, U.S. Navy Monthly Census*, Xerox copy, figures from Monthly Reports of Superintendent, Nurse Corps, to Bureau of Naval Personnel (Planning & Control Div.)
[2]   Laird, LCDR Thelma NC USNR, Jones, LCDR Dorothy NC USN, Feeney, LCDR Elizabeth NC USN, Seidl, CDR Elizabeth NC USN (Ret.), Blaska, CDR Burdette NC USN, *Chronological History NAVY NURSE CORPS*, Prepared by: Nursing Division, Bureau of Medicine and Surgery, 1 August 1962, p. 25.
[3]   Cobb, LCdr. Laura NC USN, Handwritten notes on notebook paper, reproduced at National Archives, from Navy Nurse Corps Historical Documents, Box #2, National Archives, Washington, D.C..
[4]   Nelson, Lt. Mary Rose Harrington, former Navy Nurse, *Oral History Interview Tape Transcript*, Interviewer LCdr. Alice Lanning NC USN (Ret.), 12 August 1989.
[5]   Cobb, LCdr. Laura NC USN, Handwritten notes on notebook paper, op. cit..
[6]   Todd, CDR. C. Edwina (NC) USN, "NURSING UNDER FIRE," speech presented at the annual convention of the Association of Military Surgeons, Detroit, Michigan, October 9-11, 1946, then printed in *The Military Surgeon*, Vol. 100, No. 4, April 1947, p. 77.
[7]   Nash, CDR Margaret A. NC USN (Ret.), *Oral History Interview Tape Transcript*, Interviewer Florence Alwyn Twyman NC USN (Ret.), 28 September 1990.
[8]   Todd, CDR. C. Edwina (NC) USN, "NURSING UNDER FIRE," op cit..
[9]   Nash, CDR Margaret A. NC USN (Ret.), *Oral History Interview Tape Transcript*, op cit..
[10]   Ibid..
[11]   Todd, CDR. C. Edwina (NC) USN, "NURSING UNDER FIRE," op cit..
[12]   Nelson, Lt. Mary Rose Harrington, former Navy Nurse, *Oral History Interview Tape Transcript*, op cit..
[13]   Cobb, LCdr. Laura NC USN, Handwritten notes on notebook paper, op. cit..
[14]   Ibid..
[15]   Moeller, Ruth Captain Navy Medical Service Corps, *Oral History Interview Tape Transcript*, Interviewer Doris M. Sterner Captain Navy Nurse Corps, 17 October 1988.
[16]   Ibid..
[17]   Dixon HC USN, Lt. Ben F., "The "White Lily," *Hospital Corps QUARTERLY*, Hospital Ships Number, July 1945, p. 3.
[18]   "U.S.S. `Solace' Cited For Distinguished Service," *American Journal of Nursing*, Volume 43, No. 4, April 1943, p. 400.
[19]   Newcomb, Ellsworth, "*The Solace: Mercy Ship*," *Great Adventures in Nursing*, Helen Wright and Samuel Rapport, Editors, Harper and Bros., New York, 1960, p. 274.
[20]   Mitchum, Jennifer, "Navy Medicine January-February 1943," *Navy Medicine*, Jan Kenneth Herman, Editor, Vol. 84, No. 1, January-February 1993, p. 30.
[21]   "Nurses Christen Two Navy Hospital Ships," *American Journal of Nursing*, Volume 43, No. 7, July 1943, p. 686.
[22]   Smith, Clarence McKittrick, *United States Army in World War II[:] The Technical Services[:] The Medical Department: Hospitalization And Evacuation, Zone of Interior*, Office of the Chief of Military History, Department of the Army, Washington, D.C., 1956, p. 406.
[23]   Mehes, Florence Wisneski, Lieutenant Navy Nurse Corps, *Oral History Interview Tape Transcript*, Interviewer Dorothea Short Tracy Navy Nurse Corps, 25 June 1990.
[24]   Georgiana, Charlotte Sprague Lieutenant Navy Nurse Corps, Letter to CDR Patricia Warner Navy Nurse Corps, 23 January 1991.
[25]   Hummel, Sue Smoker Captain Navy Nurse Corps, *Oral History Interview Tape Transcript*, Interviewer Lt. Helen Barry Siragusa Navy Nurse Corps, 29 January 1991.
[26]   Eubanks, Grace Smith LCDR Navy Nurse Corps, Letter to LCDR Jan Barcott Navy Nurse Corps, 20 May 1986.
[27]   Lindner, Mary J. Commander Navy Nurse Corps, *Oral History Interview Tape Transcript*, Interviewer CDR Jean E. Davis Navy Nurse Corps, 19 July 1989.
[28]   Whitehead, Helen Gavin Commander Navy Nurse Corps, *Oral History Interview Tape Transcript*, Interviewer CDR Jean E. Davis Navy Nurse Corps, 24 April 1990.
[29]   Swanson, Claire LCDR Navy Nurse Corps, *Oral History Interview Tape Transcript*, Interviewer Linn Larson Navy Nurse Corps, 15 July 1988.
[30]   Hanf, Madonna M. Timm LCDR Navy Nurse Corps, *Written Material*, written August 1990.
[31]   Swanson, *Oral History Interview Tape Transcript*, op. cit..
[32]   Hanf, *Written Material*, op. cit..
[33]   Swanson, *Oral History Interview Tape Transcript*, op. cit..
[34]   Mitchum, Jennifer, "Navy Medicine November-December 1943," *Navy Medicine*, Editor Jan Kenneth Herman, Vol. 84, No. 6, November-December 1993, p. 22.
[35]   O'Toole, Sarah Lt(jg) NC USNR, Chief Nurse, US Naval Air Station, Deland, Florida, "I'm in the Navy Now," *American Journal of Nursing*, December 1943, p. 1077.
[36]   Rubin, Jeanne Grushinski Captain Navy Nurse Corps, *Oral History Interview Tape Transcript*, Interviewer Mary Carmickle Snedeker Navy Nurse Corps, 8 August 1989.
[37]   Morris, Margaret A. Lt NC USN, Chief Nurse, Letter to Capt. Sue Dauser NC USN, Superintendent Navy Nurse Corps, 29 August 1943.
[38]   Ibid..
[39]   Ibid..

40   Ibid..

41   Ibid..

42   Dauser, Sue Capt NC USN, Superintendent Navy Nurse Corps, Letter to Lt Margaret Morris NC USN, 4 September 1943.

43   Covington, Margaret L. CDR Navy Nurse Corps, *Oral History Interview Tape Transcript*, Self interview, 22 July 1990.

44   Gaston, Nancy Aulenbach LT Navy Nurse Corps, *Oral History Interview Tape Transcript*, Interviewer Lt(jg) Helen Bowman Devlin Navy Nurse Corps, 2 August 1989.

45   George, Evelyn Hope Navy Nurse Corps, *Oral History Interview Tape Transcript*, Interviewer Lt(jg) Irene Smith Matthews Navy Nurse Corps, 17 June circa 1970.

46   Ibid..

47   Scheips, Edna Marie Lt(jg) Navy Nurse Corps, "Navy Nurse Officers Club," *American Journal of Nursing*, Vol. 43, No. 9, September 1943, p. 816.

48   Ibid..

49   Wright, Freddie Tucker LT Navy Nurse Corps, *Written Material*, written 8 August 1990, p. 3.

50   Laird, et al, op. cit., p. 25.

51   Schmidt, Esther I. Lt(jg) Navy Nurse Corps, "Training of WAVES for Hospitals," *American Journal of Nursing*, Vol. 43, No. 8, August 1943, p. 717.

52   Ibid., pp. 717, 718.

53   "Army and Navy Nurses Tell Us," *American Journal of Nursing*, January 1943, p. 103.

54   Laird, et al, op. cit., p. 26.

55   Van Gorp, Dymphna M. CDR Navy Nurse Corps, *Oral History Interview Tape Transcript*, Self interview, 25 August 1990.

56   Fuller, Bettie Eberhardt Lt(jg) Navy Nurse Corps, *Oral History Interview Tape Transcript*, Interviewer Helen Barry Siragusa Navy Nurse Corps, 12 May 1989.

57   Ibid..

58   Raborn, Mildred Terrill CDR Navy Nurse Corps, *Oral History Interview Tape Transcript*, Interviewer Mary Wing Kingman Navy Nurse Corps, 5 June 1991.

59   Typewritten transcript of an alleged Diary of a Japanese Acting Officer, May 1941. Donated by CDR Mildred Terrill Raborn Navy Nurse Corps.

60   Ibid..

61   Ibid..

62   Ibid..

63   Bullough, Bonnie, "The Lasting Impact of WORLD WAR II on Nursing," *American Journal of Nursing*, January 1976, p. 120.

64   Ibid..

65   Mullan, CAPT. Fitzhugh, M.D., Director Public Health History Project, Office of the Surgeon General, *WAR, WOMEN, AND THE CARE OF THE SICK-THE U.S. CADET NURSE CORPS*, Pamphlet issued at a reception commemorating the 50th anniversary of the signing of the Nurse Training Act of 1943, U.S. Department of Health and Human Services, Public Health Service, Washington, D.C., 1993.

66   Kalisch, Beatrice J. and Kalisch, Philip A., "The Cadet Nurse Corps - in World War II," *American Journal of Nursing*, Volume 76, Number 2, February 1976, p. 241.

67   Kalisch, op. cit..

68   Mullan, op. cit..

69   Ibid..

70   Jamieson, Elizabeth M., B.A., R.N., and Sewall, Mary F., B.S., R.N., *Trends in Nursing History*, W.B. Saunders Company, Philadelphia and London, 1949, pp. 517, 518.

71   Monlux, Irma F. Lt(jg) NC USNR, "Letter to Captain DeWitt NC USN" and "Report on the Cadet Nurse Corps Program," reproduced at National Archives, from Navy Nurse Corps Historical Documents, Box #35, Cadet NC 1944-1948, National Archives, Washington, D.C..

72   Ibid..

73   Ibid..

74   Ibid..

75   "Developments in Nursing School Programs," *American Journal of Nursing*, Volume 43, No. 11, November 1943, p. 1040.

76   *NEWS RELEASE*, American Nurses Association, 600 Maryland Ave. SW, Suite 100 West, Washington, DC 20024-2571, April 12, 1993.

77   Carnegie, Mary Elizabeth D.P.A., R.N., F.A.A.N., *The PATH WE TREAD*, J.B. Lippincott Company, Philadelphia, Penna., 1986, p.46.

78   Ibid..

79   Hine, Darlene Clark, *BLACK WOMEN IN WHITE*, Indiana University Press, Bloomington and Indianapolis, 1989, p. 151.

80   Ibid., p. 152.

81   Ibid., pp. 152, 153.

82   Ibid., p. 171.

83   Goodnow, Minnie R.N., *Nursing History*, W.B. Saunders Company, Philadelphia, London, 1948, p. 196.

84   Roberts, Mary M. R.N., *AMERICAN NURSING*, The Macmillan Company, New York, 1963, p. 321.

85   Ibid..

86   *The Manual of The Medical Department of the United States Navy*, Published by the Bureau of Medicine and Surgery Under the authority of the Secretary of the Navy, United States Government Printing Office, Washington, 1943, Chapter I, pp. 5, 6.

87   Mitchum, Jennifer, "Navy Medicine January-February 1943," op. cit., p. 32.

88   *THE NAVY NURSE CORPS*, Published by the Bureau of Medicine and Surgery, Navy Department, Printed by the U.S. Government Printing Office, Washington, 1943, p. 5.

89   Ibid., p. 11.

90   "Quotas for Assignment to Army and Navy Nurse Corps," *American Journal of Nursing*, Vol. 43, No. 2, February 1943, p. 217.

91 Kernodle, Portia B., *The Red Cross Nurse In Action*, Harper and Brothers, New York, 1949, p. 422.

92 "Married Nurses in the Army," *American Journal of Nursing*, Vol. 43, No. 3, March 1943, p. 306.

93 *Nurse Corps, U.S. Navy Monthly Census*, op. cit..

94 Mitchum, Jennifer, "Navy Medicine March-April 1943," *Navy Medicine*, Editor Jan Kenneth Herman, Vol. 84, No. 2, March-April 1993, p. 26.

95 *200 Years, A Bicentennial Illustrated History of the United States*, Joseph Newman, Directing Editor, Books by U.S. News & World Report, Inc., 2300 N Street, N.W., Washington, D.C. 20037, 1973, book 2, p. 175.

96 Ibid., pp. 174, 175.

97 Ibid., p. 185.

98 Ibid., p. 184.

99 *The World Book Encyclopedia*, Field Enterprises Educational Corporation, Chicago, Volume 20, 1966 edition, p. 385.

100 Ibid., Volume 16, p. 420.

101 Ibid., p. 422.

102 *200 Years, A Bicentennial Illustrated History of the United States*, op. cit., pp. 183, 184.

103 Wells, H.G., *The Outline of History*, Revised and brought up to date by Raymond Postgate, Garden City Books, Garden City, New York, Volume II, 1961, p. 936.

104 *The World Book Encyclopedia*, op. cit., Volume 20, 1966 edition, p. 385.

105 Ibid., p. 402.

106 Copy of Bureau of Medicine and Surgery Letter to Commanding Officers of Naval Hospitals and Commandants and COs of Naval Shore Activities and Commanding Generals and COs of Marine Corps Activities, Subject "Navy Nurse Corps; commissioned rank; laws applicable," dated 18 May 1944. Copy is courtesy of the Nursing Division, Bureau of Medicine and Surgery, Washington, D.C..

107 Laird, et al, op. cit., p. 29.

108 Ibid..

109 *Uniforms of the United States Navy 1900-1967*, text accompanying this set of color lithographs written by Captain James C. Tily, CEC, USN (Ret.) in coordination with office of Director of Naval History and Curator for the Department of the Navy, U.S. Government Printing Office, Washington, D.C. 20402. (See section 'Uniforms of the United States Navy 1918-1919.)

110 BUMED-N-MGL (OG), *MEMORANDUM*, signed by Sue S. Dauser Captain (NC) USN, dated 22 August 1944.

111 Tily, James C., *The Uniforms of the United States Navy*, Thomas Yoseloff, Publisher, 8 East 36th Street, New York 16, New York, 1964, p. 269.

112 Ibid., p. 265.

113 *History of the Nurse Corps, U.S. Navy*, 5727.1 OONCA/np, draft prepared by: Nursing Division, Bureau of Medicine and Surgery, revised 24 April 1991, p. 6.

114 Schmidt, Esther L. R.N. and Meridith, Catherine R.N., "The Senior Cadet Program in a Naval Hospital," *American Journal of Nursing*, Volume 45, No. 3, 1945, pp. 196 and 198.

115 Ibid., p. 197.

116 Laird, et al, op. cit., p. 29.

117 Ibid., p. 27.

118 Ferguson, Edith L. Colton LCdr Navy Nurse Corps, *Written Personal History*, 23 July 1991, p. 6.

119 Ibid., p. 3.

120 Ibid., pp. 1-3.

121 Gouge, Ruth L., RN, MD, JD and former Navy Nurse, *Written Personal History*, 21 May 1991, pp. 1-3.

122 Wright, Freddie Tucker LT Navy Nurse Corps, *Written Personal History*, 26 August 1990, pp. 2, 3.

123 Todd, Rachel B. LCDR Navy Nurse Corps, *Oral History Interview Tape Transcript*, Self-Interview, April 1989.

124 Ibid..

125 Wharton, Ednoa Pauls LT Navy Nurse Corps, *Written Personal History*, 24 August 1990, pp. 10, 11.

126 Walsh, Claire M. CDR Navy Nurse Corps, *Oral History Interview Tape Transcript*, Interviewer CDR Barbara (Bobbie) Ellis Navy Nurse Corps, 25 August 1990.

127 Laird, et al, op. cit., p. 26.

128 Van Gorp, Dymphna CDR Navy Nurse Corps, *Oral History Interview Tape Transcript*, Self interview, 25 August 1990.

129 "Nurses Also Teach," *Military Nurse*, Military Nurse Publishing Co., 230 W. 41st, New York 18, New York, circa. 1945, p. 22.

130 Goble, CDR Dorothy Jones, NC USN (Ret.), as written in her unpublished history research notes.

131 Laird, et al, op. cit., p. 30.

132 Goble, op. cit..

133 Laird, et al, op. cit., p. 30.

134 Listing provided through the courtesy of Norma Harrison Crotty Lt(jg) Navy Nurse Corps; one of the original Navy Flight Nurses.

135 Purvis, Emily G., R.N., "Nursing Care In Air Ambulances," *American Journal of Nursing*, Vol. 47, January to December 1947.

136 McClean, Eveline Kittilson LT Navy Nurse Corps, *Oral History Interview Tape Transcript*, Self interview, 4 July 1990.

137 Hey, Rita Reed LCdr Navy Nurse Corps, *Oral History Interview Tape Transcript*, Self interview, 20 September 1990.

138 Kelley, Sara Marcum Navy Nurse Corps, Letter to Jan Barcotte, 17 October 1989.

139 Wabeck, Mildred DeLisa LCdr Navy Nurse Corps, *Oral History Interview Tape Transcript*, Self interview, 11 June 1990.

140 Hudson, Henry W. Captain (MC) USNR, *The Story of SNAG 56*, Harvard University Printing Office, Cambridge, Massachusetts, U.S.A., 1946, pp. 19-21.

141 Ibid., pp. 69, 70, as quoted from the article "Naval Nurses Return Home From England," *Richmond Times-Despatch*, December 3, 1944.

142 Ibid., p. 70, as quoted from the article "Naval Hospital in England Treats Hundreds of Wounded First Two Weeks of Invasion," *The Journal of the American Medical Association*, Sept. 2, 1944.

143 Desmarais, Mary Virginia Ensign Navy Nurse Corps, "Navy Nursing on D-Day Plus 4," *American Journal of Nursing*, Volume 45, January -

December 1945.
[144]   Hudson, op. cit., pp. 45, 46.
[145]   Laird, et al, op. cit., p. 27, as quoted from Mutual Broadcasting System Script for Broadcast 11 November 1944.
[146]   Goble, op. cit..
[147]   "Navy Nurse Receives Medal for Work in England," U.S. Navy Magazine, Roy Jackson, Publisher and Editor (not a publication endorsed or sponsored by the U.S. Navy/Navy Department), Vol. VII, No. 6, January 1945, p. 7.
[148]   Ibid., p. 28.
[149]   Staats, Elizabeth Torrance LT Navy Nurse Corps, Oral History Interview Tape Transcript, Interviewer Mary Carmickle Snedeker Navy Nurse Corps Officer, 28 July 1989.
[150]   Ibid..
[151]   Ibid..
[152]   Blair, Margaret Jackson LCdr Navy Nurse Corps, Oral History Interview Tape Transcript, Self interview, 27 May 1991.
[153]   Fuller, Bettie Eberhardt, op. cit..
[154]   Giorgiani, Charlotte Sprague LT Navy Nurse Corps, "Written Addendum" to an NNCA Autobiographical Survey conducted in 1990.
[155]   Swanson, Claire Vecchione LCdr Navy Nurse Corps, Oral History Interview Tape Transcript, Interviewer LCdr. Linn Larson Navy Nurse Corps, 15 July 1988.
[156]   Ibid..
[157]   "Veteran Nurse," Military Nurse, Military Nurse Publishing Co., 230 W. 41st, New York 18, New York, circa. 1945, p. 28.
[158]   Ibid..
[159]   Laird, et al, op. cit., pp. 27-29.
[160]   Ibid., p. 29.
[161]   Nurse Corps, U.S. Navy Monthly Census, op. cit..
[162]   Laird, et al, op. cit., p. 30.
[163]   Nash, CDR Margaret A. NC USN (Ret.), Oral History Interview Tape Transcript, op cit..
[164]   Todd, CDR. C. Edwina (NC) USN, "NURSING UNDER FIRE," op cit..
[165]   Rudin, Emily B., "Memories of a World War II POW Nurse," U.S. Navy Medicine," Editor Jan Kenneth Herman, Vol. 73, No. 5, May 1982, p. 19.
[166]   Nash, CDR Margaret A. NC USN (Ret.), Oral History Interview Tape Transcript, op cit..
[167]   Cobb, LCdr. Laura NC USN, Handwritten notes on notebook paper, op. cit..
[168]   Todd, CDR. C. Edwina (NC) USN, "NURSING UNDER FIRE," op cit..
[169]   Evans, Jessie Fant, "Release From Los Banos," American Journal of Nursing, Vol. 45, January - December 1945.
[170]   Cobb, LCdr. Laura NC USN, Handwritten notes on notebook paper, op. cit..
[171]   Valentine, Carolyn B.S., "Nursing at Los Banos," R.N. A Journal for Nurses, Nightingale Press, Inc., Rutherford, N.J., Volume 8, Number 8, May 1945, p. 66. Magazine donated by LCdr Hazel Bennett Navy Nurse Corps.
[172]   Todd, CDR. C. Edwina (NC) USN, "NURSING UNDER FIRE," op cit..
[173]   Nash, CDR Margaret A. NC USN (Ret.), Oral History Interview Tape Transcript, op cit..
[174]   Cobb, LCdr. Laura NC USN, Handwritten notes on notebook paper, op. cit..
[175]   Kalisch, Phillip A. and Kalisch, Beatrice J., "Nurses Under Fire; The World War II Experience of Nurses on Bataan and Corregidor," Nursing Research, Volume 25, No. 6, November-December 1976, p. 427.
[176]   Nash, CDR Margaret A. NC USN (Ret.), Oral History Interview Tape Transcript, op cit..
[177]   Todd, CDR. C. Edwina (NC) USN, "NURSING UNDER FIRE," op cit..
[178]   Todd, ibid..
[179]   Nash, CDR Margaret A. NC USN (Ret.), Oral History Interview Tape Transcript, op cit..
[180]   Goble, op. cit..
[181]   Ibid..
[182]   Ibid..
[183]   Ibid..
[184]   Benner, Mary CDR Navy Nurse Corps, Oral History Interview Tape Transcript, Interviewer Irene Matthews, 6 February 1970.
[185]   Ibid..
[186]   Wright, Freddie Tucker Lt(jg) Navy Nurse Corps, Self-Written Personal History, August 26, 1990, pp. 3-5.
[187]   Gouge, Ruth L., RN, MD, JD, former Lt(jg) Navy Nurse Corps, Self-Written Personal History, 21 May 1991, pp. 3-5.
[188]   O'Toole, Sarah LT Navy Nurse Corps, "They Pioneered on Tinian," American Journal of Nursing, Vol. 45, January - December 1945.
[189]   Laird, et al, op. cit., p. 32.
[190]   Laird, et al, op. cit., p. 31.
[191]   Hinnershitz, Edna A. Lt. NC USNR, copy of a Letter to Capt. Sue Dauser NC USN, Superintendent of the Navy Nurse Corps, BuMed, Washington, D.C., 28 September 1945.
[192]   Laird, et al, op. cit., p. 33.
[193]   McCann, Dick Sp(X)1c, "Our Growing Mercy Fleet," All Hands Magazine, August 1945, p. 8.
[194]   Ibid..
[195]   Ibid. p.10.
[196]   Ibid. p.11.
[197]   "Army's Hospital-Ship Fleet," All Hands Magazine, August 1945, p. 11.
[198]   "USS Rescue Converted in Eight Weeks," Hospital Corps Quarterly, United States Government Printing Office, Washington, D.C., Volume 18, No. 7, July 1945, p. 51.
[199]   Laird, et al, op. cit., p. 32.

200   Ibid. p. 33.
201   Marks, R. Adrian, "America was Well Represented," *United States Naval Institute Proceedings*, The Institute, Annapolis, Maryland, April 1981, p. 48.
202   Ibid., pp. 48, 49.
203   Daniels, Edna Park LCdr Navy Nurse Corps, *Oral History Interview Tape Transcript*, Interviewer LCdr. Dorothea Tracy Navy Nurse Corps, 9 May 1990.
204   Ibid..
205   Laird, et al, op. cit., p. 33.
206   Bernatitis, Ann Capt. NC USN (Ret.), *Oral History Interview Tape Transcript*, Interviewer Irene Smith Matthews Lt(jg) Navy Nurse Corps, taped 19 May 1971.
207   Copy of the Navy Communique No. 347 of April 29, 1945 was graciously provided on 27 June 1993 by Beatrice Rivers Gallagher Lt. Navy Nurse Corps.
208   Goble, CDR Dorothy Jones, NC USN (Ret.), as written in her unpublished history research notes.
209   Ibid..
210   Purvis, Emily G., R.N., "Nursing Care In Air Ambulances," *American Journal of Nursing*, Vol. 47, January to December 1947.
211   Covington, Margaret Lou CDR NC USN (Ret.), *Oral History Interview Tape Transcript*, Self Interview, taped 22 July 1990.
212   Copy of Navy Department, Bureau of Naval Personnel letter, "Naval Flight Nurse - insignia for," 27 February 1945. Copy enclosed in research notes of CDR Dorothy Jones Goble, NC USN (Ret.).
213   Laird, et al, op. cit., p. 31.
214   Covington, op. cit. .
215   "Okinawa-Frisco Express," *Military Nurse*, Military Nurse Publishing Co., 230 W. 41st, New York 18, New York, circa. 1945, p. 26.
216   Urgitis, Emma E. LCdr. Navy Nurse Corps, "Air Evacuation Information," a four page typewritten account found in the research notebook of CDR Dorothy Jones Goble, NC USN (Ret.), circa 1946, pp. 1, 2.
217   Covington, op. cit. .
218   "News of the Month," *R.N., A Journal for Nurses*, Nightingale Press, Inc., Rutherford, N.J., May 1945, p. 52.
219   Covington, op. cit. .
220   Oddo, Irene Freeburger Lt(jg) Navy Nurse Corps, *Oral History Interview Tape Transcript*, Self Interview, taped 13 December 1989.
221   Bauman, Edythe May Bogie Lt(jg) Navy Nurse Corps, *Written History Material*, written 27 June 1991, p. 3.
222   Ferguson, Edith Lorene Colton LCdr. Navy Nurse Corps, *Written History Material*, written 23 July 1991, pp. 6, 7.
223   Houp, Geraldine A. Captain Navy Nurse Corps, *Oral History Interview Tape Transcript*, Interviewer Helen Barry Siragusa LT Navy Nurse Corps, 9 May 1990.
224   *The World Book Encyclopedia*, Field Enterprises Educational Corporation, Chicago, Volume 16, 1966 edition, p. 422.
225   Ibid..
226   Ibid., Volume 18, p. 382b.
227   Wells, H.G., *The Outline of History*, Revised and brought up to date by Raymond Postgate, Garden City Books, Garden City, New York, Volume II, 1961 by Doubleday & Company, Inc., p. 939.
228   *200 Years, A Bicentennial Illustrated History of the United States*, Joseph Newman, Directing Editor, Books by U.S. News & World Report, Inc., 2300 N Street, N.W., Washington, D.C. 20037, 1973, book 2, p. 208.
229   *The World Book Encyclopedia*, op. cit., Volume 20, pp. 407, 408.
230   Davis, Dorothy M., R.N., "Processing And Caring For Prisoners Of War," *American Journal of Nursing*, Vol. 46, January to June 1946.
231   Cannon, Ethel Buler, Navy Nurse Corps, *NNCA Autobiographical Survey*, Attached written addendum, 1989.
232   Price, Mary E. Commander Navy Nurse Corps, *Oral History Interview Tape Transcript*, Interviewer Rita E. Duffin Navy Nurse Corps, 8 November 1989.
233   Bernatitis, Ann Capt. NC USN (Ret.), *Oral History Interview Tape Transcript*, Interviewer Irene Smith Matthews Lt(jg) Navy Nurse Corps, taped 19 May 1971.
234   Bernatitis, Ann Capt. NC USN (Ret.), *Oral History Interview Tape Transcript*, Interviewer Doris M. Sterner Captain Navy Nurse Corps, taped 7 May 1990.
235   Bernatitis, op. cit., Interviewer Irene Matthews.
236   Bernatitis, op. cit., Interviewer Doris Sterner.
237   Bernatitis, op. cit., Interviewer Irene Matthews.
238   Copy of the communication donated by Lt. Beatrice Rivers Gallagher Navy Nurse Corps.
239   Wheeler, Marion Ceaser CDR. NC USN (Ret.), *Oral History Interview Tape Transcript*, Interviewer Anna Corcoran, Commander Navy Nurse Corps, taped 18 July 1991.
240   "Angel of the Orient," *U.S. Navy Medical Newsletter*, Captain M.T. Lynch MC USN, Editor, Vol. 55, No. 4, April 1970, p. 10.
241   Erickson, Ruth A. Captain NC USN (Ret.), *Oral History Interview Tape Transcript*, Interviewer Alice Lanning LCdr. Navy Nurse Corps, taped 9 January 1990.
242   Laird, et al, op. cit., p. 34.
243   McClean, Eveline Kittilson LT Navy Nurse Corps, *Oral History Interview Tape Transcript*, Self interview, taped 4 July 1990.
244   Larson, Margaret L. LCdr. Navy Nurse Corps, *NNCA Autobiographical Survey*, Attached written addendum, 1989.
245   Covington, op. cit. .
246   Urgitis, Copy of typewritten account, op. cit., circa 1946, p. 4.
247   Laird, et al, op. cit., p. 36 and *History of the Medical Department of the United States Navy in World War II*, U.S. Government Printing Office, Washington, D.C., circa 1950's, pp. 216, 217.
248   McEniry, Marion, Women's Editor, "Civilian Award for Heroine Lt. Cmdr. Cobb Acclaimed," *San Francisco Examiner*, 24 February 1946, reproduced at National Archives, from Navy Nurse Corps Historical Documents, Box #2, National Archives, Washington, D.C..

249	Avon Advertisement, circa 1946, reproduced at National Archives, from Navy Nurse Corps Historical Documents, Box #2, National Archives, Washington, D.C..

250	Cobb, Laura M. LCdr NC USN, Letter to CDR Nellie Jane DeWitt NC USN at the Bureau of Medicine and Surgery, Navy Department, Washington, D.C., dated 4 March 1946, reproduced at National Archives, from Navy Nurse Corps Historical Documents, National Archives, Washington, D.C..

251	Letter of recommendation with endorsements, dated 6 December 1945, reproduced at National Archives, from Navy Nurse Corps Historical Documents, Box #2, National Archives, Washington, D.C..

252	*Nurse Corps, U.S. Navy Monthly Census*, Xerox copy, figures from Monthly Reports of Superintendent, Nurse Corps, to Bureau of Naval Personnel (Planning & Control Div.)

253	DeWitt, Nellie Jane Captain NC USN, Superintendent, Nurse Corps, Copy of letter to Miss Genevieve McDonald, Commander Jean Templeman Post, No. 162, St. Paul, Minnesota, dated 15 November 1946, Part of the Navy Nurse Corps Records not yet processed, when obtained, reproduced at the Naval Historical Center, Washington Navy Yard, Washington, D.C.

254	Laird, et al, op. cit., p. 35.

255	Ibid., p. 34.

256	Ibid., entire paragraph including quote, p. 34.

257	Wharton, Ednoa Pauls LT Navy Nurse Corps, *Written History Material*, written 24 August 1990, p. 12.

258	"Points Reduced!," *The Anodyne*, 22 October 1945, page 1. "The ANODYNE [was] published by the Navy Yard Print Shop every pay day and distributed free to the staff and patients of the U.S. Naval Hospital, Charleston, S.C. . . . at no cost to the Government." This quote is from page two of the said publication which was graciously provided by LCdr Hazel V. Bennett Navy Nurse Corps.

259	DeWitt, Nellie Jane Captain NC USN, Copy of Memorandum to LT H. Browdy, MSC,USN, BuMed Public Relation Division, dated 28 January 1949, "Subj: Navy Nurse Corps, Statistics of, World War I and World War II," reproduced at National Archives, from Navy Nurse Corps Historical Documents, Box #2, National Archives, Washington, D.C..

260	"For All Hands," *The Anodyne*, 22 October 1945, page 1, op. cit..

261	Navy Department, "Change In Navy Nurse Corps Regulations," *Immediate Release Press And Radio*, 10 January 1945, copy reproduced and provided by the Naval Historical Center, Washington Navy Yard, Washington, D.C., Navy Nurse Corps documents Box 13, #34, Marriage Policies (1942-1945).

262	Laird, et al, op. cit., p. 32.

263	"Wedding Performed," *The Hypo-Herald*, 3 August 1945, Volume II, No. 31, pages one and two. The Hypo-Herald was "published weekly by and for the personnel of United States Naval Base Hospital FIFTEEN." This publication was graciously provided by LCdr Hazel V. Bennett Navy Nurse Corps.

264	Laird, et al, op. cit., p. 35.

265	Bureau of Medicine and Surgery, "News Of The Nurse Corps, U.S. Navy: Release Of All Married Nurse Corps Officers," *Memorandum To The Editor*, 17 October 1945, from Navy Nurse Corps Historical Documents, Box #11, personnel policies, marriage, National Archives, Washington, D.C..

266	Laird, et al, op. cit., p. 31.

267	"The Proposed Draft of Nurses." *The American Journal of Nursing*, Vol. 45, No. 2, February 1945, p. 87.

268	Kernodle, Portia B., *The Red Cross In Action*, Harper and Brothers, New York, 1949, p. 446.

269	Ibid., p. 447.

270	"Paradox," *Survey*, February 1945, p. 50.

271	Hine, Darlene Clark, *BLACK WOMEN IN WHITE*, Indiana University Press, Bloomington and Indianapolis, 1989, p. 181.

272	Laird, et al, op. cit., p. 32.

273	"News of the Month," *R.N., A Journal for Nurses*, Nightingale Press, Inc., Rutherford, N.J., February 1945, p. 51.

274	Laird, et al, op. cit., p. 33.

275	McIntire, Ross T. Vice Admiral (MC) USN, Navy Surgeon General, Copy of a letter to the Judge Advocate General of the Navy, dated 25 August 1945.

276	Ibid..

277	Laird, et al, op. cit., p. 34.

278	Ibid., p. 35.

279	Goble, CDR Dorothy Jones, NC USN (Ret.), unpublished history research notes.

280	Laird, et al, op. cit., p. 37.

281	Information obtained from the file cards of Miss Hogue's and Miss Hudson's assignments, Bureau of Medicine and Surgery, Navy Department, Washington, D.C..

282	Dauser, Sue Captain NC USN, Copy of Letter to Finance Division, dated 9 October 1945, Subj: Program for Cadet Nurses, reproduced at National Archives, from Navy Nurse Corps Historical Documents, #37 Education and History and Cadet Nurse Policies, National Archives, Washington, D.C..

283	McIntire, Ross T. Vice Admiral MC USN, Copy of Letter to Surgeon General, U.S. Public Health Service, dated 21 November 1945, reproduced at National Archives, from Navy Nurse Corps Historical Documents, #37 Education and History and Cadet Nurse Policies, National Archives, Washington, D.C..

284	DeWitt, Nellie Jane Captain NC USN, Copy of Letter to Finance Division dated 24 February 1947.

285	Laird, et al, op. cit., p. 36.

286	"Nurses of the Navy," *Military Nurse*, Military Nurse Publishing Co., 230 W. 41st, New York 18, New York, circa. 1945.

287	Goodnow, Minnie R.N., *Nursing History*, W.B. Saunders Company, Philadelphia, London, 1948, p. 182.

288	Ibid., p. 270.

289	Ibid., p. 273.

290	Ibid., footnote 25, p. 200.

291 Roberts, Mary M. R.N., *AMERICAN NURSING*, The Macmillan Company, New York, 1963, p. 366.

292 Roberts, Mary M., R.N., *American Nursing History and Interpretation*, The MacMillan Company, New York, 1963, p. 666.

293 Jamieson, Elizabeth M., B.A., R.N., Sewall, Mary F., B.S., R.N., *Trends In Nursing History*, W.B. Saunders Company, Philadelphia, 1949, p. 540.

294 Roberts, Mary M., R.N., op. cit., p. 469.

295 Chow, Rita K., R.N. Ed.D., Nelson, LTC Ethel A., USAF, NC, Hope, Gloria S., R.N., Ph.D., Sokoloski, LTC James L., ANC, Wilson, CAPT Ruth A., NC, USN, Ret., "Historical Perspectives of the United States Air Force, Army, Navy, Public Health Service, and Veterans Administration Nursing Services," *Military Medicine*, Vol. 143, No. 7, July 1978, p. 457.

296 Jackson, Captain W. Leona Jackson Director of the Navy Nurse Corps, "We've Reached The Golden Year," *The American Journal of Nursing*, Vol. 58, No. 5, May 1958, p. 672.

297 Laird, et al, op. cit., p. 37.

298 Moeller, Ruth Captain Navy Medical Service Corps, *Oral History Interview Tape Transcript*, Interviewer Doris M. Sterner Captain Navy Nurse Corps, 17 October 1988.

299 Ibid..

300 Ibid..

301 Ibid..

302 Ferguson, Edith Colton, LCdr Navy Nurse Corps, *Written History Material*, written 23 July 1991, pp. 7, 8.

303 Laird, et al, ibid..

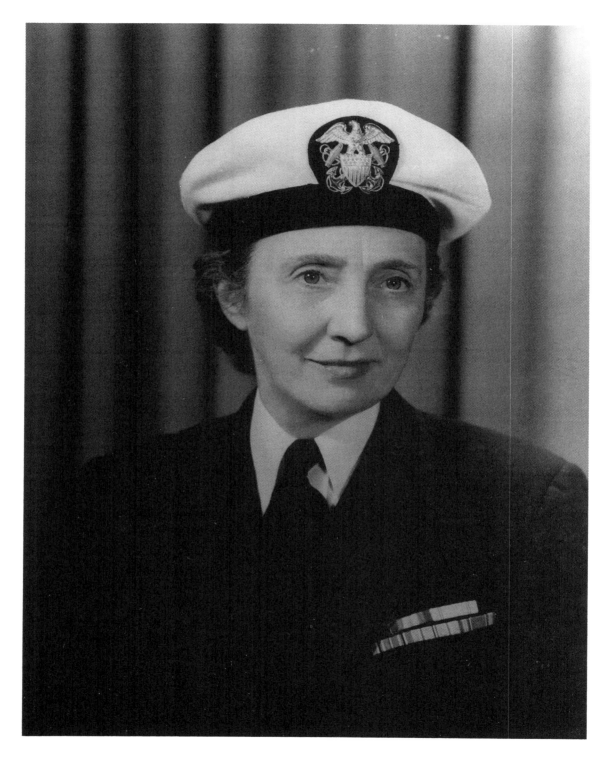

Superintendent/Director - Captain Nellie Jane DeWitt NC USN
(Official U.S. Navy photo courtesy of Nursing Division, Bureau of Medicine and Surgery, Navy Department.)

CHAPTER 7

Superintendent/Director - Captain Nellie Jane DeWitt
(1946 - 1950)

☆☆☆

On 1 April, 1946, Commander Nellie Jane DeWitt is promoted to Captain and is officially installed as the Superintendent of the U.S. Navy Nurse Corps. She had reported to the Nurse Corps Office at the Bureau of Medicine and Surgery on 10 October of 1945 in order to prepare for the position as Captain Dauser's successor.

Nellie Jane DeWitt was born in Susquehanna, Pennsylvania on July 16, 1895. (Susquehanna is a small town in the Northeastern section of the state, close to the New York state line.) She attended Susquehanna High School which was "located close to her family farm home in Jackson, Pennsylvania."[1] Miss DeWitt "became a student nurse at the Stamford Hospital School of Nursing at Stamford, Connecticut from which she graduated in 1917."[2] The next year she volunteered for the Navy Nurse Corps and entered on the 26th of October 1918. Her first duty station was the Naval Hospital at Charleston, South Carolina. In 1919 Navy Nurse DeWitt had T.A.D. orders aboard the transport ship *Martha Washington.* The ship "was engaged in taking prisoners and internees back to Europe."[3] In 1922 she transferred from the Reserve to the Regular Navy Nurse Corps and served at many of the Naval Medical facilities such as Newport, Rhode Island; Portsmouth, Virginia; Puget Sound; Washington, DC; Hospital Corps School San Diego, California; Guantanamo Bay, Cuba; to mention only a few. Also, she took three training courses in Dietetics during this time. In 1923 and 1931 she attended Miss Farmer's School of Cookery in Boston and in 1934 she went to George Washington University in Washington, DC. In February 1937, when Navy Nurse DeWitt was stationed at the Naval Hospital, Washington, DC, the Commanding Officer there received a letter from the Chief of BuMed. The subject of the correspondence was: "Nellie Jan DeWitt, nurse, U.S.N.; preparation for examination for promotion to Chief Nurse." The letter goes on to state that "

"1. A Board appointed by the Surgeon General to recommend nurses for promotion to the grade of Chief Nurse, has recommended Nellie Jane DeWitt, nurse, U.S. Navy, for promotion.

"2. It is requested that you direct the chief nurse to prepare this nurse for the necessary written examination, which will include the Navy Regulations and the Manual of the Medical Department, appertaining to the Nurse Corps.

"3. Upon receipt of the information that this nurse is prepared, the examination questions will be forwarded."

About a month later the Commanding Officer sent a letter to BuMed stating that Nellie Jane DeWitt had been prepared. One day later BuMed sends another letter stating:

"1. Inclosed in an envelope marked 'Confidential' is a set of questions covering the examination required in the case of Nellie Jane DeWitt, nurse, U.S.N., who has been selected for promotion to the grade of Chief Nurse.

"2. The questions shall be detached in rotation and shall be affixed to the paper on which the answer is to be written.

"3. The Bureau directs that these questions shall be safeguarded and the usual precautions required in examinations shall be observed. Upon completion of the entire paper, the questions with the attached answers shall be forwarded without marking to the Bureau of Medicine and Surgery, under cover marked 'Confidential'.

"4. It is requested that a physical fitness report be forwarded with this examination."

In April 1937, Miss DeWitt was notified that she had passed the test and was promoted to the grade of Chief Nurse. (This was the procedure for promotion at the time.) Then, in 1945, Commander DeWitt was Chief Nurse at the Naval Hospital, Aiea Heights, Territory of Hawaii when she was ordered back to BuMed in preparation for being the next Superintendent.

In April, 1946 Captain DeWitt takes over responsibility for a decreasing Navy Nurse Corps. Now that the war is over, demobilization is drastically reducing the ranks of the Corps. In May the strength of the Nurse Corps is about 7,500 and will go much lower. In May, Secretary of the Navy, James Forrestal, congratulates the Navy Nurse Corps on its 38th anniversary and states that, "More than 97 percent of the Navy's wounded survived [WWII], and a 'substantial share' of the credit is due the Navy Nurse Corps."[4] Further, "Mr. Forrestal said in a statement: 'Throughout the war, at advanced bases, afloat and in the air, as well as at home, Navy nurses carried on their vital work with patience, devotion, fortitude and skill in the best traditions of their profession and of the Navy.'"[5]

In June legislation is passed increasing "base pay for all ranks and grades on a percentage basis. Base pay for Ensign [increases] from $150.00 to $180.00 per month."[6] And, in July of 1946, "16 ONOP's [Office of Naval Officer Procurement billets; recruitment] open to Nurse Corps procurement."[7] On 20 September, "President Truman grants permission for women serving with the Army and Navy, to wear civilian clothing when off duty."[8] Also, in this year, the "Naval School of Air Evacuation of casualties for flight nurses is discontinued."[9]

In July, 1946, "About 42,000 servicemen and scientists were gathered at the Pacific islands cluster of Bikini Atoll for Operation Crossroads and the first postwar atom bomb tests."[10] Navy Nurse Frances V. Buchanan tells us that she had been six months at the Naval Hospital at Aiea Heights in Hawaii when she received "orders to the USN Base Hospital 21 . . . which was on the Island of Kwajalein in the Marshall Islands, to participate in Operation Crossroads for the testing of the atom bomb on the island of Bikini in the Marshall Islands [on] July 1, 1946. On this date, the island of Kwajalein was evacuated of natives and unnecessary personnel, just in case there would be an accident when the plane took off from Kwajalein to Bikini. . . . We had no special training for the duty, and since we did not fully realize the total danger of the bomb, we were not concerned, but did have fear of the unknown. We breathed a sigh of relief when all went well after the bomb was dropped on Bikini. . . . There were nine Navy nurses . . . on Kwajalein during the height of the preparation and the aftermath of the dropping of the bomb. During my last two or three months on the island, only two of us were left for a 24 hour on-call duty. My duties during the entire time consisted mainly of supervising the Central Supply Department and the Operating Room. In addition to the nurses, there was a large number of American Red Cross female personnel there who mainly staffed the American Red Cross Canteen and service units at the air terminal, especially when evacuation flights came in at the terminal. Morale on the island of Kwajalein was good but, heat and humidity consumed us at times. Therefore, on weekends, we were sent to a Hospital Ship . . . for rest and recreation and especially to enjoy the air conditioning. On the island we made our own recreation when we had time. I was asked if I was exposed to radiation and I do not believe I was . . . because, so far [1990], I have been healthy in that respect. I have contacted the Defense Nuclear Agency for atomic readings . . . in atmospheric nuclear testing from 1945 to 1962. To my knowledge, no one became ill at the time of the bombing, that I can recall. Now, when I look back and know more about the effects of the bomb, it is a bit scary to have lived through the duty . . . on Kwajalein."[11]

Back in February, 1946, Nurse Corps Officer Pauline W. Schmid flies "to Yokosuka, Japan to report for duty aboard the hospital ship USS *Bountiful*. Shortly thereafter we had orders to return to the States. We had a minimum of patients, none seriously ill or injured. Since I knew how to operate a sewing machine, I was assigned to the Linen Room to mend pajamas, sheets, etc.. When the ship rolled it was difficult to stay at the machine. . . We returned to California for supplies, then sailed for Bikini atoll in June 1946. The ship was anchored off shore. We were permitted to go ashore and roam the beaches searching for interesting shells and cats' eyes. We met officers from the other ships and had picnic lunches. Five of us were invited for lunch aboard the Admiral's Flag ship. After lunch, each of us had a helicopter ride over the entire area. 1 July, 1946 the first atomic bomb was dropped in the area from a plane. The previous day we had sailed out to sea. That morning we gathered on the open deck, backs to the drop area, head bowed, eyes closed tightly and covered by an arm. Even so, we could see a brilliant flash. When given the signal, we could look and we saw the tremendous mushroom shaped explosion rising higher and higher in the sky. That evening our ship returned to the anchor spot amid many ships that had been bombed. It was an unforgettable sight watching damaged ships sinking nearby. There were two hospital ships at Bikini. We had very few patients, none as a result of the bomb. When a second underwater test was done,

24 July 1946, we stayed close and could watch it. It caused a huge wave several stories high, but we were far enough away not to be affected. Since our ship was not air conditioned, we endured very hot weather. We wore the gray searsucker uniforms, usually two or three a day, washing them out, hanging on the open deck. They dried in minutes. Shortly thereafter we returned to the States where the ship was decommissioned."[12]

One of the other hospital ships, the USS *Repose*, is at Shanghai, China. She is attached to one of the Service Squadrons of the Seventh Fleet. In October she sails for the U.S. where she undergoes repairs. Meantime, the hospital ship, USS *Relief*, is decommissioned.

An American Journal of Nursing article of 1946, states that, "the Navy maintains several pools of nurses at various East and West Coast hospitals for assignment to transport duty during this period of transfer of military personnel and families back and forth. Describing one such trip on the `Lurline,' Lieutenant Frances A. Nelson (NC) USN, writes:

'Our Navy medical unit consisted [of] three doctors, a dentist, ten nurses, and thirteen corpsmen. Our sick bay was a large wardroom containing approximately one hundred and fifty double bunks and two small rooms, one at either end, which served as quiet or isolation rooms, as the situation demanded. Adjoining smaller rooms served as treatment rooms, laboratory, pharmacy, x-ray department, and galley. The dental department and operating room were located on lower decks. We also had a formula room where baby food and formulae were made up daily.

'We nurses worked shifts corresponding to those in our naval hospitals, but we rotated more frequently. 'As we sailed from San Francisco, we carried approximately five hundred passengers—an assortment of Army and Navy personnel and dependents, as well as several paying passengers. We encountered the usual run of patients who were seasick, along with colds and minor ailments, and the third day out we delivered a full term baby in the operating room. . . .

'At Honolulu we disembarked several passengers and took on many others, sailing for Pago Pago, Samoa. Soon after starting we admitted a woman to sick bay suffering from a cerebral hemorrhage. She became comatose almost immediately and expired in six hours, necessitating burial at sea, since the ship had no embalming facilities. The Navy chaplain conducted a very simple and beautiful funeral service.

'On arrival at Samoa, we were entranced with the tropical beauty of the small harbor and surrounding islands. A few of us had an opportunity to visit the Samoan Hospital located in Pago Pago, where we met some of our Navy nurses stationed there. At our next stop, Suva in the Fiji Islands, we were able to visit the shops and a native village. . . . Among the passengers who came aboard at this point, swelling our broad assortment of nationalities, were one hundred and fifty Indians who were to go with us to Auckland, New Zealand, where they were to get further transportation to their native land. Of this group of Indians it was necessary to hospitalize only one woman who was seven months pregnant and suffering from seasickness and acute cystitis. . . .

'At Auckland we took aboard three hundred war brides and children. . . . Colds, otitis media, and gastric upsets were the only difficulties which the children had on the way to Sydney. At that port we discharged all of our passengers and most of our patients, the only passengers remaining being the three hundred New Zealand brides, who were on their way to the United States. When we left Sydney we carried five hundred additional Australian brides, and their children, thus making a full load of over eight hundred passengers. . . . 'Our ship had no sooner left Sydney, however, than we hit a storm, resulting in a very rough sea. Practically everyone aboard became ill, and sick bay was a bedlam, day and night, for forty-eight hours. With the combined efforts of three Red Cross workers, and a few able-bodied passengers . . . we eventually were able to get things under control. . . . 'We reached San Francisco again on a Sunday, passing under the familiar Golden Gate Bridge in the morning hours.'"[13]

A Navy nurse stationed in California tells us that "Eight months after the war ended I volunteered for TAD (temporary additional duty) and left Long Beach on the USS *Charles Carrol*, a transport ship that was taking the first State Department personnel back to China. A doctor from the hospital also went. We sailed straight to Shanghai, and after discharging the passengers, spent five days anchored out so we had to go ashore in launches. This was a great experience for me. We did alot of sight-seeing and enjoyed the rickshaw rides. Next we sailed to [another port in China] where we picked up airplane parts for Hawaii. There the Marine General invited Dr. . . . and me to lunch. From [there] we sailed north to [another Chinese port} in the China Sea where we took almost 2,000 Marines for transport back to the States. I was the only female aboard. The Marines spent their days lying out on the deck playing records, occasionally dedicating one to the nurse aboard. Main deck and below were off limits to me, so I would go into one of the gun tubs and take a sun bath. On the return voyage we had one appendectomy, and in those days a patient spent up to a week in bed post-op, so each morning I would go to sick bay and give him a bath, just to have something to do. This entire trip took seven weeks and I enjoyed it very much. I finally got to go to sea, and the experience of seeing the Orient was fascinating."[14]

Even during peacetime, overseas duty can always be exciting and different. For instance, Navy Nurse Rita Rein is stationed on Guam which she says "was an interesting place. We soon learned to cope with the heat. There was always a lovely breeze in the late afternoon [and] the pretty sunrises and the colorful sunsets. . . . Guam gave me a surprise all-day ride in a PBY [plane that lands and takes off on water.] This is the story of how it happened. One morning my Chief Nurse called me to the office along with the operating room nurse and informed us that on Yap [island in the Marianas Islands southwest of Guam] they had some emergency surgery to do on a military wife who was not able to be flown up to Guam because of her illness. Two doctors, two corpsmen and a foot locker of all our supplies, along with the operating room nurse and myself, flew about six or seven hours in a PBY. It is most exciting to take off from the ocean and also to land in the water. We arrived in the evening on the island of Yap. The doctors checked the patient and the rest of us set up the operating room. Because of the heat, the operating room consisted of screening on the four sides and also across the top. Lights were available. We prepared the patient for surgery, took care of her problem and, very sleepily, crawled into bed in the early hours of the morning. The doctors stayed on the island of Yap several days in order to check the patient's health — the doctor who was assigned there [at Yap] was not a surgeon. The operating room nurse and myself, as anesthetist, had most of the time to ourselves, and the other people there [on the island] were very generous and gave us a tour of the island which had been occupied by the Japanese. There [were] still craters and much damage because of the fighting there. Needless to say, we were glad to get back to Guam."[15]

Navy nurses quickly learn to adapt to many different types of duty and circumstances that are seldom encountered in civilian nursing. One such situation is with the patient who has recently returned from the battlefield. Navy Nurse Lillian Schoonover describes the process as it affected her nursing care of Orthopedic patients, "One of the initial safety lessons to learn was a personal safety lesson. It quickly became apparent that to young servicemen with orthopedic wounds, anyone and everyone waking them from sound sleep should expect to be perceived as E-N-E-M-Y! Nurses [and corpsmen] neither took long learning [patients'] names nor how to call them awake. We began several beds away to speak their names. Depending on the time it took for the name to register on [their] consciousness, the nurse [carefully] approached the bed to do [nursing] care. They seemed to come up [awaken] fighting, nine out of ten times — having to learn all over again that they were 'home' to be cared for, not fighting to survive. We dreaded these episodes for they often injured themselves further, or even hurt one of us, during these terror-filled moments between the reality of things that had been and things as they were in the present."[16]

"If the story of Navy Nurse Sara Griffin, has not been told, I think it should be. She had a leg injury in Europe resulting in leg-loss, prosthesis, and duty on [the] West Coast in Orthopedic Rehabilitation (mid-forties or bit later, it now seems to me.) One day she had a young Marine with leg prosthesis learning to walk again between the stroll-bars. He lagged. She nagged. In angry frustration he screamed, `What-the-hell-would-you-know-about-how-I-feel?' She motivated him to finish his work-out, then [allowed him to] rest before returning to his ward. As he rested, she lifted her skirt so he could see her artificial leg and she said quietly, `This is how much I know about how you feel.'"[17]

Navy Nurse Betty A. Nimits tells us that one day in 1946 she received dispatch orders to a Navy Medical facility at Dublin, Georgia. "They said they were critically short of nurses. We got to Dublin, three or four of us who went from Charleston, and the place was filled with veteran patients; probably about 400 patients, about 50 of them were active duty military.

"My first exposure to segregation occurred there. They had a little of it in Charleston; all of our black patients were at one end of the ward. In Dublin, they were all in the same ward regardless of what their condition was, no matter what their problem was; psychiatric patient, a wound or rheumatic fever or whatever, they were all in the same ward. Periodically, they [other personnel] would make rounds in the ward and have a shake-down [search.] They came up with enough equipment [that] they could have taken on the whole hospital with all the knives and guns and hatchets and things that they had acquired. It was a very awakening situation for someone who came from northern Illinois where we went to school with blacks and never thought about Jim Crowe — read about it, but never thought about it.

"Dublin was interesting in that we saw the Klu Klux Klan in operation. We had a young Black veteran who happened to be a property owner, which was unusual at that time in that part of the south. He'd been injured in a hunting accident. He had been brought in to a civilian hospital where they were ignoring him. He developed gangrene and he was immediately dispatched over to our hospital where they had to amputate a leg. Because of all the furor that arose because of the poor treatment he had, the Klu Klux Klan got into the act. We went over and saw the burning cross and the white sheeted men and the whole thing.

"I dated a character from town for a while, a very nice young man. (His grandmother thought that I probably had to do with Al Capone because I came from Illinois near Chicago.) He gave me some moonshine. A bunch of us were sitting around [the nurses' quarters] one night . . . (I happened to live right over the chief nurse's quarters) and we wondered if this stuff [the moonshine] would explode. So we put it in one ot the Navy saucers and it exploded all right. That saucer shattered probably into nine million pieces; all little bits of fire burning all over my room. But, the noise was enought to wake Miss Orr [chief nurse] right up out of a sound sleep. Nobody got burnt or hurt, but it was a very rude awakening for her and she never got over it. (Some years later when I ran into her she said, `I remember you. You tried to blow up the nurses' quarters!'"[18]

As for world events in 1946, it is the beginning of the "vanishing of Empires. Old-style imperialism [of Britain, France and Holland] was [ending], and [eventually] in Asia and Africa independent powers replaced colonies and dependencies (except, of course, where Communism ruled)."[19] But in Great Britain, the British Parliament finds itself "with a mandate not so much for the ending of the Empire as for the establishment of a Socialist community in which the massive unemployment and the wretched poverty of the inter-war period should be unknown. They [find] themselves in charge of a nation whose financial condition [is] such that it [looks] as if grinding [poverty will] be the lot of everyone."[20] The U.S. had discontinued Lend-Lease with the end of the war so Britain no longer had that financial support. But, the U.S. comes to their aid when Congress approves a three billion seven hundred fifty million dollar loan for Great Britain.[21]

In 1947, the United Nations (born in 1945) holds its first sessions in London, England and begins the job of organizing itself to deal with world problems.[22] Even at the beginning, the Russians began disruptive protests and actions; "kidnapping by a trick sixteen Polish leaders, which resulted in there being no delegation at all from the country in whose defence the Second World War had nominally been begun."[23] But the UN does complete the business of giving the Allies its approval for the peace treaties with the Axis countries of Italy, Bulgaria, Hungary, Romania, and Finland. The Treaties are "signed in Paris in 1947. Disagreements between Russia and the West [delays] the peace treaties for Austria, Germany, and Japan."[24]

In the U.S., the Secretary of State and former General of the Army, George Marshall, explains a plan proposing "that the war-damaged nations of Europe join in a program of mutual aid for economic recovery, assisted by grants from the United States. Communist nations rejected the plan, but 16 other countries accepted it."[25] This is how the Marshall Plan comes into being. Also, in 1947, Congress passes the Taft-Hartley Labor Act. This legislation empowers "government to obtain [an] 80-day injunction against any strike endangering national health or safety"[26] and includes other business/union provisions. It is a controversial bill but passes over President Truman's veto. Another important piece of legislation taking effect this year, is the National Security Act. The "War and Navy departments [are] united with a new Department of the Air Force in the

National Military Establishment (NME)."[27] The head of the NME is called the Secretary of Defense and is a member of the President's Cabinet. The first Secretary of Defense is James V. Forrestal.[28] This new Department of the Air Force is "literally born of the Army, having been created lock, stock, and barrel out of the Army Air Force."[29] Another bill passing into law is the Army-Navy Medical Service Corps Act. This brought the Navy's Medical Service Corps into being.

In the field of Nursing, the International Council of Nurses is re-established in London and the American Nurses Association hosts the Congress of the ICN this year in Atlantic City, New Jersey. Also, the ANA begins working with the ICN and its exchange-nurse program.[30] Meantime, the American Association of Nurse Anesthetists (not associated with other nursing associations) opens its membership for men in 1947. "This is one of the many fields in which there is an urgent demand for more nurses and in which men are very acceptable. Twenty-six of the 88 schools recognized by the AANA accept men. One school for nurse anesthetists is directed by a man nurse."[31] The African-American nurses are progressing slowly since there "are now sixty-six schools taking Negro students, half of them `mixed' schools, accepting both white and Negro. . . . Two Negro nurses are on the board of the N.O.P.H.N. [National Organization for Public Health Nursing], and there are 1100 doing public health nursing."[32]

On the 16th of April 1947, Public Law 36 is passed by Congress. Title II, Sec. 201 of this law states, "A Nurse Corps, which shall be a component part of the Medical Department of the Navy, is hereby created and established as a Staff Corps of the United States Navy. The Navy Nurse Corps shall consist of officers commissioned in the grade of nurse by the President, by and with the advice and consent of the Senate, and such officers shall have the rank of commander, lieutenant commander, lieutenant, lieutenant (junior grade), or ensign: *Provided*, That the total number of officers in the permanent rank of commander and lieutenant commander shall not exceed seven-tenths per centum and one and six-tenths per centum, respectively, of the total number of officers permanently commissioned in the Navy Nurse Corps and serving on active duty. The total authorized number of officers of the Nurse Corps shall be six for each thousand of the authorized number of officers, midshipmen, and enlisted personnel of the active list of the Regular Navy and Regular Marine Corps.

"Sec. 202. There shall be a Director of the Nurse Corps appointed by the Secretary of the Navy, upon the recommendation of the Surgeon General of the Navy, from among the officers of the active list of the Nurse Corps of the permanent grade or rank of lieutenant commander or above for a term of not more than four years, to serve at the pleasure of the Secretary of the Navy. While so serving the Director shall have the rank of captain, shall be entitled to the pay and allowances as are now or may be hereafter prescribed by law for a captain of the Navy, and her regular status as a commissioned officer of the Nurse Corps shall not be disturbed by reason of such appointment."[33] On 13 May 1947 Secretary James Forrestal appoints "Captain Nellie Jane DeWitt, Nurse Corps, USN, as the first Director of the new Navy Nurse Corps. . . . The appointment was made in a directive handed Captain DeWitt by Secretary Forrestal at a ceremony attended by Fleet Admiral Chester Nimitz, Chief of Naval Operations, and Rear Admiral Clifford A. Swanson, Surgeon General, as well as other high ranking officers of the Navy Medical and Nurse Corps. . . . The ceremony highlighted the thirty-ninth anniversary of the founding of the Navy Nurse Corps."[34] What a Nurse Corps' birthday this is. This new law finally authorizes permanent commissioned officer rank for the nurses and it also allows integration of reserve Nurse Corps Officers under 35 into the Regular Navy.[35] Lt. Commander Gladys Dvorak is stationed in Washington, D.C. at BuMed on Director DeWitt's staff at this time and tells us that she was able to go to the Congressional Hearings on this legislation and found it very interesting. She says "I felt very fortunate to have been assigned to the Bureau because I found out how I could get all of these laws that pertained to the Nurse Corps. . . . I believe the last that I had was a law that was sent to me by [Senator] Scoop Jackson, along with a cover letter. . . . At that time we [had] . . . one Captain, four Commanders and I don't remember how many Lieutenant Commanders. Not very many. I was one of the very fortunate because I was Lieutenant Commander. Another very emotional thing, because there were nurses in the service many years my senior that were not selected [for promotion to Lt. Commander]. I was proud to have been selected, but I felt these other people . . . my heart ached because they had spent years in the service."[36]

Flight Nurse Dymphna Van Gorp states that the "occasion of greatest importance to the history of the

Navy Nurse Corps [occurring] during my time in the Navy, was, most surely, the granting of permanent rank. I was [stationed] in Rio de Janiero at the time and didn't know about it . . . until that evening. Among our patients was a man from the U.S.S. *Memphis* and the medical officer aboard [the ship] visited the hospital and invited me to dinner on the cruiser that evening. He was Dr. . . . who had been physician for students when I was at Marquette University. After dinner and a movie on deck in pouring rain, several of his fellow officers watched as he handed me my [uniform] hat. My little anchor [insignia] was gone and in its place the doctor had fastened his own big eagle insignia. I received congratulations from all."[37]

Navy nurses are now Navy Officers. The Navy Nurse Corps has become a Staff Corps within the Bureau of Medicine and Surgery just as are the Dental Corps, Medical Corps and Medical Service Corps. This designation means a new insignia for the Nurse Corps. "The spread oak leaf is the basic device used by all corps under the control of the Bureau of Medicine and Surgery, and is like the device prescribed for medical officers in 1883. . . . A leaf with no acorn is used for the Nurse Corps."[38] (The Medical Corps has an insignia of an oak leaf with an acorn. The Dental Corps has one of an oak leaf with two hanging acorns. The Medical Service Corps utilizes an oak leaf with a branch for their insignia.)

It is interesting to note a few sections of the new law, that the legislators evidently considered important enough to include. Sec. 201 says, "Officers of the Navy Nurse Corps shall have authority in medical and sanitary matters and all other work within the line of their professional duties in and about naval hospitals and other activities of the Medical Department of the Navy next after officers of the Medical Corps and the Dental Corps of the Navy. They shall exercise such military authority as may be prescribed from time to time by the Secretary of the Navy: *Provided*, That they shall not be eligible for the exercise of command. . . . Sec. 206. (e) Boards for selection of Nurse Corps officers for recommendation for advancement to the ranks of commander, lieutenant commander, and lieutenant shall be composed of not less than six nor more than nine officers not below the rank of captain on the active or retired list of the Medical Corps: *Provided*, That in case there is not a sufficient number of officers of the Medical Corps legally or physically qualified to serve on the selection board as herein provided, officers of the line of the active list of the rank of captain may be detailed to duty on such board to constitute the required membership. . . . Sec. 207. (b) Each officer of the Navy Nurse Corps who attains the age of fifty-five years while serving in the rank of commander or lieutenant commander and each officer of such corps who attains the age of fifty years while serving in the rank of lieutenant or below, shall be retired by the President on the first day of the month following that in which she attains such age, and, except as otherwise provided in this section, shall be placed on the retired list in the permanent rank held by her at the time of retirement."

In early July, Captain DeWitt is making an inspection at the Naval Hospital in Philadelphia, Pennsylvania. (She "is on a tour of inspection that includes the First, Third, and Fourth Naval Districts.) The inspection is devoted largely to the checking of housing conditions for nurses, general evaluation of nursing conditions in the Navy, the possible improvements of nursing care for patients, and new ideas that might add to the distinctive efficiency of the Nurse Corps.

"Upon completion of her inspection of USNHP, Capt. DeWitt stated: 'I hope the new Nurse Corps will be able to carry on in the same fine manner and tradition as the pioneers of naval nursing.'"[39]

A Navy Procurement Directive (No. 8-47) comes out this year giving the requirements for entering the Nurse Corps. The main guidelines include:

A native born or naturalized citizen of the U.S. for at least ten years.
A graduate of an approved school of nursing.
A high school graduate with at least 15 units of credit.
A graduate registered nurse in good standing.
Single at time of original appointment.
Must be 21 years old and not reached 29th birthday on 1 July of the year in which appointed.
Reserve nurses must be 21 years old and not reached 40th birthday on 1 July of the year in which appointed.

A 500 word biography must be submitted by each candidate in her own handwriting.

The pay of an Ensign, at this time, is $180 per month which also includes maintenance. Outside of CONUS (continental limits of the U.S.) she receives an additional ten percent of her base pay. For every three years of service, there is a five percent pay increase. Higher rank results in higher pay. Also, there is a death benefit of six month's pay to a dependent relative, medical and dental care plus leave time, with pay, of thirty days per year.

In December of 1947, "many of the Lt. Commanders went back in rank to Lieutenant, because the Nurse Corps was top heavy in rank."[40] This was not only because of the new law but because of the exodus of so many nurses returning to civilian life at the end of the war leaving the Corps top-heavy with Lt. Commanders. This year also sees Navy nurses permitted to move out of nurses' quarters in some places.

The educational programs of the Nurse Corps are in full swing except the courses in Occupational Therapy; they are discontinued. There are ten nurses at Columbia University for courses in Teaching and Ward Administration, twenty nurses at George Washington University for Dietetics, seven nurses at the Pennsylvania Hospital in Philadelphia for a four month course in Psychiatric Nursing, five nurses at the University of Utah School of Medicine for a twelve month course in Anesthesia, three nurses at Baylor University Hospital in Texas for a nine month course in Anesthesia and one nurse for twelve months at University Hospitals of Cleveland also for Anesthesia.[41]

Flight nurse Lt.(jg) Edythe Bogie[42] is stationed at the Naval Hospital Patuxent River, Maryland. "Her duties as a flight nurse require frequent trips to the west coast to transfer patients and she was on such an assignment yesterday [21 January 1947]."[43] The four-engined Navy plane was coming in to land at Oakland Airport "when, for the first time in more that 76,000 landings, radar-ground-control failed to guide a ship to safety.

"The big Naval Air Transport . . . plane landed 150 feet short of the fog-shrouded runway and crashed into a four-foot rock wall at the edge of the field.

"Its undercarriage sheared away and the plane skidded across the field on its fuselage for 1,000 feet, shedding wreckage and passengers as it went. Then it caught fire and burned."[44]

"Lieutenant Bogie, herself suffering from shock, said she had seen to the safety belts of the other passengers and strapped herself in her seat to wait for the landing.

"'It wasn't too long before I realized that the plane was not making a normal approach and the thought struck me that we were going to crash. The impact followed shortly afterwards and no one cried out as the plane skidded down the runway,' she said.

"The plane caught fire at the moment it came to rest, Lieutenant Bogie said, and all uninjured passengers and crew members 'pitched in' to help evacuate the injured from the danger area. . . . After ministering to the injured passengers and crew members, Lieutenant Bogie consented to be taken to the hospital."[45] According to the Oakland Tribune newspaper, "One WAVE was killed but 14 passengers and six crewmen survived."

In April 1947, at Texas City, Texas (about 40 miles southeast of Galveston) a ship loaded with highly combustible fertilizer, explodes in the harbor. The next day, a nearby ship loaded with sulphur and ammonium catches fire. A large chemical plant close by is destroyed as well. 552 people die and 3,000 are injured.[46] Truly a horrifying disaster. "Twenty-two Navy nurses from U.S. Naval Hospitals, Houston and Corpus Christi, and the Naval Station, Orange, Texas, [assist] in the care of casualties."[47]

A former member of the Cadet Nurse Corps, Ruth W. Martin, tells us that she spent her last six months in training not at a Naval Hospital, as she had requested, but at the "McCloskey General Hospital, an Army amputation center in Temple, Texas. [This was at the end of 1945 and the beginning of 1946.] Cadet nurses were granted officers' privileges and responsibilities under the supervision of the Army nurses. I enjoyed military nursing but still felt that the Navy would be more to my liking."[48] After her training and some hospital experience she applies to the Navy and is accepted. "At this time I did not know the difference between the Regular Navy and the Reserves and don't remember being given a choice. Subsequently, my physical exam was done . . . and I was told to await orders. I was sworn in the Regular Navy as an Ensign on August 21, 1947. . . . As new members of the Navy Nurse Corps we were called `indoctrinees' and were required to attend classes and to learn about the military, nursing in the Navy, customs, protocol and so forth. We even had marching practice. We were out fitted with uniforms; dress uniforms as well as ward whites. Our indoctrination officer was [a] Lt. Commander [an older Nurse Corps Officer]. Our patients: they were mostly veterans of WWII, WWI and even some Spanish American War veterans. There were not too many active duty personnel on the wards that I supervised which were mostly the medical wards. Off-duty time was the greatest. As our duty hours were 8AM to 3PM, 3PM to 10PM, and 10PM to 8AM for night duty. We had night duty once a year for a whole month without any nights off. We had plenty of time to go to the beach, we toured Hollywood and Los Angeles, and Catalina Island. We were also invited and expected to attend parties at the Officers' Club on Terminal Island for the officers of visiting ships which were in port. It was thrilling and exciting.

"Our chief nurse was Miss Sue English whom I both admired and was in awe of. Once a week she would take the new nurses in her car to an ice skating rink some distance from the hospital. Being from the South this was an entirely new experience for me. Very few of us had cars in those days.

"Everyone lived in the nurses' quarters, two to a room. The older nurses had private rooms; the rooms were comfortable [with] twin beds, 2 desks, a large closet for each girl and a lavatory. The Bath unit was down the hall and there was one telephone on each hall. We were expected to keep our rooms neat and had a weekly inspection. I believe we had maids who cleaned up our rooms. There was also a little kitchenette where we could make coffee, warm soup, make sandwiches, etc..

"We were served three meals a day cafeteria style in a lovely large dining room which was adjacent to the living room. The meals were excellent. I believe that the cafeteria was staffed with civilians and I think we paid for our meals by the month."[49]

During WWII a young lady named Dolores Cornelius worked as a civil service employee at the Naval Armory in Detroit. "My love of the Navy really started there. Each morning I would go to the sick bay office and type out the binnacle list [sick list]. I got to know the [Navy nurse] assigned there and thought how wonderful it would be to become a Navy nurse. The result was that I entered the Cadet Corps and became a student [nurse] at the Grace Hospital in Detroit."[50] Miss Cornelius finishes training in early 1947 and joins the Navy. She receives orders to report for duty in November. "My orders were for me to report to Bremerton, Washington, a place I had never heard of. My father and I looked it up of the map so I knew it was near Seattle, but I didn't realize until getting there that it was 17 miles from Seattle across Puget Sound.

"I'll never forget the day that my fellow Nurse Corps officer, June Norman and I left Detroit to start the long train journey to Bremerton. My whole family was there at the train station to see me off as was June's family. The railroad station was very crowded. June and I felt very emotional about leaving our families for the unknown in Bremerton. . . . Thus I started my Navy career at the Bremerton Navy Hospital on the third of November 1947 as a regular naval officer. This meant nothing to me at the time, but a few years later, this was changed and nurses who came into the Navy came into the reserve and had to be augmented into the regular Navy.

"At that time, new Nurse Corps officers in the Navy were indoctrinated at whatever hospital they reported to and I believe the course was eight weeks; a part-time indoctrination, perhaps two to four hours a day and then the rest of the day we were oriented on the wards.

"The Ensigns at Bremerton were a close-knit group. I was saving money to buy a car and had put in an order for one at the Oldsmobile dealer in Bremerton. One morning I received a call that the car was there sooner than I had expected. Ensign Doris Cox stopped by my room after lunch and wondered why I was looking so dejected. So I told her about the car and my keen disappointment about not having enough money to pick it up. I had wired home for the remainder of what I needed, but it would take a few days before it arrived. She left my room and within fifteen minutes Doris was back with four hundred dollars. The other Ensigns were willing to loan me until the money came from my family. When we got off duty that day, seven of us went downtown to pick up the new car. Still it just amazes me to think that the Ensigns had that much money available at the time. I'm still in touch with Doris Cox Brown."[51]

Even though the war is over, there are still Navy nurses doing overseas duty. Navy Nurse Pauline Schmid is one of five nurses receiving orders to the First Marine Division Hospital in Tientsin, China. "The hospital had been built and used by the Japanese during their occupation. It was sparse. The only heat was a Coleman stove in the middle of the wards. The winter was bitter cold and we had a lot of pneumonia patients. We were eleven nurses and lived in the former Italian consulate. There were Marine guards at the gate 24 hours a day. We could hear Communist gun fire outside the city limits. We had eleven house servants paid a total of $88 a month salary, plus each received a cupful of white flour. We wore the gray seersucker uniforms with Marine-issued longjohns and sweaters to keep warm. We had a lot of snow and it was cold. We drove our own jeeps to and from the hospital. The Marines enclosed the jeeps for the winter.

"Two nurses were given R&R (rest and recreation) at one time. Ruth Flickinger and I went on R&R in mid-December. We joined a group of Marines on a train trip to Peking for a week. It was bitter cold with strong winds blowing down from the Gobi desert. We were able to stay at the former Rockefeller Hospital run by German Deaconist Nuns and one U.S. Army charge nurse. The nuns were elderly and in the process of repatriation. They were very sad as they had lived in China most of their lives and had no one in Germany. . . . Everyday our rickshaw boys picked us up to take us sightseeing. One day we went through a narrow alley into a small courtyard. A beautifully decorated Christmas tree was in the center. The owner bowed deeply and said, `Welcome to our christian home.' We were most impressed and delighted."[52]

Norma Ellingson Bartleson says, "The highlight of my career was duty in China . . . I was able to live in Shanghai and Tsingtao and visit [Peking] and Hong Kong . . . Another nurse, May Anderson, and I arrived in Shanghai the 5th of April 1947. We were the first and only Navy nurses to serve on duty in Shanghai. We were stationed at the dispensary in a . . . building in Shanghai and lived at what had been the German school. We had heard little about communism until we reached China.

"If a Chinese person was injured in an accident and an American driver was at fault it was our [duty] to take him in and care for him. I remember one who was a University student who had been hit by a jeep operated by an American and I don't think he was very happy with us Americans, as he would give us staring glances. Often, on our way to work via jeep, we would see trucks loaded with bodies that had died during the night from starvation or exposure to bitter cold. We also saw trucks with one, two, three or maybe more persons tied to the back of the truck and taken to a place to be executed. We were told that they had done wrong. Chinese people seem different from Americans and their poverty, though appalling to us, was commonplace to them since they had never know another way of life. Their mere struggle for existence might best be explained by the phrase `survival of the fittest.' In the fall we would see men and women with sacks on their backs picking up twigs and sticks and putting them in the sacks. They mixed mud with the twigs and sticks and built huts for the winter. The huts were small, but eight or ten people, maybe more, would huddle together to keep warm. As colder weather arrived, they added layers of clothing. Then as warmer spring weather arrived they would start removing layer by layer of clothing. Weather in China can be bitterly cold in the winter and very hot in the summer. It's a humid, hot weather and in August it is called 'tiger' heat. We saw many people sleeping on the streets and with a brick as a pillow under the head. Rickshaws were many and the longevity for Rickshaw drivers was about twenty years. Health standards were poor and meats, such as chicken and other perishables, could be seen hanging at the outdoor food stand with flies swarming about. . . . dysentery was very prevalent and when on a trip we always carried 'bismuth and paregoric' in case we needed it for diarrhea. . . . We never ventured out alone at night, not even during daylight hours; it was not safe. Your purse, watch or so forth could be plucked off in a hurry."[53]

Also in the far east, is the Hospital Ship *Repose*. Navy Nurse Margaret Scott is aboard the ship as it travels to the northern part of China to take care of military dependents up there at the harbor in Tsingtao [northeastern China.] While there the ship "was sent to Japan for dry docking and half the staff went with the ship. The rest of us remained behind to tend to the needs of the families."[54] She says they set up at a local Chinese hospital where they tend to the Dependents' needs. She notes that all lights and water are turned off at midnight in the hospital so they have to do deliveries by [flash] light. They even had to do a Cesarean Section but all went well and the *Repose* returned shortly thereafter.[55]

In 1948, Norma Ellingson reports aboard the USS *Repose* in China and she notes that "the ship could handle about seven hundred patients. I had had training in dietetics and served as dietician as well as ward [nurse] on the ship. There were many babies delivered aboard the ship and we all took our turn on night calls. While in the harbor of Tsingtao, a Chinese ammunition dump exploded leveling a city block and killing two hundred and injuring eight hundred Chinese. It occurred within half a mile of the docks where the USS *Estes*, flagship of the American Western Pacific Fleet, and the Hospital Ship *Repose* were tied up. The resulting fires left a mass of black ruins in a wide sector. The *Repose* and all of the US Navy medical facilities afloat and ashore immediately gave assistance. The fire raged for several hours. The *Repose*'s staff swiftly went about the job of rescuing Chinese from falling buildings and giving first aid. We found our wards, decks and every available space filled with Chinese wounded."[56] "Everybody looked alike in quilted, padded, faded blue jackets and pants. Until we could get the clothing removed by cutting, we didn't know whether we had a man or a woman. They were with us for two days and the ship smelled of garlic from top to bottom."[57] "During this time a great number of the hospital staff contracted amebic dysentery. We had worked long hours, we were very tired and none of us were feeling up to par."[58]

(On yet another day in 1949, orders come in to the *Repose* for immediate sailing to an unknown destination. They sail south to the mouth of the Yangtze River outside of Shanghai. Up the river at Nanking, some British ships had been fired upon and there were casualties. "The casualties were brought out to us and we cared for them on the ship. We were there for about three days. I remember a British Captain coming in. He had a large bolt in his hip and he had stayed behind in Shanghai to bury the British sailors that were lost, and then we did surgery on him on the ship [the *Repose*]. . . . [then we] took the casualties down to Hong Kong to the Hong Kong British Colonial Hospital."[59] After a few days, the Repose returns to northern China. They rendezvous with a group of ships there then leave with only the embassy people remaining behind.[60] "The Communists overran this territory [in China] early in 1949 and Americans were not allowed in China for twenty-five or more years."[61])

"Between World War I and World War II the Navy operated two transports, the USS *Henderson* and the USS *Chaumont,*for the purpose of carrying the families of naval personnel to make homes on foreign shores and overseas stations. . . . Now [1948], the Navy operates nine transports in the Pacific - to China, Japan, the Philippines, Guam, Hawaii, etcetera, and one in the Atlantic to Caribbean ports. These transports have assigned to them, as part of their peacetime complement, Navy nurses, for regular duty.

"The established routes are called by various names, one of the most popular (and appropriate) being `The Diaper Run.' Assigned to the Caribbean run the U.S.S. *President Adams* . . . affectionately known to her crew as `The Blue Goose of the Mickey Mouse Fleet' and `The Galloping Ghost of the Atlantic Coast' acquired the latter appellation as a result of the natural consequence of the fact that the ship seldom stays in port for any considerable length of time. . . .

"At present there are two Navy nurses on board the *President Adams* and their work is arranged to suit the necessities of the day . . . The junior nurse . . . handles the feeding problems of the young passengers, particularly those who are still being bottle fed. The ship has a diet kitchen adjoining the children's nursery. In this kitchen the dependent nurse spends each morning, encompassed by an array of bottles and utensils, conscientiously preparing formulas for the liquid diet babies. . . . [This] normally is a routine procedure until the seas become heavy and turbulent. A peek into the kitchen in the latter circumstances frequently shows a thwarted nurse surrounded by broken glass and overturned pans. Each day on completion of her duties she prays that the rising sun will bring calm seas.

"The senior, or chief nurse, attends the sick. The *President Adams* has a small dependents' sick bay in which there are two bunks for those patients who must be interned. This sick bay is located immediately adjacent to the nurses' quarters where there is an electrical buzzer [connecting the two areas]. . . . Although the chief nurse is present at all sick call hours, both nurses are available and on call at any hour of the day or night when at sea.

"On board [the ship, the nurse] is treated as any other officer to a great extent, but her routine varies. She stands personnel inspection on Saturday morning and stands by the spaces for which she is responsible during below decks material inspections. . . . Her emergency station is the dependents' sick bay at all general drills except Abandon Ship. During the latter drill the nurses muster with the passengers at their assigned boats in order to assist as necessary. The nurses are also mustering officers for all cabin passengers at Abandon Ship stations. The special sea detail assigned to the nurses when the ship is getting underway is the patrolling and inspecting of passenger spaces for stowaways. Both nurses mess at tables with a group of male officers of the ship and are accepted as fellow officers."[62]

On 1 July 1948, the US Naval School of Nursing, Guam Memorial Hospital, Guam, M.I., publishes a Bulletin about the School. Under 'History' it states that the school is patterned after nursing schools in the U.S., that it is a three year course and that "some nine island areas of the south Pacific area are represented and it is planned that more will be included in the future." Under 'Aim' it says, in part, that the "school is an integral part of an organized plan to train people of the south Pacific islands to care for their own people." The 'Entrance Requirements' are especially interesting, "The School of Nursing requires that applicants must be between the ages of 17 and 35 at the time of enrollment, sound of mind and body and must possess a vocabulary of a minimum of one thousand (1000) English words. . . . If it is found upon reporting that the applicant's knowledge of English and arithmetic is inadequate it is necessary that additional preparation be given prior to the course in nursing and exclusive of the three year period." The bulletin goes on with 'Temperamental And Moral Acceptability,' saying, "The examiner in selecting students, should investigate facts regarding morals, family background and temperament. It should be kept in mind that this applicant is to be educated to do nursing on an island where she will have only the technical and moral supervision of a medical man and she may in some instances have little, if any, close supervision." Then it mentions that the students will receive an monthly stipend of twenty dollars as well as room, board and health care while under instruction.

In 1948 a young nurse joins the Navy after two years experience as an operating room nurse and associate instructor for Yale University's School of Nursing. Her name is Barbara Ellis and she states, "My mother had been a Navy nurse in World War I and her best friend with whom she had joined the Navy, was Nellie Jane DeWitt. All my life I'd known Navy nursing and finally I decided it was for me also."[63] Her mother's name was Pauline Huck Ellis and Barbara Ellis continues, "As I said, she was a Navy nurse during WWI, but she got out of the Navy because she married my dad. He, during WWI, was a sailor aboard the USS *Niagara*. His home port happened to be Charleston, South Carolina and she was stationed there too. So when his ship came in, they went through all sorts of jigs and reels in order to meet one another. One of her admirers was one of the Navy doctors . . . He would take my mother out and then they' meet my father some place and he'd leave them for a little bit. Then he'd meet her to escort her back to the hospital. After the war was over in 1930, he wrote a book called `Anchors Away' and, supposedly, it's the story of my mother and dad's romance.

"While I was growing up, we used to visit Nellie Jane [Director DeWitt 1946-1950] at the various Naval hospitals where she was stationed. When she was stationed in the Brooklyn Naval Hospital, she would come visit us at our summer home in Westbrook, Connecticut and bring various friends with her. By coincidence . . . my good friend that I grew up with, had an aunt who was also a Navy nurse . . . She too was stationed in Brooklyn . . . She built a home down there, too, and various retired Navy nurses would come to visit her. Among them I remember Sue Dauser [Superintendent 1943-1945]."[64]

A New York newspaper dated May 13, 1948 prints an article about the Navy Nurse Corps' 40th birthday celebration at the Naval Hospital on Long Island. The article notes that the birthday party is held in conjunction with a retirement party for the Chief Nurse, Lt. Commander Irene Shelley. The World Telegram Staff Writer writes, "How conditions have changed for Navy nurses since olden times was a main topic of conversation today at the US Naval Hospital, St. Albans, L.I., where the 40th anniversary of the Navy Nurse Corps was celebrated . . . . The celebration also marked the nurses' farewell to Cmdr. Shelley, who, after 22 years in the Navy will retire June 1.

"When Cmdr. Shelley was asked how much her Navy pension would be she was puzzled.

"'I don't know,' she replied. I really don't know. I've been too busy to figure that out.'

"The assistant chief, Lt Cmdr. Sylvia Koller, who will succeed Cmdr. Shelley, figured it out - $204 a month."[65]

1948 is also the year that Nurse Corps' educational opportunities are increased to include attending educational institutions for obtaining BA and BS degrees in Nursing. On 17 December 1948, eight Navy nurses graduate from the first combined course of flight training for Army and Navy nurses at Randolph Air Field, Texas. "Previously, all flight nurses of the Navy trained at NAS, Moffett Field, California."[66]

In April of 1948, the Bureau of Medicine and Surgery, US Navy, puts out a flyer about the US Navy Nurse Corps and Reserve Nurse Corps. (It seems probable that this was used for recruiting purposes.) In this flyer is the following on 'Living Conditions:'

> "1. NURSES QUARTERS: Nurses are furnished quarters and subsistence at most stations. All nurses during their first year in service will be on duty at hospitals which provide such quarters. Most are able to provide single rooms.
>
> 2. BACHELOR OFFICERS QUARTERS: Some of the smaller activities such as dispensaries do not have quarters for nurses. In such instances, the nurses are usually assigned a section of Bachelor Officers Quarters and take their meals in the dining room with other officers of the station.
>
> 3. If Nurses Quarters or Bachelor Officers Quarters are not provided, nurses are permitted to live out of the Naval Activity in quarters of their own choice. In this case, the nurse is paid an allowance for quarters and subsistence."

This same flyer discusses the Navy Nurse Corps Reserve saying, "Reserve nurse may be on active duty in the Navy under the following programs:

> (a) Two weeks annual period of active duty. This is a voluntary program.
>
> (b) Active duty for an indefinite period. These nurses are expected to serve not less than one (1) year. This is a voluntary program.
>
> (c) As their services are required in time of national emergency as declared by the President."

The next section is on uniforms for the Nurse Corps' reserves. "Reserve nurses have the following allowances for purchase and maintenance of uniforms:

> (a) Nurses who report for their first period of two-weeks of active duty are allowed $100.00 with which to purchase the ward uniforms, caps, cape, sweater and insignia.
>
> (b) Nurses reporting for a minimum period of one year active duty are allowed $150.00 in addition to the $100.00 initial allowance. Nurses who report for a year period of active duty must provide themselves with a complete set of uniforms. These are not to be purchased until instructed to do so after reporting to the station for assignment.
>
> (c) Naval Reserve nurses will be allowed $50.00 for each (4) year period for upkeep of uniform equipment."

This monetary uniform allowance was only for nurses in the Navy Reserve, not for nurses in the Regular Navy. Regular Navy nurses received no uniform allowance and, as could be expected, this caused a resentment between the two, in some cases.

In June 1948, the Chief of BuMed, Rear Admiral Swanson, Medical Corps, sends a BuMed Circular letter to Medical Officers in command of US Naval Hospitals. The subject is, "Training Program for members of Nurse Corps, U.S. Naval Reserve, on active duty for a two weeks training period." The letter outlines 3 hours of lectures on traditions, customs, uniforms, administrative structure of the hospital and a tour of the hospital. Then it mentions one hour with the Disbursing Officer for info on pay records. Following that, the letter suggests one week of AM duty for the two-week Reservists, on a busy military ward followed by one week in her specialty or continuance on the ward.

A "new style [of] Service Dress White Uniform [is] authorized for all women officers. [The] style of

WAVES uniform [is] adopted with white braid rank stripes and yellow silk embroidered Corps insignia on [the] sleeves. The Combination hat [replaces the] outdoor flat cap. . . . [Also, a] new style sweater [is] authorized."[67] As for the Dress Blue Uniform the "blue jacket of the WAVES was prescribed for all women, to be worn with gilt buttons, and by nurses without the WAVE insignia. All commissioned officers were to wear sleeve lace of Reserve blue [light blue], with corps devices in the same colored embroidery, except that acorns were to be white. . . . Commissioned women officers were to wear the same cap device as male officers . . . Nurses were to retain their special clothing - indoor duty whites, caps, and capes. A dress of gray and white seersucker, slacks, dungarees, raincoats, overcoats, and an exercise suit . . . were authorized for all women."[68]

Despite its new position in the Navy, the Nurse Corps is not without its problems. Captain DeWitt, Director of the Nurse Corps, notes the most serious problem in her April 1948 official correspondence, "In common with the rest of the nursing profession, our major problem is shortage of personnel. At the time of the last biennial meeting of the ANA, the strength of the Navy Nurse Corps was 2969, with approximately 300 of those nurses being in a terminal leave status. Even at this date it was apparent that demobilization had been too rapid, however, separations continued and by July 1947 the nursing shortage was acute." Captain DeWitt then gives some numbers showing the problem:

"Number of nurses authorized 1947 - - - - - 2775
Average number on duty [in] 1947 - - - - - 2723
Number of nurses authorized 1948 - - - - - 3428
Average number on duty (to 4-1-48) - - - - 1976"

It is not just the Navy Nurse Corps that has a shortage, the entire profession is under pressure for more and more nurses. "Shortage of nurses! In that irritatingly recurrent phrase, which was to be replaced by the more accurate 'increased demand for nursing service,' may be found the motivation for sharp acceleration of processes in both nursing education and nursing services which were already in existence."[69] "A well-attended National Health Assembly (1948) whetted citizen as well as professional interest in health and medical care programs. The assembly and the ten-year health program, subsequently prepared for President Truman by the Federal Social Security Administration, aroused partisanship on the highly controversional [sic] question of compulsory versus voluntary insurance as a method for paying for medical care which was steadily becoming both more scientific and more costly. . . . [This] constituted an important factor in the mounting demand for nursing service."[70]

This is the year (1948) that the ANA's "House of Delegates opened the gates to black membership, appointed a black nurse as assistant executive secretary in its national headquarters, and witnessed the election of . . . [a black nurse] to the board of directors. . . . [The executive secretary] was assigned the task of clearing the credentials of individual black nurses from the intransigent southern states of Georgia, Louisiana, South Carolina, Texas, Virginia, Arkansas, Alabama, and the District of Columbia. The decision to grant individual membership to black nurses barred from these state associations was followed by the adoption of a resolution to establish biracial committees in districts and state associations to implement educational programs and promote development of intergroup relations.

"The American Nurses' Association's individual membership program helped to bridge the way from exclusion to complete membership."[71]

1948 is an election year and President Truman is running against Republican Thomas Dewey. "Few persons beside Harry Truman himself thought that he could win election to a full term as President. Every public opinion poll predicted that Dewey would win a landslide victory."[72] "'DEWEY DEFEATS TRUMAN' bannered an early edition to the *Chicago Daily Tribune* on election night. *Life* carried a picture of the 'next President' - Dewey. Syndicated columnists, anticipating what seemed inevitable, filed election-day stories on the Republican victory."[73] It simply did not happen. They were all wrong. "When all the returns were counted Truman had 2 million more popular votes and 114 more electoral votes than Dewey. The President had pulled off the biggest political upset of American history."[74]

The rest of the world sees the British pull out of Palestine and Israel becomes an independent Jewish state in 1948. And, the world watches as communist Russia takes over Romania and Czechoslovakia. To complicate matters further, Russia then begins the blockade of Berlin, Germany. The US military governor of Germany, General Lucius Clay declares "that the Western powers [will] not be driven out of Berlin `by any action short of war.' The British foreign minister [says] Britain [is] prepared to fight. But rather than risk war by sending in supplies by armed convoy, the United States and Britain [resort] to a massive airlift that, after almost a year, [breaks] the Russian will to continue the blockade."[75] However, the Russians proceed to take over Poland in 1949 and the "United States, Canada, Great Britain, France, and eight other nations signed the North Atlantic Pact. They agreed that an attack on one member would be considered an attack on all. Other countries later joined the North Atlantic Treaty Organization (NATO) and helped group their armed forces to defend western Europe against aggression. General Dwight D. Eisenhower served as the first supreme commander of NATO forces."[76] Meanwhile, the Chinese communists drive the Chinese nationalists, under Chiang Kai-shek, out of China and the nationalists end up on the island of Formosa. Also in 1949, the Dutch are forced out of Indonesia. The world seems to be seething with disorder.

In civilian nursing, the ANA completes its first Inventory of Professional Registered Nurses in 1949. One of the interesting facts discovered is "that only 0.8 of 1 per cent of all active registered professional nurses were men. Only six states . . . had more than 100 men nurses."[77]

Moving onto the military, in 1949 the National Military Establishment (the NME) is changed to the Department of Defense. The Army, Navy and Air Force remain separate entities under the Secretary of Defense. Also, this year, the US Air Force Nurse Corps comes into being with its root "formed by 1,199 nurses who transferred from the Army Nurse Corps."[78] And, the US Congress passes the Career Compensation Act of 1949. "This increased the base pay for an Ensign from $180 to $213.75 per month with a subsistence allowance of $42 per month."[79]

On the 18th and 19th of May 1949, a Chief Nurses Conference is held at the Bureau of Medicine and Surgery in Washington, D.C.. According to a typewritten copy of her remarks, Captain DeWitt addresses the group on two subjects; one, the assignment of nurses and two, fitness reports. On the 'assignment of nurses' she urges the chief nurses to carefully consider the experience and qualifications of both the nurses (military and civilian) and the "sub-professional nursing personnel" (Captain DeWitt's terminology) when making out duty schedules. She notes, "Many of our Navy nurses while well qualified professionally lack experience and need much guidance if they are to develop into the type of nurses we need in our military hospitals." She goes on to say, "So it would seem more than ever before the senior nurse in the Navy must be both supervisor and instructor." Later in her talk she mentions some of the items that have come to her from the General Inspecting Officer, monthly reports and from staff nurses.

"1. Nurses are rotated or changed too frequently.

2. Too few nurses are assigned to P.M. and night duty.

3. The tendency to assign too high a percentage of nurses to Dependent's Units, resulting in great under-staffing of the service wards.

4. The assignment of nurses to other than professional duties—housekeeping, linen-room etc..

5. The lack of consideration given to special training and experience.

6. The lack of time off duty. Navy hours of duty should compare favorable with civilian duty hours.

7. The failure to post changes in the detail of nurses well in advance. For example: Bi-weekly, weekly, or day to day.

8. Failure to assign at least one senior nurse to both P.M. and night duty."

Then Captain DeWitt turns to the subject of 'fitness reports' and she really tells it like it is. "The value of any fitness or efficiency report is determined not so much upon the form used as upon the one who completes the form. . . . It was my privilege to talk to several members of the Selection Board after its adjournment this Spring, and my attention was repeatedly called to the fact that many fitness reports on the nurses are incomplete and that no mention was made of the ability of the nurse in respect to professional or administrative capacity." She goes over the fitness report form in detail then states, "I feel that each nurse should have her completed fitness report shown to her and the adverse comments, if any, called to her attention." (This was a bone of contention for many nurses when they could not see their fitness reports. The feeling being that of "how could you improve if no one told you what was wrong?")

Another speaker at the Conference is one of the Nurse Corps Director's staff members, LT Gladys E. Dvorak NC USN. Miss Dvorak speaks on 'Budget and Retirement' for the edification of the Senior nurses. LT Leona Jackson is Education and Uniform Officer of the Navy Nurse Corps on the Director's staff. She tells about the Nurse Corps' educational and career management program. She notes that "The program had been initiated upon the policy that nurses over 35 would be considered for further education only in unusual circumstances. That rather effectively shut out the more senior nurses. We were training junior nurses who could be only as effective in the Navy nursing situation as the understanding of their seniors permitted, while the more senior nurse was placed in the untenable position of having under her supervision nurses with superior professional preparation. Cut off from further education in the Navy, too old to leave the Navy in order to get additional education and return to Naval service, it was the occasion for considerable bitterness among the more senior group, and understandably so. It seemed that a really effective and satisfactory program needed to begin with the more senior group and work down. Accordingly, in July of 1948 a letter was sent to all lieutenants with more than ten years service, asking each to assess her needs for further training. . . . Most of this 'over 10 years in service' group who requested advanced training are either under instruction at this time or are scheduled to begin within the next year . . . . Along with this group of 'over ten years in service' nurses we are picking up those from the intermediate (six to ten years in service) group. . . . A third group, those who have no preparation beyond the nursing diploma, are entered each year in universities to complete one year of study toward the degree in nursing education. . . . The Nurse Corps educational program is designed primarily for the career nurse in the Navy . . . We are not interested in nurses who come into the Navy to get their education and leave. . . . Public Health Nursing will not in the future be awarded to nurses with ten years or more of service, but to the jg's or the newer lieutenants. Those nurses when due for foreign service will be assigned to our native hospitals and public health services on Guam and Samoa, and in the United States to dispensaries in shipyards and similar places where industrial and public health training is a factor. . . . Anesthesia has a 35 year age limit recommended by the American Association of Nurse Anesthetists. With the irregular hours and frequent 'call' this is a field for the younger nurse. Ensigns and jg's may be given preference in this specialty, provided they have had at least two years of satisfactory experience in general nursing following completion of their training. . . . Flight Nursing, too, will be awarded the more junior nurse. . . . Three per cent of the nurses in the Navy can be kept under instruction."[80]

LT Jackson also speaks to the group about Uniforms and then she hands out copies of clothing items available at the Naval Clothing Depot in Brooklyn, New York. Here are some of the ' Nurses Uniforms' items and their cost:

Uniform, Service Blue	each	$15.00
Uniform, Service White (no buttons)	"	5.00
Raincoat, Wool	"	15.00
Uniform, Indoor, white, long sleeve	"	2.95
Belt, Uniform, white	"	.30
Cap Cover, Outdoor, Blue	"	1.00
Brim Only	"	1.50
Cap, Indoor, White	"	.30
Cap Markings, Ensign	"	1.30
Cap Markings, Lt(jg)	"	2.05
Cap Markings, LT	"	2.50
Cap Markings, LCdr	"	3.25
Cap Markings, CDR	"	3.70

| Device, Pin, Miniature, Nurses' | " | .65 |
| Cape, Navy Nurse | " | 63.00 |

In March of 1949, Captain DeWitt issues a BuMed memorandum to nurses being ordered to Foreign duty. It lists the items of uniform and civilian attire that the nurse should take with her. Under 'Remarks' she says, "You will travel in your Blue Uniform. You <u>must</u> have calling cards. A charge account in a West Coast Department Store will probably be a convenience to you and it is suggested that you open one before you leave. White ward uniforms and white shoes are worn in Honolulu; seersuckers usually are worn in other stations in the Pacific. If you own a car arrangements can be made for shipping and it is a convenience to have one." At the bottom of the memo is a list of duty stations and the "Tentative Plans For Rotation Of Duty In The Pacific."

"Guam 10-12 months	Kwajalein 3-4 months
Guam 6-8 "	USS Repose 7-9 "
Guam 6-8 "	Honolulu 10-12 "
Guam 6-8 "	Japan 7-9 "
Guam 6-8 "	Saipan 7-9 "
Guam 6-8 "	Subic Bay 7-9 "
Guam 6-8 "	Sangley Pt. 7-9 "
Guam 10-12 "	Midway 3-4 " "

In early 1949, a BuMed Circular Letter[81] is sent to all ships and stations that have Nurse Corps officers aboard. It outlines an interim plan for promotion in the Nurse Corps. For promotion to Lieutenant junior grade and Lieutenant it says that the professional examination will be alike but that more will be expected of those taking the exam for Lieutenant. It says the exam will include:

"General principles of nursing.
Medical and surgical nursing.
Practical examination in general nursing procedures.
Ward Administration.
Administration of clinical nursing service.
Counseling and placement of personnel within a ward or department.
U.S. Navy Regulations.
Manual of the Medical Department, U.S. Navy."

The letter then addresses the exam for promotion to Lieutenant Commander:

"All phases of nursing and naval aspects of nursing.
Planning, organization, and administration of nursing service in dispensaries, clinics, and hospitals, ashore and afloat.
Planning nursing service for the establishment of dispensaries, clinics, and hospitals, ashore and afloat.
Counseling and placement of personnel in the nursing service in a medical activity and for medical activities.
U.S. Navy Regulations.
Manual of the Medical Department, U.S. Navy."

For promotion to Commander the letter continues, "Examination for promotion to the grade of commander shall embrace all phases of administration, personnel management, progress and current trends in nursing service, as well as:

U.S. Navy Regulations.
Manual of the Medical Department, U.S. Navy."

In April of 1950, the Director of the Navy Nurse Corps sends an official Memorandum to all officers of the Nurse Corps about forthcoming changes in Uniforms. The memo is dated 24 April 1950 and states, in part, "It is my pleasure to announce that subsequent to the survey initiated [in 1949] . . . the Permanent Naval Uniform Board reviewed the existing regulation (1947) governing uniforms for women officers in Naval service and, taking into account the results of that survey, recommended that the dress blue uniform for women officers be changed in accordance with the preference of the majority. Accordingly, the dress blue uniform for officers of the Nurse Corps and the WAVES will follow the design which has been worn by the WAVES and which by uniform regulations in 1947 was authorized for the nurses, EXCEPT that the color will be DARK BLUE instead of the navy blue [slightly lighter than the dark blue] presently authorized, and that the sleeve stripes and insignia will be of GOLD." This color, dark blue, has an interesting history that goes all the way back to the 1700's. "On a ride through the park one day, the Duchess of Bedford unwittingly established dark blue as the official color of the United States Navy. It was in the year 1746 - predating the independence of America and the founding of its sea service. It all happened when King George II saw the noble lady galloping by in an eye-catching riding habit of blue, faced in white. Taking an immediate liking to the deep blue color, the King prescribed it as the official shade for uniforms of the Royal Navy. As with so many customs and traditions, the United States Navy adopted its official color from the British."[82]

As for Navy nurses out in the field (working outside of the Nursing Section at BuMed in Washington, DC), they continue to do the unusual and continue to call it their ordinary duty. Navy flight nurse, Elizabeth M. Schwartz, tells us that, "In 1949 I was one of two nurses who received orders to Burbank, California for the commissioning ceremony of the Lockheed aircraft, 'The Constitution.' Many celebrities joined us for short flights between the forty cities visited, including Arthur Godfrey, Buddy Rogers, Alan Ladd, Robert Montgomery, [and] Bill Holden. The purpose of this trip was to recruit young men and women for the Navy Flight Program. After the completion of the tour, I returned to Honolulu for more evacuation flights.

"During one 24-hour layover, a request came in for a Hospital Evacuation plane. [The request came] from American Samoa. I asked to go. . . . [On the way to Samoa] we passed over the equator and I was duly sworn in as a `Shellfish' (no initiation aboard the plane, though.) We landed in late afternoon, and I went to the naval hospital to see my patients - two of them. A violent storm at sea had tossed a merchant ship about, causing many injuries. One patient had a broken neck and clavicle, and was in braces with possible spinal cord injury. He needed complete attention with no movement [allowed.] The second had broken ribs with his chest in a body cast and a broken left wrist, also in a cast. My corpsman and myself had constant watch during the seven hour flight. Both arrived in Honolulu in good condition."[83]

Another Navy Nurse, Geraldine Houp, speaks of her duty in Guam in 1949, "we lived in the old Butler huts . . . which were built right after WWII. . . . Shortly after I got to Guam, we had a powerful typhoon. It destroyed much of the island. We didn't have too much damage at the hospital but we had no electricity. All the food that we had in freezers had to be cooked so it wouldn't spoil. . . . Before we went to the hospital, everything in the nurses' quarters was put on shelves because we knew that it might be flooded and I think they [later] said there was about 10 or 12 inches of water that flowed through the quarters. They [the quarters] were a terrible mess by the time we got back [from the hospital] and had to be thoroughly cleaned. At the hospital, none of the buildings had any windows on them, they had screens, and the hospital itself had large porches around the wards. As the wind blew in the rain, you'd have to shove the patients from one side of the room to the other. And, in the midst of that typhoon . . . a marine ammunition depot [across the island] caught fire; in this wind and pouring rain, this terrible fire. . . . But everybody certainly worked together and I think it was experiences like that, plus meeting up with your shipmates at different places, that gives you the feeling, the close camaraderie that you have in the services."[84]

On 1 May 1950, Captain Nellie Jane DeWitt, Director of the Navy Nurse Corps, retires from active duty. (Captain DeWitt returns to her home state of Pennsylvania and an active retirement life. "She established the Hospital Auxiliary at . . . [a local hospital]. She became President of the Susquehanna County Unit of the American Cancer Society. She was health consultant for the Girl Scouts . . . In 1951, she was selected and installed as a Distinguished Daughter of Pennsylvania . . . In 1955, a chapter of the National Business and Professional Women was organized in Susquehanna and assumed as its name 'The Nellie Jane DeWitt Business and Professional Women's Club'. . . . [Then] Captain Nellie Jane returned to Washington . . . [D.C. area, where] she worked in an advisory capacity in the establishment of Vinson Hall, the Marine and Navy Retirement Center at McLean, Virginia. She finally made her residence at Vinson Hall and passed away on March 22, 1978 while living there. Burial was in the Nurses' Section at Arlington [Cemetery] with full military honors."[85]

[1]   DeWitt, Evelyn E., quotation from a three page typewritten summary of the life of Captain DeWitt, 1991. Evelyn DeWitt is an Attorney and the niece of Captain DeWitt.

[2]   Ibid..

[3]   Ibid..

[4]   "Forrestal Lauds Navy Nurses, Says 97% of Wounded Lived," Article by the Associated Press in an unknown newspaper, 12 May 1946. This news item was graciously provided by LCdr Hazel V. Bennett Navy Nurse Corps.

[5]   Ibid..

[6]   History of the Nurse Corps, U.S. Navy, 5727.1 OONCA/np, draft prepared by: Nursing Division, Bureau of Medicine and Surgery, revised 24 April 1991, p. 7. Supplied through the courtesy of Captain Margaret E. Armstrong NC USNR.

[7]   Goble, CDR Dorothy Jones, NC USN (Ret.), as written in her unpublished history research notes with a notation that this item was "found in Capt. DeWitt's report on NNC [Navy Nurse Corps] at Biennial Nursing Convention 1948."

[8]   Goble, CDR Dorothy Jones, NC USN (Ret.), as written in her unpublished history research notes.

[9]   Laird, LCDR Thelma NC USNR, Jones, LCDR Dorothy NC USN, Feeney, LCDR Elizabeth NC USN, Seidl, CDR Elizabeth NC USN (Ret.), Blaska, CDR Burdette NC USN, Chronological History NAVY NURSE CORPS, Prepared by: Nursing Division, Bureau of Medicine and Surgery, 1 August 1962, p. 38.

[10]   Bezdek, Michael, of The Associated Press, "GIs: `Why didn't anyone tell us?' of danger," The Daytona Beach Sunday News-Journal, March 27, 1994.

[11]   Buchanan, Frances V. LCdr Navy Nurse Corps, Oral History Interview Tape Transcript, Interviewer Sally Ann Buchanan, 3 October 1990.

[12]   Schmid, Pauline W. Capt. Navy Nurse Corps, Oral History Interview Tape Transcript, Self-interview, 19 July 1990.

[13]   Stotz, Evelyn T., R.N., "Transport Duty With The Navy," The American Journal of Nursing, Volume 46, July - December 1946.

[14]   McClean, Eveline Kittilson LT Navy Nurse Corps, Oral History Interview Tape Transcript, Self-interview, 4 July 1990.

[15]   Hey, Rita Rein LCdr Navy Nurse Corps, Oral History Interview Tape Transcript, Self-interview, 22 September 1990.

[16]   Schoonover, Lillian B. LCdr Navy Nurse Corps, Typewritten Personal History, 29 April 1991, pp. 2-3.

[17]   Ibid., p. 2.

[18]   Nimits, Betty LCdr Navy Nurse Corps, Oral History Interview Tape Transcript, Self-interview, 25 March 1991.

[19]   Wells, H.G., The Outline of History, Revised and brought up to date by Raymond Postgate, Garden City Books, Garden City, New York, Volume II, 1961 by Doubleday & Company, Inc., p. 944.

[20]   Ibid., p. 945.

[21]   Ibid., p. 942.

[22]   The World Book Encyclopedia, Field Enterprises Educational Corporation, Chicago, Volume 20, 1966 edition, p. 412.

[23]   Wells, H.G., op. cit., p. 941.

[24]   The World Book Encyclopedia, op. cit., p. 412.

[25]   The World Book Encyclopedia, op. cit., Volume 18, p. 383.

[26]   The Columbia-Viking Desk Encyclopedia, by staff of the Columbia Encyclopedia, William Bridgwater, Editor-in-chief, The Viking Press, New York, 1953, p. 969.

[27]   The World Book Encyclopedia, op. cit., Volume 14, p. 32.

[28]   Ibid..

[29]   Holm, Jeanne Major General USAF (Ret), Women In The Military: An Unfinished Revolution, Presidio Press, 31 Pamaron Way, Novato, CA 94947, 1982, p. 122.

[30]   Roberts, Mary M. R.N., AMERICAN NURSING, The Macmillan Company, New York, 1963, p. 667.

[31]   Ibid., p. 323.

[32]   Goodnow, Minnie, R.N., Nursing History, W.B. Saunders Company, Philadelphia, Pennsylvania, 1948, pp. 199-200.

[33]   United States, 80th Congress, Public Law 36, Chapter 38-1st Session, Army-Navy Nurses Act of 1947, April 16, 1947, pp. 1,2.

[34]   Typewritten synopsis of pictorial event appearing on the back of a released "Official Photograph U.S. Navy."

[35]   Laird, LCDR Thelma NC USNR, Jones, LCDR Dorothy NC USN, Feeney, LCDR Elizabeth NC USN, Seidl, CDR Elizabeth NC USN (Ret.), Blaska, CDR Burdette NC USN, Chronological History NAVY NURSE CORPS, Prepared by: Nursing Division, Bureau of Medicine and Surgery, 1 August 1962, p. 38.

[36]   Larson, Gladys Dvorak LCdr Navy Nurse Corps, *Oral History Interview Tape Transcript*, Interviewer LCdr. Margaret (Linn) Larson NC USN (Ret), 29 March 1989.

[37]   Van Gorp, Dymphna Cdr Navy Nurse Corps, *Oral History Interview Tape Transcript*, Self interview, 17 September 1990.

[38]   Tily, James C., *The Uniforms of the United States Navy*, Thomas Yoseloff, Publisher, 8 East 36th Street, New York 16, NY, 1964, p. 233.

[39]   "Capt. Dewitt on Tour Of District NC Staffs," *Sky-Lines*, A commercially printed publication of the U.S. Naval Hospital, Philadelphia, Pennsylvania, Vol. 8, No. 12, 15 July 1947, p. 1.

[40]   Bjornsrud, Barbara E. Dodge LCdr Navy Nurse Corps, *Oral History Interview Tape Transcript*, Interviewer Orin C. Bjornsrud, 28 August 1990.

[41]   Goble, CDR Dorothy Jones, NC USN (Ret.), information from her unpublished history research notes.

[42]   Lt(jg) Bogie eventually resigned her commission to get married. Her married name is Edythe Bogie Bauman.

[43]   "Barnet Nurse Is Heroine Of Navy Plane Crash," *Caledonian Record*, St. Johnsbury, Vermont, 22 January 1947.

[44]   Ibid..

[45]   "No Panic in Plane Wreck," *Oakland Tribune* 21 January 1947, Vol. CXLVI, No. 21, Front Page.

[46]   Floyd, Candace, *America's Great Disasters*, Mallard Press, An imprint of BDD Promotional Books Company, Inc., 666 Fifth Ave., New York, N.Y. 10103, 1990, pp. 93, 94.

[47]   Laird, et al, op.cit., p. 38.

[48]   Deus, Ruth Martin LT Navy Nurse Corps, *Oral History Interview Tape Transcript*, Self interview, 1 February 1990.

[49]   Ibid..

[50]   Cornelius, Dolores Captain Navy Nurse Corps, *Oral History Interview Tape Transcript*, Self interview, 28 December 1989.

[51]   Ibid..

[52]   Schmid, op. cit..

[53]   Bartleson, Norma Ellingson CDR Navy Nurse Corps, *Oral History Interview Tape Transcript*, Interviewer Patty Hoff, 22 August 1990.

[54]   Scott, Margaret E. CDR Navy Nurse Corps, *Oral History Interview Tape Transcript*, Interviewer CDR Marion B. Haire Navy Nurse Corps, 5 June 1990.

[55]   Ibid..

[56]   Bartleson, op. cit..

[57]   Scott, op. cit..

[58]   Bartleson, op. cit..

[59]   Scott, op. cit..

[60]   Ibid..

[61]   Bartleson, op. cit..

[62]   Wisneski, Florence M. Lieutenant NC USN, Chief Nurse USS *President Adams*, "Naval Transportation Service Nurses," *Naval Transportation Service COURIER* October 1948, Vol. 2 No. 10, pp. 2, 3 and pp. 8, 9.

[63]   Ellis, Barbara CDR Navy Nurse Corps, *Oral History Interview Tape Transcript*, Interviewer CDR Claire M. Walsh Navy Nurse Corps, 25 August 1990.

[64]   Ibid..

[65]   MacDougall, Sally, "Navy Salutes Its Corps of Nurses," *New York World-Telegram*, 13 May 1948.

[66]   Goble, CDR Dorothy Jones, op. cit..

[67]   Laird, et al, op.cit., Chronological History of Changes in Uniform Regulations section, p. 3.

[68]   Tily, James C., op.cit., p. 270.

[69]   Roberts, Mary M. R.N., op.cit., p. 469.

[70]   Ibid..

[71]   Hine, Darlene Clark, *Black Women In White: Racial Conflict and Cooperation in the Nursing Profession, 1890-1950*, Indiana University Press, Bloomington & Indianapolis, 1989, p. 183.

[72]   *The World Book Encyclopedia*, op. cit., Volume 18, p. 384.

[73]   *200 Years, A Bicentennial Illustrated History of the United States*, Joseph Newman, Directing Editor, Books by U.S. News & World Report, Inc., 2300 N Street, N.W., Washington, D.C. 20037, 1973, book 2, p. 232.

[74]   Ibid..

[75]   Ibid., p. 231.

[76]   *The World Book Encyclopedia*, op. cit., Volume 18, p. 384.

[77]   Roberts, Mary M. R.N., op.cit., p. 325.

[78]   Chow, Rita K. R.N. Ed.D., Hope, Gloria S. R.N. Ph.D., Nelson, LTC Ethel A. USAF NC, Sololoski, LTC James L. ANC, Wilson, CAPT Ruth A. NC USN Ret., "Historical Perspectives of the United States Air Force, Army, Navy, Public Health Service, and Veterans Administration Nursing Services," *Military Medicine*, Vol. 143 No. 7, July 1978, p. 458.

[79]   Laird, et al, op.cit., p. 38.

[80]   Copies of "Remarks by LT Leona Jackson, NC USN" at the Chief Nurses Conference, Bureau of Medicine and Surgery, Navy Department, Washington, D.C., 18-19 May 1949, pp. 1-4.

[81]   Pugh, H. L. Rear Admiral, MC USN Acting Chief of Bureau, "Interim Plan for Professional Examination for Promotion of Officers of the Nurse Corps," *BuMED Circular Letter No. 49-36*, 30 March 1949. Copy of letter donated by CDR Gladys Dvorak Larson Navy Nurse Corps.

[82]   Kirkland, Alma, "A salute to the Navy nurse ... Florence Nightingale in Navy blue," Independent (AM) Press Telegram (PM), Long Beach, California, Thursday, May 13, 1971, pp. 17-18.

[83]   Schnell, Elizabeth M. Schwartz LT Navy Nurse Corps, *Written History Interview*, 21 March 1994.

[84]   Houp, Geraldine A. Capt Navy Nurse Corps, *Oral History Interview Tape Transcript*, Interviewer LT Helen Barry Siragusa Navy Nurse Corps, 9 May 1990.

[85]   DeWitt, Evelyn E., op. cit..

"Navy Nurses are
now Navy Officers."

☆ ☆ ☆

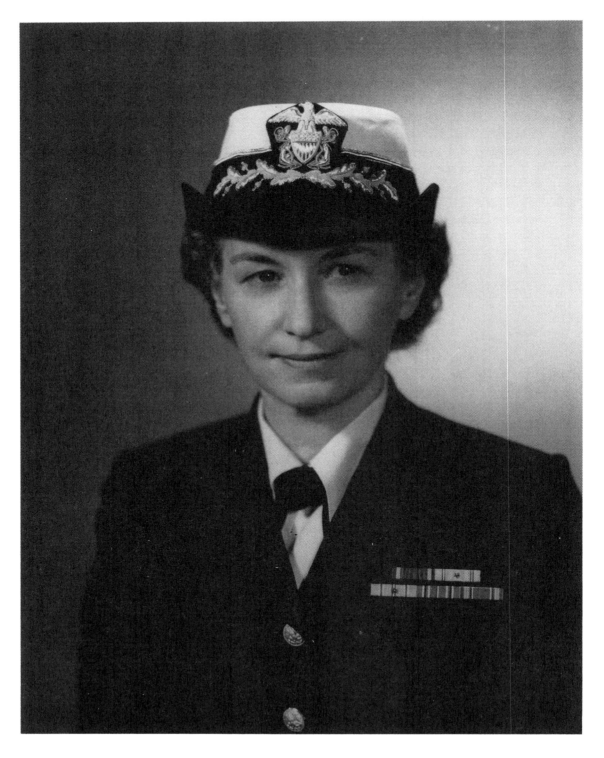

Director - Captain Winnie Gibson NC USN
(Official U.S. Navy photo courtesy of Nursing Division, Bureau of Medicine and Surgery, Navy Department.)

CHAPTER 8

Director - Captain Winnie Gibson
(1950 - 1954)

On 15 March 1950, Commander Winnie Gibson (Palmer, DeWitt) reports to the Bureau of Medicine and Surgery, Washington, D.C. where she prepares for her promotion to Captain and for the position as Director of the Navy Nurse Corps. Captain Gibson assumes office on 1 May 1950.

Winnie Gibson was born in Itaska, Texas (about forty miles SSE of Fort Worth) on December 15, 1902. She obtained her nurse's training first in Taylor, Texas then at Seton Hospital in Austin, Texas. She graduated in May of 1923 and received her RN in December of that year. Miss Gibson worked at her profession gaining experience and "Before I went into the Navy, I was working with surgeons who were operating. I did that for seven years."[1] She joined the Navy on 4 April 1930. She was stationed at the Naval Hospitals at Philadelphia, Pennsylvania and New York, New York until January 1934. At that time she went to the School of Nursing, Graduate School of Medicine at the University of Pennsylvania in Philadelphia for instruction in Anesthesia. She left there in May 1934 for duty as Operating Room Supervisor AND Anesthetist at the Naval Hospital in New York followed by the same duties at Quantico, Virginia until 1937. That year she was ordered aboard the USS *Relief*. In 1938 Miss Gibson went, as Anesthetist, to the Naval Hospital Mare Island, California then another tour as Operating Room Supervisor and Anesthetist at the Naval Hospital, Pearl Harbor. She was there on 7 December 1941.

She returned Stateside in late 1942 and was Chief Nurse at the Naval Hospitals in Jacksonville, Florida then Annapolis, Maryland and Houston, Texas. In April 1949 she had a short TAD tour at BuMed then was sent as Chief Nurse to the U.S. Naval Hospital, Naval Medical Center, Guam, Mariana Islands.[2] From Guam to the highest office a Nurse Corps Officer can achieve, Director of the Corps, and little does Captain Gibson know of the stress and turmoil she will have to face.

"At the end of World War II, forces of the United States and Soviet Russia liberated Korea from Japan."[3] "The Russians had occupied under armistice terms the half of Korea north of the 38th parallel, the Americans the southern half; the Americans under United Nations instructions had set up a formally democratic state . . . but the Russians had prevented United Nations representatives from entering the northern half and had set up the usual Communist dictatorship. In June, 1950, the North Korean armies invaded South Korea; it was immediately clear that they had been equipped by their Communist allies with all the munitions of modern war, and the South Koreans, who possessed little more than an armed police, quite unprepared for such warfare, stood no chance. Owing to the Russian absence, the Security Council of the United Nations was able within two days to resolve to come to the aid of South Korea; the aggression was so flagrant that 48 countries supported the Council's decision to authorize the raising of an army, to be led by the United States, who alone had any forces of importance in the region. Even India and Sweden sent medical units to the United Nations army."[4]

A few days after North Korea invades South Korea, U.S. President Harry Truman orders U.S. air, naval and ground troops to aid South Korea. In early July, the President names General Douglas MacArthur as the Supreme Commander of the U.N. forces in the Far East.[5] "When Harry Truman ordered U.S. ground troops to Korea without obtaining congressional authorization, he called it a police action and told his closest advisers: 'We've got to stop the sons of bitches no matter what.'. . . In the first U.S. Battle, 540 ill-trained and ill-equipped troops . . . dug in against the Soviet-made tanks of the 90,000-man North Korean army. . . . [The] task force was overwhelmed by the invaders. . . . The soldiers who followed . . . were drawn from a U.S. led coalition of 16 nations - the first time the fledgling United Nations sent an army into the field to combat aggression. The defenders were nearly pushed off the Korean peninsula, then turned the tide with a Marine landing at Inchon, history's last great amphibious assault. The allies then decided to cross the 38th Parallel and unify the country under one flag."[6] The capital of North Korea is captured and troops make it to the Yalu River which is the border of Communist China. But, at this point the Communist Chinese enter the war and by the end of the year the U.S. Army and U.N. forces are in retreat.

President Truman understands "the urgency of the situation [in Korea] and [puts] the United States on a semiwar basis."[7] Despite Korea, the Congress and most of the general public are engrossed in the antics of one Congressman. In the U.S. Congress, Senator Joseph McCarthy announces, in early 1950, that he has "a list of 205 'card-carrying' Communists in the employ of the State Department."[8] (This Senator's Communist witch hunt goes on for four long years. Even when Eisenhower comes into office, McCarthy "would not let up; he implied that President Eisenhower himself was 'soft on communism.' In the notorious Army-McCarthy hearings of 1954 - best TV show of the decade - the administration fought back by means of witty counsel . . . Finally, after the Senate censured him by an emphatic vote, McCarthy collapsed."[9] The witch hunt ends but not without shattered reputations and disenchanted viewers/listeners.)

In 1950, the Trumans are living in Blair House (across Pennsylvania Avenue from the White House) while extensive structural repairs are being made to the White House. "On Nov. 1, 1950, two Puerto Rican nationalists tried to invade Blair House and assassinate the President. They killed one Secret Service guard and wounded another. One of the gunmen was killed and the other captured. Truman commented that, 'A President has to expect those things.' He kept all his appointments that day, and took his usual walk the next morning."[10]

As for the profession of nursing, "At mid-century, although there were more registered professional nurses actively engaged in nursing than ever before, there were serious deficits in all fields of nursing. The most urgent needs were those of the hospitals although, collectively, they had added 50,000 registered nurses to their rosters in the postwar period. By 1950, according to the AMA, hospitals were augmenting the services of well over 200,000 professional nurses and approximately 100,000 student nurses with those of about 225,000 practical nurses, attendants, and nurses' aides. . . . Many nurses left the practice of nursing to become nurse anesthetists or some other type of medical technician. The American Association of Nurse Anesthetists reported a demand [for Anesthetists] far exceeding the supply in 1950. . . . [Also,] At mid-century the long-established tradition that the hospital is 'the workshop of the doctor' was giving way to the concept of patient-centered institutions. 'Consider the patient as a person,' says a report on medical education, 'was merely a platitude in medical schools until relatively recently.' . . . [Excellent] examples of medical teamwork (not to be confused with the nursing team) could be found in pediatric departments such as the one in which the order for 'TLC' (tender, loving care) first appeared on a patient's chart and in many departments caring for polio patients. . . . The broad, social concept of total patient needs has many implications for the nursing department, as to both its activities and the competence and attitude of its staff."[11] Another milestone occurs in 1950, when the "American Red Cross, Metropolitan Life Insurance Co., and John Hancock Mutual Life Insurance Co. announced dissolution of visiting nurse services to be completed by 1953."[12]

Turning to the Navy Nurse Corps; in May 1950 legislation is passed allowing reserve Navy Nurses to be integrated into the regular Navy up to the age of 40. Also in May, Navy Nurses have a new uniform change authorized. It will be in the style of the WAVES' uniform but it will be in the traditional dark blue with gold braid. In June there is the violation of the 38th Parallel by the North Korean forces and the "first involuntary recall of reserve nurses to care for Korean casualties."[13] At the end of June there are only 1510 regular and 440 reserve Navy Nurses on active duty; this was the result of the overall reduction of naval forces after World War II.[14] These 1,950 Navy Nurses are "assigned to 26 naval hospitals, 67 station hospitals and dispensaries in and outside continental United States; 3 Hospital Corps Schools; 2 Hospital Ships, and 8 Military Sea Transport Service ships [MSTS]."[15]

The Director of the Nurse Corps and her staff are having a very difficult time trying to supply Navy Nurses to meet all the needs. Navy Nurse Marion Caesar (Wheeler) is on the Director's staff at this time, and she says, "Winnie Gibson came back [to the BuMed office] one day and said to us [her staff], we'd been ordered by the Secretary of Defense to order up 125 nurses a week until we hear otherwise. So . . . McCory [Navy Nurse] was her assistant . . . and Ruth Erickson was detail [assignments] officer and I had Budget and Statistics. We went over to the Reserve Section. Well, it was a hilarious mess. Most of the jackets [folders for individual records] had nothing in them. . . . So that day we decided that the group of us would list some of those [Reserve] nurses that we had personally known, that we knew were still active in nursing. . . . So that first group of 125, were named by those people at the Bureau and I had about four of my friends [on that list]. I didn't tell them for many months that I was the one [that did this]. . . . But, we finally got it worked out a little better . . . then, of course, they worked on setting up a Nurse Corps Reserve section."[16]

But, with the involuntary recall, numbers of nurses started coming into the Corps overloading many of the nurses' quarters at the stateside naval hospitals. Also, all active duty nurses are 'frozen' and unable to leave the service. Thus, because of the large numbers, some Navy Nurses are permitted to live out of quarters for the first time, and draw subsistence pay.

July 1950 is when the responsibility for the governing of Guam is transferred from the Navy Department to the U.S. Department of Interior. This move transfers operation of the native hospital and the school of nursing on Guam from the Navy to the Department of Interior.

In July the USS *Consolation* is ordered to Korea and arrives at Pusan Harbor in South Korea on August 16, 1950. The USS *Repose* and USS *Benevolence* are pulled from the Reserve Fleet and made ready for sea duty in Korean waters. Fifteen Navy Nurses are assigned duty aboard the hospital ship *Benevolence*. They are:

> LT Eleanor Harrington, Chief Nurse
> Lt(jg) Marie Brennan
> Ensign Mary Deignan
> LT Mary Dyer
> LT Jean Fralic
> LT Catherine Harkins
> Ensign Patricia Karn
> LT Wilma Ledbetter
> LT Marie Lipuscek
> LT Josephine McCarthy
> Ensign Ruth Martin
> LT Gail Matthews
> Lt(jg) Rosemary Neville
> Ensign Dorothy Venverloh
> LT Helen Wallis

Ensign Ruth Martin (Deus) tells us, "My first impression of the ship was 'how beautiful it is - all gleaming white with several red crosses painted on her side.' The ship was moored alongside a long cement wharf which was bustling with activity. A civilian crew, members of MSTS (Military Sea Transport Service) or Navy Yard workers were de-mothballing the ship. Every day the nurses [assigned to the ship] walked to the ship, climbed aboard up the ladder, saluted the Officer of the Deck and the Quarterdeck, and asked for permission to come aboard. We wore our everyday striped seersucker uniforms, black ties, black pumps and beige stockings. Our duty hours were spent on board getting familiar with the ship and getting it ready for the impending voyage. We sat in the operating room for hours on end making bandages and assembling medical supplies. . . . On Monday, August 21st, two weeks after reporting in, we were served a delicious dinner for the first time aboard the ship. It was served in the nurses' wardroom. It was served nicely by a Negro steward, and with all the silver and china befitting a formal meal. Even the china was monogrammed with the name of the ship! . . . On Tuesday, August 22nd, the ship was taken on its first trial run without the nurses aboard. . . . On Wednesday, August 23rd, the nurses [15 in all] moved aboard the ship - two to a stateroom. The rooms were small with one porthole. The staterooms were furnished with a double decker bunk, a locker for each occupant, and a desk with a small safe for valuables. I immediately locked up some jewelry and $200 to $300 worth of traveler's checks purchased in San Diego and which I was refunded later on. Each nurse was issued a 'Mae West' life jacket, which I decided I wouldn't be needing, and to get it out of the way I stuffed it up into the small space between the top of my locker and the overhead.... On Friday, August 25th, 1950, the ship was scheduled for a second trial run. If the ship proved seaworthy then the civilian crew would turn it over to the Navy for commissioning, and we would soon be on our way.... Excitement was in the air as the ship steamed out from Mare Island Shipyard into San Pablo Bay, past Alcatraz, under the Golden Gate, and out into the Pacific Ocean. The ship was still under the command of the civilian crew. On board there were a little over 500 people - the civilian crew, some of the civilian workmen who just came along for the ride, the Navy crew, and the Medical personnel."[17] Navy Nurse Dorothy Venverloh states, "We left Mare Island about eight o'clock, 0800 . . . The ship engaged in various maneuvers to see how the engines would function at full speed and half speed and quarter speed, and tested the maneuverability of the ship. Then about two o'clock we went under the Golden Gate Bridge out into the Pacific. We went as far as the Farallon Islands [off the coast of California] then turned around and returned."[18]

Ruth Martin (Deus) continues, "That day as I stood on the top deck, I thought what a magnificent ship this is, and how lucky I am to be a part of this duty assignment. After all, wasn't this one of the reasons I had joined the Navy . . .

"Everyone was jovial and upbeat that afternoon at a brief commissioning ceremony in the Captain's quarters as the ship was officially turned over to the Navy.... [The] *Benevolence* continued cruising as dinner was to be served at 1700. About that time I went into the nurses' head which was located almost directly across from my cabin on the port side of the ship. There was no one else there. Suddenly I heard a loud crashing sound and felt a severe jolt which almost knocked me off the toilet. My first thought was that one of the boilers probably had blown up. We nurses had heard this had happened just a week or two earlier when the '*Repose*' had made her trial run. I stepped out into the passageway. Someone yelled 'a ship rammed us.' For some reason I didn't get excited nor too concerned since the ship had just been proven seaworthy and we had been told it was 'compartmentalized,' right? I dashed down the ladder to the nurses' wardroom which was on the deck immediately below my cabin. It was empty. Dishes and crockery were flying across the room from their storage places along the bulkhead and off the table which was set for the evening meal. The ship was listing noticeably to port. Something was dreadfully wrong! I hurriedly climbed back up the ladder to my cabin. About this time a call was sounded over the loudspeaker system to 'man your life jackets and man the lifeboats!' The time that had elapsed since the first jolt was felt was probably no more that five minutes. My cabin then was at about a 45 degree angle. Like a mad woman I climbed up to retrieve my life jacket and had to tug it loose from its hiding place. I put on my raincoat, (it might be cold out there,) and grabbed my uniform purse with the shoulder straps."[19]

In another cabin Dorothy Venverloh and her roommate, Rosemary Neville, had been getting ready for dinner. Ensign Venverloh says her roommate "looked out the porthole and said, 'Gee, that ship's mighty close.' And with that there was a severe bump. It knocked things over on the dresser and almost immediately thereafter, the loud speaker system came on and we were told to take our life jackets and proceed to the starboard side of the ship and prepare to abandon ship. So the ship kept tilting over and we had to climb on our chair to get our life jackets off the top of the cabinet. Rosemary put her coat on and her life jacket and her purse and said, 'I don't know what you're going to do, but I'm getting out of here.' I followed her but then I remembered I didn't have my glasses so I went back to get my glasses. As I came down the passageway, by this time it was necessary to walk with one foot on the . . . deck and one on the bulkhead, the ship was listing so much.... [By] the time I got to the cross passageway, some of the men were holding the door open and were reaching in to grasp my hand to pull me out through the doorway, and I had to hold on to the hand rail and pull myself up on the hand rail to get out on deck."[20]

Ensign Martin (Deus) says, "Everyone was gathering on the opposite side - the starboard side - of the listing ship. The angle of the list was so severe that it was difficult to climb up to reach the outer deck but with the help of strong arms I reached outer deck, got to the railing, and climbed over. Someone helped us to put on our life jackets - we had never had a drill.

"As the ship went down on its port side we gradually walked over until we were standing upright on the starboard side of the ship. The ship eventually was completely turned on its side! The ship had turned so quickly that it had been impossible to release the life boats!. Fortunately, about six life rafts were released. People jumped on them immediately even though there never was any order to abandon ship. The loudspeaker system went out almost immediately. Most of the nurses were together. Everyone was calm. I kept thinking, 'this can't be happening to me - it must be a dream.' One of the Navy Captains assured us that the ship wouldn't go down any further because at this spot the water just wasn't deep enough. So we all had visions then of standing there on the side of the ship waiting for a rescue party, but not for long. Apparently, it was high tide. The ship was going down fast - bow first. Most of the people had shoved off by this time except for the nurses, some medical officers, and the two Navy Captains. Our Medical Captain . . . and one of the Dental officers had the foresight and courage to go back into the ship before it had turned completely over and gather some rope and two or three 8 foot wooden rafters. They tied the 11 nurses together around our waists so we wouldn't get separated. They tied the rafters together. That was a wonderful idea. Sliding on our seats we shoved off into the water - 11 of us nurses plus 9 other people. While holding onto the roped rafters we paddled like 'hell' away from the sinking ship. Ten minutes after we abandoned her, our beautiful ship couldn't be seen. Bow first it went down. The time was approximately 1730. . . . It took just approximately one-half hour for the ship to go completely under.

"Visibility was poor. It was so foggy you could see only a short distance over the water. The water was very cold. I was lucky that I had put on my raincoat. I still had on my pump shoes which stayed on the entire time. The first half hour in the water I kept moving and was not too uncomfortable. It was a great feeling of security to be able to put your hands with all the other hands holding onto those rafters. . . . No one was very encouraging. One of the civilian crew who was with our group told us that they had not been able to get an S.O.S. message out. No one knew for sure how far out we were. No one knew if the ship that had collided with us had stayed around. It was getting dark and the fog was very thick. My roommate, Lieutenant Helen Wallis, was not with our group and I wondered if she was okay. . . . We wondered how far out we were. Were those sounds we heard ships or fog horns? I looked around me and everyone looked blue with cold - almost like they were in shock. Much later I realized that the blue dye from the Mae West jackets was rubbing off on our faces. The Mae West jackets were supposed to be secured by straps brought from the back between the legs. As all the nurses had on dresses I don't think this was done. Consequently, the jackets kept riding up around our faces.

"Finally we saw a little fishing boat and we all yelled to attract their attention. They went on by. Later we found out it was filled to capacity with survivors - mostly stragglers and those without life jackets who were a lot worse off than we were. The Catholic girls were saying their prayers out loud continuously. Miss Harrington, our Chief Nurse, was a great morale booster. She encouraged us to sing. . . . It was getting colder and darker, and the waves were getting choppier. You would get a mouthful of salt water that took your breath away momentarily - spitting out as much as you could, but it was impossible not to swallow some.

"Then we saw the Army tug that eventually picked us up. They somehow conveyed the message that they would return for our little group. What a disappointment that was! Could they find us again in that fog? This half hour was the longest of all as we were all so cold and tired. Finally the tug returned, threw us a life line which one of the men caught, and pulled us alongside. It was at this crucial time, so close to rescue, that one of the nurses with us, Lieutenant Wilma Ledbetter, became hysterical. She apparently could not swim. She let her head fall back in the water. Several tried to hold it up for her. Later I found out she had died (not drowned) but literally was scared to death. [She died aboard the Army tug shortly after being taken from the water.]

"The crew aboard the tug threw a ladder over the side and tried to pull us up on deck."[21] Miss Venverloh tells us, "they started pulling us out of the water, or trying to pull us out of the water, but they didn't understand that we were tied together. So finally, two of the men jumped in behind us and started cutting the ropes that held us together. When I got to the side of the ship, they reached down to grab my hands. The difficult part was with the waves. At first you'd be up near the deck, then you'd be down near the bottom of the ship. It was up and down. So finally they got a hold of me and pulled me up manually out of the water and on to the deck. One of the men said, 'Are you all right? Are you going to be able to walk?' And I said, 'Oh, I think I can.' I walked about three steps and my legs gave way. So two of the men came and escorted me down below deck where there were many other survivors who had been picked up before us."[22]

Ensign Martin (Dues) says of her rescue, "They took off our wet coats and wrapped blankets around us. Several of us nurses were put in the Captain's cabin. The clock read 1945. We couldn't stop shaking. They tried to give us hot coffee, but we couldn't even hold the cup. I got sick about then from all the salt water I had swallowed, and threw up in the Captain's lavatory. I was so embarrassed by that.

"About a half hour later we landed at Fort Mason . . . Buses, people, corpsmen, doctors, nurses, newspaper reporters and photographers, ambulances and the Red Cross were all awaiting our arrival. A hospital corpsman walked me to one of the waiting buses. The California Highway Patrol blocked off the lower level of the Bay Bridge to clear the way for the ambulances and buses racing with their loads to Oak Knoll Naval Hospital in Oakland. . . . My only casualties were a few bruises and muscular aches and soreness - I didn't even get a cold. Some of the girls had sprained ankles and stiff necks. We were all, of course, saddened by the loss of Lieutenant Wilma Ledbetter, a lovely, gentle, young lady from Chillicothe, Texas."[23]

Miss Martin (Deus) finds her shipboard roommate, Helen Wallis, the next morning. "She had been separated from the other nurses. The group she was with had been picked up by the little fishing boat that passed us by. It was returning to San Fransico loaded down with its day's catch. In taking survivors aboard all the fish were thrown overboard. . . . On Sunday morning, August 27th, the 522 foot *Benevolence* lay on her side in shallow coastal waters with the big red cross on her white hull showing through the waves washing over her."[24] (Two years later, the *Benevolence* is demolished as a menace to shipping.)

To return to the survivor nurses at the Oakland Naval Hospital; after all the survivors are put to bed, the staff of the hospital, "collected our clothing, had it laundered, took our coats to the dry cleaners, but we didn't have shoes. We lost our shoes. So within the next couple of days, Lieutenant Helen Steve [Navy Nurse Corps] came around and took all of our shoe sizes, hosiery sizes, our underclothing sizes, to order these things for each of us from one of the well-known department stores in Oakland and had it all put on her charge. Then when we could be half-way adequately dressed, we dressed in our gray seersucker uniforms. We didn't have purses, so the little money we had, which had come from a check that the nurses at one of the Naval Hospitals in the east (I don't know if it was Great Lakes or Philadelphia) - they had sent a check out [to us]. They had taken up a donation - a collection for us and sent us a check, and we each got about $25 from this check. We had this money tied in our handkerchiefs."[25] The Navy takes care of its own.

Less than a month after the sinking of the *Benevolence*, on 19 September 1950, a military transport plane is crossing the Pacific carrying eleven Navy Nurses to their new duty assignment at the U.S. Naval Hospital in Yokosuka, Japan. Korean casualties are being brought to the hospital and the staff at Yokosuka is to be augmented by these eleven Navy nurses. They are:

> Ensign Eleanor C. Beste
> Ensign Marie M. Boatman
> Lt(jg) Jeanne E. Clarke
> Lt(jg) Jane L. Eldridge
> Ensign Constance R. Esposito
> Lt(jg) Alice S. Giroux
> Lt(jg) Calla V. Goodwin
> Lt(jg) Constance A. Heege
> Lt(jg) Margaret G. Kennedy
> Ensign Mary E. Liljegreen
> Ensign Edna J. Rundell

All persons aboard perish as the plane crashes in the Pacific Ocean as it is taking off from a stopover at Kwajalein Island in the Marshall Islands. The entire Navy Nurse Corps is shaken by the two deadly catastrophes so close together. Navy Nurse Marion Ceaser (Wheeler) is stationed at BuMed on the staff of the Director when these events takes place and says, "One of the saddest times ever was when those nurses that we ordered out . . . to Japan [were killed at Kwajalein.] . . . There was a large number [eleven] because we were trying to build up [the nursing staff] at Yokosuka. It was terrible. And then Ruth Erickson, who had Details [the Assignments nurse at BuMed], said, 'I cannot go to that Board and pick out another group.' . . . I guess Leona Jackson and myself and Kay Armstrong [all Navy Nurses at BuMed], we went to the Board and went through with [selecting nurses as replacements]. . . . Everybody was broken up about [the tragedies]. They never knew what happened so it was terrible. . . . And you know, for weeks afterwards, stuff [belonging to the nurses on the plane] would wash to shore [at Kwajalein] and then it would be sent because it was tagged with so and so's name on it. And it would come to the Bureau for us to take care of. To get it to the families. So that was very hard on Winnie Gibson [Director of the Corps]."[26]

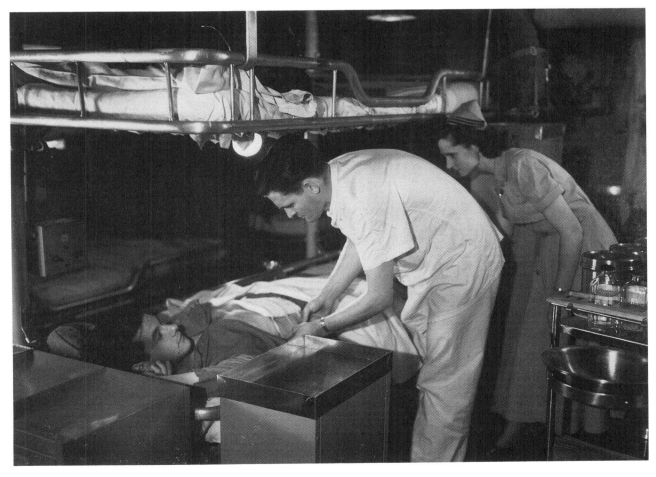

Aboard USS *Repose* Navy Nurse supervising dressing change by hospital corpsman. (Photo courtesy of NNCA Memorabilia Collection.)

Meanwhile, the USS *Consolation* is out in the Korean waters and desperately in need of additional nurses. There are six nurses ordered aboard the ship who are waiting for transportation in Oakland. They finally get aboard a plane for Honolulu where they remain overnight then the next morning they leave "in a prop plane that had seats in it. It had regular seats, not just bucket seats. We hadn't been in the air too awfully long, just to the point of no return where we would have to go on, when oil began to stream back across the windows, so someone went forward and told the pilot. He came back and checked and allowed as how we were losing oil and that we would have to return to Honolulu. This we did and found that a chain that held the cap on the oil tank had gotten caught between the cap and the tank and that's why the oil had left the motor and had we gone on much farther, it would have been bad. . . . From there we went on to Johnson Island, a speck in the ocean that was used as a stop-over for refueling. Coming down on it, it didn't look like it was any bigger than a carrier deck. [An interesting phenomenon on this island is when one stands on the land and looks out to sea, which you can see on all sides, it seems as though the sea is actually higher than where you stand. It is nice to have only a short stay there.] When we got to Guam, we were taxiing in, a truck was backing out and backed into us and tore a hole in the side of the plane."[27] But, they finally arrive safe in Japan and get to Yokosuka at two in the morning with no place to stay because of the influx of personnel, patients and others associated with the 'Korean Crisis.' An MSC (Medical Service Corps) officer and his wife ultimately take them into their home. The next day they are given transportation to further south in Japan and after another mix-up finally get to Sasebo where the hospital ship is thought to come in. To make a long tale short, the ship doesn't come in there and after about a week the six nurses finally get word that the ship will arrive in Yokosuka so back they go to Yokosuka. There they find the ship already in port. The ship unloads, resupplies and heads out for Korea with the six nurses now aboard.[28]

Navy Nurse Helen Brooks is one of the six new nurses aboard the *Consolation* and she says, "This was the old type of war-time where there would be a push [military action] and it would be very active for two to three weeks with a mass of casualties [for the ship] the second or third day. The numbers would lessen a little until a piece of real estate had been secured. Then we would begin taking care of the lesser wounded. Then there would be a low period until the Marines or the Army would do another push. . . . The operating room [aboard the ship] was a busy place. . . . The patients were brought aboard. We didn't have a holding area. We didn't have an intensive care unit and many times the most seriously wounded were lined up outside the operating room so as soon as they could get to them they would. It meant that in addition to your operating room duties, afterward you would be doing intensive care work with the patients outside the door. If a patient went sour, you would quickly have to get them into an operating room. The nurses really had a heavy responsibility, but I don't think many of us recognized it as such at that time. We did two to three patients per operating room, although three in a room was a little bit much. Two orthopedic cases were about all you could do because of the heavy casting and things that we had to do at that time.

"We had a considerable number of head wounds. Dr. C . . . was the only neurosurgeon in the Korean area so we had Army patients, Air Force from all over - there were very few casualties among the Air Force at that time. Dr. C . . . worked around the clock. He would make his rounds on his wards; he had a whole ward of head cases. Then he would come down and operate. He would finish operating and whoever was assisting him would go ahead after he got the flap in and close the scalp while [Dr. C] would go on a guerney and stretch out. The next patient would get positioned and get his head shaved and ready then we would call Dr. C . . . and he would get up and start operating. Many times we were shaving the brain as well as the hair and the scalp.

"Orthopedics were our largest number of patients. We did have two or three Orthopedists aboard, but again we had corpsmen who did all the casting. Many of these patients would have body casts on. . . . The cast would hardly be dry - not even dry - and they would be put on stretchers and hoisted off the side of the ship. They'd go to small boats that would take them ashore . . . to the airport . . . where they would be put upon planes that would evacuate them to Japan.

"Although our functioning capacity was about 700 to 750 patients, we had many more than that at times, sometimes up to a thousand or more. . . . This was a United Nations activity so we had patients from all over the globe. We had French, Greek, Colombian, Turks. . . . [Some time after] we were transferred up to Hungnam which is the farthest north we went, close to the DMZ. It was here that the so-called strategic retreat began. The hospital ship was out in the stream at anchor and during this time, which was bitterly cold, the *Missouri* was anchored not too far off . . . and would do its firing at night softening up the shore. To those of us down in the operating room, which was the third deck down, it sounded like a sledge hammer pounding on the side of the ship. At this time we were taking on casualties from the fighting . . . some of these had been wounded twice and many of them were frostbitten. At this time the helicopters, which were only one or two seaters, were bringing out more of the wounded than they had previously and the litters were strapped to the side of the helicopter; one to each side. Of course it was bitterly cold and many of these patients came in with frostbite. . . . While we were there, each night, as I mentioned, they were shelling on the shore line trying to keep the Communist forces back so that the evacuation of troops could take place. On the day before Christmas, we were still at anchor and we stayed as the rest of the ships that had been there steamed out in the final evacuation of Hungnam . . . The hospital ship stayed so as to have a more distant place in the line of ships that were leaving and so it could take the final wounded from the shore. . . . It was a magnificent sight to see these ships going out, in defeat really, but as they passed the hospital ship that was waiting at anchor for the remaining injured to come, they would all salute the ship [the *Consolation*]. Then when we did pull up anchor and leave, we passed many of them and all of them gave honors to the ship as it passed loaded with the wounded. It couldn't help but bring tears to your eyes."[29]

On Christmas eve the *Consolation* is at sea and the Chief Nurse, Estelle Kalnoske (Lange) writes a letter home saying, "This day I shall never forget and while it's all fresh in my mind, I'll try and give you an idea of what it has been. I believe I wrote you about being a spectator and today I saw the destruction of Hunguam [sic]. All last night the guns just fired away and I wondered if any Chinese Reds escaped that barrage - but from what the patients tell us - they are madmen - probably all doped up with opium. This morning our troops were evacuated - I watched them scramble up the cargo nets - the buildings on the beach were burning and every now and then an ammunition drop would blow up so that it looked as if an atomic bomb was let loose. Unfortunately one of the ammunition dumps blew up prematurely with the result that we got 25 wounded and one dead. The cruiser *St. Paul* fired all morning right over our ship and the noise was terrific.

"The *Missouri* was at the entrance to the harbor and firing away. All I could see was smoke and fire on the beach, then planes were dropping bombs and it looked like something out of this world. We finally got all the patients on board when the word was passed that we were getting underway and in no time we were out of the harbor - that was at 3 o'clock. When I looked out at 6 o'clock - we were in the lead and the rest of the ships were in back of us - that was unusual because we are always at the tail end. It's a beautiful moonlight night - it's Christmas Eve - and we are on our way to Pusan to debark our Korean patients.

"So much for Christmas Eve - and I miss you all very much. I'm going to midnight mass."[30]

Meantime, on the Hospital Ship *Repose*, a civilian MSTS crew had been manning her until she arrived in Yokosuka in early September. There a Navy crew takes over the manning of the ship and she heads to Pusan, Korea. ("At 1122 on 28 October 1950, USS *Repose* [is] officially returned to commissioned service."[31] Lieutenant Annette Baer is the Chief Nurse at this time.)

Navy Nurse Eveline Kittilson (McClean) is one of the nurses aboard the ship at this time, and she says, "We arrived at Pusan on September 20, 1950. The Army band was on the dock to greet us which made us feel really welcome, in fact, they were there and played for us each time we arrived or departed Pusan. . . . The North Koreans had pushed south to the Pusan perimeter, so Pusan had over one million people. It was overcrowded, filthy and smelly; words cannot describe the situation there. The odor even penetrated our ship. The fighting was only 20 air miles away, and sometimes we could hear the guns. An Army evacuation hospital at the front lines would administer first aid to the wounded, and then send them down to us by train, which usually took 12-24 hours. The train started arriving on the dock near the ship at about 6:00 PM and continued until almost midnight each day. There was an Army evacuation hospital in Pusan also, so they received one-half the patients, but the most seriously injured were sent to us as we had better facilities for them. We received anywhere from 100-150 patients each night, all ranging from 17-20 years of age. Everyone worked like mad until all patients were admitted and cared for. The doctors were operating almost constantly, doing only the emergency work, and when the patient was well enought to travel, we sent them to Japan by air. We usually did not keep them more than three days. Some had a leg or arm blown off, or both. Some were hit in the face, some were blinded and one had half his brains blown out. There was every kind of casualty. The patients were dirty when we received them as they were taken right out of the rice patties. Some had worms and many had lice. After their wounds were cared for, there was the job of cleaning them up. It was the first sheets they had slept on in months and they were so appreciative. . . . The UN forces had pushed the North Koreans up to the Yalu River [the border of Manchuria, China] and General MacArthur was saying we would all be home for Christmas. Well, the Chinese communists entered the picture and started pushing our troops back."[32] At this point, the *Repose* had returned to Japan to disembark her patients and then returned to Inchon, Korea. Navy Nurse Kittilson (McClean) continues, "An Australian [ship] pilot took us up the channel to Chinnanpo. The channel had been heavily mined and he had been in charge of sweeping the mines. The channel was shallow so we had to go up on high tide. It was probably 30-40 miles to Chinnanpo and took several hours. We were told later that North Koreans were on the hills watching us. We anchored a short distance off shore and had sentries on the ship at night. Also, the ship was blacked out at night, which is something hospital ships never do. We were anchored here about a week before we received any patients, so we had a lot of leisure time. The doctors played volleyball on the boat deck, and we played cards and so forth. Then, suddenly, the patients started coming. We admitted 780 in three days. We filled every bed, including the iron lung. Most were ambulatory, as the most seriously injured were air evacuated to Japan. . . . The patients told us the Chinese communists were well organized and kept charging against them, regardless of strong gun fire; that they wore some sort of metal armor under their clothes so the bullets just bounced off. One patient said he hit a Chinese 39 times with his machine gun before he finally fell. I was never afraid or worried while we were there. . . . One of the nurses went berserk and we had to send her to Japan, but she was afraid that the North Koreans were going to attack the ship any night.

"When we left Chinnanpo, we went to Inchon where we transferred 300 of our patients to the Army hospital. They were patients who would soon be ready to return to duty. We spent the rest of December anchored in Inchon, along with many other ships."[33]

In September 1950, another hospital ship, the USS *Haven*, was recommissioned with Lieutenant Ruth Cohen to be the Chief Nurse. The *Haven* is to replace the lost *Benevolence*. (The *Haven* doesn't arrive in the far east until 1951.)

In August of 1950, Navy Nurse Dolores Cornelius is one of two Navy nurses aboard the MSTS ship USS *President Jackson* when it leaves "San Diego for Kobe [Japan] with a shipload of Marines. . . . The other Navy [nurse's] . . . tour of duty was coming to an end . . . but she was experienced and gave me an excellent orientation. The first night out at sea was rough and that night [we] assisted the two surgeons, with the Marines, with three appendectomies. Not only was the sea rough, but the operating room air conditioning was not working and it was like an oven in there. Also, [the other nurse] and I had taken anti-seasickness pills so we were trying our best to keep alert as the situation warranted. Everything turned out well.

"On the ship I met some of the corpsmen that I had worked with at Bremerton. [Corpsmen are assigned to Marine Units.] A few of them were later killed in the Korean Conflict. . . . Only [the] Captain of our ship and a few others knew where we were going and what the purpose of our mission would be. When we got to within 15 miles of Inchon Harbor [Korea], we joined hundreds of other Navy ships. It was 15 September 1950. At dawn I watched out on deck as the Marines went over the side into boats to take part in the Inchon landing. Then the battleships started their big guns, the noise was deafening. . . . Our ship was designated as a temporary hospital ship and on 'D Day' plus one or two we started to receive casualties. We also had a surgical team report aboard to assist us with the casualties. . . . A few days [later] we rendezvoused with two hospital ships in port; I believe this was in Pusan. One was the hospital ship *Repose* . . . We transferred our casualties to the hospital ships."[34] They then returned to Yokosuka, Japan.

Also in 1950, Esther Ramsey is a Reserve Navy Nurse on active duty aboard the MSTS ship the *Daniel I. Sultan*. "Our next trip was to Japan and then to Korea, sailing mid November. The ship was loaded, not with dependents and transferring personnel, but with Army troops and officers. . . . We debarked them in Yokohama, waited for about three days and boarded all of them again with combat gear. . . . We sailed, very carefully, in the late afternoon (the Captain did not know whether the channel had been mined or swept) and were ready to debark the troops at the harbor north of the 38th Parallel by evening the next day. The seas were rough and there was no pier so the debarkation was accomplished by lowering the cargo nets and letting the troops descend to the waiting LCM's below. It was growing dark and the rough seas caused the nets to present a serious hazard so debarkation was postponed until the following morning. Within three days we began to board the Marines who had returned from the Reservoir. . . . The hospital ship *Consolation* was hanging on the hook in the harbor and had received many of the more serious frost bite and wound cases, though many had been air evacuated from the area. We sailed down from Hungnam Harbor to Pusan with some 5,000 Marines on board and debarked them at Pusan, some with bandaged and frost bitten feet. . . . Our ship returned to Hungnam Harbor to await the evacuation. We hung on the hook for several days and watched the battleship *Wisconsin* bombard the beach, and the *Philippine Seas* as she pursued her mission. We boarded . . . [patients] from the *Consolation*, who was carrying a full load. The evacuation was on Christmas eve . . . The *Sultan* was the first ship to leave the harbor on evacuation day and she sailed to Pusan. . . . Although this evacuation from north of the 38th parallel goes relatively unnoticed in the history of the military and of the Nurse Corps, I felt that though there were only two Nurse Corps Officers on the *Daniel Sultan*, that we had participated in an important operation."[35]

Navy Nurse Florence Alwyn (Twyman)is one of the staff at the US Naval Hospital Yokosuka, Japan. She says," I was one of the great horde of nurses that were recalled and we went to Oak Knoll and I was there for 10 days and we immediately went to Yokosuka, Japan. That was in November of '50. . . . When I arrived in Japan, we got there just before Christmas, and that was just at the time when the Marines broke out of the . . . Reservoir. So we were getting patients in so fast that when we left our quarters in the morning, we didn't know whether we had a bed to sleep in that night because they kept moving us around to take in patients. Our census at . . . one point got up to around 5,000. This was [on] a large naval base that had previously been the 'Annapolis' of Japan. . . . I think the top census of [Navy] Nurses there at one point was 205 or something like that. So we were moved around depending on where they needed to put patients. And we had patients in triple decks."[36]

Navy Nurse Barbara Ellis is also at Yokosuka at this time and states, "Yokosuka was quite busy because it was the peak of the fighting in Korea. On an average we had 191 patients admitted daily. During the 48-hour period of 6 to 7 December, a total of 2022 patients were received by air and hospital ship from Korea. . . . I was in the operating room at that time and we were so busy that we had two OR [Operating Room] tables in one room working simultaneously."[37]

Back in the Hawaiian Islands on Oahu is Tripler Army Hospital and several Navy Nurses are stationed there. "When they closed Aiea Naval Hospital they transferred some of the nurses down there [to Tripler]."[38] "The most memorable duty I had in the Navy I suppose was at Tripler Army Hospital when . . . [we] began receiving the casualties of the Korean War. They came in by the huge plane loads. We took care of thousands of them from the field hospital in Korea. . . . Ruth Houghton was the [Navy] Chief Nurse there . . . and, of course, they had the Army equivalent. I came there from Guam. some of the nurses were transferred from Guam to Tripler or some of them would go on to Japan to finish their [overseas] duty. When I went there . . . there was an air-evac ward being set up. I had requested outpatient department but they needed people in the air-evac and I went there. . . . Shortly after we had the ward set up, we received the first casualties. . . . Many of them still had the dirt from the battlefield on them. . . . They received hot meals, they had baths, and had all the dressings changed. It was a hectic, hectic time, but it was a very rewarding experience."[39]

Navy Nurse Eveline Kittilson (McClean) also speaks of Tripler, "In the middle of October, 1951 I received orders to Tripler Army Hospital in Hawaii. I think this was my most unique experience, because I was a Navy Nurse assigned to an Army Hospital. However, somehow the Army and Navy decided on an exchange program, whereby 36 Army nurses were assigned to the U.S. Naval Hospital in St. Albans, New York, and 36 Navy Nurses were assigned to Tripler Army Hospital. This was a beautiful modern hospital with seven miles of tubes [probably pneumatic tubes], so one could send messages to any department in the hospital. I had never seen anything like this before. The nurses' quarters were very modern and lovely, built on the hillside behind the hospital with a beautiful view of Honolulu, Waikiki and Diamond Head. Duty here was quite different from the Navy. We worked different hours, had different days off during the week, so I didn't have as many week-ends off. At first I was assigned to a medical-surgical ward. There were several nurses on the ward, each of us being assigned to three or four patients that we bathed, gave medication to, did dressings and all treatment, unlike the Navy where the corpsmen do most of these duties. The OBGYN [Obstetrics, Gynecology] clinic had a Navy Captain in charge, so Navy Nurses were assigned to this clinic. After a couple months at Tripler, I was assigned Head Nurse in this clinic and had one Navy Nurse working with me, as well as three native attendants. This was the busiest place in the hospital. Some days we would see over 400 pre-natal patients, but I enjoyed the work. I had my evenings free and every week-end off."[40]

In 1951, the hospital ships *Consolation*, *Haven* and *Repose* continue to rotate as station hospitals in the Korean waters. Yokosuka Naval Hospital continues to receive many of the battlefield patients throughout the year. The Korean conflict wages on.

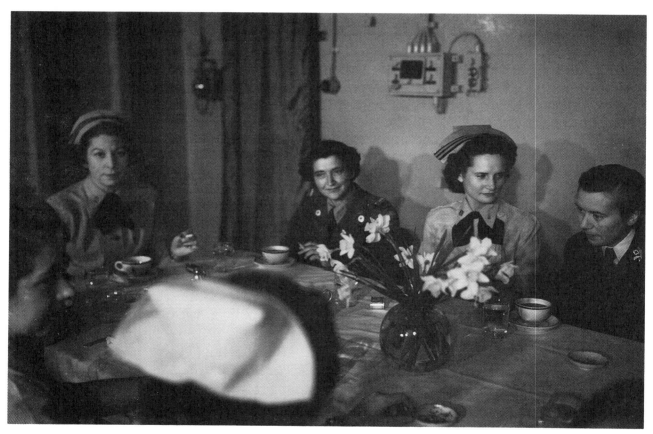

Nurse Corps officers from United States, Sweden and Denmark aboard USS Repose - Korea. (Photo courtesy of NNCA Memorabilia Collection.)

The *Repose* is in Pusan in September and celebrates her first year of Korean service with a ship's party. The *Haven* then joins with the *Repose* to give "a party for 500 orphans at Pusan's 'Happy Mountain Orphanage.'"[41] Occasions such as these help ease the strain, pain, and the horror of battle casualties. Make no mistake, these nurses (and all medical personnel aboard the hospital ships) worked long hours. At Hungnam [Korea], for example, more than one nurse worked around the clock with only time out for a catnap. When one nurse was ordered below by her supervisor, she replied, 'Oh, I couldn't sleep as long as I knew there were patients to be taken care of.'

"At Inchon and Wonsan [Korean waters] it was the same way. Says Captain Robert E. Baker, (MC) USN, commanding officer of Consolation's hospital. 'They worked days and night on end. They did everything they could.'"[42]

With the advent of the Korean crisis, Navy Nurses have a multiplicity of assignments in the Far East, in addition to the hospital ships. At Yokosuka, what had been a Naval Dispensary has grown into "a full fledged hospital with a staff which would include 200 nurses (compared to a mere six at the outbreak of the war) and capable of handling 6,000 casualties. Other nurses had been shifted from Stateside duty to ships of the Military Sea Transportation Service, ships which would carry troop replacements into Korea and transport wounded men back to Japan or the U.S.. Still other nurses were ordered to duty as flight nurses to serve aboard air evacuation planes shuttling between the war-torn peninsula and Japan."[43]

Meantime, back in the States, not all Navy Medical facilities are affected by the Korean situation. Navy Nurse Geraldine M. Carey (Thom) reports in to the US Naval Infirmary, NAOTS, Chincoteague, Virginia. She says, "When Addie Nicora and I reported at the same time in 1951, the only comment the CO [Commanding Officer] of the station had for us was, 'I told the Bureau not to send Ensigns here!' The six nurses [stationed at Chincoteague] lived in a nice little house. We staffed the infirmary around the clock. Two doctors delivered babies, did some surgery and manned the out-patient clinic. The mosquitos were the biggest and most vicious I've ever encountered! The Navy was not allowed to spray because of the famous Chincoteague oyster beds. [Nearby] Assateague Island was not yet a National Park and the wild ponies swimming [from Assateague] to Chincoteague once a year was a major event. We were far from any large cities (it took a ferry to get us to Washington, DC) but, needless to say, we had a ball with all the young bachelor aviators!"[44]

At a Marine Air Station in North Carolina, Navy Nurse Helen Barry (Siragusa) tells us, "About six weeks after I arrived at Cherry Point in March of 1951, we had a severe measles epidemic with a very rare strain of measles. We had to open an extra ward for just measle patients, many of whom had post-measles complications. One of our nurses had the mumps, our female physician had the measles, and I also got the measles.... Since we were short of nurses, I asked Captain . . . if I could stay in my room in the nurses' quarters in isolation. He thought that was a good idea and Eleanor Harrington, our Chief Nurse, and Dr. . . . made a sick call together after duty. I was fine for a few days and then I developed what turned out to be a strep throat and so I had to be admitted into the hospital. In another week or so I developed swollen joints and abdominal pains and I was diagnosed as having Rheumatic Fever. Within a few weeks I developed a Mastoiditis and I was to lie flat in bed for a month. I stayed in the infirmary at Cherry Point for three months. During that time, [Chief Nurse] Eleanor Harrington, who was very good to me and visited me daily, told me that we were having a visit from the Chief [Director] of the Nurse Corps, who was Winnie Gibson from Washington. She said she would bring her in to visit me. A few days later, Winnie Gibson came into my room and said, 'I had to come and see what you look like and see how you were doing because all this time I've been picking up the sick list every morning and seeing your name at the top of the list.' She told me that if I ever needed her help or if she could ever do anything for me to call on her. Winnie Gibson was a dark haired, smiling, pretty woman who personified the Navy Nurse Corps admirably.

"While I was a patient at the Marine Corps Air Station at Cherry Point, [Chief Nurse] Eleanor Harrington had the Marine bakers bake me a birthday cake for my birthday. The base of it was three feet wide. It fed every patient and staff member in the infirmary with almost a whole layer left over.... I was taken by air to Philadelphia Naval Hospital in June 1951. [Chief Nurse] Eleanor Harrington accompanied me. A Marine Colonel volunteered to fly the plane.... After three months they had a medical conference and . . . decided that I should be given a medical discharge which I really didn't want. By this time I was seriously considering making a career of the Navy Nurse Corps. I asked if I could go back to limited duty, to see if I could do my work. They agreed that this was feasible and recommended that I return to limited duty for six months after which I was to receive orders to a Naval Hospital for a reevaluation. As soon as they released me, I went home to await orders. . . . I remembered

Winnie Gibson's promise, so I went to her Washington office to see if I could speak to her. She was not there the day that I went so I spoke to her Aide and explained to her that she had said that she would be happy to help me if I ever wanted her help. I explained that my [purpose] in coming was to request orders back to Cherry Point, since I was there only six weeks when I became ill. In a few weeks I had my orders back to Cherry Point."[45] Navy Nurse Helen Barry (Siragusa) goes on to note about the Cherry Point Chief Nurse, "Eleanor Harrington was a caring, efficient, authoritative Chief Nurse. She was small in stature, but she was intimidated by no one." (This Chief Nurse is the Navy Nurse who was Chief Nurse of the *Benevolence* when it sank near San Francisco. Also, Chief Nurse Harrington, while at Cherry Point, requests duty as Chief Nurse aboard the *Haven*. Her request is granted.)

The large Naval Hospitals in the states, are the ones receiving patients from the Korean conflict. Attempts are made to see that patients are sent to the large hospitals nearest their homes, as much as is possible. At the Philadelphia Naval Hospital, Navy Nurse Evelyn Hope (George) says that patients "came in drafts, sometimes at night and we didn't know how many we were getting. . . . We would get these drafts in at night by plane or ship and . . . maybe we'd get 50 in all at one time. We had to break out beds and break out the cook and get food for them. Usually it was around one or two o'clock in the morning. We had them in the hallways, we had bunks, beds, everything . . . Most of our cases were frostbite cases or psychiatric."[46]

The recall of Reserves for the Korean Conflict created many a hardship on some of these recalled nurses; upsetting their civilian plans and careers. For instance, Margaret Larson had been a Navy Nurse in WWII. When she was released from active duty she utilized the G.I. Bill to achieve her Baccalaureate degree and obtained a position at Menninger's Clinic in Topeka, Kansas to "pursue a career in psychiatric nursing. I couldn't believe it. I just couldn't believe that the Navy still had a grip on me."[47] She had received orders to the Naval Hospital Oakland, California. Menninger's was "writing letters to try and get my orders rescinded and so on. Nothing happened and nothing happened. So I decided that was it and I was on my way. Then when I got to Idaho [home] I got this letter saying I really didn't have to go. But, I had come this far and I decided I would follow through on my orders. So, by January 1, 1951 here I was back in Oakland again. [She had been there in WWII.] . . . By that time ['51] Oakland was a psychiatric center for the Pacific area and for the West Coast so that psychiatric patients were transferred to Oakland. We would get admissions, we'd have maybe 25-30 admissions. They'd bring them up especially from San Diego. A lot of them [were] recruits; six months, three months active duty and they would be having acute psychotic breaks."[48]

In January of 1951, a "course in Aero-Medical Nursing (Flight Nurse Training) is made available to Reserve Navy Nurses on active duty. This training had, to date, only been available to Regular Navy Nurses since WWII."[49] In February, a Memo signed by the Surgeon General is sent out to Medical facilities 'urging' that Navy Nurses be utilized for professional duties only; another attempt to get Navy Nurses out of the Linen Room detail in the Naval Hospitals.[50] This particular detail was a sore point to many nurses. It involved counting linen received and linen given out. Dirty linen is replaced with the same amount of clean linen. Torn linen is repaired (at times the nurse had to do the sewing). Any and all chores associated with linen; hardly, a professional job.

In April the U.S. Naval Hospital at Bainbridge, Maryland is commissioned again and the Hospital Corps School is re-established there.[51]

In July 1951, American Samoa is released from the US Navy's stewardship and placed under the supervision of the Department of Interior. Also, in July, the Director of the Nurse Corps, Captain Gibson, goes on an inspection trip with the Surgeon General. They visit medical facilities in San Francisco, Honolulu (Tripler, Barbar's Point and VR-8 with its flight nurses), the Dispensary at Kwajalein, Naval Hospital Guam, Philippines, Japan, Korea, USS *Haven* and USS *Repose*, as well as some small activities along the way.[52]

The census of the Navy Nurse Corps reaches a peak of 3,328 nurses on 1 July. 1,515 are Regular Navy and 1,723 are Reserve. These nurses are "serving in 29 naval hospitals, 78 station hospitals and dispensaries at home and abroad; 4 Hospital Corps Schools and more that 8 Military Sea Transport Service ships."[53] Plus, let us never forget, the three hospital ships rotating in the Korean waters.

In September, a new Naval Hospital is commissioned at St. Alban's in New York.[54] Then in October the US Naval Hospital at Corona, California is re-established.

December 1951 and the Reserves with WWII service (those who were recalled involuntarily) are released from active duty when they have completed seventeen months of active service. Also, on December 14, Lieutenant Commander Maxine Moesser is the first Navy Nurse Corps Officer to recommission (or commission) a naval vessel; the USS LST664 at the Naval Air Station, Jacksonville, Florida.[55]

As for Nurse Corps' Uniforms, the Director of the Nurse Corps sends a Memorandum, dated 19 February 1951, to all Nurse Corps Officers. It is a five page memo that describes in detail each type of uniform and each article of the uniform, including insignias, shoes, handbags and all other accouterments. Sections of the memo provide clear descriptions of the new uniform regulations passed last year, as follows:

"2. Uniforms for all women of the naval service have been standardized. Articles of uniform previously authorized may be worn until 1 July 1952, or until the articles in question are no longer serviceable, whichever is earlier. However, the new style uniform should be procured if buying a new one.

3. Authorized naval uniforms for members of the nurse corps are listed below for your information and guidance in accordance with US Navy Uniform Regulations.

(a) The service dress blue uniform will follow the single breast design which has been worn by the Waves, except that the color will be dark blue instead of the navy blue and that the sleeve stripes and corps insignia will be gold.

(b) The white service dress uniform will be the present Wave white uniform with gilt buttons, the sleeve stripes will be white braid, the corps device will be yellow embroidery.

(c) The Indoor White Duty Uniform as prescribed.

(d) When authorized by the Commanding Officer, the gray indoor duty uniform may be worn by personnel while on duty in areas outside the continental limits of the United States where difficulty is experienced in the maintenance of white starched uniforms.

(e) The gray indoor duty cap, like the regulation white ward cap, will be worn when the gray seersucker dress is ward uniform. This will be worn with the present gold and velvet rank insignia. WHEN WORN AS A WARD UNIFORM THE TIE WILL BE OMITTED.

(f) The blue raincoat (dark blue with set-in sleeves) has been modified to provide shoulder straps, OPTIONAL UNTIL 1 JULY 1952, and MANDATORY ON AND AFTER THAT DATE. Effective 1 July 1952 the metal shoulder rank insignia will be worn on the shoulder strap of the raincoat AND NOT BEFORE. The old style raincoat may be worn with the new style uniform until 1 July 1952. .

(h) The combination hat will be the present Wave officer hat. It is well to remember that white gloves are worn with white hat covers and black gloves with black hat covers."

Further on in the memo, the manner of wearing the metal corps device is specified, "The corps device shall be placed in a position such that the longer dimension is at right angles to the upper edge of the collar with the stem of the leaf pointing down and curving slightly to the front.
WHITE SHIRT (when coat is not worn) and GRAY DRESS: Worn on the left collar tip so that the center of the insignia is approximately 1" from the bottom edge and 1" from the upper edge of the collar.
WHITE INDOOR DUTY UNIFORM: Worn on the left collar tip with the center of the insignia approximately 1" from the outside edge and 1" from the bottom edge of the collar."

The metal rank device then is allocated a similar position on the right collar tip. But when it comes to the garrison caps, "metal pin-on rank devices shall be worn on the right side of the garrison caps with the center of the insignia approximately 2" from the front edge and 1 1/4" from the bottom of the cap. The device shall be vertical. The miniature cap device is worn on the left side NOT THE MINIATURE NURSE CORPS DEVICE."

Under 'Neckties' the memo states, "Shall be one piece; of rayon or silk, black in color. They shall be tied in a square knot in front, under the collar opening, so that the two tie-ends are even in length and fall naturally. (The four-in-hand tie is worn with the double breasted suit [the previous official uniform].)"

Then, under 'Pins, Pencils, Jewelry' appears, "No pencils, pins, pens, handkerchiefs or jewelry shall be worn or carried exposed upon the uniform by any naval personnel except cuff links, as prescribed and authorized decorations, medals, ribbons, and insignia. No eccentricities of dress, such as earrings, shall be permitted." The memo also details the specifics of the green and the khaki uniforms of the Navy Flight Nurses.

Additionally, in 1951, General George C. Marshall establishes 'DACOWITS' which stands for Defense Advisory Committee On Women in The Services. This is a committee of notable civilian women, within the Department of Defense, responsible for policies pertaining to women in the military. The committee members are from high positions in the fields of religion, national organizations, health, education, professional services and the media. Generally, the Directors of the military Nurse Corps meet with the committee at least once a year.

By 1951 the needs for nurses are increasing. The "low birth rate of the depression years was seriously affecting the potential supply of student nurses. Then, too, as the need for nurses increased, competing opportunities for young women were also increasing."[56] The nationwide shortage of nurses is severe and despite the needs for professional nurses in the military, men nurses are still not eligible to join the Nurse Corps. "Men nurses were encouraged, however, by a memorandum sent to local draft boards early in 1951 by the director of the Selective Service System. It calls attention to 'the dire shortage of male nurses . . . especially in our state mental institutions. This communication points out that, although no blanket deferment is possible under existing law, . . . it would be advisable that male student nurses continue their training so that upon graduation they can help fill the large number of vacancies resulting from the [nationwide] critical shortage.'"[57] But, "The picture of nursing as a profession for men is changing. This is partially revealed by the enrollment for January, 1951. There were . . . more that 1000 men in 181 nursing schools, only three of which restricted enrolment to men. In a 10-year period the number of schools admitting men had almost trebled."[58]

1951 sees the end of the National Association of Colored Graduate Nurses. A "press release painstakingly enumerated the successes realized by the NACGN and thus attempted to justify its demise. The number of state associations prohibiting black nurses from membership had been reduced from a high of seventeen to five. The number of schools admitting all qualified students had risen from approximately 28 prior to World War II to 330 by 1950. It also emphasized that an unprecedented number of black nurses had been integrated into the staffs of hospitals, public-health agencies, and military and veterans' services."[59]

Over in Korea, "A huge new Chinese offensive began New Year's Day [of 1951]. The U. S. Eighth Army fell back to positions some seventy miles below the thirty-eighth parallel, again abandoning Seoul to the Communists. Criticized for miscalculating Chinese strength and intent, MacArthur lashed back at the administration for making him fight a limited war."[60] "But Truman believed that the fighting must be confined to Korea, and not be allowed to spread into a possible global war. Truman become angry when MacArthur made several public statements criticizing this policy. In April, 1951, Truman dismissed MacArthur, creating a nationwide furor."[61] "MacArthur returned to the United States and was wildly greeted. He addressed Congress and drew tears when he quoted an old army song saying, 'Old soldiers never die, they just fade away.'"[62] Despite all of this, armistice talks begin in July of 1951 and that's all that occurs as far as armistice goes; a lot of talk.

"Representatives of 52 countries met in San Francisco in September, 1951, to draw up a peace treaty with Japan. On September 8, diplomats from 49 of these countries signed the treaty. Czechoslovakia, Poland, and Russia opposed the terms of the pact and refused to sign."[63]

Despite the attempts at peace and talks on armistice, the world of 1952 is further in turmoil with countries struggling with new independence and self-government; the Mau Mau atrocities in Africa and middle East unrest and alienation. In the fall of 1952, the UN breaks off truce talks in Korea "because the Communists would not agree on one point insisted upon by the Allies. This was *voluntary repatriation of prisoners*. . . . The UN negotiators believed many North Koreans and Chinese had been forced into Communist armies and would prefer to live in South Korea."[64] So the battles and killing of this unpopular 'war' goes on. In addition, the Communists inflict Americans with "a technique that came to be known as 'brainwashing.' . . . Seventy-eight captured American airmen were subjected to psychological and physical torture in 1952 to make them confess to having waged germ warfare against North Korea, and thirty-eight of them did so. After the germ warfare charges were unsuccessfully brought to the United Nations, the U.S. delegate, Dr. Charles Mayo, described the brainwashing technique:

> The total picture presented is one of human beings reduced to a status lower than that of animals, filthy, full of lice, festered wounds full of maggots, their sickness regulated to a point just short of death, unshaven, without haircuts or baths for as much as a year, men in rags, exposed to the elements, fed with carefully measured minimum quantities and the lowest quality of food and unsanitary water served often in rusty cans, isolated, faced with squads of trained interrogators, bulldozed, deprived of sleep, and browbeaten with mental anguish."[65]

Back in the U.S., 1952 is another Presidential campaign year. President Truman announces that he will not run for another term. So, the Democrats choose Adlai E. Stevenson as their candidate and the Republicans select the popular General Dwight D. Eisenhower of the U.S. Army with Richard M. Nixon as Vice President. The Republican ticket wins, overwhelmingly.

As for the nursing profession in 1952, the Men's Nursing Section of the ANA is disbanded because, finally, "The interests of men members had been integrated in the total program of the association."[66] Also, in this year, the "National League for Nursing [is] organized;" and the National League of Nursing Education, the National Organization for Public Health Nursing and the Association of Collegiate Schools of Nursing are all dissolved.[67]

In May, Congress passes legislation for a 4% base pay increase and a 14% raise in allowances. For example, the base pay of an Ensign with less that two years service now becomes $222.30 per month and the base pay of a Captain with over 22 years service becomes $666.90 per month. Also, in May, for the second year in a row, a Senior Navy Nurse Corps conference is held at the National Navy Medical Center, Bethesda, Maryland. Senior nurses are able to discuss mutual problems and different solutions as well as meet with the Director and/or her staff members to learn more about policies and procedures.

June of 1952 brings out a Nurse Corps policy change that directs all initial appointments to the Navy Nurse Corps to be in the U.S. Naval Reserve (NC USNR.) No longer will a newly appointed nurse be able to join the Navy as a Regular Naval Officer (NC USN.) However, an Augmentation Program is established whereby the Reserves can become Regular Navy by way of a Permanent Augmentation Board. This Board decides which USNR officers, with several years of service, qualify for becoming USN. The decision is partially based on who can serve for twenty years of active service by the time they reach fifty years of age.[68]

On 11 July 1952, a "Nurse Corps' Indoctrination Center is established at the U.S. Naval Hospital, St. Albans, New York. All Nurse Corps officers reporting for active duty are ordered to attend this 5-week indoctrination course before reporting to their first duty assignment. LCDR Rita V. O'Neill NC USN is the Senior Nurse Corps Officer"[69] for the indoctrination. One of the new Navy Nurses for the first indoctrination course is Rachel Fine. She travels all the way from the West Coast and says, "The long train ride was and still is very vivid. Alone, away from home for the first time was frightening. First stop was Chicago, a change of trains on the other side of Chicago and on to New York City. Grand Central Station completely overwhelmed me. What was I doing here and where was St. Albans? The shore patrol didn't know but a Red Cab did. Boarding the Long Island railroad train . . . and arrival at St. Albans. On to the main gate with two over-loaded suitcases and a bus ride around the base [then] I was mistakenly let off at the WAVES quarters. I was informed the nurses quarters were across [the way.] So, with suitcases in hand, I finally arrived; late for the group meeting of the indoctrination class.

"The quarters had long passageways and many, many individual rooms in several wings. Meals were served at the hospital, about a half a mile away. Uniform fittings took place at the Naval Shipyard in Brooklyn.

The white civilian uniforms were worn until the ward whites were ready. . . . The main hospital was permanently constructed and leading off from the hospital was a long winding rampway with numerous wings jutting off. These were temporary wards used for the heavy influx of patients during WWII and the Korean Conflict. At the end of the rampway was the dependents' wards and clinics. During my tour at St. Albans, I was assigned to the temporary wards which we called 'splinterville'. . . . We attended classes to learn the Navy ways and language, how to march, and to qualify for the Red Cross course in swimming. The Quick magazine [a small weekly news magazine] published a picture of us jumping into the pool in our gray seersucker uniforms during the survival course."[70] (They had to learn how to abandon a sinking ship while fully clothed.[71])

Meantime, Navy Nurse Estelle Kalnoske Lange, Chief Nurse aboard the *Consolation*, receives her orders to the National Naval Medical Center at Bethesda, Maryland. (She and the Consolation's Captain, Captain Lange, had just married.) While at Bethesda, she works "in the 'tower' (which was the entire hospital in 1952)" where they occasionally had a VIP patient. "'I remember when President Truman was in the hospital and we couldn't find any bed long enough to fit him. I never knew he was so tall,' she said. 'All I can remember thinking is how embarrassed I was that his feet were sticking off the end of the bed. I mean, this was the President of the United States.'"[72]

On the Island of Guam, out in the Pacific, Navy Nurse Iris M. Stock says, "USNH Guam, at the time I had duty there, was still located in Butler Huts on Agana Point. Guam proved to be one of the most fun duty stations. We worked tropical hours and enjoyed our time off duty exploring the Island, going to the beach, and enjoying a social life. The squadrons were sent there for training and we often were allowed to go flying with the pilots.

"Two memorable experiences happened while I was stationed there, as far as nursing duties were concerned. My first experience in evacuating a hospital happened. I do not remember the name of this particular hurricane, but since the hospital was located in Butler Huts, we were directed to evacuate early one morning, to the Marine Barracks located at the naval supply depot. I was on night duty at the time, and when we went to Condition 2, I had the responsibility of packing equipment we would need to set-up a ward at the supply depot. Having no written directive at the time, it was a challenge to decide what would be needed, and to get it into a crate the dimensions of a . . . sea chest. The next morning we were ordered to evacuate the hospital. Patients that could be discharged were sent back to duty or, in the case of dependents, were sent home. I was assigned to the dependents' ward and I remember we had one patient in active labor. . . . [so] they took a delivery table with us.

"It was quite a sight seeing patients with IV's and drainage bags climbing on buses. We remained at the Marine Barracks until 2100 that night. By that time . . . everyone was glad to get back to our usual quarters. I remember the dependents' ward was a sea of water and the nurses' station was wet and soggy looking. The ward was built with a large overhanging roof and a screened veranda went entirely around the ward. Otherwise there was no protection from the weather. . . . (The woman [in active labor] did deliver a small girl while at the naval supply depot and I had the honor of carrying the infant home in the ambulance on our return.)"[73]

Navy Nurse Carolyn Shearer has duty at a two nurse duty station also out in the Pacific. "My most memorable duty. It was probably Midway Island. Midway is 136 miles east of the International Date Line. . . . It's located almost in the center of the Pacific. It's the home of the famous Gooney birds and Moaning birds. . . . At night, these Moaning birds . . . burrow and nest in the ground and they cry in the night like a tortured human being. So when we first arrived there we had to get used to the squalling and carrying on in the night. . . .

"The island is approximately two and a half square miles long versus one and a half miles wide. When landing on the island, they said, 'Look down there, nurse, there's your new home.' It looked about the size of my little finger . . . it had water all around, beautiful reefs, but it was mighty small. I used to walk around the island everyday just for exercise. It was a small place.

"This island was used as a refueling base for aircraft that needed refueling or if they had trouble. . . . Our [the medical personnel] main reason for being on Midway was to care for the few wives that needed periodic medical attention. There were not that many there because of the [lack of] housing. [Also, the MATS planes with flight nurses stopped there with their wounded from Korea, at times.] . . . We also gave a hand to the flight nurses because at that time they were pretty worn out. . . .

"If there was a plane that was going to be grounded for a while, . . . we'd know the plane was coming in and, God bless those wives [at Midway], . . . their husbands would call and they would start to bake cookies. When the plane would land, they would take the cookies. . . . I always thought it was a wonderful gesture that they would do this. [These wounded were from Korea and some were serious cases.] . . . We had, as far as staff goes, two Navy Nurses, one doctor and one dentist and a group of corpsmen." They helped the flight nurses as much as they could and gave the worn out flight nurses some respite.

"I think Midway Island was thirty feet above sea level; that was the highest spot on the island. If there was any kind of a question of there being a tidal wave, we had to run up to the top of this hill. This did actually happen one night. We were told there would be a tidal wave. The Marines came by with their loud speakers and told us to go immediately. We ran to the top of the hill about three o'clock in the morning. The tide did come in high but it was not as bad as expected."[74]

Navy Nurse Rita Beatty, recalled to active duty, has duty aboard the USS *Consolation*. "When I arrived a big communist offensive was under way. During the first four days, nurses, doctors and corpsmen worked around the clock getting as little as eight hours sleep for the entire four day period. In one 24-hour period, as many as 62 helicopters were landed on the small flight deck located on the ship's fantail.

"The mobility of a floating hospital ship, plus the use of helicopters enabled a casualty to receive comprehensive medical and nursing attention within minutes after being wounded. No one can say exactly how many lives had been saved by this new and extraordinary method of casualty evaluation, but many critically wounded patients would not have lived without the prompt treatment.

"Not only did the ship's nursing and medical staff care for casualties but, having been exposed to the poverty, the homeless and orphans in Inchon [Korea], community health service also become part of their focus. They provided care to the sick babies and children at the Star of the Sea Orphanage at Inchon.

"Occasionally children and adults were brought to the *Consolation* with wounds as battles raged through their villages. They were brave children and adults who suffered stoically and smiled rarely. As a result of the invasion of South Korea by the communists, this action was not officially designated as a war. The realities of the casualties and the devastated Koreans were nonetheless harsh. . . .

"I had the privilege of having duty with Captain Edwina Todd, who was my Chief Nurse aboard the USS *Consolation*. She impressed me as a woman of courage. During World War II having been a war prisoner for 37 months in a civilian prison camp in the Philippines, near Manila, where she endured many hardships and suffering and provided nursing care to inmates under the poorest conditions, she returned to the invasion scene without fear, bitterness or hostility to care for and ensure that casualties and others received the nursing care needed to save their lives. She was a courageous woman."[75]

Navy Nurse Nancy Crosby is aboard the USS Haven in the waters off Inchon. She says, "Periodically the battles intensified and we were working around the clock with four hours off. We were caring for over 575 patients with about 30 nurses, 30 doctors and [many] corpsmen. When the fighting subsided, several of the nurses, including me, were invited to visit three of the forward Medical companies. Two large copters flew us North to the 'A' Medical company six miles from the front lines. Navy corpsmen and doctors cared for the Marine Corps wounded here. It closely resembled the `MASH' TV series without nurses. The Marine Corps was responsible for the western sector and the Army held the area further east.

"At the front it seemed 110 degrees in the shade but no one seemed to mind our damp seersucker uniforms and dusty high heeled shoes. The men at the front had not seen American women for many months. Patients even wore pajama bottoms in our honor.

"Jeeps then moved us to 'E' med. The beds in these forward areas were only stretchers with wool blankets used for padding. And over the loud speaker someone was playing music from 'South Pacific.'

"On our way to 'C' med unit, three miles from the front, we drove past the United Nations' camp, housing our conference teams near Panmunjom. 'C' med had just received eleven patients so their operating room teams were busy.

"We walked to the copter landing pad atop a hill and watched an American air attack 5-6 miles north. Large clumps of smoke/dust were visible and the deep `thump' sound soon followed. It seemed so odd to be so close to the enemy. . . . The helicopters landed and we were returned to the ship.

"The most frightening experience of the entire day was having to climb the 'Jacob's' ladder from the barge [copter landing pad] tied alongside the ship. Your feet swung 3 feet toward the side of the ship while you hands reached up and back beyond your head. It was about a two story climb - in high heels. No one fell.

"In mid August, Dr. . . . was killed. He walked into the spinning rear blade of a small helicopter delivering patients. He died within twenty minutes.

"The hospital ship '*Repose*' eventually arrived to relieve us. We transferred the less seriously wounded, received the sickest patients from the '*Jutlandia*' [Danish hospital ship] and left for Japan."[76]

"In March of 1953, the *Repose* is back in the States for repairs and renovations, then she returns to the Korean waters in June. She sails for Yokosuka, Japan on 1 August, arriving on 2 August and transferring 350 patients to the Naval Hospital there. And what is it like at the hospital when massive numbers of casualties start arriving? From personal experience I recall the patients from a hospital ship coming in to the Yokosuka Naval Hospital, one after another and in groups. I remember, on one occasion, that it is getting dark when word is passed for all off-duty nurses to report to the hospital at once. We are given assignments as we report in. Most of us are sent directly to the wards where the patients are being admitted. These are all battle casualties and they are all bloody, muddy and still in battle fatigues. Their wounds are covered but the ship personnel had not had time to clean the patients and the battlefield mud is still on them. The patients had come to the ship directly from battle and with so many patients at once, only the wounds could be cared for. The Yokosuka Naval Hospital operating room is already taking care of the most urgent cases; two operating tables - two surgeries - in the OR rooms that can accommodate them. On the wards, most of us who had been off duty are put to work cleaning the mud and blood and getting the patients into clean hospital pajamas. We have no time to talk or even think, we just keep going; the only thought being to get these patients and their wounds clean and cared for. At one point, late in the night, I look across the open ward and there is the Chief Nurse, Minnie Overton, bending over a bed cleaning the mud-caked feet and legs of a young Marine. We are all in this together; this is why we are here. These patients are so exhausted they sleep while we clean them and those that are somewhat awake are so weary they can't talk. Sometime, just before dawn, it is done. Only now, at this point in time, are we tired and aware of our surroundings."

The USS *Haven* is doing the same type of work in the same areas. The Chief Nurse at this time is Lieutenant Eleanor Harrington; the Chief Nurse of the *Benevolence* when it sank. In an article for the American Journal of Nursing, Chief Nurse Harrington gives a brief description of her ship, "The USS *Haven* is a floating hospital that can accommodate 795 patients. She can be moved to any port where her facilities are needed. Besides the nursing staff [30 nurses], she carries a staff of 25 doctors, 3 Medical Service Corps officers, 194 hospital corpsmen, 3 dental officers, and 6 dental corpsmen in addition to the line crew, whose teamwork is always at our service. . . . The 18 wards aboard the ship vary in size and will take from 26 to 58 patients. The double-decker bunks have comfortable mattresses, and the orthopedic wards are equipped with fracture beds which have appliances for any necessary traction. All the lower bunks have regular standard hospital frames and can be adjusted to the patients' needs. Small trays fastened to the bunks replace the more familiar bedside stands and help to keep the patients' personal belongings within reach. Each bunk is equipped with a bedside lamp as well as earphones over which the patient can hear the transcribed programs from the Armed Forces Radio Service and the religious services from the ship's improvised chapel.

"Most of the wards have their own diet kitchens, equipped with electric food-warming tables from which piping hot food can be served. Also included in the hospital spaces are three large operating rooms, pathology laboratory, and x-ray and physiotherapy departments. An EENT clinic is equipped with its own operating room and optical laboratory. A complete dental clinic and the latest electrocardiographic and encephalographic machines complete a modern general hospital."[77]

One of the nurses aboard the USS *Haven*, Reinelda Vickey, says, "We shared duty with the USS *Consolation* and the USS *Repose*. Our ship was more unique as it had a neon red cross. One ship was always in the States for overhaul maintenance and the other two alternated tours in Inchon, Korea and Yokosuka, Japan. Sometimes the Danish ship, *Jutlandia*, shared duty with us. She was a beautiful sailing ship and was the envy of the fleet when all her sails were unfurled. . . .

"The truce delegates had been struggling for two years to achieve peace in the Korean war. Finally the truce was signed on 27 July 1953 in Panmunjom, Korea. Operation 'Big Switch' began and the flight deck was busy receiving wounded POW's. Flight quarters were a constant echo. Some of the POW's were from the Turkish Army. All had black hair and mustaches and they all looked alike. All of our fighting forces said they were fierce fighters. We had a Chinese POW with a head injury. The doctors thought he died mainly from fright as the ambulatory Turkish patients kept walking by his room. A Marine guard was assigned to keep the Turks from harming him. . . .

"I was in charge of the operating room and we operated day and night for 48 hours. The ship's crew and many of the ambulatory patients assisted with minor chores - folding linen and running errands. The laundry personnel collected and delivered clean linen throughout the crisis. This was usually the job of the operating room corpsmen. It was wonderful to have so much help even though the linen was folded wrong or other simple tasks were not done properly. The patients were grateful to be aboard the ship and needed to express their gratitude. The corpsmen and nurses in the operating room appreciated the assistance given by the patients and the ship's personnel.

"The ship received orders to leave Inchon, Korea on 20 August 1953. The ship's crew were at their stations and anxiously awaiting the arrival of our sister ship. As the ship came into the harbor we were ready to depart before she dropped anchor. Salutes were exchanges, as always. We departed for Yokosuka, Japan . . . before sailing nonstop to the USA. . . .

"We approached the Golden Gate Bridge after midnight and dropped anchor. We waited for the port pilot to complete our journey. On the morning of 4 September, we sailed under the Golden Gate Bridge for Alameda, California. Arriving in the USA and sailing under the Golden Gate Bridge gives one the same thrill as seeing the lighted torch in the hand of the Statue of Liberty. Both are the gateway to the USA and each a symbol of America.

"We debarked all our patients. It was a wonderful day for all of us, but especially for the POW's. We were greeted with much fanfare. The USS *Haven* then sailed to San Pedro, California for her yearly overhaul. The medical personnel were given TAD orders to other hospitals or dispensaries. I stayed at the dispensary at Long Beach, California."[78]

Lt(jg) Rachel Fine tells us of receiving orders to Guam in 1953. She says, "It was during the Christmas season that a troop plane carrying servicemen who were going home on leave, left Anderson Air Force Base [on Guam], only to fly out over the water and turning back, crashed into the housing area at Anderson. It was a horrible accident. The plane took out three rows of housing. At 0500, patients began to arrive, some hemorrhaging, others badly burned."[79] "As we were the only military hospital, we got all the survivors; approximately twenty. Most of [the casualties] had died from third degree burns over most of their bodies. The majority of the nurses volunteered for special duty, as each survivor required at least one nurse and two corpsmen on each shift. This meant sixteen to twenty hour duty for most of us. Tragically, only a very few survived due mainly to the severity of their burns, and lack of a modern burn center, not to neglect or effort. The unselfish devotion of nurses, doctors, and corpsmen was wondrous to behold."[80]

Back in the States, nurse Miriam Sherman states, "I came into the Navy on May 1, 1953 and reported to St. Albans [New York] for indoctrination. One of the things that they had us do, which was compulsory, was survival at sea . . . I don't believe they do this anymore in orientation, and if they did, they wouldn't have to do it like we did; in the white ward uniforms. They took us to the pool - we reported to the indoor pool - you wore your white [ward] uniform. You didn't wear your girdle but you put a bathing suit on under your uniform. Our white ward uniforms were [fastened] two thirds with buttons and the lower third was sewed up. You wore your white stockings and your white shoes. Of course, at that time we had long sleeves. We did not wear a cap for this performance. The idea was that you jump off the high diving board at the deepest end of the pool, you swim a little way out and you take off your uniform. The whole idea is that if the ship is going down and you're at sea, you know how to jump off of the ship, land in the water and save your life. The instructions were; jump off of the diving board, swim half way down the pool, first remove your shoes, once you tread water then remove one shoe, hold it in your mouth with the shoelace . . . remove the other shoe . . . tie the shoelaces together and then put the shoes around your neck. The reason for that is, after you abandon ship you swim to shore and you have shoes because of coral or anything else [necessitating] . . . shoes.

"The second thing is to take off your stockings (mine landed in the pool) but you had to take off your stockings treading water. Then you took off your uniform. . . . You must step out of the uniform because if you slip it over your head, you could hang yourself and drown. . . . Then when you get out of the uniform you swing the uniform around and you get air in the one sleeve and you tie the cuff together so you have an air pocket. Then, you swing the other sleeve around and you tie that cuff together. Then, you swing the uniform around up in the air and with the two cuffs [individually] tied, you have air wings and it really works. [Supports you in the water.] Well, I jumped off the diving board and I've never jumped off a diving board that high in my like, and that deep of water. I jumped off the first time and I forgot to hold my breath. I jumped off the second time and I held my breath but I forgot to hold down my uniform. When you jump in the water you are supposed to balloon out your uniform - it will help you float. So, I forgot to balloon out my uniform and I landed in the water. The third time I was scared because I couldn't get my shoes off. . . . The fourth time . . . I managed to get my shoes off, tied together around my neck, and I forgot to balloon out my uniform again. The fifth time, I did everything right but my nylon stockings landed in the bottom of the pool and I never bothered retrieving them. But, I think it is important that we know about this survival. . . . I did say to one of my classmates, 'look, if that ship goes down, I'm not going to waste any time thinking about doing all of this, I'm just going to jump and swim as fast as I can.'"[81]

In March of 1953, the first Navy Nurse is assigned to a Naval Dispensary in Izmir, Turkey. In May the Congress passes legislation that provides "for direct appointment of qualified nurses to the Nurse Corps, U.S. Navy in the grade of Ensign between ages of 21 and 27; in grade of Lieutenant junior grade between ages of 28 and 30 years."[82] June 1953 sees an age increase for the Nurse Corps' Augmentation program. Reserve nurses up to age 55 can now apply for transfer to the Regular Navy.[83] In July the census of the Nurse Corps is 2600; 1292 are Regular Navy and 1308 are Reserve nurses on active duty.[84] In September, Lt(jg) Gizella Papp (NC) USN is the flight nurse selected to represent the Nurse Corps at the National Aircraft Show in Dayton, Ohio. (Miss Papp, a flight nurse, had her picture on the cover of Newsweek in 1950 as she was the first nurse to accompany patients in the C47 plane.)[85] Then on 31 December, the Augmentation "program for reserve nurses to regular Nurse Corps is discontinued."[86]

Navy Nurses served with honor and distinction during this Korean war time. (True, it was not to be labeled a 'war' but it certainly had all the ingredients of one and the casualties would undoubtedly agree with that.) Three Navy Nurses receive the Navy Bronze Star medal for their service during this time; LCdr. Estelle Kalnoske (Lange) as Chief Nurse on the *Consolation*, Lt. Ruth Cohen as Chief Nurse on the *Haven*, and Lt. Eleanor Harrington as Chief Nurse aboard the *Haven*. Six other Navy Nurses receive a Commendation with Ribbon; LCdr. Alberta S. Burk as Chief Nurse at the Yokosuka Naval Hospital, Lt. Althea Allegier for duty at the Yokosuka Dispensary, Lt. Edna Daughtry for duty aboard the *Repose*, Lt. Annette Baer for duty aboard the *Repose*, Lt(jg) Barbara Taurish for duty in Navy Flight Nursing, Lt. Sarah J. Griffin (Chapman) for duty in the Rehabilitation Unit at Oakland Naval Hospital.[87] (Miss Griffin (Chapman) was "an amputee (left foot) as a result of an accident in June 1947, while on active duty . . . [she] volunteered and returned to active duty to work in the program for rehabilitation of amputees at U.S. Naval Hospital, Oakland, California during the Korean Conflict. She was released from active duty on 8 January 1953 following her marriage."[88]) And, there are ninety Navy Unit Commendations awarded during this time.

The Korean truce was signed on the 27th of July 1953. "The armistice was accepted as a stalemate, the first war America didn't win."[89] "An exchange of 88,559 prisoners of war was completed in September. The Neutral Nations' Repatriation Commission forces took custody of prisoners who refused to return home. The armistice agreement provided that delegates from home countries could visit these prisoners and persuade them to return. But after the talks, 14,227 Chinese, 7,582 North Koreans, 325 South Koreans, 21 Americans, and 1 Briton still refused repatriation."[90] "As peace came to the war-torn land [of Korea] and bewildered prisoners were exchanged . . . Americans assessed the 'police action' in which they suffered 140,000 casualties."[91] A little over 54,000 Americans died in two and one-half years. It was an unpopular war. The American public did not, as a whole, give its support and the service people felt it. As quoted in a newspaper article, another veteran says it for all of us, "'We came home with all the emotional scars war puts on a man [or woman] and families looked at us as if we'd been nowhere at all.'"[92]

President Eisenhower begins his term in office in 1953 by setting "up a staff system based on that of the Army. He made each Cabinet officer or other executive responsible for an area of government affairs. Sherman Adams, Assistant to the President, was 'chief of staff.' He coordinated the work of all these officials, freeing the President of many routine jobs. Several weeks after Eisenhower took office, the Department of Health, Education, and Welfare was created. . . . Mrs. Oveta Culp Hobby became the first secretary of the department."[93] Mrs. Hobby had organized and directed the WAC in WWII.

As for other affairs of the world, in March 1953 the Russian Premier and Communist dictator, Joseph Stalin, died suddenly. In June, "the East German workers rebelled against their 'peoples' government'; they were put down by Russian tanks."[94] The Russians, in August 1953, detonated a hydrogen bomb and in the spring of 1954, the U.S. explodes a bomb "100 times more destructive than any previous man-made blast."[95]

Over in Southeast Asia, events are building to a boiling point. To explain; back in 1945, at the Potsdam Conference between President Truman, Premier Stalin and Prime Minister Churchill, and "just before the Japanese defeat, the question of who would take control of Indochina and accept the Japanese surrender was resolved by a secret decision of the Allies that the country below the 16th parallel would be placed under British command and that north of the 16th under Chinese. Since the British were obviously dedicated to colonial restoration, this decision ensured a French return. . . . A week after the Japanese surrender in August 1945, a Viet-Minh congress in Hanoi [north of the 16th parallel] proclaimed the Democratic Republic of Vietnam and after taking control in Saigon [south of the 16th parallel] declared its independence, quoting the opening phrases of the American Declaration of Independence of 1776. In a message to the UN transmitted by the OSS, Ho Chi Minh warned that if the UN failed to fulfill the promise of its charter and failed to grant independence to Indochina, 'we will keep on fighting until we get it.'"[96] The French eventually take charge and, no surprise, fighting takes place. "Conclusion of the Korean armistice in July 1953 had raised a new alarm that China might transfer its forces to aid a Communist victory in Vietnam. The Viet-Minh had succeeded in opening supply lines to China and they were receiving fuel and ammunition that had risen from a trickle of ten tons a month to more than 500 tons a month. . . . It was recognized that the French could win only if they gained the genuine political and military partnership of the Vietnamese people; that this was not developing and would not, given French reluctance to transfer real authority . . . In the meantime, in proportion as a French slide appeared imminent, American aid [to the French] increased. Bombers, cargo planes, naval craft, tanks, trucks, automatic weapons, small arms and ammunition, artillery shells, radios, hospital and engineering equipment plus financial support flowed heavily in 1953."[97] "By 1953 French domestic opinion had grown weary and disgusted with an endless war for a cause unacceptable to many French citizens. . . . Although the United States was paying most of the bill, the French people, assisted by the Communist propaganda, were increasing clamor against the war and mounting heavy political pressure for a negotiated settlement."[98] This, then, is the Vietnam situation in early 1954.

To return to the U.S. Navy; on 8 January 1954, the Navy Department issues an ALNAV that permits resignation from active service "upon completion of four years active service plus any additional service obligated by assignment under instruction."[99] (If the Navy sends you to school, you are obligated pay back with a certain number of years of active duty.)

In the Navy Nurse Corps, a large event takes place: the Director of the Corps (Captain Winnie Gibson) is placed on the retired list as of 1 May 1954. When asked what she feels was her greatest achievement during her term as Director, she answers, "My greatest achievement was promoting the increases in ranks of the nurses in the Nurse Corps."[100] She doesn't mention the trials and tribulations of being Director during the Korean Conflict and all that entailed.

During her career Captain Gibson received the American Defense Service Medal, Base Clasp; the Asiatic-Pacific Campaign Medal; the American Campaign Medal, and the World War II Victory Medal. Captain Gibson retired to live in Ohio but, as of this writing, now lives in the state of Texas.

[1]   DeWitt, Winnie Gibson Palmer Capt. Navy Nurse Corps, *Oral History Interview Tape Transcript*, Interviewer LCdr Barbara Thomas Tucker Navy Nurse Corps, 16 July 1989.

[2]   Information prepared by the Navy Nurse Corps Officers on the staff of the Director of the Navy Nurse Corps, 1991.

[3]   *The World Book Encyclopedia*, Field Enterprises Educational Corporation, Chicago, Volume 11, 1966 edition, p. 297.

[4]   Wells, H.G., *The Outline of History*, Revised and brought up to date by Raymond Postgate, Garden City Books, Garden City, New York, Volume II, 1961, p. 959.

[5]   *The World Book Encyclopedia*, op. cit., Volume 11, p. 298

[6]   Dvorchak, Robert, "Lessons of Forgotten War still learned today," Daytona Beach Sunday News-Journal, 25 July 1993, p. 7A.

[7]   *The World Book Encyclopedia*, op. cit., Volume 18, p. 386.

[8]   Tuchman, Barbara W., *The March of Folly From Troy to Vietnam*, Ballantine Books, New York, 1985, p. 247.

[9]   *200 Years, A Bicentennial Illustrated History of the United States*, Joseph Newman, Directing Editor, Books by U.S. News & World Report, Inc., 2300 N Street, N.W., Washington, D.C. 20037, 1973, book 2, p. 235.

[10]   *The World Book Encyclopedia*, op. cit., Volume 18, p. 384.

[11]   Roberts, Mary M. R.N., *AMERICAN NURSING*, The Macmillan Company, New York, 1963, pp. 485, 488, 489, 490.

[12]   Ibid., p. 668.

[13]   Laird, LCDR Thelma NC USNR, Jones, LCDR Dorothy NC USN, Feeney, LCDR Elizabeth NC USN, Seidl, CDR Elizabeth NC USN (Ret.), Blaska, CDR Burdette NC USN, *Chronological History NAVY NURSE CORPS*, Prepared by: Nursing Division, Bureau of Medicine and Surgery, 1 August 1962, p. 39.

[14]   "Navy Nurse Corps - A Pictorial Review," *Navy Medical Newsletter*, Captain M.T. Lynch MC USN, Editor, Vol. 55, No. 5, May 1970, p. 8.

[15]   Ibid..

[16]   Wheeler, Marion Caesar Captain Navy Nurse Corps, *Oral History Interview Tape Transcript*, Interviewers Cdr Anna Corcoran Navy Nurse Corps and Cdr Irene Sullivan Navy Nurse Corps, 18 July 1991.

[17]   Deus, Ruth Martin LT Navy Nurse Corps, *Oral History Interview Tape Transcript*, Self interview, 1 February 1990.

[18]   Venverloh, Dorothy J. LCdr Navy Nurse Corps, *Oral History Interview Tape Transcript*, Interviewer LCdr Kathleen Laughlin Donnelly Navy Nurse Corps, 17 April 1990.

[19]   Deus, op. cit..

[20]   Venerloh, op. cit..

[21]   Deus, op. cit..

[22]   Venerloh, op. cit..

[23]   Deus, op. cit..

[24]   Ibid..

[25]   Venerloh, op. cit..

[26]   Wheeler, op. cit..

[27]   Brooks, Helen Louise Captain Navy Nurse Corps, *Oral History Interview Tape Transcript*, Self interview, 27 July 1990.

[28]   Ibid..

[29]   Ibid..

[30]   Yates, Bill, Journal staff writer, "Veteran nurse reminisces," The Journal, National Naval Medical Center, Bethesda, MD 20814-5000, Vol. 2, No. 18, May 10, 1990, p. 4. The article contains a copy of this letter written by Cdr Estelle Kalnoske Lange while on the USS *Consolation* (AH-15) and is dated 24 December 1950.

[31]   Code 15, BUMED, "Angel of the Orient," *Navy Medical Newsletter*, Captain M.T. Lynch MC USN, Editor, Vol. 55, No. 4, April 1970, p. 11.

[32]   McClean, Eveline Kittilson LT Navy Nurse Corps, *Oral History Interview Tape Transcript*, Self interview, 4 July 1990.

[33]   Ibid..

[34]   Cornelius, Dolores Captain Navy Nurse Corps, *Oral History Interview Tape Transcript*, Self interview, 2 January 1991.

[35]   Ramsey, Esther Captain Navy Nurse Corps Reserve, *Oral History Interview Tape Transcript*, Self interview, 26 June 1992.

[36]   Twyman, Florence Alwyn CDR Navy Nurse Corps, *Oral History Interview Tape Transcript*, Interviewer LCdr Dorothea Short Tracy Navy Nurse Corps, 9 August 1989.

[37]   Ellis, Barbara CDR Navy Nurse Corps, *Oral History Interview Tape Transcript*, Interviewer CDR Claire M. Walsh Navy Nurse Corps, 25 August 1990.

[38]   Houp, Geraldine A. Captain Navy Nurse Corps, *Oral History Interview Tape Transcript*, Interviewer LT Helen Barry Siragusa Navy Nurse Corps, 9 May 1990.

[39]   Ibid..

40   McClean, op. cit..
41   Code 15, BUMED, "Angel of the Orient," *Navy Medical Newsletter*, op. cit..
42   "'Women In White' Help Guard Your Health," *All Hands* (a magazine for Naval Personnel), February 1953. This quote is from a reprint of said article.
43   Ibid..
44   Thom, Geraldine M. Carey LCdr Navy Nurse Corps, *Written Personal History*, 18 June 1991.
45   Siragusa, Helen Barry LT Navy Nurse Corps, *Oral History Interview Tape Transcript*, Self Interview, 25 April 1990.
46   George, Evelyn Hope Navy Nurse Corps, *Oral History Interview Tape Transcript*, Interviewer Lt(jg) Irene Smith Matthews Navy Nurse Corps, 17 June circa 1970.
47   Larson, (Linn) Margaret LCdr Navy Nurse Corps, *Oral History Interview Tape Transcript*, Interviewer LCdr Jan Barcott Navy Nurse Corps, 1 April 1990.
48   Ibid..
49   Goble, CDR Dorothy Jones, NC USN (Ret.), as written in her unpublished history research notes.
50   Ibid..
51   Ibid..
52   Ibid..
53   Laird, et al., op. cit..
54   Goble, op. cit..
55   Ibid..
56   Roberts, Mary M. R.N., op. cit., p. 471.
57   Ibid., p. 322.
58   Ibid..
59   Hine, Darlene Clark, *Black Women In White: Racial Conflict and Cooperation in the Nursing Profession, 1890-1950*, Indiana University Press, Bloomington & Indianapolis, 1989, p. 185.
60   *200 Years, A Bicentennial Illustrated History of the United States*, op. cit., p. 239.
61   *The World Book Encyclopedia*, op. cit., Volume 18, p. 386.
62   *200 Years, A Bicentennial Illustrated History of the United States*, op. cit., p. 240.
63   *The World Book Encyclopedia*, op. cit., Volume 20, p. 412.
64   Ibid., Volume 11, p. 303.
65   *200 Years, A Bicentennial Illustrated History of the United States*, op. cit., p. 241.
66   Roberts, Mary M. R.N., op. cit., p. 319.
67   Ibid., p. 668.
68   Goble, op. cit..
69   Laird, et al., op. cit., p. 40.
70   Fine, Rachel A. Captain Navy Nurse Corps, *Oral History Interview Tape Transcript*, Self Interview, 29 August 1989.
71   Noble, Bob, of the N.Y. Herald Tribune, "Girls Overboard!," *Quick*, Cowles Magazines, Inc. Publisher of Quick and Look, Des Moines, Ia., Vol. 7, No. 8, 25 August, 1952.
72   Yates, Bill, Journal staff writer, "Veteran nurse reminisces," op. cit..
73   Stock, Iris M. LCdr Navy Nurse Corps, *Oral History Interview Tape Transcript*, Self Interview, 25 June 1990.
74   Shearer, Carolyn Jean LCdr Navy Nurse Corps, *Oral History Interview Tape Transcript*, Interviewer LT Helen Barry Siragusa Navy Nurse Corps, 12 March 1991.
75   Beatty, Rita T. LT Navy Nurse Corps, *Oral History Interview Tape Transcript*, Self Interview, 26 February 1990.
76   Crosby, Nancy CDR Navy Nurse Corps, *Oral History Interview Tape Transcript*, Interviewer CDR Joan McIntyre Navy Nurse Corps, 24 November 1990.
77   Harrington, Eleanor LT Navy Nurse Corps, "Aboard A Hospital Ship," *The American Journal of Nursing*, Vol. 53, Mo. 5, May 1953.
78   Vickey, Reinelda E. LCdr Navy Nurse Corps, *Oral History Interview Tape Transcript*, Interviewer Captain Rose Marie Lochte Navy Nurse Corps, 9 March 1991.
79   Fine, R., op. cit..
80   Eberhardt, Marie CDR Navy Nurse Corps, *Oral History Interview Tape Transcript*, Self interview, 19 May 1990.
81   Sherman, Miriam CDR Navy Nurse Corps, *Oral History Interview Tape Transcript*, Self interview, 7 August 1990.
82   Laird, et al., op. cit., p. 41.
83   Goble, op. cit..
84   Laird, et al., op. cit..
85   Goble, op. cit..
86   Laird, et al., op. cit..
87   Goble, op. cit.
88   Laird, et al., op. cit. p. 40.
89   Dvorchak, Robert, op. cit..
90   *The World Book Encyclopedia*, op. cit., Volume 11, p. 304.
91   *200 Years, A Bicentennial Illustrated History of the United States*, op. cit., p. 243.
92   Hill, William D.A., "America's forgotten soldiers," Daytona Beach News-Journal, 25 May 1992.
93   *The World Book Encyclopedia*, op. cit., Volume 6, p. 108.
94   Wells, H.G., op. cit., p. 960.
95   *200 Years, A Bicentennial Illustrated History of the United States*, op. cit., p. 244.

96   Tuchman, Barbara W., *The March of Folly From Troy to Vietnam*, op. cit., pp. 239, 240.

97   Ibid., pp. 254, 255.

98   Ibid., p. 257.

99   Laird, et al., op. cit. p. 41.

100   DeWitt, Winnie Gibson Palmer Captain Navy Nurse Corps, *Oral History Interview Tape Transcript*, Interviewer LCdr Barbara Thomas Tucker Navy Nurse Corps, 16 July 1989.

". . . On Sunday morning, August 27th [1950],
the 522 foot *Benevolence* lay on her side
in shallow coastal waters
with the big red cross on her white hull
showing through the waves washing over her. . . ."

☆ ☆ ☆

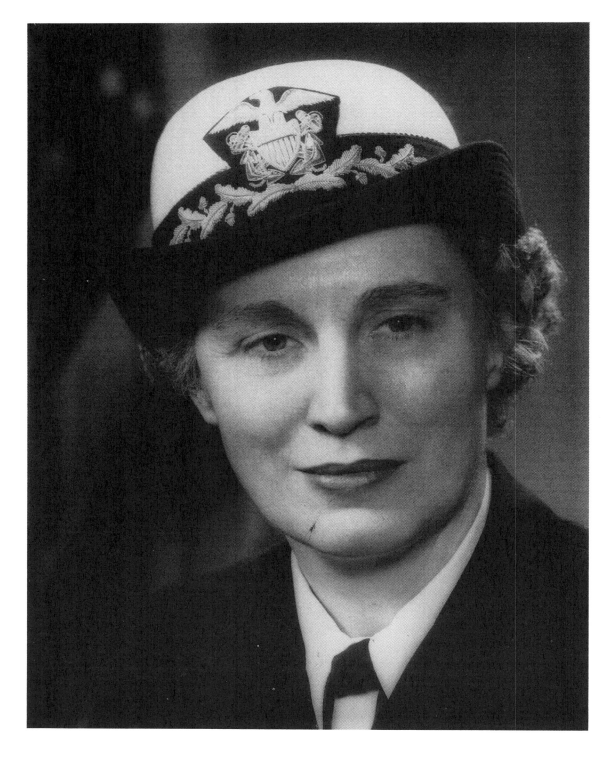

Director - Captain W. Leona Jackson
(Official U.S. Navy photo courtesy of Nursing Division, Bureau of Medicine and Surgery, Navy Department.)

CHAPTER 9

Director - Captain W. Leona Jackson
(1954 - 1958)

☆☆☆

Commander Leona Jackson is Chief Nurse of the Naval Hospital at Portsmouth, Virginia when she learns of her selection for the top position in the Navy Nurse Corps. On 1 May 1954, Captain Leona Jackson takes the position of Director of the U.S. Navy Nurse Corps. This is the same Navy nurse who was captured by the Japanese on Guam during World War II then became a Prisoner of War in Japan.

Leona Jackson was born in September 1909 at Union, Ohio. She graduated from Butler Centralized School in Vandalia, Ohio in 1927. From there she went into nurses' training at Miami Valley Hospital, Dayton, Ohio. She graduated in September of 1930. On 6 July 1936 Miss Jackson was appointed to the Nurse Corps. Her first duty station was the Naval Hospital, Philadelphia, Pennsylvania and on 5 July 1939 she was transferred to the Naval Hospital in Brooklyn, New York. From there she went, briefly, to the Naval Hospital, Mare Island, California in late 1940, then to the U.S. Naval Hospital, Guam, Marianas Islands. When the Japanese came ashore, in December 1941, the Naval Hospital personnel were taken prisoners of war. All of the Navy nurses were taken to Japan in January 1942 then repatriated in August of 1942. On the 29th of August 1942 Ensign Jackson reported to the US Naval Hospital Bethesda, Maryland. From there she reported to the Office of Naval Officer Procurement, Washington, D.C. for duty in public relations and nurse procurement. She was promoted to Lieutenant (junior grade) in February 1943. In April 1944 she began eight months of duty at the Bureau of Medicine and Surgery in the Nurse Corps' Personnel Division. In November 1944 she was promoted to full Lieutenant. The next month Lt. Jackson reported to Fleet Hospital #103 on the island of Guam, then from January to December 1945 she was the Senior Nurse Corps Officer in the Island Command. "She received a Letter of Commendation, with authorization to wear the Commendation Ribbon, from the Commander in Chief, Pacific Fleet, as follows:

> 'For meritorious service while serving as Supervisor, U.S. Navy Nurses, Guam, Marianas Islands, from 19 January to 2 September 1945. Lieutenant Jackson was of outstanding assistance in solving many trying problems in a period of unsettled conditions during early hospital construction and development on Guam. She rendered valuable service in the supervision of assignment of nurses to U.S. Navy and Military Government hospitals, the efficient coordination of Nurse Corps activities in those hospitals and the liaison established between the Island Medical Office and the four U.S. Army hospitals on Guam. Her initiative, sound judgment and professional knowledge were important factors during the Iwo Jima and Okinawa Campaigns when large numbers of casualties were received on Guam, severely taxing the available hospital facilities. Her conduct and devotion to duty were an inspiration to all with whom she served and at all times in keeping with the highest traditions of the U.S. Naval Service.'"[1]

When Lt. Jackson returned to the States, she was assigned to the Navy Department at the Naval Dispensary in Washington, D.C.. In April 1946 she was promoted to Lieutenant Commander. In June of 1950 she had new duties as Education Officer in the Nursing Section of BuMed. From July 1950 to June 1952 the Navy assigned her to 'duty under instruction' at Columbia University in New York City. She received her Bachelor of Science and Master of Arts in Nursing Administration degrees. Then LCdr. Jackson served at the Naval Hospital, Oakland, California where she received her promotion to Commander. On December 29, 1953 she reported into the Naval Hospital, Portsmouth, Virginia as the Chief Nurse.[2]

The day following the new Director's appointment, 2 May, the Officer Grade Limitation Act of 1954 (Public Law #349) is passed. It provides "for an increase of temporary Commanders and Lieutenant Commanders in the Nurse Corps."[3] This is the legislation that Captain Winnie Gibson DeWitt fought for and perceives as her main accomplishment for the Nurse Corps.

But, back in Vietnam, events are taking place that will have long range effects on the world, the U.S. and on the Nurse Corps itself. "Early in 1954 forty B-26 bombers with 200 United States Air Force technicians in civilian clothes were dispatched to Indochina, and Congress appropriated $400 million plus another $385 million to finance the offense planned by General . . . in a last fevered burst of French military effort. By the time of the terminal catastrophe at Dien Bien Phu, a few months later, American investment in Indochina since 1946 had reached $2 billion and the United States was paying 80 percent of the French expenditure for the war . . . Like most such aid, the bulk of it trickles away into the pockets of profiteering officials. . . . On 7 May, Dien Bien Phu fell, giving the Viet-Minh a stunning triumph to support their claims at Geneva."[4] At Geneva, an international conference has been set for a settlement of the Indochina crisis. "Bargainings and bilateral conferences took place behind the scenes. The Soviet Union, moving toward detente after Stalin, exerted pressure on Ho Chi Minh to settle. Chou En-lai, China's delegate, told Ho that it was in his interest to take half a loaf in order to get the French out and keep the Americans out, and that he would gain the whole eventually. He was prevailed upon very unwillingly to settle for the 17th parallel and a two-year lapse before elections. Settlement was reached in time for a final declaration on July 21 that brought the French war to an end. . . . The Geneva Accord declared a cease-fire, confirmed under international auspices the independence of Laos and Cambodia and partitioned Vietnam into separate North and South zones, under the specific provision that 'the military demarcation is provisional and should not in any way be interpreted as constituting a political or territorial boundary.' . . . The settlement at Geneva ended a war and averted wider participation by either China or the United States, but lacking satisfied sponsors anxious to sustain it, and including dissatisfied parties looking to reverse it, it was born defective."[5]

Navy Nurse Marie Eberhardt is stationed at the U.S. Naval Hospital at Yokosuka, Japan at this time. She notes that, "when France was forced out of Vietnam, all of the U.S. ships in Yokosuka took off to aid the evacuation. They took most of the doctors and corpsmen from the hospital. I was Charge Nurse of the general surgery ward, and when I reported for duty that morning I had only two corpsmen left and no doctors for about eighty patients. I appointed some of the up-patients to help with nursing care, and acted as nurse/doctor for the day, extending antibiotic therapy at that time, as was required every forty-eight hours, etc.. At three in the afternoon, a Nursing Supervisor finally paid a visit to the ward and asked if I needed any help. By then everything was taken care of and the ward was all ship-shape. This lasted about a week before the doctors were flown back, although the Commanding Officer and the Executive Officer of the hospital finally issued some of the medical care of the patients in the doctors' absences. All of the patients survived my ministrations, and the experience was good for my self-esteem."[6]

The hospital ship, USS *Haven*, also plays a role in this turmoil and the aftermath of Dien Bien Phu. The tale is best told by two of the Navy Nurses aboard the ship. One of the nurses is Reinelda E. Vickey. She says that the *Haven* is "in Yokosuka, Japan on our routine R&R [Rest and Recreation] in August 1954. We were to sail on 1 September for Vietnam's 'Paris of the East,' Saigon. We made preparations to embark over 700 patients. We arrived in Saigon on 8 September 1954 after a winding trip up the Saigon River. All the camera freaks were busy and I was one of them. We embarked 721 patients. These included members of the French Army and Navy, the French Foreign Legion, Germans, African natives with the scars of puberty ritual, and Moslems who covered their beds like tents and bowed to Mecca each day. There were probably other nationalities that I did not know. Needless to say, it was an unusual group of patients. The majority of these men were not injured. We were just transporting them closer to their home countries. We departed at noon on 10 September for our refueling point, Port Said, Egypt. . . . The French official and Drum and Bugle Corps gave us a splendid departure. . . .

"We entered the Suez Canal on 26 September and had to anchor overnight as the ship's winch had to be repaired. Ships were not allowed passage if any mechanical problems prevailed. We were besieged by natives in small boats selling their wares. I still have a red fez that I purchased. The natives who helped to repair the winch slept on deck. They also stayed on board while we went through the Canal. We left Port Said on 27 September.

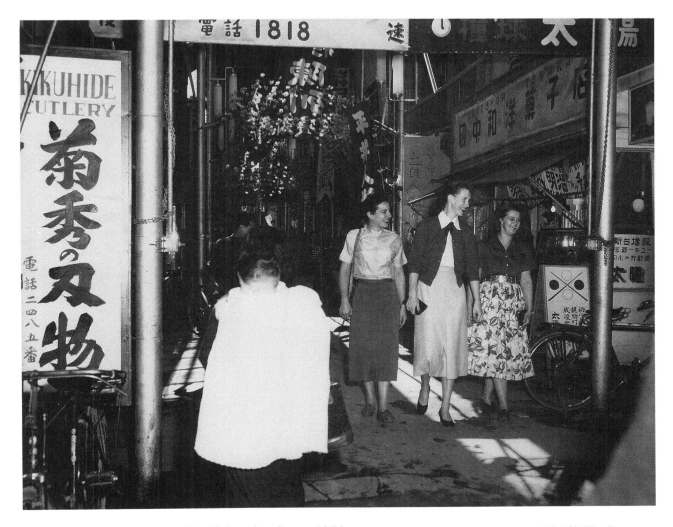

Navy Nurses on R & R in Yokosuka, Japan 1954. (Photo courtesy of Captain Rachel Fine NC USN (Ret.))

We arrived in Oran, Algeria on 2 October 1954 and debarked 420 patients. . . . We had been at sea for 22 days. Some of the ship's crew were given two hours liberty. The ship's crew was doing all the hard work.

"We sailed for Marseilles, France in the late afternoon of 2 October, just prior to mealtime. During the meal we heard the cry of 'man overboard.' We all rushed on deck. One of the ship's crew had jumped overboard. He refused to grab hold of the life-ring that was thrown into the water for him. A boat had to be lowered and he was finally rescued despite his refusal to cooperate. He was court martialed.

"We arrived in Marseilles, France on 4 October and were greeted with the usual fanfare. Listening to the French play their national anthem was almost as thrilling as hearing our national anthem. They probably played ours too. The last patient was carried off at 1105 and we breathed a sigh of relief. We could all relax and not be afraid of causing any international incidents by our talk or actions. We stayed in port for four days but we still had to stand watches on the ship. Some of the doctors and nurses went to Paris but the time limit was too short to enjoy the journey. . . .

"We departed on 8 October and passed the Rock of Gibraltar on 10 October. . . . On 16 October, a medical SOS was received by the USS *Haven* from [a] Swedish tanker. . . . She was in the Caribbean Sea and the course of both ships had to be changed so that we could rendezvous in the Mid-Atlantic to execute a rescue at sea. A German sailor was seriously ill. The weather was stormy and the ocean was very rough. The sailor had to be transferred to the *Haven* via a 'highline.' It didn't look very high to me. An emergency appendectomy was performed. The sailor was released to the authorities of the Canal Zone Immigration in Balboa, Panama for repatriation. We arrived at Balboa, Panama on 22 October, traveled through the Canal and left Colona, Panama on 24 October. . . . We arrived in Long Beach, California on 1 November 1954. Many relatives and friends were waiting at the municipal pier. My mother was among them. It was great to see a familiar face from home after such a long journey that took us halfway around the world. I am sure that we were greeted by the Navy Band but I don't remember. Getting on land again was especially great for me, as I would not have to take any more medication for seasickness. No more ships for me was my motto!"[7]

The other Navy nurse aboard the *Haven*, during this trip, is Anna Corcoran. This is her recall of the same voyage. "The last week in August [1954], the Chief Nurse [of Yokosuka Naval Hospital in Japan] called six of us, who were due to rotate [back to the States], to her office and asked if we would like to go home on the USS *Haven*. . . . The *Haven* had just received orders to go to Vietnam (in those days we called it French Indochina) . . . Dien Bien Phu had fallen and the U.S. government had offered assistance and the assistance [the French] requested was a hospital ship to take the people who had been prisoners, some of them for two years or more, and bring them back to . . . Iran, Algeria and, the French Troops, to Marseilles, France. The *Haven* [had been] all ready to return to the states and, consequently, [had] sent many of her nurses to other places to finish their tours of duty. So, four of us (Ruby Brooks, Martha Bruce, Harriette Johnson and myself) said we would take the orders. . . . The ship sailed from Yokosuka on September first. . . . We had no patients aboard at the time.

"On September 8 we arrived in Saigon. . . . It was a gorgeous city and had a very European flavor and a very Far Eastern flavor. The buildings were all white, typical of the tropics as I later learned . . . very wide streets, of course all of the roads had been built by the Foreign Legion . . . and the streets were lined with lovely trees, and there was no indication, as we [sailed into Saigon] and went ashore, that there had really been some bad fighting there . . . On the morning of September 10th, we boarded patients starting at two a.m. and we boarded 753 patients. We never did find out why we boarded them at night. There were many reasons given. One was because of the heat of the day . . . and the other was that they didn't want the, what we later called, the North Vietnamese to know how many patients we actually took out. Whatever the reason, we started to board at two a.m. and we had them all boarded by seven a.m.. We sailed that day, September 10th. I was assigned on the D ward, we had 87 patients in each ward, and they all had to be able to go to the dining room because the [ship's] elevator did not come down to our section of the ship, so that [meals could not be brought down]. . . . The bunks [on the ward] were not double bunks but were triple bunks. One of the most interesting things was when we would make sick call and we would have the doctor standing on the second bunk examining the patient in the third bunk and the interpreter would be perched on top of one of the bedside cabinets. If the patient spoke French, that was fine because [the interpreter] spoke French, German and English. If [the patient] didn't speak [these languages], then [the interpreter] would have an Arab down there who could translate for [the patient] so it was really a league of nations . . . Most of the patients were malnourished. They had been prisoners and had not been fed well. As we later learned, many of them had body lice and most of them had worms, so along with treating the acutely ill patients, everybody on the ship got sprayed every night. The corpsmen stood them in the heads and sprayed them with DDT powder from top to bottom and, of course, those of us who worked in the wards worried all the time about whether or not we would get a little 'itchy' from all this going on. One of our corpsmen who had long hair on his arms, did in fact get them, but he did okay.

"Because [the patients] weren't used to having any water, the Arabs particularly (which most of our patients down there were), they were great at turning on the water, so we had to have only one shower and that was controlled by a corpsman who would go in there with them and only let them stay in there for so long. . . .

"Two days out from Saigon we crossed the equator and those of us who, of course were Pollywogs, had never crossed the equator before, had to be initiated into the crossing by the Shellbacks. The Shellbacks were a lot of these old Chiefs who had been around the Navy for a long time . . . They were very nice to the nurses and we didn't have to put up with as much as a lot of the other people who were being initiated. We all got our Shellback certificates saying we had crossed the equator. . . . We arrived in Oran, Algeria on October 2nd and we off-loaded the French Foreign Legion. . . . The majority of the Foreign Legion troops that we had were Arabs from the many Arab countries. Iran, of course, was [French Foreign Legion] headquarters . . . so we off-loaded 400 Foreign Legion troops. . . . We left Iran around supper time and shortly thereafter, the bell was sounded for man-overboard. One of the sailors, who had convinced his buddies to let him have their liberty time, [had been ashore and] had come back having imbibed in a little in beer and decided he wanted to go back [ashore]. He had wrapped his wallet in plastic, put on a life jacket and jumped overboard. . . . They put the boat in the water to go pick him up. . . . We took him aboard and later on . . . we had a Court Martial, for him, [aboard the ship]. . . . Then we went into Marseilles, France and the Catholic Chaplain aboard, Father Frank O'Leary, had asked if any of us wanted to go to Rome while we were in Marseilles. I think about 30 of us wanted to go so we boarded the night train and arrived in Rome the next day. We were met by the Catholic USO group who took us where we could shower and get dressed and we went out in uniform to see Pope Pius XII. . . . We went out to Castle . . . which was the Pope's summer residence and saw him and that was probably one of the most impressive things in my life. Here was a man who spoke perfect English, spoke seven languages perfectly, that day, to people who were in the audience. In his presence you felt like you were in the presence of a Saint. We then went back into Rome, had dinner and boarded the train and went back to Marseilles. We took aboard patients . . . who were from the 6th Fleet."[8] From there the ship went back to the States.

A young Lt(jg) stationed at Portsmouth, Virginia, almost made that trip to France. Her name is Anna Ehrlinger (Peterson) and this is how it happened: "I had made Lt(jg), when stationed at Portsmouth, and my Reserve time [active duty] was just about up. The Chief Nurse called me in to see if I was going to sign up for more [active duty], and I told her I wanted sea duty. I requested the 'Diaper Run' from Germany to the U.S. on MSTS and she said she would see what she could do. . . . Within a week I received a phone call from the [Director] in Washington. She [Captain Leona Jackson] had been stationed in Portsmouth before going there and she knew me. Here I was, standing in the nurses' station, with everyone standing around, and she said `Ann, I can't get you on MSTS, you have to be a full Lieutenant, but I can get you on the *Consolation*, a hospital ship, in the States right now and sailing for Korea in August. Will you sign over, if I get you on that?' I, of course, said, 'Oh yes, and thank you.' Didn't know a thing about it, but was thrilled. She told me to order a foot locker or sea chest from maintenance and that my orders would be on the way, giving me leave at home, and then on to Long Beach [California] to catch the ship. Our new chief nurse at Portsmouth was Edwina Todd and she had just left the 'Connie' [nickname for the *Consolation*]. She got word of my orders and immediately called me to her quarters to give me advice on sea services; what to expect, how to behave and how not to behave. She was a godsend. But even with all of her help, I still arrived aboard that ship as green as grass. My husband tells me, when I came aboard, they all eyed me and said, 'there is one unknowing nurse.'

"When I arrived at Long Beach, the ship was not there. It had gone on sea trials to San Diego. So the OOD [Officer Of the Day] at the Naval Station sent me to the . . . Hotel in Long Beach, to stay until they returned in two days. There I met two other nurses who had to same thing happen. So we got together and on the second morning while sitting in the dining room, we saw that white wonder coming into the harbor. What a thrill that was. And off we went on our adventure. We left Long Beach August 10th in route to Pearl Harbor. There I had my first sad and emotional experience. Entering Pearl with all hands standing and saluting the *Arizona*, one of my corpsmen was crying. He told me both his father and brother went down with that ship. . . .

"From there we were off to Subic Bay, Philippines on August 18. We arrived August 31st and stayed until September 2nd. During that time we received orders to . . . French Indochina to help the French. We hit a typhoon in the China Sea and all the nurses were sick and many others, but fortunately, I was not. For 32 hours I had the duty. It was like a ghost ship in the passageways; everyone in their bunks or on the wards, except, most importantly, the Line officers on the bridge. . . . We reached [Indochina] on 4 September. . . . It had been scheduled for us to pick up the French and take them to Le Havre, France but our orders were changed and we were ordered to stand by to care for the French until the *Haven* arrived to pick them up. . . . We were disappointed, but we were needed in Korea as a hospital ship for the 1st Marine Division. . . .

"We left [Indochina] on September 27 and went to Hong Kong for R&R. Loved it; the shopping, treated like queens. The British were invited aboard ship for dental and medical problems . . . and we were all, officers and nurses, invited to the Foreign Correspondence Club for a party. It was a beautiful place in the high hills, overlooking Hong Kong and Kowloon. From Hong Kong we proceeded to Sasebo, Japan for supplies. We were there two days. There, five of the young Line officers asked one of the nurses and myself to go to a Japanese restaurant to see what Japanese culture was really like. We accepted and took a taxi up the hill overlooking Sasebo, to the White Cloud. When we arrived we had to take off our shoes and put on their slippers, and we were then shown to our dining room. Low tables and pillows to sit on . . . We were entertained by Japanese girls singing songs and offered sake [liquor]. 'No, thank you.' The walls were paper thin and you could hear others in the private rooms, easily; many Navy officers, mostly from other ships. Anyhow, as my history goes, I had to excuse myself, and Mary, the other nurse, and I went where [one of] the entertainers indicated, and we went to the ladies' room. . . . I was looking for the 'john' ['head,' in navy language]. I tripped over a hole in the floor and lost one of my slippers, and said loudly `Oh, my God - I've lost one of my slippers down this hole.' Then we figured out, the hole (those of you who have been to Japan will know) was the 'john'! Going back to the dining room was very embarrassing as everyone had heard me and all were looking out to see who had lost their slipper. Many good laughs were had."[9]

Meantime, the USS *Repose* leaves the Korean waters in January 1954 carrying some patients to Pearl Harbor then heads for the U.S.. "She arrived home on 11 February, served briefly as a pier-side hospital on the west coast [Long Beach], and was decommissioned on 21 December 1954 at Hunter's Point Naval Shipyard [San Francisco]."[10]

Navy Nurse Norma Ellingson (Bartleson) is on duty at the Naval Hospital at Bremerton, Washington in January 1954 when she receives TAD orders. She says, "I was assigned temporary additional duty to the Military Sea Transportation aboard the transport *M.M. Patrick*. I was to replace a nurse who had become ill and was unable to make the voyage. This was a routine trip between Seattle and Yokohama, Japan and Pusan, Korea, carrying one thousand troops and approximately two hundred and sixty women and children. We encountered rough seas and many were seasick. It was about a two week trip to Yokohama. We were sailing off the coast of Honshu [Japan] when a Japanese pilot was taken aboard as we entered the straits of Japan. I was comfortably seated in my stateroom about eight p.m., when I suddenly felt a thud, then heard the sounding of waves breaking against the hull of the ship. Immediately thereafter there was a continuous blast of the ship's whistle and the ringing of the general alarm bell . . . summoning all persons aboard to their collision stations. On hearing the signal of collision, I hurriedly donned my raincoat and life preserver and proceeded to my designated life boat. It was evident by the debris (life rings, wooden splinters) and oil in the water, that the ship had collided with another vessel. It was a Japanese oil tanker with about fifteen people onboard. It was cold and snowing. Shouts and screams of desperation came from an area of approximately one quarter of a mile from the ship. It was easy to detect the shrill screams of a woman and the hoarse shouting of at least two men. Due to darkness and heavy flurries of snow, our vision was impaired and being unable to give aid to the helpless people struggling in the water, created a feeling of anxiety and helplessness to everyone aboard. Soon after, the command was given to lower the lifeboats and to proceed to rescue the survivors in the icy waters. Searchlights were spotted on the area nearby and as the two lifeboats went bobbing over the waves we could see that they were nearing the victims. One man and a woman were holding on to each [other] in an attempt to keep from drowning. A little further away, another man clung to an oil barrel while awaiting rescue. By the time the lifeboat had reached the people they were in a state of exhaustion and unable to grab the oars that were held out to them. As the boat moved, the men aboard used a grappling hook to lift them into the boat. The boat carrying the survivors returned to the ship while the other boat continued the search for the remaining ones, which proved futile. The two survivors were hoisted aboard the ship on a stretcher and taken to the sick bay where they were administered first aid and treated for shock. One man and one woman were most thankful to be alive. Another man collapsed and died as he was being hoisted aboard the ship. The next morning, a Japanese Coast Guard boat came along our ship to take the Japanese survivors to the port . . . They transferred to the boat and as they were leaving, the man who had survived bowed and continued to bow until the boat was out of sight. He was saying 'thank you' and we knew he was thankful to be alive."[11]

Back in the States, Navy Nurse Barbara Ellis is stationed at the Naval Hospital in Newport, Rhode Island. She tells us about the USS *Bennington* disaster occurring on 26 May 1954. It seems that while this aircraft carrier is conducting some routine operations in nearby waters, a tremendous explosion takes place on the second and third decks of the ship in the officers' wardroom and the enlisted mess. "Ninety one persons were killed outright and twelve died later of injuries. Once again we saw around-the-clock duty and you wouldn't know what race, color or creed the patients were. They were mostly burnt to a crisp. It was quite, quite awesome. It was as bad as anything I saw over in Korea. . . . The smell and the stench of the whole thing was just awful."[12]

The Chief Nurse of the Newport Naval Hospital, Frances Quebbeman, says, "We received word early in the day . . . about the explosion aboard the USS *Bennington*. A meeting of department heads ensued where the decisions were made about where the patients would be placed and the method of treatment for burns, which was the major injury. Nurses were assigned to each unit to organize their duties and have beds and supplies in readiness. The first casualties arrived via helicopters by 1000 and we were ready. Fortunately, a number of nurses had experience in casualty management from WWII. The junior nurses learned quickly. We had much volunteer help from the Newport nurses and doctors. The [Red Cross] worker at the hospital organized a group of women to assist feeding the badly burned and in forcing liquids. After the first hard week we were able to manage with our own staff. Again, I witnessed nurses working tirelessly without thought to time off or what day of the week it was."[13]

Also in Newport is former Navy Nurse Marion C. McKenna Humphreys. "After I got out of the Navy, I was out for about two years and I had a little girl. One morning I heard on the radio that the *Bennington* had caught fire . . . and they were asking for volunteers. . . . I called up and volunteered my services. I went into the hospital and was assigned to Ward G which . . . was all severe burn cases then. The boys were put on Stryker Frames and we had five or six doctors assigned to the wards and several corpsmen and nurses. . . . I just felt as though I was back in the Navy again."[14] Once a Navy Nurse, always a Navy Nurse.

In July 1954, the census of the active duty Nurse Corps is 2345; 1151 are USN and 1194 are Reserve Navy nurses. In October, the transfer program (augmentation) is reopened for Reserve nurses to become Regular Navy. Also in 1954, the U.S. Navy commissions its "first nuclear-powered ship, the submarine *Nautilus*."[15]

On 15 October 1954, Hurricane Hazel roars into Myrtle Beach, South Carolina and rushes on through North Carolina leaving debris and devastation in its wake. It goes on up to Washington, D.C. with 50 to 60 miles an hour winds and leaving many downed trees in its path. From there it follows the coast through Maryland, Delaware, New Jersey (the Atlantic City boardwalk is extensively damaged), and New York. Then it proceeds toward the Great Lakes and slams into Toronto, Canada killing fifty-six people.[16]

The world continues on its course in 1955. West Germany becomes an independent republic while East Germany continues under communist Russian domination. This is the year that "British influence secured the signing of the 'Baghdad Pact' by Britain, Irak, Turkey, Persia, and Pakistan, to erect a Near Eastern barrier against Communism. France granted freedom to Morocco."[17]

In the United States, 1955 finds something to really celebrate; a "Polio [poliomyelitis or 'infantile paralysis'] vaccine, developed by Jonas E. Salk [a research scientist], was declared safe . . . [and] millions received anti-polio shots."[18] Then, the entire country receives a shock when "On Sept. 24, 1955, President Eisenhower suffered a heart attack while vacationing in Denver. He was taken to a hospital, and . . . The doctors reported that the attack was 'moderate.' . . . [The President] returned to his desk in December."[19]

Following the Korean Conflict, the "U.S. Army found that 15 percent of its men taken prisoner actively collaborated with the enemy, 5 percent resisted, and 80 percent were in the gray area of signing peace petitions and such. Perhaps even more shocking was that not one American had tried to escape. . . . seventy-five American soldiers had agreed to become Communist spies after returning to the U.S. and twenty-one others refused to return home at all. . . . It was the worst showing by prisoners in the history of America. A result was that President Eisenhower issued a new Code of Conduct for Members of the Armed Forces of the United States in 1955. The code, to be memorized by every American serviceman, confined them to providing only their name, rank, serial number, and date of birth if questioned while a prisoner."[20] And that included all Navy nurses.

To date, men nurses had not been able to join any of the military Nurse Corps but, in August 1955, [because of legislation] they are finally able to receive commissions in the Army Reserve.[21]

In January 1955, the Bureau of Medicine and Surgery changes the Nurse Corps Branch (in BuMed) to the 'Nursing Division.' In March, Congress passes 'The Career Incentive Act' which provides "career incentive for members of the uniformed services by increasing pay and allowances."[22] And speaking of career incentives, one of the most successful, motivating educational programs for Hospital Corps WAVES begins in July 1955; the Navy Enlisted Nursing Education Program (NENEP). This Nursing Education Program was developed in the BuMed Nursing Division and it allows a "limited number of Hospital Corps WAVES [to be] selected yearly to attend a four-year professional nursing program in collegiate schools of nursing with expenses paid by the Navy. Upon successful completion of the program, nurses are commissioned as Ensigns in the Nurse Corps, U.S. Naval Reserve."[23] Patricia Luenberger (Shields) is among the first group of Hospital Corps WAVES selected for this program. "I first entered the Naval Service as a WAVE in June of 1954. I had hoped to work in a hospital and save money enough to help me become a registered nurse after I completed my active duty tour of four years. After going through Bainbridge, Maryland for boot camp and Hospital Corps School, I was assigned to the Naval Hospital, Corona, California. It was there, during my first year as a Hospital Corps WAVE, that I was selected as one of the first ten women to participate in NENEP, which was . . . open, at that time, to females only. This was an opportunity of a lifetime for me, as this was a dream come true. . . . Four of us went to the University of Colorado in Boulder [in 1956] and six others were assigned to the University of Boston. [Eight of the original ten actually graduated.] We [at Colorado] were rated OCHN, Officer Candidate Hospital Nurse. Some of us had to drop a pay grade in order to be E3 while going to school. We had our WAVE uniforms, with new arm patches to designate our new rate. We lived in boarding houses with other non-Navy students on the Boulder campus and lived in the student nurse's dorm while at the medical center in Denver. We were known at the Navy students but we lived like all the other student nurses during the school program with the exception of our free summers which we spent at the Naval Hospital, Great Lakes. We wore our student nurse's uniforms and were a bit of a novelty. We were under the supervision of a Navy nurse."[24]

Another of the first selectees for the NENEP program, is Corpswave Joan McIntyre. She is one of those sent to Boston University to gain her B.S. degree in nursing. "At the beginning we weren't accepted very well among the other students. Later, I learned that alot of the impressions they had about women in the military were based on what their parents had told them. They had had no experience themselves in relationship to us. So, there for a while people kind of shied away from us. A polite call now and then but other than that we were pretty much on our own. What we had to do was prove ourselves. And, that's what we did. In the four years it was interesting to see what did occur and in the long run I did become president of the student body in the school of nursing. . . . One of the things that we felt so strongly in going through the program was that the Navy was sending us and therefore we had to do the best we could. We had to put our best foot forward so that we were good representatives of the Navy and the Navy Nurse Corps."[25]

In 1955 at the Chelsea Naval Hospital in Massachusetts, a Navy nurse with special qualifications is at work on the wards. Her name is Maxine Conder (destined to be a Director) and her qualifications include a special course in 'Polio' nursing taken at her last duty station in Guam. "Guam had high incidents of polio and so I took the course over there. . . . [At Chelsea] I had the usual assignments as Charge Nurse, Staff Nurse, but one day the Chief Nurse walked into the ward that I was working on and said that she was relieving me and that I was to go over to the dependents' area to a closed ward, open it up for polio patients and I'd better hurry because the first patients were, then, in the emergency room. I reported to the ward. It had been cleaned but in the middle of the entry area were large boxes full of supplies. I remember quickly emptying some of those boxes in order to find thermometers in order to admit the first two patients on the polio ward. This was in 1955 and the United States was experiencing the last large polio epidemic in the United States. It was in the northeast. If I remember correctly, they said there were about 20,000 paralytic cases. Because of the magnitude of the problem, the State of Massachusetts requested from the Navy Department, that the Naval Hospital there in Chelsea open the ward [to] take care of our own people, both dependents and active duty. And this was unique because all contagious patients, infectious disease patients before then, had been sent to county hospitals for treatment. But, we did open this ward up. It quickly filled up. We were very, very busy. This was in the days of the 'iron lung' and it seemed as though there was another iron lung being wheeled onto the ward hourly. It got to the point, when I was the Charge Nurse, that I was allowed to call the company over in Cambridge [Massachusetts] directly to order another iron lung. At the same time, the Navy sent five or six nurses from Chelsea, to civilian hospitals nearby (Beth Israel, and Massachusetts General are two that I remember) to help with the polio patients that they were taking care of. It was a really, terrible, terrible situation. Everyone was involved. We had our ward open for perhaps four months. One of our staff doctor's wife was a patient who was totally paralyzed. It was quadriplegic. She had given birth to a new baby about 10 days before being diagnosed with polio. This was quite a common occurrence. She remained in the hospital, at Chelsea, for nearly a year in her iron lung with round-the-clock specializing [nursing care] before she was transferred to a rehabilitation center somewhere in a nearby city. But it was a unique experience. It demonstrates that Navy Nurses were very flexible and we were assigned to a number of assignments that perhaps we weren't always prepared for, but we worked hard and we did a good job."[26]

Navy Nurse Kathleen M. Laughlin (Donnelly) is in Guam in 1955 and says, "When we first got there, we were living in 'Quonsets' and they had 'Quonsets' for the hospital as temporary buildings. They had built this beautiful new Naval Hospital which was dedicated while we were there."[27] After Navy Nurse Laughlin (Donnelly) returns home from overseas, she is interviewed for the newspaper in Kansas City, Missouri about her service in Guam. In the interview she describes "the concern of the military service toward its members. 'There was the case of a young man [active duty] who was critically injured in a swimming accident at Okinawa,' she says. 'They brought him to the new and modern hospital at Guam where I was assigned.

"'The young man was paralyzed below the shoulders, and surgery was necessary. The Navy flew the parents from the United States to Guam, to be at their son's bedside.'

"Operations were performed, and when the patient reached a stage of recovery permitting travel he was transferred to this country. The transport plane which brought him to America was equipped with an iron lung. A select team of medical personnel was aboard.

"'The last I heard of the boy was that he was slowly improving.'"[28] (LCdr Donnelly had a commendation placed in her jacket for her work.[29])

As for hospital ships, the USS *Consolation* is in Korean waters early in 1955. Navy Nurse Anna Ehrlinger (Peterson) is still aboard and says, "It was here on this tour that there were several memorable cases. . . . First, the sailor they brought in a totally unconscious condition and we could not find a thing wrong. Breath smelled fine, no injury, and we checked everything. Finally, found out in time, it was alcoholic poisoning from Vodka. Luckily we saved him in time. The second [case] was a Korean woman who was shot accidently and had a newborn. We set up one of our small wards for her and her baby. I was assigned to her and the baby, and had to round up diapers and so forth. Had to hand wash the diapers. Our inspections were every Saturday morning and my corpsman was having a fit because I had diapers all over the place. I assured him I'd take full blame if we didn't pass inspection. Our Captain came in and looked around and grumbled. I said, 'Sorry, sir, this is the best I can do.' He turned to his Yeoman and told him to give us a passing grade. After all, they were clean diapers. The third case was the challenge of my career. A 90 percent burn case was flown in by helicopter and the doctors ordered a Stryker frame. Our Chief Nurse came in the wardroom and asked if anyone had ever used or knew how to use one. Out of 16 nurses, I was the only one. So I was assigned to this boy [the burn patient]. I had to teach the corpsmen how to use the Stryker frame. (I give credit, not to myself, but to St. Lukes [School of Nursing] in Denver for this as they didn't leave a stone unturned in their training. My last case before I graduated [from training] was a burn case on a Stryker frame.) I followed that boy [the burn patient on the *Connie*] through four weeks of sheer 'hell.' Then helped him on his transfer to the hospital in Yokosuka and kept track of his progress. He finally made it to Oak Knoll - Naval Hospital in Oakland, California - but he passed away, shortly after his transfer, with uremic poisoning. What a waste. He was only 19."[30]

During this year, 1955, the *Consolation* takes a Good Will Tour to Hiroshima. Navy Nurse Ehrlinger (Peterson) says, "We were the first American hospital ship to call there since the war. And, we saw, first hand, the destruction of the atomic bomb. We were guests of the ABBC, Atomic Bomb Casualty Commission. They had set up a complete hospital and we toured this. The staff consisted of doctors and nurses from all over the world. The work they were doing was fascinating - following up on the wounded from the atomic bomb."[31]

Over in the Atlantic Ocean, Navy Nurse Anna Byrnes is on the MSTS ship, *General H.W. Buckner*. There are two Navy nurses aboard and Anna is the Senior Nurse. "We carried troops and dependents to South Hampton, England and Bremerhaven, Germany. We went to Casablanca one trip and we accompanied the ship when we went to 'under-way' training . . . in Cuba. . . . We had friends at the hospital in Guantanamo Bay, Cuba. They were having some kind of an epidemic at the time and they requested if we could come ashore and help them with the inoculations. We did. That was interesting and fun. [Everyone was restricted to the base at that time.]

"We had storms. We had some rough [seas] with the ship [taking] a pounding. At the time, in the North Sea, there were still mines. There was a channel that was cleared but there was always a 'lookout.' There were reports of mines that had broken loose so somebody was watching for that kind of thing. . . . We just kept going back and forth across the ocean. . . . My first morning on the ship I heard them announce, about five o'clock in the morning, about a 'clean sweep down fore and aft' and `such and such company of troops lay down to the mess deck' and all that kind of thing. Never heard it again. One day I said, 'You know, I remember hearing all kinds of announcements when I first came on board and they don't do it anymore.' They said, 'Of course they do. You just don't' hear them.' I had gotten so used to it, I guess.

"While I was on the ship, I was in charge of 'welfare and recreation' funds which was an experience for me. (I wasn't too swift at balancing my checkbook.) It was turned over to me in Germany. I really didn't know exactly what the job meant but when we got into New York, the auditors came on board to audit the books. They were not in very good shape from my predecessor. He had failed to get permission from the Captain to have parties, for example, . . . or buying records. (They didn't have tapes then, it was records and a lot of athletic equipment.) So they informed me of what my responsibilities were and they gave me two books to read. So I was conscientious and I read the books and discovered that a lot of funny things had been going on. The officers were having a party every time we went to Germany and the enlisted were not having any. They were entitled to a certain amount of entertainment too. So when we were going back to Germany, in the wardroom some of the fellows said, 'Well, where are we going to have our party this time?' And I said, 'Well, you are not going to have a party. The enlisted people have to have several parties to catch up with you.' They were just shocked and disappointed. I think they thought that perhaps I wouldn't pay much attention. But, I said I wasn't going to go to jail for problems. And, we had a lot of money, sometimes as much as twenty and thirty thousand dollars in welfare and recreation funds because we got the money from our ship's store. And then a certain percentage of that money had to be shipped to the general recreation fund and then another percentage went to some other fund. I can't recall now. Then the money that was left was to be used for the ship's company, not just the officers. So we ended up with a big party in Brooklyn after a trip and everybody went. . . . I just almost died when they ever gave me that assignment. . . .

"I was the Catholic chaplain also, on board. There's another [collateral duty]. The Protestant chaplain was Baptist and he would have a hymn session at three o'clock and I followed at three-thirty in the library with the rosary, after which I would go back up to the wardroom and make tea. Everybody who was coming off duty would have tea instead of coffee. And we'd have buns until they were all eaten. Then on Sunday I conducted my own idea of a service and that was really very traumatic because in those days women just didn't do that kind of thing. I was really kind of scared. It was in the main dining room and all these people came in; troops, officers, wives, kids and all and I'd come out in my 'blues' [blue dress uniform] and proceed. I was a deacon, I used to say. We did have - twice, I think - a Catholic chaplain make Reserve [duty] trips with us. Then we would have Mass. But, I told them what I did and they said it was fine. After all, it was better than nothing. But I still felt very strange. I'm sure women today wouldn't feel that way."[32]

In Portsmouth, Virginia at the Hospital Corps School in 1955, is stationed Navy Nurse Alene Duerk (a future Director.) She had been one of the recalled Reserve nurses in 1951 and had first been assigned to Portsmouth Naval Hospital. She was at the Hospital only a short time when asked to transfer to the Corps School because of her civilian nursing experience. "I thought that would be a great opportunity, and it was. I was there five years. We had classes at that time of about 80 students [student Hospital Corpsmen]. I can't remember if [the course] was eight weeks or ten weeks because they would change the curriculum. When the need was great, the curriculum got shorter and when the need wasn't quite so great, the curriculum was lengthened out a little bit. But anyhow, I worked with the Hospital Corpsmen. One nurse had eighty students and they came into these classrooms right from boot camp, or from the fleet, no more interested in being a Hospital Corpsman than the man in the moon. They said it was the farthest thing from their mind, but the need was great [especially during the Korean Crisis] and there they were. It took you about four to six weeks to get them interested. You did everything you could. It wasn't dry, believe me, because you had to demonstrate all these [nursing] procedures and you demonstrated on the kids and you had return demonstrations. But it was fun. It was really very rewarding. And, about the sixth week, suddenly the lights came on and they just were all enthusiastic. By the time they graduated, they were out there ready to go and save the world. Then you'd start back with another group. Those large groups were hard to take care of. We were out in this temporary building, no air conditioning, maybe you had a fan or two, and it was hot. In Portsmouth, Virginia it gets very hot. Even to keep them awake was difficult. Well, that was five years and then [in 1956] at the end of the period, I guess about the last six months I was there, I was at B School. Now those were the people who had gone through Hospital Corps School, had duty aboard ship and they came back for advance training. They were the fellows who were going to go back out there on the ships with no doctor and were going to do all these different treatments and make all these diagnoses and everything. They were very interesting because they were motivated to begin with or they wouldn't have been there. That was an interesting group to teach."[33]

In March of 1956, a Naval Medical activity is first established in Nice, France and a Navy Nurse Corps officer is assigned there.[34] Also, in 1956, legislation permits any Nurse Corps officers, regular or reserve, "qualified in dietetics, physical therapy or occupational therapy, and not above permanent grade of Lieutenant, to transfer to and be appointed in the Medical Service Corps of the Regular Navy. As a result of this legislation, 46 Nurse Corps officers" are appointed to the Medical Service Corps.[35] One of these nurses is LCdr. Ruth Moeller. "This was a time of decision for nurses trained in these fields; to transfer to the Medical Service Corps or to return to nursing duties. Those who chose not to transfer to MSC would no longer be used in physical therapy departments [or the other two specialties]; they would be used by the Nurse Corps in nursing duties specifically. Some chose nursing, others chose the MSC. For those who chose to transfer, the decision was not necessarily easy or simple. Some Chief Nurses encouraged their transfer as they needed all their Nurse Corps billets filled by full time nurses. Some MSC officers welcomed the nurses to their Corps, some did not because most of the nurses, while younger, would out-rank the MSC officers.

"Some of the senior MSC officers, men specifically, advised the nurses to apply for transfer under Code 5590 which would have markedly limited they career opportunities, even forcing some of them out of the Navy in a few years. [In 1952, the Women's Specialist Section of the Medical Service Corps had been established which is what Code 5590 evidently refers to. But, this new, 1956 legislation allows the Nurse Corps specialists into the all-male MSC.] The highest grade achieved under Code 5590 would be Commander and they would be in competition for promotion with only women and, under the other code (which some male MSC officers discouraged) it permitted promotion to Captain and also the rank on the retired list would be the highest rank, permanent or temporary, and the competition for promotion would be with men of the Corps. In other words, with everyone within the MSC.

"So, having received a letter from the Chief of Naval Personnel dated 23 November 1956 regarding this program, I submitted my request for transfer to the MSC and on June 9, 1957, I resigned from active duty in the Navy Nurse Corps and on 10 June 1957, executed oath of officer in the MSC."[36] (LCdr. Ruth Moeller goes on in her career in the MSC to make Captain and to serve as 'Head of Women in the MSC' at the Bureau of Medicine and Surgery in Washington,D.C.. She retires on 1 September 1969.)

In 1956, 9 percent of newly commissioned Nurse Corps officers have baccalaureate or higher degrees and 16 percent of the Navy Nurse Corps (approximately 346 Navy Nurses) have degrees. "1.6 percent of the corps members were in full-time baccalaureate programs; another 6.5 percent were studying part time, quite a number of them toward a masters degree."[37] And, Captain Jackson notes that, "The trend toward growth and improvement in professional qualifications can be expected to continue."[38]

1956 is another election year in the U.S. and President Eisenhower decides to run for another term. He had another bout of illness necessitating an emergency operation but quickly recovers without changing his mind on running for election. The President and his Vice-President, Richard Nixon are campaigning against the Democratic Nominees Aldai E. Stevenson and Senator Estes Kefauver. President Eisenhower and V.P. Nixon win by a landslide and are "the first Republican President and Vice-President to be re-elected as a team. . . . [And,] Eisenhower became the first President in more than a hundred years to take office without a majority of his party in either house of Congress."[39]

Across the globe in communist Hungary in October 1956, the Hungarian people revolt against the communist government. In November, Russian troops and tanks pour into the country and crush the revolt "with massive slaughter. No assistance to the Hungarians, despite appeals, came from the West."[40] However, from December 1956 to February 1957, six Navy "Nurse Corps officers [are] temporarily assigned to the 'sea lift' bringing Hungarian refugees to the United States."[41] Aboard the MSTS ship *General Randall*, at this time, is Navy Nurse Betty A. Nimits and one other Nurse Corps Officer. (They are there on permanent, not temporary, duty orders.) Betty Nimits says, "Word had gotten to the Hungarian people if they could get to ports where American ships came in, they would be brought to the States. The *Randall* picked up some of these political refugees in Bemerhaven, Germany. A lot of them were professional people (medical, educators, etc.) bring with them only what they could carry."[42] "The people we evacuated were people just like us. They were very nice, average people. They were not the wealthiest, or the poorest. They came out to the ship and everything they owned, that they were taking with them, was on their backs or in their arms. . . . Those that had some good jewelry probably had it on or had it in a bag wrapped around their waists. They had two or three changes of clothes [and] they were wearing them! And that was it. They hadn't even been able to change money. We did a money exchange on the ship for them. They were allowed to use the ship's store to buy soap, toothpaste and toothbrush and combs and that sort of thing. . . . We carried navy denims and quite a few of the men - these are well-dressed men in tailor-made suits - were running around in denims. It was an interesting situation."[43]

1957 and President Eisenhower begins his second term in office. In September he is forced to send federal troops into Arkansas when the Governor refuses to end segregation of Little Rock's Central High School. In October, the Russians launch "Sputnik I, man's first artificial satellite. On Nov. 3, 1957, they launched a second satellite, Sputnik II. It carried a dog named Laika, the first animal to soar into space."[44] Then in November, the President is taken ill with "a mild stroke that affected his speech for a short time."[45] But, he recovers rapidly and resumes his Presidential duties.

Congress passes legislation, in July 1957, that provides a continuing program for Navy Nurse Corps augmentation; transfer from Reserve to Regular Navy. Heretofore, it had been an 'on again, off again' program. Then in August, Congress passes a Public Law that markedly improves career opportunities for the "Nurse Corps and Medical Specialist Corps officers of the Army, Navy and Air Force. For the Navy Nurse Corps it provides:

a. An increase in promotions by removing the limitations in selection in the grade of lieutenant commander; increasing selection in the grades of commander to 5 percent of Nurse Corps officers on active duty and selection, for the first time, in the grade of captain; the number limited to .2 of 1 percent of the officers on active duty.

b. One third of the membership of selection boards for promotion of Nurse Corps officers, to be Nurse Corps officers.

c. Mandatory and statutory retirement."[46]

Finally, Nurse Corps officers can be on the selection board for choosing their own. And, on 17 October 1957, Commander Ruth A. Houghton NC USN is the first Navy nurse to be selected for Captain in a competitive selection![47]

On 28 September 1957, the Nurse Corps Candidate Program begins. This is, essentially, a student nurse recruitment program. Student nurses already in collegiate schools of nursing can apply for the program. If accepted, the students are enlisted into pay grade E-3 for their final year in the college. In addition to the E-3 pay, the students' tuition, fees, books and any other approved expenses for their last year are paid by the Navy. After graduating the nurses become Ensigns in the Nurse Corps, U.S. Naval Reserve. The collegiate school must be accredited by the NLN (National League for Nursing) and the students incur an obligatory amount of active duty time after graduation.

Meantime, back in January, Nurse Corps officers are first stationed at the MAAG (Military Assistance Advisory Group) Dispensary in Taiwan, Formosa, Republic of China. Navy Nurse Virginia Eberharter is not among the first Navy nurses to report in but does arrive in December 1957. She says that there are six other Navy nurses aboard with her and that the doctors are Navy and Air Force and Army medical officers at this tri-service medical facility. "At the [medical facility], we had Chinese nurses working for us. When we were on night duty, they would bring us different kinds of Chinese food to eat. I managed to eat everything they brought except the black eggs that were hundreds of years old. So when they brought the eggs, I always managed to send them on an errand when we began to eat. The eggs were deeply disposed of by the time they returned. It wasn't in my stomach, I can assure you. . . .

"During the time that I was in Taiwan, we could hear continuous bombardment of [a nearby] Island by the Communists. [This] Island was just off the main land of China and 90 miles from Formosa [Taiwan]. One morning when I went on duty, I was told we just missed getting bombed last night by the skin of our teeth. The Chinese were after the airport and the [medical facility] was in line with it. I never did know why the Chinese changed their minds, but thanked God they did."[48]

Then in September two naval hospitals are closed; the one at Mare Island, California and the other at Corona, California. In October, Navy nurses are stationed at the Naval Air Facility in Rota, Spain.

Also, in 1957, a former Army nurse decides to join the Navy Nurse Corps. Her name is Mary Cannon and she explains, "in 1950 when the Korean War of Police Action, whatever it was called, went into being, . . . I went down to the recruiting office . . . an Army recruiting office. . . . Since I had been working as a nurse for some time, I went on active duty as a Captain in the Army Nurse Corps. I remained in the Army on active duty for four years. During that time one of my duty stations was in Korea. I spent twenty-two months over there. In late 1951, all of `52 and part of 1953 I was assigned first in an evacuation hospital . . . then was assigned in one of our POW camps; one in Pusan. That was only a very short assignment for two months, and the third assignment was a MASH up in the furthest east and north part of Korea. . . . This was a most interesting assignment and, as you know, the Korean War was not a popular one. However, we didn't know too much about that nor did, from my own experience, find out too much about it until I got back to the United States and started reading the papers.

"Following my tour in Korea I was assigned to Fitzsimmons Army Hospital in Denver, Colorado which was a beautiful part of the country. And at that time I started going to classes at Denver University. That was kind of something to do. I found I had a lot of extra time on my hands. Eight hour duty I wasn't quite used to after Korea, so I started going back to school and found that I rather liked it. So, I decided to leave active duty, remain in the Reserves and use the Korean GI Bill to go back to school. . . .

"I had every intention, when I left the Army, of going back in. However, during the time I was in school, my father died very unexpectedly. And my mother being alone in Chicago, I felt that I should be back in that area. So, while I was mulling this over, there were fifteen Navy nurses who were attending Indiana University while I was there, and if you wanted to know anything about heavy recruiting they were certainly doing it. I was hearing a great deal about the Navy. So much so that the more I thought about it, and they made me realize that the Navy had Great Lakes [Naval Hospital and Corps School] which was certainly near Chicago, and I knew that the Army had almost nothing in Chicago except a small dispensary at Fort Sheridan. Well, they so convinced me, I wrote a letter to Captain Leona Jackson who was the Director of the Navy Nurse Corps at this time, told her of my thoughts, and asked if I might be able to see her. I received a letter from her in which she invited me to come to Washington, at my convenience, and she'd be glad to discuss this with me. . . . I flew to Washington, was met by Mrs. Jackson and spent a delightful hour or more at her home. She was most gracious. I was very thrilled to meet her. She is a lovely lady. Mrs. Jackson assured me that with active duty I would be able to be assigned to the Naval Hospital at Great Lakes. I returned to Indiana [and] the brain-washing continued by the fifteen nurses. I must admit that I didn't need too much brain-washing. Meeting with Mrs. Jackson certainly convinced me. . . . So in 1957 I was commissioned in the Navy Nurse Corps, went to St. Albans for my basic training and then to Great Lakes as planned. One of the things that did bother me when I was first in the [Naval] service and periodically from then on; most people felt because I had been Army and then switched to Navy that I was discontented with the Army or upset with the Army. This was far from true. I had very, very fine duties in the Army and met a lot of wonderful people and I rather resented the fact that people just seemed to think I'd changed because I didn't like it. My hope was as time went by I was able to convince people that the transfer was for personal or humanitarian reasons. But it took a long time. It certainly was a natural thing for people to feel, but I must say I had excellent assignments in both services."[49]

Also entering the Navy in 1957, is Lucille Emond. After indoctrination she reports to San Diego Naval Hospital, California. She tells us, "All the nurses were initially assigned to the nurses' quarters except for the married ones. Requests to move out [of the quarters] were approved [for an individual with rank] of the length of time on board the duty station. The availability of civilian housing was quite limited. Junior nurses had to find two or more roommates to be able to afford an apartment. At that time it was very difficult, if not impossible, for a single woman to get a home mortgage loan. Not only that, not too many women made enough money to be able to make mortgage payments.

"Life in the nurses' quarters was fun for junior nurses. There were up to 75 Ensigns and JG's when I was there. We were assigned to one of two section duties. We worked a six day week. We had every other weekend off. We were on a.m.'s one week and p.m.'s the next. We worked nights every eight weeks. So, we got to know the nurses in our [duty] section quite well. There was always someone available (or several people available) to do things with, regardless of the shift we worked. . . . A couple of months before I reported aboard, one of the nurses' quarters' traditions had be eliminated; that of serving meals in the dining room of the quarters. The meals [had been] served by stewards. The nurses had their own napkin rings. We were told that the nurses sat at the table according to rank, descending in order from the chief nurse. They had formal china and silverware and all nurses' quarters had lovely silver tea and coffee service [sets]. During my tour in San Diego, the nurses' quarters were closed so all the nurses had to move to civilian housing. And that held true, pretty much, over the next few years at all the nurses' quarters except for some [places] overseas. . . .

"At that time, nurses were pretty much generalists and had hardly any specialty training. Therefore, nurses, particularly those who came from hospital training schools, . . . could, pretty much, work in any of the clinical areas. . . . It was rather frightening , at first, to realize than in many instances we were assigned to more than one ward. However, the circumstances and the types of patients, in those days, were quite different. We had some patients that were acutely ill. There were many that were convalescing. Some were kept in the hospital for weeks and even months at a time during convalescence. [Active duty patients were kept in Navy Hospitals until able to return to full duty.] So it was possible for nurses to be assigned to several wards at one time. . . .

"The types of nursing procedures that were performed in those days seem, in retrospect, quite simple compared to today's very sophisticated medicine. For example, intravenous solutions were limited to probably four or five. We gave few medications intravenously . . . CPR [Cardio Pulmonary Resuscitation] was unknown. We had no intensive care units of any kind. Patients [after surgery] spent a period of time in a recovery room and then were sent to the wards. . . . Many days, it was a constant shifting of patients as they convalesced [on the open wards], they were moved farther and farther away from the [nurses'] desk. The wards at that time were 'open wards.' There were as many as . . . forty beds [on a ward]. [Twenty beds on the starboard or right side of the large ward and twenty more beds on the port or left side.] That seemed to generate [a supportive] type of atmosphere where patients looked out for each other's interests. If, for instance, a patient needed a glass of water or something, and some of the other patients noted that the nurse or corpsmen were . . . [busy], the other patients frequently would assist and give that patient whatever was needed.

"We had ward 'Master-at-Arms' who were convalescing senior enlisted people who would assume responsibility for assignment of the other convalescing, lower rated enlisted men, to keep the ward clean. All the cleaning in those days was done by a combination of patients, the corpsmen and the nurses. There was no housekeeping department, as such. Every Thursday evening and Friday morning were spent in frantically getting the ward ready for the weekly [Captain's] inspection. [This is when] a Senior Officer accompanied by a Senior Nursing Supervisor, would visit each ward and . . . inspect them for cleanliness, need for maintenance; a variety of items. . . . The particular ward . . . that received the highest mark . . . would receive what we called the pennant. In some instances the 'pennant flag.' Sometimes the Commanding Officer would award the patients that were eligible, a couple of hours of extra liberty for gaining the pennant for their area."[50] The 'Captain's Inspection' or the 'Commanding Officer's Inspection' is usually started at ten hundred hours (10 a.m.) and every hospital area is supposed to be in readiness at that time. The Ward Nurse and the Senior Corpsman are to be at the entrance to the ward to meet the inspection party (usually we stood, more or less, at attention.) The senior corpsman is to carry a flashlight (for checking any dark corners the inspection team may require), a towel that is dampened on one end and a bottle of alcohol (if the inspector gets dirt on his hands, although some inspections are done with the inspecting officer using white gloves.) The nurse walks to the left of the Captain and answers any questions. Every other corpsman, and the ambulatory patients stand at attention. The 'up' patients stand at attention beside and at the foot of their beds. All beds not occupied are fully and tautly made. Even the bed-patients' bunks are without wrinkles, as much as humanly possible. The nurse and senior corpsman remain with the inspection party until they leave the ward.

"[At that time] hospital food was not served on trays prepared in advance. The food arrived in [a food warmer] cart. [The food was in large containers on the cart.] And the nursing staff, corpsmen and nurse, would serve the food to the patients.

"There were not televisions nor any radios to keep the patients entertained in those days. Sometimes special services would have a movie, perhaps once a week. And sometimes there were small groups of musicians that would visit the ward and sing and play musical instruments."[51] Also, there were Red Cross personnel to visit the patients and provide them with some 'occupational therapy' such as, leather work (many a patient made himself a wallet) or putting together a model airplane or even a jig-saw puzzle to work on or a book to read. There really was life before television.

Another Navy Nurse speaks of the 'open wards,' "the patients didn't get nearly as lonely. They had someone to communicate with. They had someone to commiserate with and it's a whole lot easier [for the nursing personnel] to see what's going on with open wards. You can look down that ward and you know what's going on immediately."[52] Every afternoon for one hour (usually from 1300 to 1400, there was the 'Quiet Hour' as part of the ward routine. All the shades on the ward windows were pulled down, all lights (except the one at the nurses' desk) were turned off and patients either napped or simply rested, and silence reigned. Also, as a routine, every ward has their patients placed in a 'patient classification' by the Ward Medical Officer. (All patients when admitted, are put into class 4 or 5.) The classes are:

> 5 - Bed patient.
> 4 - Bed patient with head privileges.
> 3 - Ward privileges only.
> 2B - Placed on a ward detail (a cleaning job), compound privileges when detail completed, liberty by special request (approved by doctor.)
> 2A - Compound detail as assigned by Hospital's Master-At-Arms, liberty Tuesday and Thursday and the weekend from 1500 Friday to 0600 Monday.
> 1 - Compound detail and liberty every night.

(Those big 'open' wards and their routines may be long gone but they are not forgotten.)

It is now 1958 and this is the year that Captain Leona Jackson retires from the Navy and her position as Director of the Nurse Corps. On 14 April Captain Jackson writes an official letter "To All of Our Navy nurses."[53] Among several things, she states in this letter, "I wish, as I write this letter, that I could take each of you by the hand and somehow let you know what our association has meant to me. My years in the Navy have been rich in professional and human experience, and in the fullness of living, and the culmination of it all has been these four years as your Director. . . . As I look back on almost twenty-two years in the Navy, I am more sure than ever that if I could live those years over again, I would not change them. . . . I cannot imagine having missed the opportunity to grow individually and professionally, and to participate in the finest kind of patient care.

"Some of that growth for me was bitter - and the circumstances in which I gave that care were adverse . . . . the news of Pearl Harbor on December 7th - and watching the Rising Sun ascend the flagstaff at Government House on Guam on December 10th . . . . . caring for patients under the hostile eyes of the World War II Japanese . . . . . But from the bitter experiences we learn to separate the wheat from the chaff in life. . . . I want to assure each of you of a warm welcome at Lilac Hill, my old house at Union, Montgomery County, Ohio, where the cat family and I shall at last have room for all of our treasures. . . . May God keep you each in His care."

As Director, Captain Jackson "proposed a reorganization of the Nurse Corps Division of the Bureau of Medicine and Surgery, recommending the establishment of three branches: Professional Branch, Personnel Branch and Nurse Corps Reserve Branch. She further proposed the assignment of an Assistant Director for the Reserve Branch responsible for keeping the Director advised on current policies and legislation affecting the Nurse Corps Reserves. In addition, Captain Jackson started the Nurse Corps Candidate Program."[54]

Captain Jackson, during her career, "was awarded the Commendation Ribbon, American Defense Service Medal, Asiatic Victory Medal and the National Defense Service [Medal]."[55]

[1]   Information prepared by the Navy Nurse Corps Officers on the staff of the Director of the Navy Nurse Corps.

[2]   Ibid..

[3]   Laird, LCDR Thelma NC USNR, Jones, LCDR Dorothy NC USN, Feeney, LCDR Elizabeth NC USN, Seidl, CDR Elizabeth NC USN (Ret.), Blaska, CDR Burdette NC USN, *Chronological History NAVY NURSE CORPS*, Prepared by: Nursing Division, Bureau of Medicine and Surgery, 1 August 1962, p. 42.

[4]   Tuchman, Barbara W., *The March of Folly From Troy to Vietnam*, Ballantine Books, New York, 1985, p. 257 and p. 266.

[5]   Ibid., p. 267.

[6]   Eberhardt, Marie CDR Navy Nurse Corps, *Oral History Interview Tape Transcript*, Self interview, 19 May 1990.

[7]   Vickey, Reinelda E. LCdr Navy Nurse Corps, *Oral History Interview Tape Transcript*, Interviewer Captain Rose Marie Lochte Navy Nurse Corps, 9 March 1991.

[8]   Corcoran, Anna CDR Navy Nurse Corps, *Oral History Interview Tape Transcript*, Interviewer LCdr Ann P. Connors Navy Nurse Corps, 7 August 1991.

[9]   Peterson, Ann Ehrlinger Lt(jg) Navy Nurse Corps, *Oral History Interview Tape Transcript*, Self interview, 11 March 1990.

[10]   "Angel of the Orient," *Navy Medical Newsletter*, Captain M.T. Lynch MC USN, Editor, Vol. 55, No. 4, April 1970, p. 11.

[11]   Bartleson, Norma Ellingson CDR Navy Nurse Corps, *Oral History Interview Tape Transcript*, Interviewer Patty Hoff, 22 August 1990.

[12]   Ellis, Barbara CDR Navy Nurse Corps, *Oral History Interview Tape Transcript*, Interviewer CDR Claire M. Walsh Navy Nurse Corps, 25 August 1990.

[13]   Quebbeman, Frances, CDR Navy Nurse Corps, *Written Personal History*, 13 May 1991.

[14] Humphreys, Marion McKenna LT Navy Nurse Corps, *Oral History Interview Tape Transcript*, Interviewer CDR Lucy Ann Job Navy Nurse Corps, 13 February 1990.

[15] *The World Book Encyclopedia*, Field Enterprises Educational Corporation, Chicago, Volume 14, 1966 edition, p. 83.

[16] Floyd, Candace, *America's Great Disasters*, Mallard Press an imprint of BDD Promotional Books Company, Inc., 666 Fifth Avenue, New York, N.Y. 10103, pp. 72, 73.

[17] Wells, H.G., *The Outline of History*, Revised and brought up to date by Raymond Postgate, Garden City Books, Garden City, New York, Volume II, 1961, p. 960.

[18] *The World Book Encyclopedia*, op. cit., Volume 6, p. 109.

[19] Ibid., pp. 109, 110.

[20] *200 Years, A Bicentennial Illustrated History of the United States*, Joseph Newman, Directing Editor, Books by U.S. News & World Report, Inc., 2300 N Street, N.W., Washington, D.C. 20037, 1973, book, book 2, pp. 242, 243.

[21] Schwartz, Linda Spoonster, R.N, M.S.N., "Our Unknown Veterans Emerge From The Shadows," *Yale Medicine*, Alumni Bulletin of the School of Medicine, Volume 26, Number 3, Summer 1992, p. 15.

[22] Laird, et. al., op. cit., p. 42.

[23] Ibid..

[24] Shields, Patricia Luenberger CDR Navy Nurse Corps, *Oral History Interview Tape Transcript*, Self interview, 30 September 1990.

[25] McIntyre, Joan CDR Navy Nurse Corps, *Oral History Interview Tape Transcript*, Self interview, 12 October 1989.

[26] Conder, Maxine Rear Admiral Navy Nurse Corps, *Oral History Interview Tape Transcript*, Self interview, July 1991.

[27] Donnelly, Kathleen M. Laughlin LCdr Navy Nurse Corps, *Oral History Interview Tape Transcript*, Interviewer LCdr Dorothy J. Venverloh Navy Nurse Corps, 17 April 1990.

[28] "Nurse Reviews Trip to Far East," *Kansas City Star*, Kansas City, Missouri, 1955. Article provided courtesy of LCdr. Kathleen Donnelly Navy Nurse Corps.

[29] Donnelly, op. cit..

[30] Peterson, op. cit..

[31] Ibid..

[32] Byrnes, Anna M. Captain Navy Nurse Corps, *Oral History Interview Tape Transcript*, Interviewer Captain Madeline Ancelard Navy Nurse Corps, 11 May 1990.

[33] Duerk, Alene B. Rear Admiral Navy Nurse Corps, *Oral History Interview Tape Transcript*, Interviewers Captain Doris M. Sterner Navy Nurse Corps and Dr. Lynn Dunn, 12 July 1988.

[34] Laird, et. al., op. cit., p. 42.

[35] Ibid..

[36] Moeller, Ruth Captain Medical Service Corps, *Oral History Interview Tape Transcript*, Interviewer Captain Doris M. Sterner Navy Nurse Corps, 17 October 1988.

[37] Jackson, W. Leona Captain, Director Navy Nurse Corps, "We've Reached The Golden Year," *American Journal of Nursing*, Vol. 58, No.5, May 1958, p. 672.

[38] Ibid..

[39] *The World Book Encyclopedia*, op. cit., Volume 6, p. 110.

[40] Wells, H.G., op. cit., p. 961.

[41] Laird, et. al., op. cit..

[42] Nimits, Betty A. LCdr Navy Nurse Corps, telephone conversation with Captain Doris M. Sterner Navy Nurse Corps, 28 June 1993.

[43] Nimits, Betty A. LCdr Navy Nurse Corps, *Oral History Interview Tape Transcript*, Self interview, 25 March 1991.

[44] *The World Book Encyclopedia*, op. cit., Volume 17, p. 572e.

[45] Ibid., Vol. 6, p. 110.

[46] Laird, et. al., op. cit., p. 43.

[47] Ibid..

[48] Eberharter, Virginia M. CDR Navy Nurse Corps, *Oral History Interview Tape Transcript*, Self interview, 5 August 1990 and telephone conversation with Captain D. Sterner on 17 July 1995.

[49] Cannon, Mary F. Captain Navy Nurse Corps, *Oral History Interview Tape Transcript*, Self interview, 8 January 1990.

[50] Emond, Lucille G. Captain Navy Nurse Corps, *Oral History Interview Tape Transcript*, Self interview, 1 May 1990.

[51] Ibid..

[52] Nimits, op. cit..

[53] Jackson, W. Leona Captain NC USN, Department of the Navy, Bureau of Medicine and Surgery, BUMED-32-ils, Letter dated 14 April 1958.

[54] Information prepared by the Navy Nurse Corps Officers on the staff of the Director of the Navy Nurse Corps.

[55] Ibid..

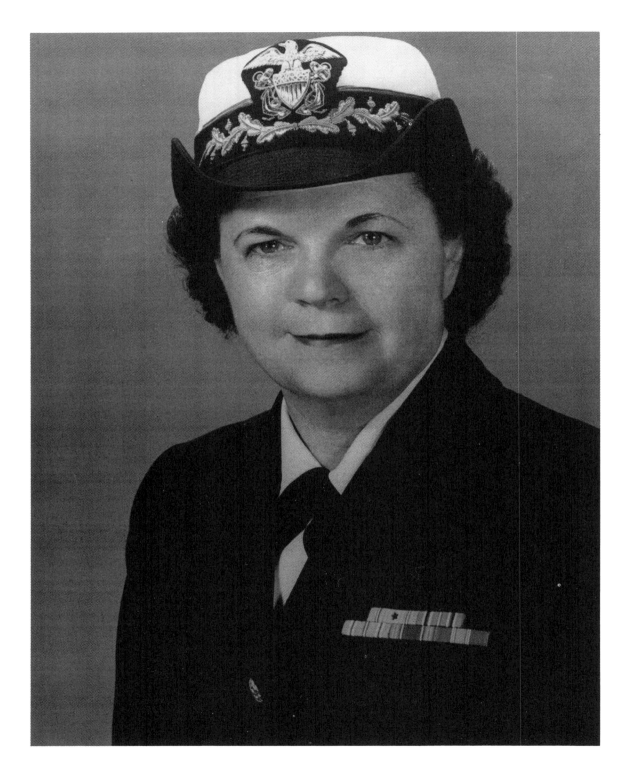

Director - Captain Ruth A. Houghton NC USN
(Official U.S. Navy photo courtesy of Nursing Division, Bureau of Medicine and Surgery, Navy Department.)

CHAPTER 10

Director - Captain Ruth A. Houghton
(1958 - 1962)

☆☆☆

Captain Houghton is Chief Nurse at the Naval Hospital, National Naval Medical Center at Bethesda, Maryland in 1958. On 7 February 1958, the Chief of the Bureau of Medicine and Surgery (the Surgeon-General of the Navy) writes a letter to the Secretary of the Navy by way of the Chief of Naval Personnel. Part of that letter reads:

> "1. Reference (a) [Title 10 of U.S. Law] provides for the appointment of a Director of the Navy Nurse Corps by the Secretary of the Navy, on recommendation of the Chief of the Bureau of Medicine and Surgery, for a term of office of four years. The term of office of the present incumbent, Captain W. Leona Jackson NC, USN, expires on 30 April 1958. Captain Jackson . . . has requested voluntary retirement on 1 May 1958, upon the completion of her four year term of office.
> 2. I, therefore, am recommending Captain Ruth Agatha Houghton NC, USN, for appointment as Director of the Navy Nurse Corps to succeed Captain Jackson on her retirement."

The Chief of Naval Personnel forwards the letter to the Secretary of the Navy with this remark, "Forwarded, readdressed and recommending approval." Captain Houghton is approved by the Secretary of the Navy and receives orders to report for duty on 3 March 1958 at the Bureau of Medicine and Surgery, Navy Department. She is appointed and becomes Director of the Navy Nurse Corps on 1 May 1958.

Captain Houghton was born 29 June 1909, at Methuen, Massachusetts which is north of Boston near the New Hampshire-Massachusetts border. She graduated from St. John's Hospital School of Nursing (Lowell, Massachusetts) in February 1932. On 1 June 1935 Ruth A. Houghton was commissioned an Ensign in the Navy Nurse Corps and reported to the Naval Hospital, New York, NY. From 1936 to 1942 she was stationed at four other Naval Hospitals: Newport, Rhode Island then Coco Solo, Panama Canal Zone followed by Puget Sound, Washington then Corona, California. During WWII she was sent as Chief Nurse to the Naval Training School, Cedar Falls, Iowa. In July 1943 she reported, as Chief Nurse, into the U.S. Naval Hospital Echo Base Hospital #10 in Sidney, Australia where she is promoted to Lieutenant Commander. In August of 1944 she is Chief Nurse at Base Hospital #13 in New Guinea. In 1945, LCdr. Houghton is Nurse Indoctrination Instructor at the Philadelphia Naval Hospital. Then follows duty at Klamath Falls, Oregon and Portsmouth, New Hampshire. In 1946, she is assigned to the Nursing Division of the Bureau of Medicine and Surgery with duty as the Detail Officer for the Nurse Corps. (The Detail Officer has the task of assigning change-of-duty orders.) Meantime she is taking off-duty courses at George Washington University in D.C.. In 1949 she is sent to Boston College, in Boston, Massachusetts where she obtains her Bachelor of Science Degree in Nursing Education. From there she heads overseas as the Senior Nurse Corps Officer in the Navy Medical Unit at Tripler (Army) General Hospital in Hawaii.[1]

In a letter to LCdr. Houghton, dated 19 December 1950, Captain Winnie Gibson (Director at that time) writes that, "A letter from the Commanding Officer of the Navy Unit of that hospital [Tripler] has urgently requested that a nurse in Lieutenant Commander rank be assigned to the hospital to take care of Nurse Corps matters for the Navy Nurses. You will be under the Chief Nurse of the Army, who is a very fine person I understand, and I am confident that you will work with her in complete harmony." There was a comparatively small contingent of Navy Medical personnel at this large Army medical facility and the Army was, of course, in charge. While she was at Tripler, Miss Houghton is promoted to Commander. In 1952 CDR Houghton received orders as Chief Nurse of the San Diego Naval Hospital and in 1954 she goes to Bethesda Naval Hospital as Chief Nurse. She also obtains a Master of Science Degree in Nursing from the Catholic University of America in Washington, D.C..[2] Now, she is the Director of the Navy's Nurses.

In the world of 1958, Khrushchev is the strong man of communist Russia and the United Arab Republic (Egypt, Syria and Yemen) is the source of unease among the other Arab nations and in Washington. In 1957 President Eisenhower had introduced a doctrine for the Middle East in which U.S. military help would be supplied to any nation requesting "help against communist aggression. In July, 1958, Eisenhower used the doctrine to send troops to Lebanon to protect the government from rebel forces."[3] "Eisenhower, assured that the Russians would not attack, ordered American troops into Lebanon. The same morning that [Lebanon] asked for help, Lebanese at the beach watched three battalions of [U.S.] Marines wade ashore. The crisis was ended."[4] Then in August, the President orders the U.S. Seventh Fleet to help the Chinese Nationalists on Taiwan (Formosa) take supplies to the Nationalists' Islands (located between Taiwan and the Chinese mainland) which are being bombed by the Chinese communists. This all dies down come October.[5] As to the space program, the U.S. launches its first satellite into space in January and in March the second one goes up. In December the first communications satellite is launched by the U.S..[6]

Congress passes new legislation in June of 1958 that provides "for an increase of pay for officers with more than two years of service on active duty . . . [It is] designed to reduce . . . turnover and give the Armed Forces greater selectivity in retention of highly qualified personnel."[7]

As for the Nurse Corps in 1958, May the 13th is its Golden Anniversary. Fifty years old and most Nurse Corps Officers the world over, take some time to celebrate. It is a strong and vibrant Corps that has more than proved itself.

In August 1958, the nurses' quarters are closed "at U.S. Naval Hospitals: San Diego, California; Key West, Florida; and Bremerton, Washington."[8] Then when October comes, a 'five-day' work week with an improved staffing design begins at the St. Albans Naval Hospital in New York.[9]

On the 3rd of September an in-service course in 'Nuclear Nursing' is begun at the Department of Nuclear Medicine at the Naval Medical School of the National Naval Medical Center, Bethesda, Maryland. Lieutenant Commander Lenore Simon and Lieutenant Sarah McGinness have been assigned to direct the course. The Director of the Nurse Corps, Captain Ruth Houghton, addresses the first class of students. "It is a pleasure to be asked to greet you today as members of the first class in Nuclear Nursing, not only in the Navy, but as far as I know, in the world. You are making history. . . .

"As we stand on the threshold of another decade in the history of the Navy Nurse Corps, we find a changing Navy - a nuclear Navy, to meet the pressures of a changing world. . . .

"Only a week or so ago our eighth nuclear-powered submarine - the largest ever built - was launched when the 447-foot `TRITON' slid down the ways at Groton, Connecticut. Congress has now provided funds for a total of 33 nuclear-powered submarines - including 9 to be equipped with the Polaris missile. The men who man these submarines must be specially selected and trained - they are schooled to be sonar operators, radar technicians, missile men and engineers specifically qualified in the new science of nucleonics. . . .

"The Navy Nurse Corps is meeting the challenge of a nuclear Navy by the establishment of this course in Nuclear Nursing. Not only will you gain an understanding of atomic radiation in mass casualties, but also the value of radioisotope in diagnostic and therapeutic techniques. . . .

"Because of the small numbers of personnel prepared in this specialty, your responsibilities will be great. I envision your work under the peacetime atom in clinical radioisotope laboratories, supervising therapeutic radioisotope wards, in teaching all levels of personnel, and in research. It is difficult to envision your role under the war-time atom, but with your knowledge you must constantly teach all levels of personnel through in-service educational programs in mass casualty procedures. The responsibilities of every single nurse will be far too great to ever measure. They tell me that in the event of an atomic disaster, each nurse will have at least 300 critically ill patients to care for with little or no equipment available. You will be in a position through your knowledge of alpha, beta, and gamma rays to determine which patients can be saved.... I envy each of you the opportunity to take this course and I wish that I could be one of the group. The future of nuclear nursing rests in your hands."[10]

Meanwhile, the Nurse Corps' one and only Indoctrination Center at the Naval Hospital, St. Albans, New York, is celebrating its sixth year of existence. Before 1947, Nurse Corps members were mainly indoctrinated at their first duty stations. "From 1947 to 1950, one Nurse Corps officer on the East and West Coasts, traveled to the various hospitals to initiate a uniform program for indoctrination of newly-commissioned nurses. By 1950, the Naval Hospitals at San Diego, Bethesda, St. Albans, Camp Pendleton, Oakland, Bremerton, Great Lakes, Chelsea, Philadelphia, Portsmouth, and Jacksonville were receiving the majority of the newly-appointed Nurse Corps officers. In each of these hospitals a senior Nurse Corps officer was assigned as Indoctrination Officer. The period of indoctrination varied in length from four to six weeks and included both theoretical aspects of naval procedure and supervised clinical and ward administration practice."[11] Then in 1952 St. Albans became the only Nurse Corps' Indoctrination Center. The 1958 Nurse Corps staff consists of Commander Ann Poytress as Officer In Charge and three instructors; LCdr Dymphna Van Gorp, LCdr Mary Fraser, and LCdr Elizabeth St. John.[12]

Out on the west coast, the USS *Haven* is no longer sailing the seas but is tied up to a pier at the Long Beach Naval Shipyard. Ltjg Edith L. Colton (Ferguson) is there in 1958 and says, "On the *Haven* (the ship always remained stationary), we ran many outpatient clinics. Since, at that time, we had no Naval Hospital in Long Beach, the *Haven* provided hospitalization for active duty and retired Navy.... We had all services except for female dependents because we could not keep women aboard; just strictly men."[13]

Over in Yokosuka, Japan, at Christmas time in 1958, Navy Nurse Miriam Sherman is once again getting ready to play Santa Claus. "I played Santa Claus for an orphanage in Japan when I was stationed in Yokosuka. I went down to [an alley] in Yokosuka and bought some beautiful velvet material to have a Santa Claus suit made. They didn't know anything about Santa Claus in Japan ... I got some rabbit [fur] for trimming, which I had put on as the trim of the jacket. Made the hat. Bought some buckram [stiffened cloth] as a backing to make a mask, the mustache and the beard. Sewed the rabbit fur on that. In Japan we [the nurses] had personal maids who did sewing and stuff for us. We shared them with other nurses. My personal maid made the Santa Claus outfit. She had no idea what she was doing [since she had no concept of Santa Claus]. I still have [that suit].

"We nurses got together and decided we didn't want to throw a cocktail party [for Christmas] and spend all that money when there were so many parties in Japan at that time [i.e. ships in port giving parties] ... we would rather spend our money for somebody else, preferably an orphanage. So, Ann Ballard and Mary Lally and a couple of others formed a committee to find an orphanage where nobody had anything for them [the orphans]. They found one in Yokohama, in the outskirts somewhere ... It was operated by the Japanese government.... We got a list of the ages of the boys and girls and the sizes [of clothes that] they wore. The money [to be donated for the party] was pro-rated ... according to the rank [of the donating nurse]. A lot of them gave much more money than they were pro-rated for. We had a good collection of money.... We [bought] something to wear, an article of clothing for each child and a toy or a [personal] article for them.... There were a couple of boys and some girls that were sixteen and seventeen [they had to leave the orphanage when they were eighteen]. We gave the girls compacts and stuff like that but then they [also] got mittens and gloves and socks.... We had so much money that we bought a basketball and a hoop, a baseball set for the kids to play (gloves, bats, balls) and we bought toys and games for the younger children for group play. We had a great big cake baked, we got the special services' bus and a whole gang of us went over to the orphanage. We had popcorn, candy, punch, a lot of food. All of this came out of the nurses' pockets.

"We had to take our shoes off as we entered [as one does on entering any Japanese house] ... I had tabbies [Japanese footwear similar to soft slippers] on under my boots [but the boots were left outside].... They [the orphans] just didn't know what Santa Claus was, but one of our personal maids that went with us on the bus, interpreted ... the kids just had a marvelous time. When we were leaving, this little girl that was hanging around me, she wanted my boots. I couldn't ... [give them to her] because there was snow on the ground and I couldn't do without my boots. But, I took my tabbies off and I gave them to her and she was absolutely thrilled."[14] And thereby, an orphanage of Japanese children is introduced to the legendary Santa Claus.

In 1959, Navy Nurse Ruth Halverson is teaching at the Hospital Corps School at Great Lakes, Illinois. She speaks of the Navy course in teaching that she had to attend before she could begin working with her first class at the Corps School. "I think that [Instructors School] was more difficult than any college course I had taken at Marquette University. Because it was so condensed; in one month. It was from 8 a.m. until 4 p.m. and then you sat about four to five hours in the evening, doing all of your class work for the next day because you had to do all your lesson plans and give demonstrations. And everything that you learned there, you had to present to the group. It was really a very condensed, difficult course. It was teaching me how to teach; how to write lesson plans. It was taught by several Chiefs at the school, and this was at the Great Lakes Training Center. The course was actually called the Instructors School. It wasn't just nurses, it was all Navy personnel that they were teaching to teach. They kept the classes at a minimum . . . because there was so much classroom work that they felt they could not be effective if they had too large a group. I have always been very grateful for that course. It was an excellent course and, I must admit, at first I had misgivings about being taught by a Chief, but those certainly were thrown out very shortly because those men were excellent. They had been well selected for their position. . . .

"We taught all the basic nursing arts to the corpsmen [at the Hospital Corps School, after the Instructors School] . . . you are supposed to have a class of twenty or twenty-five. Well, they had lowered the time period to ten or twelve weeks [for the corpsmen's course] in Hospital Corps School, and . . . I think my largest class was ninety. When you have to get up and teach somebody how to do a blood pressure with ninety students, and then have them demonstrate it, that's quite a job. But, that's the way it was.

"[The purpose of what the corpsmen were being taught was] so that they could go out into the field and into our Naval Hospitals and assist our nurses, work as corpsmen and do patient care. These men had no previous nursing background . . . you saw many of these youngsters coming directly to us from boot camp and they went there directly from civilian life . . . but, you could see them all grow and kind of meld into this [being a corpsman] and really make something out of themselves . . . they really made you proud."[15]

On 4 January 1959, "Ten newly commissioned Nurse Corps officers and one instructor attend an 8-week indoctrination course at the U.S. Naval School, Officer (Women), U.S. Naval Schools Command, Newport, Rhode Island to conduct a pilot study of the program. LCdr Dymphna Van Gorp NC, USN is the Senior Nurse Corps officer."[16] The pilot study is obviously positive because on the 30th of April the Chief of Naval Personnel approves an eight week indoctrination program for all newly commissioned Nurse Corps officers. More instructors are ordered in and classes soon begin. Navy Nurse Dolores Cornelius is one of the instructors and she tells us how it begins, "In May of 1959, I was stationed at Great Lakes Hospital Corps School and had been there just over a year. The Chief Nurse, LCdr Linnenbruegge called me and told me that I had orders to Newport but not to the hospital. We were somewhat baffled by where I was going to be assigned in Newport. LCdr Linnenbruegge suggested that since I knew her, I should call Captain Houghton . . . directly to find out what my next duty was going to be. When I called Captain Houghton, she said, 'Oh, you didn't receive my letter.' (The letter arrived the following day.) Captain Houghton told me that I would be the third Nurse Corps officer assigned to the Woman Officers School at Newport to start a new program there, where all Nurse Corps officers [coming] in the Navy would be indoctrinated with all other female officers in the Navy. . . . Captain Houghton told me that a lot of background work had been done to accomplish this. She was very excited about it and interested in its success. She felt strongly that nurses as Naval officers should have a basic Naval indoctrination rather than a hospital-type indoctrination to the Navy. She said the Surgeon General . . . felt the same way.

"The other two nurses, LCdr Dymphna Van Gorp, the senior nurse, and LCdr Aline Morin, had already reported in when I arrived at Newport on a beautiful Sunday afternoon in June of 1959. When I entered the large lounge, a Line [officer] indoctrinee was sitting with her male guest in the middle of the room. Upon seeing me, they immediately stood at attention. I was so startled and non-plussed that I forgot to say `carry on' to release them from their frozen position. To my great relief I found a door and quickly left the room. I didn't think that was a very good beginning for me at the Women Officers School.

"The three of us on the Nurse Corps staff got along well with the Line staff instructors. In fact, they appeared to be somewhat in awe of us. We were Lieutenant Commanders; they were Lieutenant(jg)'s or Lieutenants except for the Officer-in-Charge, Commander Kathleen Zeigler. I had been stationed on a ship, the USS *President Jackson*. None of them had been stationed on a ship. So, considering the fact that the three of us newcomers had invaded their territory in an established program, I thought we got on very well with the Line officer staff. There was little, if any, friction that I can remember. . . .

"The indoctrination was purposefully difficult. And, I believe, was similar or based on the program at the Male Officer Candidate School, also at Newport. Some of the nurses, as well as the Line students, felt they were treated like children when many of them are college graduates. This was expressed in their evaluations at the end of the program. Although there could have been a little more flexibility, at times, in dealing with the students, I believe it was a very effective and worth while indoctrination, especially when I compare it to my own [indoctrination] at the Naval Hospital in Bremerton.

"I think the emphasis on leadership as a Naval officer was very important. I did not really become secure as a Naval officer until I became an instructor at the Woman Officers School.

"Before starting [duty] at the Hospital Corps School at Great Lakes in February of 1958, I was sent to a four-week course at Instructor Training School on the [Great Lakes] base. This was an excellent course and prepared me well for my assignment, not only at Hospital Corps School, but also for any future teaching position. Another thing which helped me considerably was taking a course at the Catholic University of America called `The Fundamentals of Oral Communication." . . .

"Concerning the curriculum for the nurses, my memory is a bit hazy about the subject. My recollection is that LCdr Van Gorp, LCdr Morin and I, all had some involvement developing the curriculum for the nurses. I can't recall, however, whether the curriculum was the same for the Line and the nurses except for the medical department [material]. I do know that LCdr Morin did a lot of work on the leadership course, which she taught, and I developed the medical department course, which I taught.

"One of the Line officers had taken a John Robert Powers Modeling Course and taught some of us how to help her to give this [information in a] short course. It was amusing because the male officers in other commands would ask me . . . when was the day for the 'make-over' because they really looked forward to that day at the Officers Mess; the female officers looked so attractive [that day].

"During my tour of duty at Newport at the Woman Officers School, the indoctrination course was eight weeks. I understand [that] later it was shortened to four weeks. For the first two to three weeks, learning what was expected of the students and the fact that they had not experienced anything like this before, put them in a kind of state of shock. Many of them had spent the weeks, between graduating from the University and reporting at Newport, at home eating more than they should. I was assigned the collateral duty of `weight-control' officer by Commander Zeigler. At one time I was following about 70 young women who had to lose varying degrees of weight, or wanted to anyway. . . . It really took discipline for them to eat in the officers Mess and lose weight.

"The first six months of my tour I was very busy and just a few hours ahead of my students. The large classes, the problems with uniforming [the new Navy Nurses], the inspections, making out watches [duty lists], working on the curriculum, all of these kept me busy [as did the] counseling that was a part of my job as Company Officer.

"The staff instructors were models for the students in how to wear the uniform, our appearance, and Navy etiquette. We were constantly on stage . . . It was the only duty I had where we could go to have our hair done during regular working hours if we did not have a class or a scheduled appointment. . . .

"Graduation at the Woman Officers School was held on Thursday morning and was always an exciting event, especially when it was my company graduating. I was so proud of them. The graduates looked so sharp in their uniforms, in particular those who had lost excess weight during the last eight weeks. It was hard to believe at times that these were the same young women who reported to the Woman Officers School just eight weeks ago.

It had been a lot of work but this was the reward."[17]

One of the first small group of WAVES to enter the NENEP (Navy Enlisted Nursing Education Program) at the University of Colorado, graduates in 1959. Patricia Luenberger (Shields) is one of this group. "At graduation we received our commission from the CNO [Chief of Naval Operations] . . . Also present for our graduation was Captain Leona Jackson who was instrumental in getting the NENEP program into action. Also, Commander Vera Thompson was present who was another person who worked hard for this great educational opportunity. I may mention here that the program paid all educational expenses, plus E3 pay, and our obligation was to give back four years of nursing service upon graduation. When we graduated from the University of Colorado with a BSN, we were commissioned as Ensigns in the U.S. Navy Nurse Corps. After graduation we were ordered to report to officer's indoctrination in Newport, R.I. for six weeks orientation. We were part of the first all-nurse WN1 orientation class."[18]

Another member of the first Nurse Corps class at the Woman Officers School, was a 1959 graduate from the University of Alabama School of Nursing, Ann Currie (Gilfillan). She had been a participant in the Navy Nurse Corps Candidate Program. "We were paid $99.00 a month during our senior year because that's what hospitalmen made at that point and time. And, the Navy picked up the expense of our books and tuition, so it was very nice, really. We graduated and took our state boards, then the Navy had requested that they be sent the results of our state boards early so that we could be commissioned and participate in the orientation at Newport. So we went and took our state boards with the rest of our class and we did, we got the results of our state boards two weeks early and then we sent those to the Navy and we wound up with orders to report the 1st of July to Naval Schools Command in Newport, Rhode Island. So, off we went. . . . Our class was the very first class . . . there were about 60 of us from all over the United States; all bright-eyed, ready to go, we went over and got uniformed. Every conceivable uniform that we would need. We were told how to put insignias on and how to sew patches on, and learned how to spit-shine our black boon dockers. We were told how to form up when we marched to class because, when we marched to class, we had a Marine drill Sergeant. We were told, we didn't believe it at first, but they made believers out of us, that this was orientation to the Navy and to the military. . . .

"The two months we spent at Newport were purely military. We learned nothing about the Navy Nurse Corps other than it was a branch of the military. We spent our time learning about military justice, we had a class on ships, aircraft, and weapons; where we learned how to identify silhouettes of aircraft and ships. We learned about Naval history, we learned about Naval courtesy, we learned about Navy lingo, we had vocabulary tests . . . so that we could talk to the guys from the fleet when they were our patients. They would need us to be Naval officers first. . . . As I said, [we] marched to class, we had inspections, our rooms were inspected. If our blinds weren't vertical we got points off, if our drawers weren't exactly straight . . . and all of our clothes . . . in a group, we got points off. . . . If our slips were showing . . . we'd have points off and when you had so many points off then you'd have to march, just like everybody else, which was quite a shock to us nurses, but we all survived. We developed a real camaraderie. We also had [another] taste of [the] military in that we all got to stand [watch] after we had been there for a while. We began standing OOD [Officer Of the Day] watches. We all had our OOD patches on and we had to make rounds and log things into our little log book, and be very military and very proficient. . . .

"One of the other things . . . really valuable, I think, in our . . . orientation . . . [was the group of] ten former Navy WAVES who had been commissioned through the NENEP program. They were absolutely great; they were really the finest of the fine. They welcomed us to the Navy and they told us wonderful war stories about being WAVES and they added realism to our orientation. They were a great deal of help for inspections and for learning how to spit-shine because they knew all the tricks. They also gave us a realistic appreciation for what life as an enlisted corpsman was. I learned from them how to relate better to the corpsmen that I would be supervising when I took over my duties as charge nurse on one of the military wards and I found that, throughout my Navy career, to be invaluable information. Plus, they were just super, super human beings but, then again, I think that everybody in our class was. It was a very unique experience and one that I have always cherished and appreciated."[19]

After indoctrination, Ensign Ann Currie (Gilfillan) reports to her first duty station, the Naval Hospital at Great Lakes. She says, "So, when we got to Great Lakes, what we found . . . was there were no other Ensigns there at Great Lakes. So now there were . . . going to be two Ensigns at Great Lakes. . . . At the time I came into the Navy, Captain was as high a rank as you could go in the Navy Nurse Corps. And the only Captain that we had, was the Director of the Navy Nurse Corps. . . . But anyway, our chief nurse [at Great Lakes] . . . was a great role model for any Nurse Corps officer. She met with us individually over the next couple of weeks while we were being oriented. Sat down and chatted with us, and found out what we wanted to do for the rest of our lives; how we thought our careers might be mapped out. . . .

"Our [Naval Hospital] orientation; we had a two month orientation after we got there to learn how to become Navy Nurses. We finally got to wear our nursing white uniforms. The same thing that was true with our Navy blue uniforms and our gray uniforms, was true about our white uniform; you wore your rank insignia on your right because 'rank is always right' and your corps device on your left collar. We got to wear the full nurse's hat with the black band on it and with my gold [stripe] . . . and I was very proud of that."[20]

Another Nurse Corps Candidate that was in the first Nurse Corps class at the Newport Woman Officers School, is Beverly Brase (O'Dell). After finishing the new indoctrination at Newport she travels to her first Duty station. "I arrived at my first duty station (Oakland, California) in September, 1959. At that time, the hospital was located on the hills in Oakland in WWII wooden barracks buildings, and the buildings were connected by ramps. All of them were separate with a census of about 40-60 patients per building. Night duty consisted of covering a whole area, and my first experience with night duty was on the special surgery wards. There were six buildings, and at night time you had to go from one building to another, and you never knew what you were going to encounter when you got outside. It might be a skunk, a deer, or raccoons (all sorts of wildlife were around at night) so you always took you flashlight and looked carefully where you were going before you went there.

"One of the things that I remember very vividly, was that graduates from collegiate programs were not very highly thought of at all. The students that had graduated from Hospital Schools of Nursing were considered to be much better nurses and much better qualified. The program at the University of Colorado, I think, was a little different than some of the other collegiate programs, in that, we had a lot of ward experience and hands-on nursing experience during the program, and I felt that I was pretty well qualified and had done lots of treatments and things. . . . I remember one time I did something and the nurse said, 'I can tell you're from a Hospital School of Nursing because you know how to do the procedures,' and I have always kind of smiled to myself and never really admitted that I was a collegiate graduate.

"One of the things that I found a hard adjustment, was the equipment and supplies. Some of the things were quite different. I remember my first insertion of a Foley Catheter. I had put in many Foley Catheters during nurses' school, and I felt well-qualified to do it. The Senior Nurse that I was with asked if I had ever put in a Foley before, and I said yes, I had and I had done many and that I didn't feel it would be a problem. So, I collected all the equipment and went in to insert the Foley. Got everything ready, inserted the Foley, got ready to inject the fluid (the 5cc's to . . .[fill the bag and hold the catheter in place]) and there was no stopper in the end of the Foley Catheter. I was at my wits end, I didn't know what to do. I finally got the patient to ring for the nurse to come in and help me. [The nurse] said, `you just double up the end of the catheter and tie it off with a string, and then you take the needle and inject the fluid in through the wall of the catheter.' I remembered after that not to say I knew how to do something until I actually watched somebody do it with equipment that they had in the Navy because it was very different than what we had in school.

"Another adjustment that I felt was very hard for new nurses coming in, is supervising the corpsmen. At that time, the corpsmen were as old, or a little older than I was. They always tried very hard to establish a personal relationship rather than a professional relationship. It seemed when I first came in that the corpsmen really knew how to do a lot of things, but I found out, not too much after, that they knew how to do it but they didn't know why. So, I enjoyed teaching and working with them and found that very rewarding. I felt they were like sponges and they were interested and bright and would learn anything that you took the time to teach them."[21]

In February 1959, there is approval for Nurse Corps officers of the Regular Navy to attend full time duty under instruction for a Master's degree. However, the applicants must be able to complete the requirements for the degree in one semester or one semester and a summer session. In other words, the applicant must have completed some of the educational requirements, on her own, before applying.[22] And, in September, the Naval Medical School at Bethesda Naval Medical Center in Maryland, establishes an "annual ten-week orientation course for military nurses from friendly allied countries."[23] Also, in September 1959, the Indoctrination Course for Nurse Corps Officers at the St. Albans Naval Hospital in New York is discontinued since the Newport Woman Officers School now has that assignment. In October a Nurse Training Branch opens at the Naval Medical School at Bethesda. The mission of this Training Branch is "to develop and conduct inservice . . . short courses, institutes, and workshops to improve patient care and personnel practices."[24] The Head of this Training Branch is Cdr Rita Clarke and the Assistant Head is LT P. Hope McIntyre.[25]

In 1959, another uniform is authorized for Navy women; "a light blue uniform for both officers and enlisted personnel. The light blue and white striped, corded dacron/cotton uniform was to be used as a counterpart of the khaki service uniform worn by male officers and chief petty officers. The short sleeved jacket was worn open at the neck with the collar and lapels turned back. No shirt was worn with this jacket which was trimmed with navy blue piping and closed with four blue Navy eagle buttons. Women officers wore pin-on insignia of grade and/or corps on the collar points . . . The skirt, of the same material as the jacket, according to the regulation, was to come to the middle of the calf of the wearer's leg. The shoes were black and the stockings the usual beige. The cap is very similar to that introduced for wear by officers of the newly created WAVES in 1943 and was worn with a cover to match the jacket. . . . A plain black handbag of leather or synthetic material was carried when the blue uniforms were worn. . . . The bags had detachable shoulder straps so they could be slung from the shoulder or carried in the hand."[26]

Also authorized, in the uniform instruction of 6 April 1959, is "'Service Dress Blue C' . . . now known as 'Service Dress, Blue, modified'. The blue coat is worn with a white skirt, hat with white cover, white dress shoes, beige stockings and a black handbag. Grade is indicated in the same way as for male officers, by gold lace on the sleeves, with a . . . corps device above the lace. . . . [The cuff] stripes of gold lace. . . . The white summer coat is similar in cut to the blue one . . . but instead of gold sleeve lace, white braid is used with the device embroidered in yellow. The hat is the basic one for all Navy women. Officers display the standard cap device, two crossed gold foul anchors, surmounted by a silver shield with a silver spread eagle above. The white shirt has short sleeves and is worn with a black tie, tied with a square knot."[27] Both the blue and the white service coats "prescribed for all women of the United States Navy, both officer and enlisted [are] single-breasted, straight backed, easy fitting in front, with a rounded collar which overlaps the half-peaked lapels."[28]

In July 1959, "Nurse Corps officer representation [begins] on the Inspector General's Survey Party for inspection of Naval Medical activities."[29] And, in November, the requirements for joining the Navy Nurse Corps are changed by the Secretary of the Navy. From this time on all incoming selectees must be able to complete twenty years of active duty by the time they reach 55; by the 'fiscal' year that they reach 55. Also, rank on entering will be determined not only by age but by education and experience. All Ensigns cannot be over 28, all Lt(jg)'s must not be over 32, and the maximum age for incoming LT's is 35.[30]

As for national events, the United States and Canada celebrate the opening of the Saint Lawrence Seaway, in 1959. The seaway, itself, "extends for 182 miles from Montreal to the mouth of Lake Ontario."[31] The importance of this seaway is that it "permits large ocean-going ships to sail from the Atlantic Ocean to ports on the Great Lakes. . . . [A distance of over] 2,300 miles inland from the Atlantic Ocean."[32] Also, in 1959, the U.S. produces 'synthetic penicillin.'[33]

As for the 'space program' in 1959, Russia launches a rocket probe to the moon; it passes the moon and goes into orbit around the sun. The U.S. soon follows with its own moon probe, Pioneer IV, that also ends up in orbit about the sun. Then in September, Russia launches yet another probe but this one crashes on the surface of the moon.[34]

Down in Cuba, Fidel Castro and his followers, force out the incumbent President and declare Castro the new Premier, then the victorious revolutionaries proceed with a large number of in-country executions. Over in Russia, Khrushchev accepts President Eisenhower's invitation to visit the U.S.. He comes and agrees to a meeting next year with the heads of the U.S., Great Britain and France.[35] The U.S. visit seems to warm the 'cold-war' tensions for a bit; even though Khrushchev is not permitted to visit 'Disneyland.' However, Khrushchev manages to destroy the 1960 Summit meeting (being held in Paris), when the Russians shoot down an American U-2 'spy' plane over Russia. "On May Day, 1960, Eisenhower's framework of world peace collapsed. For [the U-2 pilot] Francis Gary Powers, flying over Sverdlovsk in the Soviet Union, it was a dull thud and a lingering orange glow; then his U-2 high-altitude photo reconnaissance plane began to fall apart. With the crumbling plane went Eisenhower's dream for a breakthrough at the summit meeting in Paris."[36]

"The international situation continued to deteriorate after the Paris fiasco. Eisenhower journeyed to the Far East as scheduled in June, although anti-American feeling in Japan forced him to cancel his visit to that country. Relations with Cuban Premier Castro became more strained and Eisenhower ordered the training of Cuban exiles in Guatemala."[37] What Castro did was seize "all property owned by American companies in Cuba. He later [charges] that the U.S. embassy in Havana [is] the center of `counter-revolutionary activities' against Cuba."[38] But, there is another chaotic dilemma that has been and keeps on brewing in the Far East; Vietnam. "By 1960 between 5,000 and 10,000 guerrillas, called by the Saigon government Viet-Cong, meaning `Vietnamese Communist,' were estimated to be active in the South [of Vietnam]. While the Vietnamese army, under American advice, was mainly stationed along the partition line [of Vietnam] to guard against a Korea-style attack, the insurgents were spreading havoc. . . . `The situation may be summed up,' reported the American Embassy in January 1960, `in the fact that the [Vietnamese] government has tended to treat the population with suspicion or to coerce it and has been rewarded with apathy and resentment.' . . . In September 1960 the Communist Party Congress in Hanoi called for the overthrow of the Diem regime and of `American imperialist rule.' Formation of the National Liberation Front (NLF) of South Vietnam followed in December. Though nominally native to the South, it echoed the call for the overthrow of Diem and the `camouflaged colonial regime of the American imperialists' and announced a ten-point program of Marxist social reforms dressed in the usual garments of `democracy,' `equality,' `peace,' and `neutrality.' Overt civil war was thus declared."[39]

Despite the growing turmoil tormenting the rest of the world, in the States 1960 is an election year and that takes precedence. "In March, 1960, four months before the Republican national convention, Eisenhower announced his support of Vice President Nixon to succeed him as President."[40] The Democrats choose 43 year old Senator John F. Kennedy with Senator Lyndon B. Johnson as his running mate. At the election, the popular vote is extremely close with Kennedy winning by a mere 118,449 votes but the electoral vote gives 303 to Kennedy and 219 to Nixon.[41] The new President will be the youngest ever to hold that office.

The Navy Nurse Corps, in 1960, finds its officers "serving in 36 of the 50 United States; on the continents of Europe and Africa; on islands in the Atlantic and Pacific oceans and off the coast of Asia; and on ships of the Military Sea Transportation Service."[42] In January, Navy Nurses receive orders to the Naval Air Station at Sigonella on the island of Sicily. In April Navy Flight Nursing becomes history. The flight nursing course is discontinued and assignments are ended. Then in September, Navy Nurses have a new assignment with the Naval Advisory Group at the Chinhae Detachment (near Pusan) in South Korea.[43]

This is the year, 1960, that more emphasis is placed on education in the Nurse Corps. In May, billets are opened for Nurse Corps officers at the United States Naval Postgraduate School in Monterey, California. The course being offered is a one-year, highly qualified and very concentrated, course for a Master of Science degree in Management. In August, a Nursing Research Branch is initiated in the Naval Medical School at the Naval Medical Center in Bethesda, Maryland. Then, in September the time restriction placed on Navy Nurse applicants for graduate study, is removed. (Just last year, graduate full-time-duty-under-instruction was approved but restricted to one semester or one semester and one summer session.) And, in December 1960, the NENEP (Navy Enlisted Nursing Education Program) is opened to all enlisted women instead of only the Hospital Corps WAVES.[44]

283

In May there is a small change in the Nurse Corps' service dress white uniform but, it is one that is more in keeping with a Naval officer's uniform; gold braid is authorized to replace the white braid (denoting rank) on the sleeves of the jacket and a gold embroidered Corps device is approved to replace the yellow silk one on the sleeves above the braid.[45]

To return to the every day affairs of the Nurse Corps; Ensign Ann Currie (Gilfillan) at Great Lakes Naval Hospital in 1960, tells us, "It wasn't too long after I started at Great Lakes that we all formed real good friendships (the younger nurses did) and we decided we would like to move off base. We were living in the nurses' quarters with a whole bunch of older nurses, and having to be very quiet. Having to abide by all the rules of the nurses kind of really cramped our style, so we started looking for apartments off base. That was when I realized that there were two different worlds. There was the world of the nurse who lived off base, which all the young nurses did, and [there was the world of] the married nurse. Married nurses were still a phenomenon in the Navy at that point in time; there weren't too many of them. . . . I think it had probably been maybe only five years that Nurse Corps officers could be married, up to that point. [Before that] if you got married, you resigned your commission. Strangely enough, a lot of the elder nurses were married. They had kind of courted and, I guess, held on to their boyfriends until the Navy came around, and then they got married. The Navy loved to send them to places like Kwajalein and Midway, places like that, that were one year tours with no dependents. A lot of the girls had married old boyfriends who had been in the Navy, but the Navy had a real tough 'no fraternization' rule at that point in time, and if you got caught dating an enlisted, they made life really rough for you. You were ostracized and you knew that it was not the thing to do. If you were working on a military ward and you were caught dating a corpsman, you got sent to the dependent wards, and that was considered punishment."[46]

Meantime, a young civilian nurse, Rose Marie Lochte is about to join the Navy. She had her training at a hospital school of nursing in Baltimore, Maryland. She graduated in 1953 and had continued to work there. She says, "working conditions at the hospital declined due to the critical shortage of nurses [that was country-wide] which required us to work eighty plus hours in the operating room. We were on a straight salary and were paid the same whether we worked forty or eighty hours. I decided I needed a change. However, most of the hospitals in the area had the same problems and friends who were working at some of these hospitals were not happy.

"One day, on my way to work for a sixteen hour PM and night shift, I passed by the main post office where a Navy recruiting sign was prominently displayed. The next day I stopped in the recruiting office for information. Unfortunately, everyone in the office was enlisted, from the fleet. No one knew anything about the Nurse Corps, but I was given an address in Washington, D.C. where I could write for information. I read the information, submitted my application, quit my job and waited. Finally, I was called for a physical exam. I was commissioned in July 1960 in Washington, D.C. and reported to Newport, RI on 28 August 1960. . . . I was commissioned as a Lt(jg) because of my six and a half years of experience. . . . After OIS [Officer Instruction School] at Newport, I reported to Philadelphia for my first duty in a Naval Hospital. There were many LCdr Nurse Corps officers but very few junior nurses. The expectations of these nurses were very high. There was no formal orientation to the hospital. We were assigned to work with a Senior Nurse and reported directly to the ward. I had worked in the Operating Room for six years and had to do a lot of quick thinking to meet the everyday challenges. Everyone seemed to be talking in code: 'get me four 518's; have you completed the 24 hour report; when Big Bertha comes, be sure the list is ready; put all those chits in the daybook; give Chief Jones a Texas special.' The cryptic messages and orders never seemed to stop. Everyone expected us to know the Navy way of doing things. When I asked for an interpretation, the comment was often, 'What are they teaching at Newport? It's just a charm and finishing school.' Since I was from the 13th class that went through OIS at Newport, I think that the curriculum was still being developed. All we learned about the medical department was the organizational chart, that requests for diagnostic studies were called `chits,' and that in every hospital were these perfect assistants called Corpsmen with whom we were not to fraternize even if he was your own brother. Thank goodness for Marie Knouse. She was an outstanding nurse and really tried to help the new nurses. If she had not been my mentor, I doubt if I would have made the Navy a career. After a month I learned the ropes and was able to successfully meet all the challenges thrown my way: night duty on nine wards on three floors in both wings of the hospital; working a different ward every day both on the AM and PM shifts; relieving the civilian nurses on the dependent wards when they called in sick or got snowed in."[47]

And then there is 'Recruiting Duty.' From the Great Lakes Naval Hospital, Navy Nurse Ruth Halverson is assigned to recruiting duty in the city of Chicago. "That was a totally different and challenging experience. I must say it was very rewarding from the stand-point of seeing a part of the Navy that I had never been exposed to, and learning to work with Line officers, aviators and all the others . . . that you normally don't encounter in the hospital situation. They were counterparts in our recruiting office, and you have to work with them, and you have to go out and give presentations and travel with them. . . . We covered the states of Wisconsin, Illinois, Indiana, and that included 90 nursing schools which we corresponded with every year and set-up appointments (hoping that we could get appointments) to go in and speak to their students about the military. Most of them were very receptive, I must admit. It was very gratifying to meet many of the Directors and Instructors and tell them about our programs."[48]

Navy Nurses are also stationed in Newfoundland in 1960. Carolyn Jean Shearer says, "Out of St. Albans I went to Argentia, Newfoundland. That was a small station hospital. One of the highlights there was when I was issued a 'heavy-duty' coat. I got there in June but by the time I left there, in October of 1960, I found out what that coat was for. It was to get me from quarters over to the station hospital. It was just so cold . . . The winds were so bad blowing across the air strip when we would leave to go to work, we had to hold on to a rope to get us across or we'd blow away. In fact, we would have 'white-outs' with the snow. When we got off duty at night, we'd call the quarters and ask which door was open; there were three doors. The way the snow would blow, it would seal the door off in a certain direction so we'd have to take the door where there was no snow. . . . In the white-outs (and the bad winds that would come across the peninsula) we had our parkas on and the hoods over our heads, but we had to protect our face and be able to see where we were going. So we used old x-ray film and made small slits in it, enough so we could see out to walk. That way we were able to hang on to the rope and make it over to our station hospital. Sometimes it was so bad that, God bless the corpsmen, one would get on each side of you to walk you along that rope and get you back. But the airplanes would go off on schedule; you could set you watch by them. (We were near the airport.) . . .

"We ate lobster there by the bucket load! It was nothing for me to come by the mess hall over in the hospital and they would cook too many lobsters and they would give me as many as 15 lobsters to take over to the nurses' quarters. . . . We had wonderful food.

"[As for the nurses' quarters] we had a real nice building. . . . Our building consisted of about seven or eight bedrooms, a large living room and a large kitchen. We always ate in the kitchen at a table that had benches along either side of it. We had a large dining area too; a dining room. We had a Chief Nurse who was real sweet. She always remembered our birthdays. . . . [Two of the nurses,] for lack of something to do when the winters were really bad, decided to build a boat in the basement part [of the quarters]. There was a large rec room down there. What they didn't realize is the way they built it, they couldn't get it out the door! So they had to tear it [the boat] down and rebuild it. These are two Navy Nurses. One was an anesthetist and the other was a good little nurse . . . . They put the boat in the water and brought a bottle of champagne and christened it and everyone had a wonderful time that day. They [took] it out in the sea lane where they had no business to be and the first thing they knew, along came the security and told them to 'get that thing out of there.' That was more or less the end of the boat. They put the boat in dry dock then."[49]

At the Medical facility on the Naval Station in Rota, Spain, the Navy Nurse Anesthetist is Katherine A. Howard. "In 1960 one of the cases was quite an emergency. We had a 'walking blood bank' [for this case] and fortunately all of our dependents and active duty [personnel] were typed and cross matched. This young man [the patient] had been on the fantail of a submarine when one of the rockets was fired. This rocket was about two feet long and about eight inches in diameter. Somehow the rocket turned around and had just spiraled and hit him in the thigh. The big end of it came out his right iliac crest [hip] and it had entered below his left iliac crest. Well, that happened to be a Sunday afternoon and I was down on the beach in my sandy bathing suit when the Shore Patrol came and got me. . . . [He said], `You have to come [to the Operating Room] right now!' So that was the only time I gave an anesthetic in a sandy, wet bathing suit and my bare feet with a robe around me. [The patient had] lost a great deal of blood, but we had people lined up and donating [the 'walking blood bank'] and I'd hang up the blood that was still warm (which is the best you could get), on the patient's I.V.. . . . He finally came out of shock. He had several holes in his iliac artery on one side but [the rocket] had missed most of his intestines (just pushed them out of the way) and it missed his bladder. But, [it was] decided we could not remove this missile because he would probably go into deep shock then and bleed . . . We prepared to Air Evac him to Wiesbaden [Germany] to the Air Force Hospital [a larger medical facility with the capability for handling the more serious cases]. We heard that they sand bagged the operating room at the time they removed the missile from him. . . . The young man developed gangrene and the only decompression chamber was down in our [nearby] sub tender . . . so the Air Force sent a surgical and nurse team to come down with him to go into the Hyperbaric chamber. During the time he was in the Hyperbaric chamber, he ruptured one of his iliac artery grafts and started to bleed all over again. This was three months later. Again, I was called from home to work on this same fellow but we got him out of shock, again, and had the 'walking blood bank' donating, profusely. He did well. [However,] he eventually died about a year later; stress ulcers."

In 1961, Navy Nurses are stationed all over the world in the practice of their chosen profession. A large part of their duty as Navy Nurses, is the training and education of the hospital corpsmen (and corpswaves.) After their basic education as corpsmen and after some ward experience, qualified corpsmen can go on to 'specialty' training. At several of the larger Naval Hospitals, a Nurse Corps officer is assigned the specific duty as instructor of a specialty course for the corpsmen. One such course is in 'Operating Room Techniques.' A corpsman successfully completing this course is then known as an 'Operating Room Technician.' The Philadelphia Naval Hospital is one of the hospitals that conducts such a course. It is taught in the Main Operating Room suite by a Navy Nurse Corps officer with an Operating Room specialty education. It is a six month course and generally the class has eight to ten students. BuMed requires 135 hours of theoretical education and 825 hours of practical education for the prospective 'O.R. techs.' In actuality, these students receive slightly more than the set requirements during their six months. These corpsmen specialists have a very important niche in Naval medical care because all mobile hospital units sent overseas include O.R. techs who, under the surgeon's supervision, organize and set up an operating room until Navy Nurses arrive, if nurses are sent. If nurses are not sent then the 'tech' must train others to help him and then carry on under the supervision of the surgeon. On the Navy's ships, these O.R. techs are vital in war or in peace because Navy Nurses are not presently assigned aboard these ships. (Even if they were to be assigned there are not enough Navy Nurses available to fill such billets.) Many of the smaller ships do not carry doctors, so these techs must know how to do emergency procedures of all kinds even to the extent of giving an anesthetic or doing some emergency surgery in dire circumstances. That is why their O.R. course includes lectures and hands on experience with surgeons, anesthesiologists and other medical personnel. They learn how to prepare casts and how to apply them, they learn about sterile techniques and the workings of autoclaves, how to act as 'scrub nurse' or 'circulating nurse' during operations, what to do in a 'cardiac arrest,' and much, much more. One of the more senior (not a student) O.R. techs in the Operating Room at Philadelphia, is on call for a special medical team that is flown to Florida each time a 'Manned' space flight is made. He and the rest of the team go aboard the Navy ship that is positioned near the estimated 'splash-down' site of the returning spacecraft. These techs and all corpsmen are vital components of the Navy and Navy medicine as are all of the corpsmen (read also, corpswaves.) They are well trained.

Up in Newport, Rhode Island at the Woman Officers School, Navy Nurse Dolores Cornelius begins an exciting New Year. "In January 1961, I had made a trip to Washington, D.C. to visit friends and made an appointment to see Captain Houghton, the Director of the Navy Nurse Corps, about my next assignment. She told me that she would like me to stay in Newport for the summer which is a very busy time there with all the new indoctrinees. Then after that, in the fall, I could plan on orders to Iwakuni, Japan. That was the only billet available. I would have preferred Yokosuka but was happy at the prospect of going anywhere in Japan. So I left Washington, D.C. happy in the knowledge that towards the end of the year I would be going to Japan.

"Later that month I took my company to visit the submarine base . . . [in] Connecticut. When we arrived at the main gate, I was handed a note. It was a message to call Captain Houghton as soon as possible. I could hardly wait until we got to the Officers Club where I could make the call. Captain Houghton told me that when I got back to Newport that afternoon, TAD orders would be ready for me to go to Washington, D.C.. She could not tell me anything except that it was concerning my next assignment. She also asked if I would like to stay with her. On the bus trip back to Newport, I kept thinking about my conversation with Captain Houghton. This TAD was about my next assignment which I thought had been arranged. Then I was asked to stay at the home of the Director of the Navy Nurse Corps! It was very exciting as well as puzzling. In Newport, LCdr VanGorp had my TAD orders and I was supposed to leave on . . . Sunday; this was Friday. However, a snow storm was forecast so I discussed the possibility of whether I should leave that same day. We decided to wait. During the night we had a blizzard with snow drifts up to 17 feet high. We were completely snow-bound. Afraid that I would not be able to leave on Sunday, I called Captain Houghton. She told me to come when it was possible to travel and not to worry about it. Somehow, on Sunday morning, a taxi was able to make it to where I lived and took me to the bus station. I took a bus to Providence then boarded a train for Washington, D.C.. Many people had been stranded or delayed by the blizzard. The train was crowded with people relieved to be on their way. There was a lot of singing, laughing, and camaraderie during the trip which ended at Union Station in Washington, D.C. at 2300 [11 p.m.].

"A friend picked me up at the train station and we had a quick snack, because I was starved, before he drove me to Captain Houghton's home. (There had been no eating facilities on the long train ride.) Sitting in Captain Houghton's kitchen, eating a late supper, because I hadn't the nerve to tell her I had a snack before coming over, she said she was sure I was wondering why I was here. `It is about an assignment in the White House,' she said. 'In the morning you have an appointment with Dr. Travelle, physician to President Kennedy, and Captain . . ., a Naval Medical officer and assistant physician to the President, at nine o`clock.' The reason for the secrecy was in consideration of me, should I not be selected. I thought I would be too excited to sleep, but was exhausted by the day's events and slept like a baby. . . .

"Captain Houghton was already gone when I got up. A Navy car and driver took me to the main Navy Dispensary where the Medical Service Corps Officer-in-Charge greeted me with, 'So here is the jewel from Newport.' I suspect the 'jewel' part referred to the fact that I could take shorthand and type, a requirement for this assignment.

"A Navy car took me to the White House where I had tea with Dr. Travelle and . . . [the Navy doctor] in her office. After we had talked a short time, Dr. Travelle asked me if I could report for work on Wednesday; this was Monday. I told her that I had an apartment in Newport. So, it was agreed that I would start the following Monday. This gave me about a week to get back to Newport, move out of my apartment, find an apartment in Washington, D.C., if possible, and report for work. The only restriction on where I would live was that it had to be within a ten minute drive of the White House. Fortunately, with the help of Captain Houghton and some of the other nurses at the Bureau of Medicine and Surgery, I found a very nice one on Massachusetts Avenue that met this requirement.

"The beginning of the Kennedy Administration was a period of transition and adjustment. The days were long and sometimes difficult, but I would not want to have missed that experience. It was Captain . . ., assistant physician to President Kennedy, who wanted a Navy Nurse in the White House. He also requested two Hospital Corps Chiefs - one was in administration and the other a physical therapist. . . . I think that as a Navy Medical officer, Captain . . . wanted some Navy medical people working with him. Dr. . . . and the two Chiefs were three of the finest people it was my pleasure to work with in the Navy. They worked in the White House clinic which was located in the East Wing. I believe that Dr. Janet Travelle was the first female physician to a President. She was responsible for his medical care and anyone who was referred to her by him. Mrs. Kennedy and the children had their own physicians.

"Dr. Travelle's specialty was orthopedic medicine and she had had success in treating John F. Kennedy's back problem before he was elected President. Her appointment received a lot of publicity and she received a tremendous amount of mail. People writing to congratulate her but also seeking advice about their back problems or other medical problems.

"The first few weeks I was busy organizing my office where Dr. Travelle saw patients; ordering furniture, supplies, learning the ropes of how to get things done in the White House. Dr. Travelle taught me how to give some of her injections. It was a very busy time. I mentioned that Dr. Travelle had received a tremendous amount of mail and she answered every letter. Typing and dictation were qualifications for this position because I helped her answer the medical-type letters she received. Dr. Travelle also had a secretary who took care of her other correspondence.

"Dr. Travelle's suite was in the main part of the White House across from the elevator which went to the First Family's private quarters. It consisted of three rooms - the secretary's office, Dr. Travelle's office and my office/treatment room. Because of the location, President Kennedy often stopped by with VIP's to say hello to Dr. Travelle. Like other military personnel assigned in the Washington, D.C. area, I wore civilian clothes on duty as did . . . [the Navy doctor] and the two Chiefs.

"I left the White House to attend graduate school [the Navy sent her there for 'duty under instruction'] at the Catholic University of America in Washington, D.C. and received my Master of Science degree in nursing with a major in administration of nursing services. My relief at the White House was [Navy Nurse] LT Elizabeth Chapowicki."[50] (Though her tour at the White House was fairly brief, Captain Dolores Cornelius NC USN (Ret.) holds the distinction of being the first Navy Nurse Corps officer assigned to White House duty.)

In September 1961, hurricane 'Carla' slams into the Texas coast causing "hundreds of millions of dollars in damage with prolonged winds, high tides, and floods over most of the Texas coast."[51] Four Navy Nurse Corps officers from the Naval Hospital at Pensacola, Florida, participate in the Navy's hurricane disaster relief mission. LCdr Miriam Frank and Lt(jg) Joan Helgendorff have TAD aboard the aircraft carrier *Shangri-La* while LT Janice Langley and Lt(jg) Mary Freeman are assigned TAD aboard the carrier *Antietam*. These ladies are the first Navy Nurses to ever be assigned TAD aboard combatant Naval ships. The ships load supplies, equipment and personnel then head to the Texas coast. "Even though the ships were only down in Texas for two days, what was accomplished did lighten the burden of the disaster victims. The sanitation work that was done . . . gave the people fresh water and some sanitation facilities. The shots that were given [6,000] probably saved many lives and might have stopped an epidemic. The supplies that were brought were a welcome sight, as many places had no medical supplies or had run out. In conclusion, the trip was a success and did accomplish what it set out to do."[52]

Then on 31 October another hurricane, 'Hattie,' crashes into British Honduras with deadly results. (British Honduras is located in Central America, at the very southern tip of Mexico on the eastern coast facing the Caribbean Sea.) This hurricane leaves the capital of this country [Belize], "standing Wednesday night 'like a pile of matchsticks' without power or fresh water, little food to feed its 32,000 residents . . . Authorities said 62 dead had been counted along the British Honduras coast where the hurricane hit Tuesday morning with winds in excess of 150 miles per hour and tidal waves that rolled water 10 feet deep through the streets of Belize."[53] "On November 1, 1961, Lieutenant Commander Audrey Fellabaum, Lieutenant (junior grade) Mary McArdle, Lieutenant (junior grade) Patricia Cope, and Ensign Joan Beasley, all from the Pensacola Naval Hospital, reported aboard the *Antietam* to sail for British Honduras."[54] "Medical personnel aboard include 48 doctors, four nurses and 87 medical corpsmen drawn from Pensacola stations, plus 23 helicopters and pilots. . . . The *Antietam* left under orders to proceed at full speed to the disaster area, from which came the report much of the low-lying capital city had been destroyed. However, other reports indicate loss of life has been low due to the warning which sent residents to high ground."[55] "En route to the disaster area in British Honduras, briefing on the general conditions existing in the area were received via short wave radio. Medical personnel were divided into three groups by the Senior Medical Officer - pool, shore party, and ship's party, with an officer and deputy officer-in-charge of each group. The shore party was sub-divided into two groups with two nurses assigned to each group. All medical personnel were briefed on endemic diseases in that area, languages spoken, supplies available, mode of communication and reporting of operations carried out."[56] "Before the ship arrived, Nurses Fellabaum and McArdle left by helicopter for Stann Creek, Honduras, where they set up a typhoid immunization station. Treatment units were also set up for leprosy, malaria, tropical skin diseases, infections, puncture wounds, gangrene and fractures. By the end of the first day, 2800 typhoid immunizations had been administered. On the following day, with the assistance of two American school teachers and an Episcopal minister's wife - a pediatric nurse from England - 5000 immunizations were administered."[57] Lt(jg) Cope and Ensign Beasley are "assigned to the Bliss Institute in Belize to assist at the Memorial Hospital in that area. Emergency treatment of wounds and infections, and tetanus and typhoid immunizations were administered in cooperation with the British Medical team, upon request by them."[58]

Lt(jg) McArdle gives an account of her TAD assignment in the December issue of Pensacola Naval Hospital's news publication. "At 0630 on 3 November, LCDR Fellabaum, Dr. McKnight, HM1 Evans, and I departed from the USS Antietam on the Third Helicopter to the disaster area. From the air we saw debris floating in the water, roads blocked, houses damaged almost completely beyond recognition, and jungles of trees blown down. A few natives in small boats were the first signs of life or activity. They were waving up to us. After receiving permission our planes landed on the beach in Stann Creek. This city of 8,000 sustained 90 percent damage and was the hardest hit area in British Honduras. Capt. Lautzenheiser, Medical Officer-in-Charge of our group, made arrangements with Dr. Becker, a British doctor, for us to be taken to the Hospital. The hospital conditions were deplorable. Sick and injured lay on beds and cots, and in instances on the floor. . . . LCDR Fellabaum and I were provided with a small room at the entrance to the hospital and set up for typhoid inoculations. This room was covered with mud and blood and we had no facilities to clean. Our only help was two native girls who had to be trained to sterilize the equipment. As all the electricity was out, Miss Avril Mahea, a Public Health Nurse and the only professional woman in the area, provided us with a kerosene burner and wash basin for sterilization. Our presence was announced to the natives by a town crier. We had difficulty maintaining order and looked to the British Infantry for help. . . .

"After inoculating for [seven-and-a-half] hours we were relieved for 15 minutes. I was extremely dizzy and thirsty and drank four quarts of water, a can of juice produced in the Stann Creek Valley, and ate a spam and cheese sandwich. . . . We worked late into the evening until all the typhoid had been used and gave a total of 2,800 injections. . . . Late [the next morning], LCDR Fellabaum and I went to the Convent to inoculate the sick aged, orphaned children, and Nuns. The school teachers told us that when we landed natives had been informed that we were sent by Castro or by Russia. In order to dispel this, they draped an American flag from the convent railing, and we made certain that all the natives we contacted knew we were from the UNITED STATES and the purpose for which we came. . . . [Later that second day] Capt Lautzenheiser summoned us to return to the Antietam. On the way the Sisters of the Holy Family Convent stopped us and gave us some shells they had washed out as souvenirs. The British soldiers presented me with a flag from their jeep and a package of cigarettes. Two small boys gave LCDR Fellabaum flags. Some orphans carried our gear to the helicopter. As the plane rose I gazed at the beautiful water on the coral reefs but could only think of the destruction the storm had left."[59]

As for other happenings in 1961, "Billets for Nurse Corps officers [are] established at Lemoore, California; Keflavik, Iceland; and Roosevelt Roads, Puerto Rico."[60] In Congress, a law is passed that authorizes "the President to order units and members in the Ready Reserve to active duty for not more than 12 months, and for other purposes."[61] In view of the present country-wide shortage of nurses, this may have implications for the Navy Nurse Corps if billets cannot be filled and the shortage becomes acute within the Nurse Corps.

1961 sees the first manned space flight and it is the Russians doing the deed. A Russian cosmonaut makes one orbit around the earth in a Russian spacecraft in April. In May, an American astronaut, Alan Shepard, rockets into space but does not orbit the earth. Then in July, U.S.A. astronaut Virgil Grissom also goes into space but does not orbit. In August, the Russians send one of their cosmonauts up and he makes 17 orbits around the earth.[62]

To return to more earthly matters, back in "the summer of 1960, Congress cut American imports of Cuban sugar. Immediately, the Soviet Union offered to buy the excess sugar and increase trade with Castro. In return, Cuba would support Soviet foreign policy in Latin America. Eisenhower, furious that Castro could agree to this, severed diplomatic relations with Cuba just two weeks before he left office [January 1961]."[63]

On January 20, 1961, John F. Kennedy becomes President of the United States. He brings an aura of vitality and hope with his presence and he calls his political program 'The New Frontier.' In March, President Kennedy signs an executive order that begins the U.S. Peace Corps. "The corps sent thousands of Americans abroad to help people in developing nations raise their standards of living. The Peace Corps seemed to carry the enthusiasm of the President to the people of other countries."[64] In April, the Cuban problem escalates when "three American-made B-26s bombed Cuba. . . . Two days later 1,500 men [CIA trained anti-Castro exiles training in Guatemala] landed at the . . . (Bay of Pigs) [in Cuba]."[65] It was a disaster. They were expected and completely defeated. Then in June, President Kennedy has a two-day meeting with Khrushchev in Austria and there is no meeting of the minds. The atmosphere becomes colder and in August "the East Germans began erecting a wall between the eastern and western sectors of Berlin, and within two months the Berlin Wall was effectively blocking further escapes by East Germans to the West."[66] "In September, 1961, the Russians resumed testing atomic weapons. The tests broke an unofficial test ban that had lasted nearly three years. The United States began testing shortly after the Russians resumed their tests, but the U.S. conducted its tests underground, which created no dangerous fallout. But in March, 1962, Kennedy announced the U.S. would resume testing in the atmosphere."[67]

Over in the far east, another country [Laos] is being targeted by the Communists while Vietnam is still boiling and stewing as the U.S. government tries to devise ways to halt the advance of Communism. It is a puzzlement. "Without any clear-cut decision or plan of mission, the troops began to go. United States instruction teams required combat support units, air reconnaissance required fighter escorts and helicopter teams, counter-insurgency required 600 Green Berets to train the Vietnamese in operations against the Viet-Cong. Equipment kept pace - assault craft and naval patrol boats, armored personnel carriers, short-take-off and transport planes, trucks, radar installations, Quonset huts, airfields. Employed in support of ARVN (South Vietnamese Army) combat operations, all these required manning by United States personnel, who willy-nilly entered a shooting war. When Special Forces units directed ARVN units against the guerrillas and met fire, they returned it. Helicopter gunships, when fired on, did the same.

"Increased activity required more than a training command. In February 1962 a full field command under the acronym MACV (Military Assistance Command Vietnam) superseded MAAG [Military Assistance Advisory Group] with a three-star general . . . in command. If a date is needed for the beginning of the American war in Vietnam, the establishment of Mac-Vee, as it became known, will serve."[68]

But, to return to the States and the Navy Nurse Corps; in April 1962 the Nurse Corps receives another uniform authorization. The "Dinner Dress Blue and White Uniforms [are] authorized for women officers; mandatory for those in the grades of Commander and Captain after 1 July 1964."[69] And then, on 1 May 1962, the Director of the Navy Nurse Corps, Captain Ruth A. Houghton, retires.

During her career Captain Ruth A. Houghton Tayloe was awarded the American Defense Service Medal with a star, the American Campaign and Asiatic Pacific Medals, the World War II Victory Medal and the National Defense Service Medal. After retirement and until her death, she lived in Massachusetts. She is buried in Arlington National Cemetery.[70]

1   Information prepared by the Navy Nurse Corps Officers on the staff of the Director of the Navy Nurse Corps.
2   Ibid..
3   The World Book Encyclopedia, Field Enterprises Educational Corporation, Chicago, Volume 6, 1966 edition, p. 111.
4   200 Years, A Bicentennial Illustrated History of the United States, Joseph Newman, Directing Editor, Books by U.S. News & World Report, Inc., 2300 N Street, N.W., Washington, D.C. 20037, 1973, book, book 2, p. 255.
5   The World Book Encyclopedia, op. cit..
6   Ibid., Vol. 17, p. 572e.

7   Laird, LCDR Thelma NC USNR, Jones, LCDR Dorothy NC USN, Feeney, LCDR Elizabeth NC USN, Seidl, CDR Elizabeth NC USN (Ret.), Blaska, CDR Burdette NC USN, *Chronological History NAVY NURSE CORPS*, Prepared by: Nursing Division, Bureau of Medicine and Surgery, 1 August 1962, p. 44.

8   Ibid..

9   Ibid..

10   Houghton, Ruth Director of the Navy Nurse Corps, "Nuclear Nursing Students," Speech to Students, 3 September 1958, Records of the Office of the Director, Navy Nurse Corps, Box 14, #43, Operational Archives, Naval Historical Center, Washington Navy Yard, Washington, D.C..

11   "NC Indoctrination Center 6 Years Old," St. Albans Naval Hospital News, 5 September 1958, Nurse Corps Indoctrination Center Anniversary Edition, p. 3.

12   Ibid., p. 8.

13   Ferguson, Edith L. Colton Lt(jg) Navy Nurse Corps, *Written Personal History*, 23 July 1991.

14   Sherman, Miriam C. CDR Navy Nurse Corps, *Oral History Interview Tape Transcript*, Self interview, 7 August 1990.

15   Halverson, Ruth E. Captain Navy Nurse Corps, *Oral History Interview Tape Transcript*, Interviewer Captain Doris M. Sterner Navy Nurse Corps, 10 July 1990.

16   Laird, et.al., op. cit., p. 44.

17   Cornelius, Dolores Captain Navy Nurse Corps, *Oral History Interview Tape Transcript*, Self interview, 28 December 1989.

18   Shields, Patricia Luenberger CDR Navy Nurse Corps, *Oral History Interview Tape Transcript*, Self interview, 30 September 1990.

19   Gilfillan, Ann Currie LT Navy Nurse Corps, *Oral History Interview Tape Transcript*, Self interview, 25 April 1991.

20   Ibid..

21   O'Dell, Beverly Brase Captain Navy Nurse Corps, *Oral History Interview Tape Transcript*, Self interview, 22 May 1991.

22   Laird, et.al., op. cit., p. 44.

23   Ibid., p. 45.

24   Ibid..

25   Ibid..

26   *Uniforms of the United States Navy 1900-1967*, text accompanying this set of color lithographs written by Captain James C. Tily, CEC, USN (Ret.) in coordination with office of Director of Naval History and Curator for the Department of the Navy, U.S. Government Printing Office, Washington, D.C. 20402, See year section 1961.

27   Ibid..

28   Ibid..

29   Laird, et.al., op. cit., p. 45.

30   Ibid..

31   *The World Book Encyclopedia*, op. cit., Vol. 17, p. 38.

32   Ibid..

33   *Great Events of the 20th Century*, Editor: Richard Marshall, The Readers' Digest Association, Inc., 1977, p. 439.

34   *The World Book Encyclopedia*, op. cit., Vol. 17, p. 572e.

35   Wells, H.G., *The Outline of History*, Revised and brought up to date by Raymond Postgate, Garden City Books, Garden City, New York, Volume II, 1961, p. 962.

36   *200 Years, A Bicentennial Illustrated History of the United States*, op. cit., p. 255.

37   Ibid., p. 256.

38   *The World Book Encyclopedia*, op. cit., Vol. 6, p. 111.

39   Tuchman, Barbara W., *The March of Folly From Troy to Vietnam*, Ballantine Books, New York, 1985, pp. 281, 282.

40   *The World Book Encyclopedia*, op. cit..

41   Ibid., Vol. 11, p. 212g.

42   Laird, et.al., op. cit., p. 46.

43   Ibid., pp. 45, 46.

44   Ibid., p. 46.

45   Ibid..

46   Gilfillan, op. cit..

47   Lochte, Rose Marie Captain Navy Nurse Corps, *Written Personal History*, 20 May 1991.

48   Halverson, op. cit..

49   Shearer, Carolyn Jean LCdr Navy Nurse Corps, *Oral History Interview Tape Transcript*, Interviewer LT Helen Barry Siragusa Navy Nurse Corps, 12 March 1991.

50   Cornelius, op. cit..

51   *The World Book Encyclopedia*, op. cit., Vol. 9, p. 401.

52   "Antietam Goes To Texas," *WHITE CAPS*, Publication of the U.S. Naval Hospital, Pensacola, Florida, Vol. 2, No. 10, October 1961, pp. 1 and 4.

53   "Hurricane Kills 62 In Smashing Belize," *Pensacola News Journal*, Pensacola, Florida, Thursday Morning, November 2, 1961.

54   Kenney Rear Admiral, MC USN Surgeon General and Chrisman, A.S. Rear Admiral MC USN Deputy Surgeon General, *Bureau of Medicine and Surgery News*, Department of the Navy, Bureau of Medicine and Surgery, Washington 25, D.C., 6 December 1961, p. 1.

55   "Hurricane Kills 62 In Smashing Belize," *Pensacola News Journal*, op. cit..

56   Kenney Rear Admiral, MC USN Surgeon General and Chrisman, A.S. Rear Admiral MC USN Deputy Surgeon General, *Bureau of Medicine and Surgery News*, op. cit..

57   "Nurse Corps Officers Serve on 2 Carriers," *Navy Times*, Army Times Publishing Co., 6883 Commercial Drive, Springfield, Virginia 22159-0260, 24 February 1962.

58   Kenney Rear Admiral, MC USN Surgeon General and Chrisman, A.S. Rear Admiral MC USN Deputy Surgeon General, *Bureau of Medicine*

and Surgery News, <u>op. cit.</u>.

59   McArdle, Mary C. Lt(jg) NC USNR, "An Account Of Two Days In Storm [Stann] Creek, British Honduras," *WHITE CAPS*, Publication of the U.S. Naval Hospital, Pensacola, Florida, December 1961, pp. 5,6.

60   Laird, et.al., <u>op. cit.</u>, p. 47.

61   Ibid., p. 6 of the Chronological History of Public Laws Governing Nurse Corps Personnel.

62   *The World Book Encyclopedia*, <u>op. cit.</u>, Vol.17, pp. 572e, 572f.

63   *200 Years, A Bicentennial Illustrated History of the United States*, <u>op. cit.</u>, p. 260.

64   *The World Book Encyclopedia*, <u>op. cit.</u>, Vol.11, p. 212g.

65   *200 Years, A Bicentennial Illustrated History of the United States*, <u>op. cit.</u>.

66   <u>Ibid.</u>.

67   *The World Book Encyclopedia*, <u>op. cit.</u>, Vol.11, p. 212j.

68   Tuchman, Barbara W., *The March of Folly From Troy to Vietnam*, <u>op. cit.</u>, p. 298.

69   Laird, et.al., <u>op. cit.</u>.

70   Information prepared by the Navy Nurse Corps Officers on the staff of the Director of the Navy Nurse Corps.

13 May 1958. The Navy Nurse Corps celebrates
its Golden Anniversary.
". . . It is a strong and vibrant Corps
that has more than proved itself."

☆ ☆ ☆

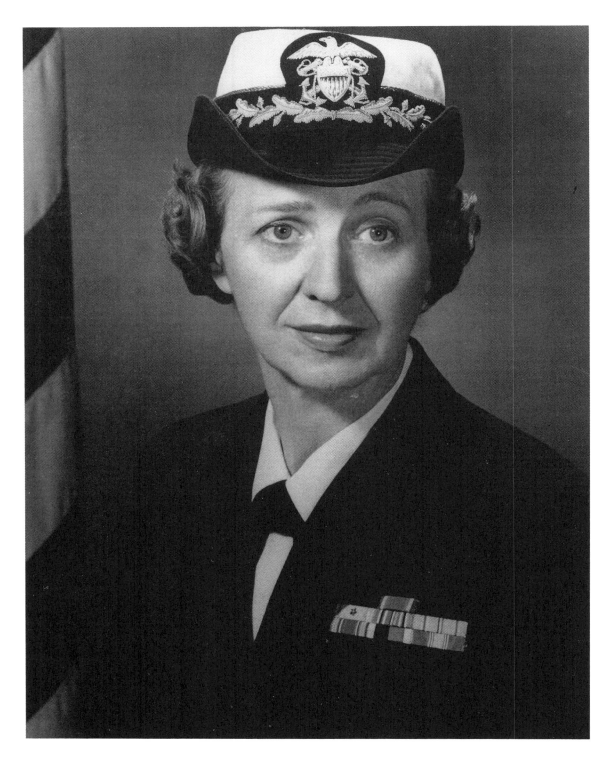

Director - Captain Ruth A. Erickson NC USN
(Official U.S. Navy photo courtesy of Nursing Division, Bureau of Medicine and Surgery, Navy Department.)

CHAPTER 11

Director - Captain Ruth A. Erickson
(1962 - 1966)

Captain Ruth A. Erickson NC USN is Chief Nurse at the Bethesda Naval Hospital in Maryland when she is selected to be the next Director of the Nurse Corps. She receives orders to report to the Bureau of Medicine and Surgery at 23rd and E Streets in Washington, D.C. on 10 March 1962. She is appointed Director on 30 April 1962.

Ruth Erickson was born in Virginia, Minnesota which is about sixty some miles NNW of Duluth. After high-school she went into Nurses' Training at the Methodist-Kahler School of Nursing in Rochester, Minnesota. She graduated in 1934 and practiced her profession for two years in Rochester, Minnesota before joining the Navy in July of 1936. Ensign Erickson went to San Diego Naval Hospital as her first duty station. She says, her "family couldn't understand it, being ordered to San Diego. That was the other side of the world. They felt it was really in Mexico rather than just a few miles from it."[1] She leaves San Diego late in 1938 for duty aboard the hospital ship, USS *Relief.* Then two years later, "I was detached from the ship out there in the port in Honolulu in May of 1940. Joined a staff of eight nurses; seven nurses and myself. Delightful quarters and had very lovely duty until December 7th, 1941."[2] She was promoted to Lt(jg) in 1943, and to LT in 1944. She served as Chief Nurse aboard the USS *Haven* and as Supervisor or Senior Nurse or Assistant Chief Nurse at Corona, California; Farragut, Idaho; St. Albans, New York; Brooklyn, New York; and Great Lakes, Illinois. From 1947 to 1949 she was the Nurse Corps' representative in the District Medical Office of the Twelfth Naval District at San Francisco. From that assignment she was assigned as Senior Nurse Corps officer in the Port Office of the MSTS in Seattle, Washington until April 1950. During this time she was promoted to Lieutenant Commander. Then for the next two years she was assigned to BuMed as Nurse Corps Personnel Officer on the staff of Captain Winnie Gibson. From there she went on DUINS (Duty Under Instruction) to Indiana University where she received a Bachelor of Science degree in Nursing Education. Thereafter, she was assigned as Chief Nurse to Naval Hospitals at Camp Lejeune, North Carolina; Portsmouth, Virginia; and Bethesda, Maryland. She was promoted to Commander in 1955 and to Captain in January 1960.[3]

The staffing of the Nursing Division of BuMed, besides the Director, consists of the Deputy Director of the Corps (Captain Dorothy Monahan), the Navy Nurse Head of Nurse Corps recruiting, the Navy Nurse Education officer, the Navy Nurse Assignment officer, and the Navy Nurse Personnel Planning Officer plus the civil service staff of typists, secretaries, and clerk. In July of 1962, for the first time, a Nurse Corps officer is assigned to the Bureau of Naval Personnel in the Staff Corps Liaison Section of the Officer Distribution Division.[4] She acts as liaison between the Nursing Division and the Officer Distribution Division, in Naval Personnel, concerning assignment orders for the Nurse Corps officers.

The next event is in July of 1962 when the Navy nurses' pin-striped, one piece, seersucker working uniform is discontinued. Then in September 1962, an Anesthesia "program for Nurse Corps officers [is] established at the Naval Medical Center [at] Bethesda, Maryland, under the aegis of George Washington University."[5] Navy Nurse Katherine Howard (a Navy nurse anesthetist) tells us, "the Navy had been training just a few nurse anesthetists in civilian schools for, usually, eighteen months to two years. The programs were shorter then . . . when we'd get these girls [after graduation] . . . we found that they were not really adequately trained and lacked a lot of experience. So we felt that it would be best for the Navy to have the use of our own students and for our own facilities as well as being able to train them the way the Navy would like to have you trained. So this program was finally set up in conjunction with the school. [Navy Nurse Corps officer] Teresa Butler was in charge, at the time, to set this up. We established a collegiate program. We wanted to have a degree program, if possible."[6] This became "the first program for nurse anesthetists in which university credit was awarded. Officers completing the program are examined by the American Association of Nurse Anesthetists for certification as registered nurse anesthetists."[7] For years recruitment has been unable to provide the numbers of nurse anesthetists needed for the Nurse Corps. (This innovative and well-designed Navy Anesthesia program would help meet some of the need for these specialists and, eventually, become renown for its educational success.)

Another first for the Nurse Corps is the first Navy Nurse Corps officer to graduate from the Naval Post Graduate School at Monterey, California. Her name is Commander Veronica M. Bulshefski. The course she attended is a very rigorous, condensed, less than one-year, course for a Master of Science degree in Management. After applying for the course and being selected she reported to the Post Graduate School on 21 July 1961 and graduated on 1 June 1962. In August of 1962, the next two Nurse Corps officers selected for this course report aboard. LCdr Marie Eberhardt is one of these officers and she says, "Another interesting experience was my experience at the Naval Post Graduate School in Monterey. I went there in August 1962 with Captain, then LCdr, Doris Sterner. While at Great Lakes [Naval Hospital] I had received a phone call from the Bureau [BuMed], in January 1962, asking if I would be interested in going to the Post Graduate School. It was a particularly cold winter, and also my first long-term experience in snow and ice and minus temperatures. My only question was `is that in Monterey, California? I'll go.' I had absolutely no idea what I was letting myself in for, but at least it was in the right section of the country. The ten month experience was like hitting myself over the head with a hammer, it felt so good when it was over. For instance, after two weeks in accounting, the instructor announced, `we have now completed the material covered in the under-graduate courses in accounting at college. We will now start on post-graduate material.' When I started, I didn't even know debit from credit, and then we started in [Bernoulli probability] statistics. The instructor asked `do you want a fast review of calculus?' I raised my hand and said `don't bother reviewing, I've never taken calculus.' I didn't even know how to use a slide ruler. So, I struggled doing all math in long-hand and my high school algebra taken in 1942. I barely squeezed through the course with a D, but managed to average that out with good marks in all other subjects, especially personnel management and economics. I received my Master of Science degree in Management in May, 1963. I never used statistics or accounting in my future work, but the course in personnel management and executive leadership helped in making decisions and managing personnel in my later assignments."[8]

And speaking of education, Navy Nurse Marie T. Gendron notes that out at the Bethesda Naval Medical Center, "all courses such as education for the corpsmen and nurses, those who were teaching, and then the courses for those who were Commander selectees and different courses like that, were being held at one week or two week institutes and seminars. . . . [Senior Nurse, Commander Rita Clark, and LT Hope McIntyre staff the Nurse Corps Training Division at the Medical Center and Miss Gendron is newly assigned there.] They were going to try sending out a team to the different hospitals to teach these courses and see how that worked out. . . . The first course [to be tried out this way] was in disaster nursing. This was during 1961 and 1962 . . . the Cold war was in full swing, shall we say, and the people were talking about their own shelters and things like that, so they got the course together and . . . I was just an onlooker, because Rita Clark and Hope were the ones who were teaching. . . . I remember that after the first couple of times, they decided so much more could be done with this disaster nursing course, as far as visual aids were concerned. So then we went to work and put [together] a real (I think it was two eight hour days) of a very intensive course. . . . We went . . . to many duty stations . . . some were just small stations, others were large ones like San Diego, Great Lakes and [the course was] two days but we sometimes gave as many as three [courses] in one week, which was a very taxing schedule. As far as the program content, we taught triage (which is sorting [patients]) and we taught first-aid; a very drastic sort of first-aid with what you have on hand, like we would have newspapers and a few boards and things like that, and they [the students] had to kind of gather things that we had scattered around and see what they could work with; what would they do for blocking a chest wound or something like that. We taught them, also, how to think disaster because it's very difficult not to panic when you have an emergency situation. So, one of the methods we used was in suggesting that they read the papers every morning and read-up on accidents that had happened . . . and to ask [themselves], 'Alright, this person has this, this and this wrong with them, what would I treat first, and what would I do to treat those injuries?' We said, 'if you do that often enough, then it will be almost an instinctive reaction that you will be doing instead of thinking, 'Oh, what do I have to do now?''. . . We also had had a one hour film that had been made especially for us by one of the Pediatricians at Bethesda on the treatment of burns particularly and the fluid therapy that is still required in burns; burn therapy. Of course, they would expect a lot of burns in nuclear war so he had made up this film for us to teach others how to judge, without an awful lot of fancy equipment, how far behind a person was in fluids and how much would be needed, and how to replace the fluids. . . . We were almost the first ones in the country, besides those at John Hopkins where it originated, who taught CPR [Cardio-Pulmonary Resuscitation]. We probably had one of the first 'Recessing Annie's' [resuscitation dummy for practicing CPR] in the country . . . and we almost had to have an act of Congress to bring it into this country because everything in 1961 was 'buy American, buy American' and the Army did have a doll, but it was a very clumsy thing and it was about three times the price and it was very inept for what we wanted it for. A funny thing did happen though, I remember Hope was giving one of the sessions and I had gone out into one of the other rooms and I had 'Recessing Annie' sitting on the floor, sort of deflated, but I had her head in my lap and I was combing it and somebody walked in and almost fainted. She [the doll] was very realistic.

"[The program] was very hard on us physically because one of the sessions we taught was on evacuation of patients from the hospitals, and this was one of the things that was badly needed in every hospital. Most people did not have a good evacuation plan, and I'm talking about evacuating patients out of their beds. How do you get them down on the floor and on a blanket and drag them . . . like in fire evacuation procedures? I had been fortunate enough to work with a very good fireman in Jersey City who had taught me these carries, and I guess he had originally learned from the father of hospital evacuation procedures who was a Lt. McGraw from Chicago. You remember the tremendous Chicago fire back in 1954 and so many deaths? It was after that, that he developed a carry. I later had the good fortune of meeting him, but I worked with . . . from the Jersey City Fire Department and we developed quite a few different carries and it didn't matter what size you were, you could handle nearly anything."[9] Again, Navy nurses are in the forefront with innovative programs such as this one.

Meanwhile, the Russians and the U.S. have been sending men into space to orbit the earth. In February 1962, the first American astronaut, John Glenn, goes into space and orbits earth three times. The country is fascinated. In May the next American astronaut, Scott Carpenter, is sent aloft for a trip of three orbits. The Russians send up two manned flights in August; one for 64 orbits and one for 48 orbits. In October another American goes into space for six orbits of the earth.[10]

At this point, we're going to turn from outer space down to the Naval Hospital at Philadelphia (now there's a jump). A new graduate nurse, a new Navy nurse, is just reporting aboard and how she arrives here is worth telling. Her name is VaLaine Pack and she is no stranger to the Navy. "I joined the Navy on a dare. A friend of mine from high school was joining and she dared me to go along with her, which I did. So in March of 1957, I was sworn into the Navy as an HN (E3) at the Fort Douglas, Utah Naval Reserve Unit. The friend of mine, who had dared me to join, subsequently only lasted for six weeks before she was discharged for medical purposes. I enjoyed the time at the Naval Reserve Unit. During that period of time, I was introduced to the program . . . which was called the Navy Enlisted Nursing Education Program (NENEP). The Navy Hospitalman Chief at the Reserve Unit was the one that showed me the literature on the program and he recommended that I give it a try. . . . 'However,' he said, 'try boot camp first; go to your two weeks of active duty for boot camp and see if you can tolerate it and then take it from there.' I went to boot camp in May, came home and filled out the papers to change over to the regular Navy so that I could go on active duty. . . . I reported to boot camp in Bainbridge, Maryland in August of 1957 and had my 21st birthday in boot camp. This was an adventure. Boot camp was no easy thing in those days. Bainbridge was hot and sticky and muggy, and rainy, had no air conditioning. There were many mosquitoes around since we were located near the Susquehanna River and we were very, very uncomfortable.

But, my goal was to qualify for the NENEP program. Now, perhaps I was a little bit naive because I have since learned that not very many people qualified for it at that time. But determined as I was, that was what I wanted to do. I finished boot camp and went to Great Lakes, Illinois for Corps School, still . . . trying for the NENEP program. I had to be in at least a year before I could apply for it. So I completed Corps School and while there, became engaged to a Marine. . . . I finished Corps School, was sent to Pensacola, Florida for duty in March of 1958. My fiancee subsequently got out of the Marine Corps that summer and went to . . . [Netherlands] for two years for a mission for the Church. . . . I decided to apply for OR Tech School. I applied for it and my name was put on the waiting list. In the meantime, my fiancee and I had a falling out and I decided . . . I would go ahead and apply for the NENEP program, just in case he and I did not stay together. So, I applied for it and was interviewed by my Chief Nurse, Commander Rita Clark, and then was interviewed by Captain Ruth Houghton, who was then the Director of the Navy Nurse Corps. She asked the question as to why I wanted to return to the University of Utah, as indicated on my application form [VaLaine had been taking courses there, before enlisting], and I told her that if I went back to the University of Utah, I could go back there as a sophomore in the school of nursing and that would cut off one year that the Navy did not have to pay for me to go to school. So, she said they would get back to me. This was in March of 1959. In April of 1959, I received orders to OR Tech school in Bethesda. Now, I really was in a quandary, because I didn't know if I were to take those orders, whether they were going to let me quit OR school and go to nursing school. If I didn't take the orders and then didn't get nursing school, I'd be stuck in Pensacola for another two years. So I decided to take a gamble and I accepted the orders to OR Tech school at Bethesda.

"I landed there in April of 1959 and began a very rigorous program in OR Tech school. Now Captain Doris Sterner, who was then Lieutenant Doris Allen, was my instructor, and I'll never forget that first day in class. I was the only girl in the class and it was very intimidating. But, as time went on during the summer, I grew to love the whole program. It was interesting, it was a challenge, it was exciting and it was an opportunity to serve in a manner which I had never had before. There were several friends that I made there, and, of course, the renowned Alice Reilly, who was the OR supervisor. I don't really need to say a whole lot about her because her reputation throughout the Navy Nurse Corps is well known. [Very strict but a strong, most knowledgeable OR supervisor. In this particular era when many doctors/surgeons still believe nurses are `hand-maidens,' these traits are a positive in the OR but, sometimes makes it difficult for the OR staff.] Then in July of that year, I had a letter from a friend of mine in Pensacola congratulating me on being selected for the NENEP program. That was the first indication that I knew that I had been accepted. Actually, I didn't know, I was dumbfounded. So I went down to the personnel office and had the Chief call down to the Bureau to see if indeed I had been on the list, and I was, and they'd sent my orders to Pensacola because they didn't know that I had been transferred to Bethesda. I never could figure that one out! So they did take me out of the OR Tech school one month short of graduating, and I ended up back at the University of Utah College of Nursing in 1959. There, I completed my three years and graduated, as I said before, on the 11th of June, 1962.

"The highlight of my time there, aside from my nursing experience, was when I was allowed to be commissioned with the Navy Cadets that were there with the Navy Reserve at the Navy Reserve Officer Training Unit. This had never happened before either, and I was the only woman that had been commissioned at the ROTC Unit up to that point in time. . . . And then that night at graduation . . . all of the people that had been commissioned in their respective [branches of the] Armed Forces (Navy, Air Force, Army, Marine Corps) were at graduation. We were in uniform; we wore our uniforms under our caps and gowns and after . . . [we had] gotten our diplomas, we shed our caps and gowns, we put on our dress hats, then the remainder of our uniforms and went back through and received our commissions officially by our Commanding Officer. That was a thrill of a lifetime. It was interesting to see the reaction of the crowd when a woman stepped down to the podium. I went through Newport, Rhode Island for officer indoctrination and began my first tour of duty as a Navy Nurse Corps Officer. In 1962, October, I was stationed in the Navy Hospital in Philadelphia."[11]

Meanwhile, over in the Far East in Japan, Navy Nurse Kathleen Martin is on duty at the Navy Medical facility at Sasebo, Japan. Sasebo is located on the western portion of Kyushu Island in the southernmost region of Japan. She says, "Sasebo, Japan was a city of about 250,000 people at that time. It had been a hidden Naval base for the Japanese during World War II. . . . One of the interesting things about Sasebo, was the living quarters. In San Diego, we all had to live out of quarters, but in Sasebo everyone was required to live in. We were in a four-story building. It was very large and the first floor was the nurses quarters. The top three floors were condemned, sealed and locked off and no one was able to get up there. [On] the first floor, everyone had their own bedroom and shared a sitting room with another nurse. There was a very, very large living [room] and many of our social activities took place there. We had two dining rooms, two kitchens; one was for the Senior Nurse or Chief Nurse, and the other was for the remaining seven nurses. We had one nurse who was an anesthetist who was on almost 24-hour-a-day duty. The only relief she got was if the physician covered for her for a weekend or a few hours.

"We were there to provide medical service to the Fleet and to the dependents of the Fleet. It did keep us busy at times, but [we had] probably no more than 100 or 110 patients at any given time. Our hospital was rather unique, because it had been a Japanese Naval Hospital during World War II. It also had a series of caves that the people could escape to any time there was an air raid warning. The Japanese were very thorough. In their caves they had facilities for housing the entire staff of the hospital and its patients. Even in 1962, we still had monthly drilling on Friday afternoons at 3 p.m.. The siren would sound and we would all take off to the caves. There were supplies. There were beds. There were medical supplies, food supplies and water. This would last for about 45 minutes to an hour, and then we'd wait for the next month.

"The hospital itself had a suite for the Emperor, if he should be there during a visit in that particular area. It was rather interesting that even the head [bathroom] that was built for him had to be at a level where, as he was sitting, he was still above the rest of the people in his country. He had an elevated bathroom that went up about three steps before he could sit. Very, very interesting. . . .

"Two other Navy nurses and myself ventured out to different little ports around the area. We even had a Japanese fisherman. He came over and spoke to us after several times of watching him unload their fishing boats. And this particular fellow had been a Japanese Naval pilot during World War II. The pilot had been shot down in the Philippines during World War II and, unfortunately, lost his right leg. However, he was picked up by the Japanese, brought back to Japan, and recovered from his loss. The government had provided him with a very good prosthesis and provided him with a pension for the rest of his life. However, he wasn't satisfied. He was a busy man and he became a commercial fisherman. He had a young family. His son was barely two years old, his youngest. He had an older son who was almost 16. His oldest son studied a great deal of the time, because in Japan, if they studied well enough in high school, the government would provide them with a college education. Many of these youngsters would be studying till one or two o'clock in the morning every single school night. It was not unusual. Far different from what we have in the United States. His youngest son, the two year old, spoke much of our English very well. Unfortunately, his wife could not speak any English, but she was a very, very wonderful hostess. . . .

"We got to know some other Japanese families in the area as well. One of them was a ring maker. He made two styles of gold rings. One style would take him an entire day and the other style, which was a bit more complicated, would take him a day and a half to make. It was so interesting to see him sitting cross-legged in front of a little small table by a window. When he actually started to use the gold and grind it down, the window was closed and a felt cloth was placed over everything to collect all the little gold flecks that would come off in the grinding process. He had managed to put four of his five children through college at the time that we knew them. His fifth child was in high school studying hard in order to be able to go through college. One of his sons was a lawyer, one was a physician, another was an engineer, and his girl had become a teacher. . . .

"Sasebo's very, very interesting for many different reasons. The countryside itself was just lovely. There were mountains all around. There were many places where you take a boat to go out and explore various islands. Frequently we would get a weekend off and have a Japanese fisherman take us out and leave us and spend a weekend just camping on one of the beautiful islands out there.

"Of course we did visit Nagasaki and the shrine [near] where . . . the American [Atom] bomb casualty personnel [worked, in a separate building] and [were shown] the various museums that had these horrible moulages [molds of body parts; arms, legs, torsos, ears, etc.] from the results [casualties] of the bombing of Nagasaki. Also, . . . in Sasebo, there were several nurses, Japanese nurses, that worked at the U.S. Navy Hospital, that had been Japanese Navy nurses during the Second World War. Frequently they would explain how they would go by train down to the outskirts of Nagasaki after the bombing, to pick up these burn patients to take them by train all the way to Tokyo. They would describe the horrors that they saw, the poor patients, how badly burned they were and many of them expired before they ever reached their destination and the great amount of pain and suffering that these people went through. . . .

"While at Sasebo, we had our monthly inspections. The Commanding Officer of the base would have everyone, including whatever nurses who weren't on duty early Saturday mornings, down on the hot tarmac for our dress white inspection. Having arrived there in June, it was very warm to begin with and as the summer progressed it became more so. As the four or five Navy nurses stood out there for these Saturday morning inspections, which lasted an hour to an hour and 15 minutes, our high heels, white high heels, would gradually sink down into the hot tarmac. As we would go to take a step forward, we'd be stuck. After a few weeks, someone came up with an lovely idea. We arrived one morning to find these boards, about two inches wide, all in a line where the nurses were to stand with our heels on the board and our toes, of course, on the tarmac. From then on, we had no more problem of sinking into the hot tarmac."[12]

In June of 1962, two Lt(jg) Nurse Corps officers are given TAD to a U.S. Navy Medical Mission to Honduras; a country just north of Nicaragua in Central America. The two Nurse Corps officers are: Jessena E. Paradis and Lois L. McCue. The assignment of the Medical Mission is "to assist local health personnel in combating an epidemic of gastro-enteritis."[13]

Let's move now, across the waters from Honduras to the island of Puerto Rico. On the northern shores is a U.S. Naval Dispensary at San Juan. (In October of 1962, a Nurse Corps officer is assigned duty there.) On the eastern shores is the U.S. Naval Hospital at the Roosevelt Roads, Naval Base. Two islands west of Puerto Rica sits Cuba where there is another U.S. Naval Base and Naval Hospital at Guantanamo Bay, near the eastern tip of the island. In October 1962, the U.S. discovers that Russia has placed missiles in Cuba and those missiles are capable of hitting the U.S.. Also, Russian ships are already at sea heading for Cuba with more weaponry aboard. President Kennedy orders the U.S. Navy to blockade Cuba and turn back those Russian ships. The whole country, the whole world is holding its breath at this point. The two strongest nations in the world are eyeball to eyeball. Just two days later, the Russians blink and the Russian ships alter course away from Cuba. Four days after that, the President and Khrushchev reach a settlement and the missiles are removed from Cuba.

Nurse Corps officer Margaret L. Covington is stationed in Puerto Rico during this world-shaking event. She says, "I don't consider my tour of duty at Roosevelt Roads unique, but it certainly could have been if the events had turned out differently. The Cuban Missile Crisis occurred just less than a year after the Navy nurses were assigned there. The hospital had been built in increments and the dependents' units had just opened up in the summer of `62. For a small base, Roosevelt Roads, which was a Naval Air facility, was in a very strategic location for the approach by air and water. In the fall of `62 when it seemed that the U.S. invasion of Cuba was a real possibility, plans were being made by the command on the base because Roosevelt Roads would surely be very much involved. Plans were that if there was an invasion, the hospital at Guantanamo Bay would be evacuated and patients would be moved to the hospital at Roosevelt Roads. Also, we could plan on receiving casualties. There followed a few weeks of suspense. I remember looking out the back door of my apartment over into the Caribbean and seeing numerous, it seemed like hundreds, of ships of the U.S. Fleet. I understood at that time there were some 10,000 Marines aboard ships in the Caribbean. Of course, our problems were resolved as history will have it, but it was some weeks before we were back to normal in the Roosevelt Roads area."[14] Meantime, in Cuba itself, at the Guantanamo Bay U.S. Naval Base, all patients and all dependents are evacuated. They leave by Military Air Transportation Service and by Military Sea Transport ship to Portsmouth, Virginia. (The dependents do not return until December.)[15]   During this time, Navy Nurse Dorothy Eaton (Root) is stationed at Gitmo (Guantanamo Bay nickname) and she says, "We [the Navy nurses] were the only women left in Guantanamo Bay during the Cuban Crisis. It was a difficult experience. There were ten Navy nurses and one Red Cross worker left down there. We had been practicing weekend after weekend on how to evacuate the dependents and children, and when the time came for evacuation, everything went smoothly. Our nurses did an excellent job. We had the underground hospital ready for any problems that might come up."[16]

   Turn your thoughts now to the far east and Vietnam. "By mid-1962 American forces in Vietnam numbered 8000, by the end of the year over 11,000, ten months later, 17,000. United States soldiers served alongside ARVN units at every level from battalion to division and general staff. They planned operations and accompanied Vietnamese units into the field from six to eight weeks at a time. They airlifted troops and supplies, built jungle airstrips, flew helicopter rescue and medical evacuation teams, trained Vietnamese pilots, coordinated artillery fire and air support, introduced defoliation flights north of Saigon. They also took casualties: 14 killed or wounded in 1961, 109 in 1962, 489 in 1963. . . . With ARVN under American tutelage, increasing its missions, with the Viet-Cong defection rate rising and many of its bases abandoned, confidence recovered. Nineteen sixty-two was Saigon's year, unsuspected to be its last. American optimism swelled. Army and Embassy spokesmen issued positive pronouncements. . . . At the ground level, colonel and non-coms and press reporters were more doubtful. . . . [Premier] Diem's mandate to govern [South Vietnam], never thoroughly accepted by the mixture of sects, religions and classes, was finally shattered by the Buddhist revolt in the summer of 1963. . . . In May, when Saigon prohibited celebrations of Buddha's birthday, riots followed and government troops fired on the demonstrators, killing several. Renewed riots and martial law were given a terrible notoriety by the desperate act of self-immolation by a Buddhist monk who set himself on fire in a public square of Saigon. The protest spread . . . culminating in a raid on the main Buddhist pagoda and the arrest of hundreds of monks. The Foreign Minister and the Ambassador to the United States resigned in protest; Diem's government began to crack. . . . In the army too Diem had enemies. A generals' coup was simmering. . . . On 1 November the generals' coup took place successfully. It included, to the appalled discomfort of the Americans, the unexpected assassinations of Diem and [his younger brother] Nhu."[17] In Saigon, at the time of this coup, are seven Navy nurses; in harm's way.

   In early 1963, two Navy nurses ,on duty in the States, had received 'dispatch' orders for duty in Saigon; CDR Florence Alwyn (Twyman) and Navy Nurse Penny Kauffman. The Army was transferring a military activity, in Saigon, to the Navy and the Navy nurses are to take over the medical area from the Army nurses stationed there. CDR Alwyn (Twyman) is to be the Senior Nurse. A Senior Medical officer and several Navy corpsmen were already there when the two Navy nurses arrive in Saigon for duty at the dispensary clinic that had been the Army's. CDR Twyman tells us, "our main mission . . . was to spot out a locale whereby we could start a hospital [she is to be the chief nurse there]. . . . A couple of times we thought we had a site all sewed up and then it would fall apart."[18] They finally find a site with an old apartment house on it. Meanwhile, back Stateside, five more Navy nurses receive dispatch orders to Saigon. In September 1963, the five all meet at Travis Air Force Base in California where they board a flight for their new duty station. The five Navy nurses are: Owedia (Tweedie) Searcy (nurse anesthetist), Vila (Bobbi) Hovis, Elaine King, Carleda Lorberg, and Jan Barcott. When they arrive they begin their duty at the clinic. Jan Barcott says, "At first we just worked in the clinic and then they had a French hotel that was converted into a hospital and we literally had to scrub it from head to toe and we had no equipment to work with. I can remember using toothbrushes and mops that had about six or seven of those strands on them."[19] Bobbi Hovis, in her book, notes that, "There were neither cleaning agents nor a profusion of rags. After two days we were ready to turn in our mops and board the first aircraft out. Instead, we became masters at improvisation. As a Navy Seabees' expression put it, `We have done so much with so little for so long that now we can do anything with nothing forever.' . . . Still, we persevered. We cleared the trash from, swept, and swabbed five stories of decks. Space for 100 beds had been cleaned and sanitized to the best of our ability. The hospital furnishings . . . had been wiped down, hauled in, and put in place. . . . But by 1000 hours on 1 October 1963, a formerly dilapidated apartment building had been transformed into a respectable medical-treatment facility. It was commissioning day.

"Our official title was the U.S. Naval Station Hospital, Saigon, Republic of Vietnam, under the command of Headquarters Support Activity, Saigon. . . . The entire hospital staff, for the first time dressed in white uniforms, mustered in ranks for the ceremony. . . . We sparkled in our ward-white uniforms (for nurses) and tropical-dress whites with service ribbons (for men)."[20]

Then, on 1 November, the day of the coup d'etat in Saigon, Jan Barcott is in the quarters that she shares with two other Navy nurses, in the 'Brink' junior officer's BOQ [Bachelor Officers Quarters]. She is the only one home. "The day of the coup d'etat I was assigned to P.M. duty along with a Thai nurse. Late that morning, one of the Army officers came by. We three [Navy nurses] all dated Army guys and it [the quarters] was kind of a hang-out for a lot of them. So we went up to the roof to have coffee. There was a lounge up there and a spectacular view of the city. There was something going on but we had no idea what [it was]. He had his transistor radio on, trying to get some news from the Armed Forces station. All of a sudden there was machine gun `ack-ack.' He said, `Hit the deck!' Boy, did I. We were lying next to each other and I swear I could hear his heart beat - thud, thud, thud. I was too dumb to be scared. Shortly after, I returned to the apartment and all these [American] dependents started coming through the door. These people, mothers and kids, had been shopping, or whatever, and were [told] to get off the streets and get into these military quarters. . . . We started putting the [furniture] cushions on the floor and around the walls, setting up a kind of barrier in case of more gun fire. . . . An hour or so later my roommate came flying in the door, her eyes were just like saucers. She had been shopping up in town and she said they were closing off parts of the town and people were told to get off the streets. She started running and she said she was so frightened because she didn't know why [they were told that] but she knew that something was wrong. . . . So I thought, well I guess I'm not going to work; I'm not going out into that street. Then I received a phone call from the Chief Nurse to stay where I was and for the time being I would not report for duty.

"Eventually the dependents were escorted home and I finally got a call to come to work. About 6 p.m. I went down to the foyer and the little civilian nurse that I was going to be [working] with was there already. [A car was sent to pick them up.] Usually those streets in Saigon are just wall to wall with bikes and vehicles, [but this time] it was almost total silence. People had just disappeared and all of the shops were closed and everything. So off we go and we get to the hospital and everybody who had been on day shift were waiting to be relieved. . . . We started doing whatever we had to do and, I think it was just as it was starting to get dark when the shooting started and flares went off and all this stuff, and we wondered what was happening; are the South Vietnamese soldiers shooting at us or who's shooting who? . . . This went on until 1 or 2 in the morning . . . and I looked over toward town where the nurses lived, and I thought, dear God, they're going to get killed. I was so worried. We even had a bullet hit the hospital and it ricocheted into one of the patient's room. . . . About 2 in the morning everything was just dead silent. I was looking out the window and I heard this strange noise. Up the street came all these Army tanks; tank after tank after tank. There must have been about 13 or 14 tanks and soldiers walking behind them. Soon they stopped and they sat down. It was south Vietnamese soldiers and they wore little red kerchiefs. They took their kerchiefs off and they had little pots they cooked on. They sat down and cooked their rice and rested for an hour. Then they all got up and off they went and continued down the road. It wasn't until early the next morning that we found out that was when the President was assassinated and that's what all the shooting was about.

"The A.M. staff arrived about 7:30 and I was relieved (in more ways than one!) of my duty. The drive back to quarters was unbelievable. It was just another typical day! Traffic was the same, the shops open - it was crazy. In our quarters were our Army buddies, all wearing their guns and waiting to see what was happening next. Soon the streets were full of tanks again and people were jubilant as they tossed flowers at the soldiers. They hated the Diem regime (especially Madame Nhu, his wife.) She and her children escaped. There was a huge statue of two famous sisters (supposedly Madame had posed for one) and one of the first things the people did was to topple this monument. Dancing had been forbidden by Madame and everyone was dancing again.

"Later in the morning, an Army officer and I went to view the damage. The palace complex had been cordoned off with barb-wire, but they would allow the Americans in. Across from the palace was the Vietnamese soldiers' barracks. We walked through and found photos of the Diem family. They had been confiscated from the palace. . . . The palace was riddled with holes as were the surrounding buildings. Some had huge gaping holes. We were not allowed in the palace. . . . Everyone was relieved and happy - but not for long."[21]

In 1963 Navy Nurse Beverly Brase (O'Dell) is stationed in Yokosuka, Japan at the U.S. Naval Hospital. She is finishing the second half of a split overseas tour of duty. (She had spent the first year in the Philippines.) She says, "The Japanese people were absolutely great. They were kind, considerate, and enjoyable, but we also had demonstrations. I have tapes of the Communist demonstration walking in front of the base screaming 'Yankee go home.' That was the first time I had ever been involved in a foreign country where it seemed they did not appreciate our presence. The duty in Yokosuka was a little hard, as far as duty hours. We were on what was called, at that time, a six-day-week, which was actually twelve days on and then a Saturday and Sunday off. It would start PM's on a Monday and work through the week-end, double-back Monday morning on AM's through Friday, and then would have Saturday and Sunday off and come back to work on PM's again. That was a little difficult, and it seemed like we were tired most of the time. . . . We traveled a lot in Japan. We had bicycles and we bicycled all over with the rest of the Japanese. We traveled by train. We traveled all over the Orient from the also, when we were on leave."[22]

Back in Washington, D.C., in May of 1963, the Nursing Division of BuMed has received approval for a revision of the Navy Nurse Corps Candidate Program. Instead of subsidizing qualified nursing students for just their last year of training, now the last two years can be subsidized. Also, the program now includes qualified "registered nurses matriculating in University programs approved by the National League for Nursing. Participants in the program are commissioned as Ensign, USNR, six months prior to completion of degree requirements."[23]

As for the Space Program in 1963, one American and two Russian manned spaceships split the heavens this year. In other U.S. happenings, prayers and Bible reading in public schools is deemed unconstitutional by the Supreme Court. The U.S. and Russia set up the 'hot-line' between Moscow and Washington.[24] But, probably the hottest issue in the country is "Negro demands for equal civil and economic rights. . . . Racial protests and demonstrations took place in all parts of the United States, in the North and the South. . . . On Aug. 28, 1963, about 200,000 persons staged a *Freedom March* in Washington, D.C., to demonstrate their demands for equal rights for Negroes."[25] Over the past two years and in this year, rioting has broken out necessitating the use of Federal forces. Then on Friday the 22nd of November 1963 at 12:30 p.m., the nation and the world come to a halt with the immensity of a singular and awful tragedy brought about by an assassin's three bullets in Dallas, Texas. Our President, John F. Kennedy, is dead. Camelot is no more.

Within two hours of the President's death, Vice President Lyndon Baines Johnson is sworn in as President. This takes place aboard Air Force One, the Presidential plane, at the Dallas airport. Lady Bird Johnson and the shocked widow, Jacqueline Kennedy, stand at his side. President Kennedy's coffin is in the rear compartment of the plane. After the swearing in, the plane takes off for Washington, D.C..

In Bethesda, Maryland, at the National Naval Medical Center, Commander Marion Caesar (Wheeler) is the Chief Nurse and her Assistant Chief Nurse is Sally Smith. CDR Caesar (Wheeler) says, "On that fateful day, November 22, 1963, during lunch hour, [Navy nurse] Pat Brennan came in looking quite shaken up and said, 'the President's been shot.' . . . We went around the corner [of the hallway] to where the administrative offices are. We put the radio on and sure enough it was coming through. . . . Things sort of stood still for a long while. . . . Around three o'clock, [the Commanding Officer of the Hospital], came in [the Nursing Office] and said, 'We're going to have to open up the tower on 17th [the Presidential suite on the 17th floor], because the President's body is going to be brought here for an autopsy. And, I'd like you to get it opened and assign nurses up there.' I said, 'Well, I think I'll assign myself up there and Sally.' . . . They thought the First Lady would be flown by helicopter from Andrews [Air Force base where Air Force One will land] and so they had me out at the helicopter pad [at the hospital], and then someone came out and got me and said they were coming by ambulance. I don't remember the name of the Catholic Chaplain, but he and I met at the ambulance. In the meantime, Sally Smith was getting the family organized up [on the 17th floor]. There was the First Lady's mother and step-father, sister and - well, there were all sorts of people up there.

"Finally, they came and I remember when she, Mrs. Kennedy, got out of the ambulance. [She came in the Navy Ambulance with her husband's body.] We were more or less going to [help] her out and she said, 'No, I must walk by myself. No one must touch me.' So we went in and up the elevator to the top floor. And her mother came forward to greet her and she said, 'Do not touch me. I must not cry.' And so from then on it was a horrible thing.

"By this time, of course, all the Secret Service men that were involved were up there and Bobby Kennedy had arrived and there was - I kind of forget all the men that were on his staff. And of course, Hill. I think Hill was the Secret Service man that was assigned to the First Lady. He was all covered with blood. But he came out of the room and I said to him, 'How could this happen?' He said . . . they never expected anything like that [the assassination] because the reception [in Texas] had been warm. . . .

"I went into the galley to get some sandwiches and things ready and the First Lady came in. She wanted to know if she could sit down on that little stool. She sat there and she kept rubbing all that blood [she still had the same clothes on as when the President was shot] and she kept saying, 'The President's brains are in my lap.' . . . It was very sad. But, she was very stoic. Then McNamara came in, the Secretary of Defense, and he said, 'We'll have to be talking now about the funeral. Will he be buried up in Massachusetts?' She said, 'No. There is a spot over there [in Arlington National Cemetery] on the hill below the mansion [of General Robert E. Lee]. He used to say, 'I'd like to think I could be laid to rest here.' I would really like him to be buried there, if the two children that are buried in Boston could be moved down.' . . . and finally, that decision was reached. . . . Nothing could get her to rest. And I was in and out of the galley. . . . Then I was warming up milk at the stove and Bobby [Kennedy] came in and he had no place to sit. . . . She had the only thing to sit on; the stool. He said, 'I think I'll sit on the refrigerator.' I said, 'You'll never get up there.' Well, one hop and he was up there. So that's where he sat while I was making the warm milk for everybody.

"Finally, Dr. Walsh came over. The White House had sent over a change of clothing [for the First Lady], but she would not change. Her obstetrician came and we finally got her to lie down. She wouldn't take any medication. Finally she said to Dr. Walsh that she'd have a little scotch and water. She didn't really drink. She toyed with it. She kept talking. And when Dr. Walsh came out of the room, her mother said to him, 'Is my daughter drugged?' He said, 'No, she never cries. . . . When the little baby Patrick died, she was very stoic. She only cried when she was alone.' He said, 'The President went to pieces when that baby died.' So she was a very stoic woman. And, I thought she was able to do this because she removed herself from the role of the wife. She always referred to him as 'the President,' 'the President.' We will take the President back to the White House in the hearse so I may go with him.' That wasn't the plan at all. They were going to have him go back with the undertaker. She told her mother, 'You must tell the children. They must not cry.' And I think that was proven when we watched it [TV] through those horrible days. . . .

"There were some amusing things that happened. Someone answered the phone and they wanted to talk to Bobby and Bobby said, 'What Johnson?' They said, 'President Johnson.' 'What Johnson?' 'President Johnson.' 'Oh-h-h-h.' It was as though you can't believe we've got a new President. Then he came back and he said to Mrs. Kennedy, 'President Johnson wants to know if you would like to have a portrait of the President displayed with the casket?' She thought a while and she said, 'No. We'll take care of that later.' . . .

"So when I left there, it was in the morning. [The Commanding Officer] said, 'I think I'll drive you home. You can walk over for your car in the morning. I [lived] that close. I said to him, 'If I had spent the night with the Queen of England, I couldn't have been more impressed with this decorum of this lady. They were planning the whole funeral, you know. They're going to walk.'"[26]

Navy Nurse Winifred L. Copeland is a Nursing Service Supervisor at Bethesda Naval Hospital at this time. She says, "I was assigned to one of the ambulances that was to stand by as [President Kennedy's] body was brought down the avenue to the Capitol Rotunda to lie in state. The crowd was massive. The doctor, corpsman and I were standing alongside the ambulance. The crowd watching the procession was like a huge tidal wave being swept along as it followed the funeral cortege. Soon we were surrounded by the crowd which swept over the ambulance in its attempt to follow the cortege. It was an unforgettable experience. The whole nation seemed in a state of shock from grief and disbelief."[27]

Navy Nurse VaLaine Pack is stationed at the Naval Hospital in Philadelphia. "When President Kennedy was assassinated, I felt really, as if I had lost somebody that I knew. He had been such a powerful figure. [He had] come to Newport, Rhode Island during the time I was in Officer Indoctrination up there and we followed his activities quite closely. The mourning that went on was just really mind boggling, not that it wouldn't go on for any President, but it just - I had never been exposed to anything like that before. We all were very, very sad, very unhappy when this happened, and very devastated for a period of time. That weekend, the four days that took place for his funeral, the viewing, and all of the honors that were paid to him, we were glued to our televisions. Even at work we would have one on in the back room and go peek in at it every now and then and take care of patients."[28]

Navy Nurse Kathleen Martin is across the Pacific, stationed in Japan. "In November of 1963, I was on leave with some nurses from Taiwan and a couple of other nurses from [the U.S. Naval Hospital at Yokosuka]. We had stayed at the Tokyo hotel for military personnel and early in the morning about six o'clock, the group that had been on the second floor came down to the first floor where we were staying, knocking on our door very excitedly. We opened up and they said, `We don't know what's wrong, but something's happened. There's a lot of Generals and Admirals and high ranking officers out in the lobby. They're all around the TV and some of them are even crying.' So we sent them out to find out what it was as we jumped out of bed and got dressed. Well then, in a very short time, back came our friends with one of the Colonels that we knew from the Marine Corps and he informed us that President Kennedy had been assassinated. We were about 18 hours in time difference, I guess, time difference from the States and you just couldn't believe this. No one knew what had happened except for the fact that he was dead; our Commander-in-Chief. We all tried to call our base hospital and find out what would happen. We thought maybe we should all report back immediately. But, they said no, just stand by and if we hear anything, then to come back. But in the meantime, continue on our leave and we had been. After all of the nurses were able to call and talk to their chief nurses and Commanding Officers, we decided we would go into the city of Tokyo anyway. So we got a Taxi cab and for the first time, apparently, in the history since the end of World War II when they first turned the Ginza lights on [the Ginza district is Japan's entertainment center], that day there were no Ginza lights. They kept them off for 72 hours in honor of President Kennedy. Taxi cab drivers that we had jokingly called the 'kamikaze pilots,' were so sad and were so apologetic to us. They just couldn't believe that our President Kennedy was dead. It was a very, very quiet Tokyo, not like the city that we had known before. We went to several of the memorial services that were held for President John F. Kennedy, then later we did return [to their duty stations]. Our vacations ended a bit early and still not knowing what had caused the loss of our Commander-in-Chief."[29]

In Saigon, Vietnam, three Navy nurses are gathered in one of the quarters at the Brink BOQ. They are; Chief Nurse Florence Alwyn, nurse anesthetist Tweedy Searcy and surgical nurse Bobbi Hovis. The previous day they had learned of President Kennedy's assassination. In her book, Bobbi Hovis writes, "The twenty-fourth of November began bright and sunny. At noon, Thi Cong [Vietnamese laundress] summoned us to the balcony. Flo, Tweedie, and I looked down upon a remarkable sight. Thousands of Vietnamese students, five abreast and carrying English-language placards, formed a procession that moved along Ham Nghi Street toward the Central Market. Banners eulogized Kennedy in what was the first pro-American demonstration we had witnessed since arriving in Vietnam. At the height of the march, the sky opened and a deluge poured down. The marchers continued. It was a poignant, unforgettable sight."[30] 1963 closes on a somber note.

Lyndon B. Johnson takes a firm hold on the reins of the Presidency and soon has "bills `coming out of Congress like candy bars from a slot machine.'"[31] "The President pushed hard for legislation that had been proposed by President Kennedy. He urged quick passage of a tax cut and a strong civil rights bill, both Kennedy measures. . . . Johnson also proposed a national 'War on Poverty.'"[32] The term 'Great Society' "was used to describe many of the President's domestic programs. Those programs included continuing the war on poverty, improving the nation's educational system, providing for the nation's elder citizens, rebuilding cities, and preserving the American countryside."[33]

As for the Space Program, in 1964, the U.S. finally develops a more powerful space vehicle, the Saturn I, which is "a giant step in developing rocket power."[34] Then on the 27th of March 1964 at 5:36 p.m., the earth moved in Alaska. "Within minutes on that Good Friday afternoon, 118 Alaskans were dead and 4,500 were left homeless."[35] The quake measured "at between 8.4 and 8.6 on the Richter Scale, making it the largest quake on record in America. The shocks were felt as far away as Houston, Texas."[36] In Anchorage, the "new J.C. Penney Co. store crumbled to the ground . . . the main thoroughfare in Anchorage sank twenty feet below street level, taking a row of parked cars with it."[37]

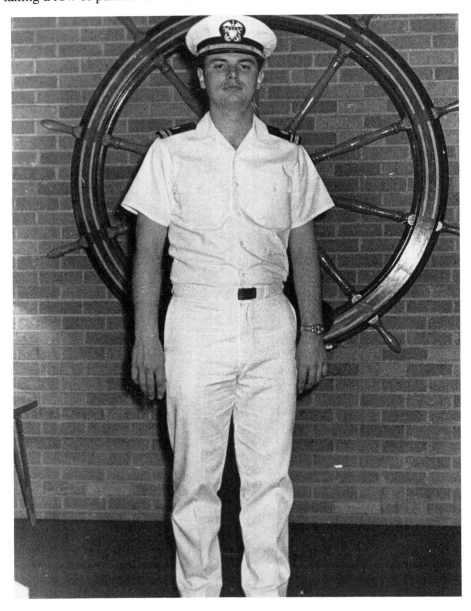

As for the status of professional nursing, there is still a drastic shortage of nurses throughout the country and, moreover, the numbers of student nurses are not sufficient to fill the foreseen needs. Congress has been made aware of the difficulties and President Johnson signs legislation called the Nurse Training Act of 1964. Among other things, the legislation provides low-interest, long-term loans for nursing students.

Also, in November 1964, the Secretary of the Navy signs an approval that finally allows male nurses in the U.S. Navy Nurse Corps. He does this by approving a change in the requirements for a commission in the Navy Nurse Corps. The change also allows qualified enlisted men of the Hospital Corps to apply for the NENEP program. This is the program that provides for up to four years of "duty-under-instruction at a university

Male Navy nurse. (Photo courtesy of LCdr. Lynn Day NC USN (Ret.))

conducting a Baccalaureate degree program in nursing."[38]

Navy nurses are still serving aboard MST ships in 1964 and Navy Nurse Iris M. Stock is one of the nurses aboard the USS *General W.A. Mann*. She gives us an in-depth description of such duty. "As the ship was a U.S. Navy Ship, we had an all Navy crew as opposed to some of the other M.S.T. ships which were manned by civilian crews, complimented by Naval personnel. The medical and dental department consisted of two medical officers, two nurse corps officers, a chief hospital corpsman and eight corpsmen. We had one dental officer and one dental technician. . . . Morning started with morning quarters when the whole department stood-to, in front of the sick bay, and the medical officer gave us a rundown on the plan of the day and other pertinent data. . . . I was the Senior Nurse and so my duties, other than overseeing that nursing care activities were carried out for the day, was responsibility for dependent sick call. We usually departed our home port of Oakland around mid-day or by early afternoon. On the day of sailing we, with the medical officer, were responsible for checking all dependent passengers aboard. We would check their shot records and try to determine that everyone was physically well enough to board. It was on embarkation you had a chance to first meet the passengers and get some inkling of possible future problems or medical needs.

"Our busiest time was always shortly after getting underway. A general briefing was given the passengers by the ship's department heads and, as Senior Nurse, I was required to give a short briefing on our sick call hours and the formula room hours for those passengers traveling with infants. Entering the Pacific [Ocean] from under the Golden Gate Bridge is always rough, even for a ship as large as the *Mann*. It was unfortunate as few passengers had time to get accustomed to the motion of the ship before we hit rough water. The largest percentage became immediately sea sick and our first duty was to make rounds of the cabin area to distribute Dramamine and crackers and encourage people to get up and try to eat and get medication down. Sick call the evening of sailing was always a mad house. For uncontrollable vomiting we gave Thorazine IM [IntraMuscularly]. We almost always found one or two children with high temps and URI's [Upper Respiratory Infections/colds]. The first night at sea was usually a wakeful night for the nurse on call as people would report for treatment throughout the night. Morning sick call was again a repeat of the previous night, with numerous nauseated, vomiting passengers. Following sick call, we would again make rounds with the ship's transportation officer, getting people up to sick call for treatment. Usually, after the first twenty-four hours at sea, sick call settled down and life settled down to leisurely days.

"Life aboard ship was generally uneventful but when things happened it was always exciting. . . . We had drills but, while I was aboard, we had at least two men overboard drills that proved to be the real thing. The first time this happened we were entering Pearl Harbor and were going up the long channel approach to Pearl Harbor when, suddenly, the ship's whistle blew and we heard `man overboard.' A Marine prisoner, who had been brought on deck for his morning exercise, decided to make an attempt for freedom, jumping overboard and narrowly missing the pilot boat escorting the ship up the channel. Luckily, the pilot boat picked him up and we did not have to attempt rescue efforts in the channel.

"Another instance of man overboard ended also with less than tragic results. One evening, near dinner time, we were about four hundred miles from Wake Island, a soldier decided life was not worth living, and jumped overboard. Luckily, some of his buddies saw him, and while one came racing to sick bay, another buddy started throwing life vests to the man in the water. Immediate rescue procedures were initiated. A dye marker is cast into the water, the boat crew races to the lifeboat and the ship starts to turn to retrace its course. For a ship as large as the *Mann*, I was told that it takes approximately one mile to slow and return to the spot where the turn was initiated. As it was winter and dark was upon us, finding this man would prove to be tricky. By the time we had returned to the spot, the lifeboat was in the water and a search was started. On all rescue attempts of this nature, a hospital corpsman and a man with a gun accompany the boat crew. The corpsman to render first aid and the man with the gun to shoot sharks, if necessary. Fortunately, the seas were relatively calm that night, and the man was found fairly quickly. Apparently, after jumping, he realized what a terrible decision he had made and grabbed a life vest, plus he did call for assistance, which greatly helped in finding him. On return to the ship he was taken to sick bay and given the necessary first aid and placed under psychiatric observation until we could transfer him to the nearest medical facility at our next port of call. One cannot realize how vast the Pacific is until you are trying to search for a human being out there.

"Other rescues that the ship was involved in, directly affected the medical department and our antiquated OR. One morning I arose and went to the ward room for my morning coffee. The engineering officer was there and said, `Have you heard about the SAR?' Having been aboard only a short time, I was soon to find out SAR meant Sea Air Rescue. During the night, our Captain had been contacted and medical assistance had been requested by a Chinese freighter for one of their crew members who was ill. No other information was given. Because the nearest ship always renders assistance, if possible when at sea, we were retracing our course to rendezvous with this Chinese freighter. We finally made contact . . . mid-morning. The seas were rough and a boat was put over the side with our senior medical officer along. It was nerve racking watching the little boat appear and then disappear as they made their way through the rough seas to the bedraggled, grubby looking Chinese freighter. After what seemed like years, we finally saw them reach the ship and saw them being assisted aboard. After approximately thirty minutes we saw them disembark with . . . the patient along. We all strained anxiously as the boat made its tortuous way back to our ship. On disembarking, the medical officer escorted the patient to sick bay. The patient proved to be the ship's cook, a wizened little Chinese man appearing acutely ill. After further examination we found him to be in the terminal stages of pulmonary TB [Tuberculosis]. He was very anemic and highly contagious. We really had almost no place to isolate this man, but did have a small room [that could be used to] set-up and isolate him.

The man spoke nothing but Chinese so communication became a real problem. After canvassing the ship's passenger list, we found a Chinese diplomat on his way to Hawaii. Though he did not speak the man's particular dialect, he was helpful in getting across to him basic information and relaying to us some of the man's requirements. Fearful that our patient would not survive the next twenty-four hours until we reach Hawaii, because of his severe anemic condition, our medical officer decided he must some how transfuse the man. We did not have the necessary lab supplies to perform a proper type and crossmatch. Medical authorities were contacted in Hawaii and at about 2200 that night we received a delivery of the necessary supplies by air. An airplane flew over the ship and dropped, by small parachute, the needed equipment onto the flying bridge. The senior medical officer again came to the man's rescue, as he was the person most compatible for [the patient's] blood type. The transfusion was given and . . . the next day was disembarked in Hawaii and turned over to Chinese counselor officials. I should add, these were all Chinese from Taiwan. We later heard that the man succumbed to his disease. I remember the medical officer stating his surprise that he [had seen] no rats aboard the Chinese freighter, though it was filthy aboard the ship. He said, `I think they must have been eating the rats.' . . .

"One voyage, we had another unusual event. My attention was first peaked by a conversation between the Executive officer and the Chaplain at lunch one day shortly after we had put to sea from Oakland. It went something like this: Executive officer, `Did you get him aboard OK?' The Chaplain responded, `Yes, he's on board.' `Where did you put him?' `Well, he's in the drawer under my bunk for now. There wasn't any place else that I could find where he would be safe.' It later developed that a retired Naval officer had requested burial of his ashes at sea somewhere off the Hawaiian chain. . . . Lunch time and dinner conversation were a change from the norm for the ensuing five days, as they were involved with the preparations of the ceremony to take place at the appropriate place and time. Our sailing schedule had to be altered somewhat because, as originally scheduled, we would have arrived at the designated point at 2400 hours. Time was finally altered enough that with our departure from Hawaii we would arrive at the appointed place at 1000 hours on the designated day. The next detail to be settled was who would be in the burial detail and what the uniform of the day would be for the ceremony. Also, black crepe arm bands had to be secured for all of the burial detail. . . . Finally, the momentous day arrived. In addition to the detail itself, the department heads were the only other portion of the ship's company taking an active role in the ceremony. Our Senior Medical officer had not been in the Navy long, and the medical department turned out in mass to check his uniform and sword to help see that he was properly attired. He did look impressive with the dress whites and sword, and the black arm band. Prior to 1000 hours, the remainder of us went to the flying bridge so that we could observe the ceremony. It was a beautiful day with a blue sky and with the sparkling blue waters and the warm trade winds blowing gently. The ceremony went off flawlessly as a short internment ceremony was given and the ashes were gently tipped over the side. . . . Old Glory was carefully folded for later presentation to the family, none of whom were present. `Taps' floated over the quiet sea. With the final notes the service was over and normal shipboard activities again resumed. Many times since, I have remembered that service and the beauty of it and the day. Certainly a fitting manner in which to end a life spent in the Navy."[39]

"On August 2, 1964, the American destroyer *Maddox*, patrolling off the North Vietnam coast [in the Gulf of Tonkin], was attacked by three torpedo boats. They inflicted no damage and were driven off. A second attack was alleged to have taken place on the night of August 4 against the *Maddox* and her sister ship, the *Turner Joy*, although evidence of this attack consisted of only a few mysterious radar blips. Shots in the dark from the destroyers apparently hit nothing but salt water.

"Although ambiguous reports from the scene cast doubt on the entire episode, President Lyndon Johnson ordered retaliatory air strikes `against gunboats and certain supporting facilities' in North Vietnam. . . .

"Johnson, as Vice President in 1961, had told President Kennedy that `the participation of American ground troops in the war in Vietnam is neither desirable nor necessary.' He said it again, a few weeks after the Tonkin incident, while campaigning for a full term as President: `We are not about to send American boys nine or ten thousand miles away from home to do what Asian boys ought to be doing for themselves.' He ran as the peace candidate, promising `no wider war.'"[40]

President Johnson and his Vice Presidential candidate, Senator Hubert H. Humphrey run against the Republican candidate, Senator Barry M. Goldwater in the 1964 Presidential election. "Johnson won re-election in a landslide. He received 486 electoral votes to only 52 for Senator Goldwater."[41]

Once the election is over, the focus of attention is again (or is still) turned to Vietnam where things have been warming up even more. Back in August, on the 13th, the Saigon Naval Station experiences an episode that demonstrates the strain and anxiety placed on the personnel there. Navy Nurse Bobbi Hovis writes, "I was in the ICU [Intensive Care Unit], facing windows that overlooked the Operating/Emergency Room area. Just as I inserted tubing into an IV (intravenous) bottle, there was an enormous explosion. The windows blew in, glass shattered, the IV tray crashed to the deck. Patients who could jumped from their beds and crouched under them.

"For a few anxious moments I thought Duong Duong [Station Hospital Saigon] was under attack. . . . We had all been on edge during August. An incident involving U.S. Navy ships in the Tonkin Gulf had occurred on 2 and 4 August; a state of national emergency had been declared on 8 August. All R and Rs [Rest and Recreation time] had been canceled in case planes were needed to evacuate civilians. We were packed and ready to leave Saigon if so ordered. . . .

"No one in the ICU was hurt from the blast. There was no smoke or fire. I hurried to the Operating/ Emergency Room area, the source of the main blast. There was no outside damage, no smoke, and no fire. But the inside was a mess! Windows were cracked, and an operating light in the ER [Emergency Room] fell from its overhead attachment, crashing and exploding onto the table. . . . I thought of the jets [planes] and the possibility of a sonic boom - my hunch was right. Minutes later, a call from General Westmoreland's office confirmed that a jet descending over the city had exceeded the sound barrier. A call went out to the squadron commander: no more sonic booms over Saigon."[42]

During September and October the Navy nurses who were the first ones assigned to Saigon, are in the midst of packing and saying good-byes. Their orders to new duty assignment have been received and their Nurse Corps replacements have arrived or are arriving. In her book, 'Station Hospital Saigon,' LCdr Bobbi Hovis states, "The second week of September . . . one of Tweedie's [Navy nurse anesthetist Tweedie Searcy] OR techs, decided to surprise Tweedie, . . . [two Navy Medical Corps surgeons], and me with a party, which was held on the hospital's fifth deck. . . . The highlight of the surprise party occurred when Generals Westmoreland and Throckmorton arrived. Both generals expressed gratitude for the care we gave their men. We were overcome that the commanding general and his deputy found a few minutes, despite enormous responsibilities, to visit us one last time. We were almost too overwhelmed to speak. The relationship between Army and Navy was indeed special. Providing the best possible medical care for American personnel in Vietnam was a cooperative and rewarding effort."[43]

The Brink Hotel in Saigon, is the BOQ (Bachelor Officers Quarters) for some of the Navy nurses stationed at the Navy Station Hospital. The rest of the Navy nurses live in another quarters. Neither the nurses nor the doctors all live in the same place in case of bombing or other catastrophic occurrence. The Brink is a seven story building with a garage underneath and an Officer's club on the top floor. Four nurses live in quarters, on the second floor, which consists of two baths, two living rooms, and four bedrooms. One other nurse lives on one of the upper floors. On Christmas Eve of 1964, four of the Nurse Corps Officers that live at Brink, are off duty. Lt Ruth A. Mason (Wilson) had been out Christmas shopping, had just entered the Brink's lobby and is standing by the stairs and elevator talking to another occupant of the BOQ. Lt Frances Crumpton had just walked in the front door of the Brink and is about ten feet across the lobby from Ruth Mason (Wilson). Lt Barbara J. Wooster is in her room on one of the upper floors and Lt(jg) Ann Darby Reynolds is on the second floor where she shares rooms with Ruth Mason (Wilson), Frances Crumpton, and another Navy nurse who is presently on P.M. duty at the Navy Station Hospital.[44] Navy Nurse A. Darby Reynolds tells us, "I was standing in our apartment looking out . . . we had glass french doors, and I had my face up against the cold glass because it was so warm. Lo and behold, an explosion went off and the door blew in and the glass shattered all over my face. It was such a blow it threw me back a few feet. I didn't realize until after that I had been cut; until I looked down. I had a laceration on my leg. I was thrown back from the door. . . . Of course at that point I knew exactly what had happened, that a bomb had gone off; I didn't know exactly where in the building. And then, another explosion followed. Then all I could remember was I had the OR call [was on call for the Hospital's Operating Room]. . . . I knew it was going to be a long evening. Now that I think, I was probably in a state of shock because I went back from the living quarters to my room . . . and started looking for my shoes; I had my sneakers on. The next thing I remember was a couple of the fellows came in and got me and said, "You've got to get out of here. The building's on fire." They escorted me down the stairway to the bottom floor. . . . At that point I could hear the sirens going and it was just mass confusion in the courtyard. When you looked over to the side, all the jeeps and cars that were over there were on fire and a couple of them had exploded from the gasoline. We found out later that there was a 200 pound explosive that was put in one of the cars and set off. That's what caused it. The building was in shambles."[45] The Navy nurses all came together to check on one another then as Darby says, "We started to take care of [the injured] down in the courtyard as the men all started coming out of the building. [This despite the fact that all four of these Navy nurses suffered lacerations from glass fragments and had been knocked to the floor by the explosion.] I guess your initial thing is, as a nurse you have to go to work, and that's what we started doing. Since I had OR call, the first jeep that came by, I told one of them that I needed to get to the hospital, 'cause we had to set up for the folks [injured] that would be coming. . . . There were a couple of patients in the back [of the jeep] that we took with us."[46] All four of the nurses are taken to the hospital where they start working in the Emergency room and outside doing triage and/or inside doing triage and taking care of the casualties. Darby Reynolds notes that, "When I got to the hospital I went right into the operating room to start getting ready. Then I noticed that I was bleeding from my leg and one of the corpsmen came up and put an Ace bandage around that. . . . After the casualties started coming through, a couple of the corpsmen came up and told me that they had put away a suture set for me. They knew I was going to have to be sutured. They were afraid supplies were running too short and they said they were going to be sure that I got the equipment. I always remember that from the corpsmen who had tucked away the instruments for that. The OR suite was quite busy that night. After everybody had cleared out, one of the physicians sutured my leg. . . . We spent the whole Christmas Eve, December 24, at the hospital; it was after midnight before we were able to leave."[47]

All four of the Navy nurses had facial and other lacerations. Darby Reynolds not only had facial and leg lacerations but was off duty for a few days due to a concussion. Navy Nurse Francis L. Crumpton was med-evacuated to Clark Air Force Base Hospital in the Philippines for ear surgery. She had a cold at the time of the explosion and suffered ruptured ear drums as a result.

All four of the Navy nurses receive the Purple Heart Medal as a result of their selfless service that fateful night. They are the first Navy nurses to receive this decoration. At an awards ceremony in Saigon on 7 January 1965, they are presented with their medals. Only three of the nurses are present. Lt Crumpton is still in the hospital in the Philippines. The nurses choose to wear their ward white uniforms for the ceremony. As all the participants stand at attention, the Commanding Officer of the U.S. Naval Support Activity, Saigon, pins on the medals. The Commanding Officer delivers a speech at the occasion and says, in part, "Before making the awards this morning, I would like to say a few words about the medal you are about to receive. In a sense, it is the most meaningful and the oldest award for personal sacrifice in the service to our nation. It was first authorized by George Washington during the Revolutionary War to recognize the suffering at Valley Forge. It is presented to service men and women who have suffered physical injury or death as a result of hostile action.

"The Purple Heart is given by the President on behalf of the people of the United States in gratitude for your sacrifice in the defense of freedom. . . .

"Among you are three of the four nurses that were wounded in the Brink explosion. The fourth, Lieutenant Frances Crumpton, is in Clark Air Force Base Hospital for treatment of her wounds. These four will be recorded by historians as the first women members of the United States Armed Forces to receive the Purple Heart in Vietnam.

"I should also like to make special note of the fact that, although wounded in the Brink explosion, these women disregarded their own wounds to care for other casualties, both at the scene and later at the Station Hospital. Their actions in this regard were beyond the call of duty and in keeping with the highest traditions of the United States Navy and the Medical profession."[48]

The Director of the Navy Nurse Corps, Captain Ruth Erickson, sends a letter to LT Ruth Mason that says, in part, "You, Miss Wooster, Miss Reynolds and Miss Crumpton now hold the unique distinction of being the first women to receive a meritorious award in this conflict. It symbolizes to me and to all Navy nurses the dedication and valor of all our Nurse Corps officers who are serving in an area of international strife. Personally I am very pleased and proud of each of you. You and your colleagues have made outstanding professional and personal contributions and performed superbly under all conditions."[49] In her reply to Captain Erickson, Miss Mason says, "At the time of the explosion I had just returned from Christmas shopping and was in the lobby of the BOQ. It seemed for a few seconds that the sky had fallen on us, but then, running outside of the building, I realized for the first time the full impact of the situation, as men came from the building wounded and bleeding. My first concern was for the other Navy nurses still in the building and when I found them to be all right, we all decided we had much work to do—and so went the remainder of the evening.

"One thing that I remember so clearly was the great feeling of relief and comfort at the sight of our U.S. Navy ambulance driving up and our corpsmen running to the scene. We knew that help was at hand and we could leave for the hospital to do our part.

"We were so grateful not to be seriously injured that it was difficult to accept the Purple Heart and recognition from only doing the job for which we were professionally trained."[50]

(In a letter to the author, dated 29 August 1995, Captain Ruth Mason Wilson reiterates what she said in her letter of 1965. It is the same statement that Navy nurses have been making since 1908. She says, "I always felt that I only did what any other [Nurse Corps] officer in the same position would have done. In time of war one does what is expected of them at that time and moment and goes on from there." To you who read this, if you are looking for heroes, male or female, here they are; in the Nurse Corps.)

All four of the wounded Navy nurses are offered the opportunity to leave Saigon and return to less hazardous duty. All four refuse the offer and remain until their regular duty rotation occurs.

Navy Nurse Darby Reynolds tells us more, "At the end of January towards the close of my tour in Vietnam, the fighting had increased. There were only two hospitals really in country at that time. Saigon was the

Navy hospital . . . [and there] was the Army hospital . . . about 200 miles north. When the casualties increased - they had mass casualties up there - they requested assistance from the Navy. So Fran Crumpton and myself and a couple of the Navy corpsmen were put on a plane and sent up there. When we arrived, it was night time. This was in January of 1965 after Fran had come back from the Philippines. Our injuries were doing well and we were off at that particular time [and] we were the first available.

"When we arrived at the air strip [where the Army hospital is located], the base was in a complete blackout and the only way you could get from the strip back to the hospital was to wait for the flares to go up. We had fatigues on at this time and I remember when we got off the plane, they asked us if we wanted a `45.' Fran and I looked at each other and said, `A 45 what? What are we going to do with that?' We weren't into handling weapons at that point so we said no. They proceeded to lead us off the strip back to the hospital compound. There were trenches all along the area. I felt myself slipping into one of the trenches and somebody . . . grabbed my shoulder and pulled me back up. We continued on and got to the hospital. It was set up in Quonset huts. They were so busy that some of those patients hadn't received antibiotics for over 12 hours. So Fran and I split up; she took one ward and I took another . . . and started giving them all their antibiotics. One thing that really made an impression on my mind at this particular time was that the Army corpsmen, or medics [as they are called], were not giving out injections. [The Army does not teach them to do this.] They didn't know how to do that. Of course, our Navy corpsmen were so surprised . . . The reason they [the patients] didn't have their antibiotics was the nurse was too busy in the OR and didn't have time. So this is when we went to work. They [the medics] had instructions right off on how to give injections. We just had too many of them [injections]. There was no way you could give them all. So one of the things that really set in all our minds was how much we depended on our Navy corpsmen. I'll always remember them and how much they could do. They were life savers. [There is a very special bond between Navy corpsmen and Navy nurses.] . . .

"We stayed up there for three or four days. We tried to sleep during the day, but again, the shelling was going on and your nerves were almost shot, I guess, at this particular point. The fighting . . . increased down in the southern part [of Vietnam] towards Saigon, so we were requested to head back. We hopped on the plane again and went back down into Saigon."[51] Shortly thereafter these nurses received their orders and returned to the States for their next duty station.

Early in 1965, the Director of the Nurse Corps, Captain Erickson, is notified that two surgical Navy nurses are needed for loan to the State Department and will be going on a surgical team to Vietnam. She alerts her staff in the Nursing Division of BuMed and soon two nurses are selected. They are given orders to come to Washington, D.C. for a briefing of about two weeks. In February of 1965, the two Navy nurses are loaned and assigned to the State Department for duty as nurse advisors in Vietnam. They are Bernadette A. McKay and Ruth M. Pojecky. Both are surgical nurses. Navy Nurse Bernadette McKay says, "the Navy and the State Department had agreed that the Navy would send one surgical team to Vietnam to work in Vietnamese provincial hospitals as part of the USOM program, United States Operation Mission, which is now called US AID [Agency for International Development]. We went there in 1965, and we went in civilian clothes and we went reporting to the State Department and not to the organized United States Military . . . my line of control was directly to the State Department. . . . We got our supplies from anywhere we could get them but, we had a unique opportunity because we knew the Navy system. If we couldn't get it through the State Department or USOM system, then we always relied on the Navy, because they were family and that's the way they treated us; the Navy treated us as family although we did not, at that point, work in family business, if you will. . . . We were in the Mekong Delta in Rach Gia. [Rach Gia is located about 200 miles west-southwest of Saigon.]"[52] They are to advise the Vietnamese on surgical nursing and operating room nursing "while assisting with the Health care of Vietnamese villagers."[53]

Navy Nurse Ruth Pojecky tells us, "[it] was a most peculiar assignment. Number one, we had to . . . not resign from the Navy, but all of our records up in Washington, our pay records, our health records . . . nothing was in our possession and nothing was in the Navy's possession over in Saigon. All we had was our little I D cards [military Identification cards] and they almost didn't give that to us. Well, . . . when we did arrive in Saigon if we hadn't had that little I D card, we never would have gotten any food because the State Department wasn't prepared for us and you had to have a certain amount of money [Vietnamese money] when you got there; we had none. . . . So we went to the naval hospital in Saigon and luckily we could show our I D cards to get in and get something to eat."[54]

Miss Pojecky tells us that the surgical team consists of two doctors, the two nurses, one corpsman (who was also a lab tech and an X-ray tech), a male Air Force nurse who was the anesthetist, and the seventh member is an Army "logistics man. . . . On our first day of arrival [in Rach Gia], dignitaries met us [and with] two or three riding down the road - red lights flashing - sirens going - people on the roads couldn't imagine what was happening. . . . The policemen wear white outfits down there [in Rach Gia] and this one guy was standing up in the jeep and he's waving his arms, 'Get off the road! Get off the road! The American team is coming.' They were so happy to see us. Then when we got into town, we were like a parade. People lined on the sides of the streets . . . waving at us. . . . So we had a big luncheon, we had a tour of the hospital and . . . then we were on the welcoming stand. . . . They [had] built it out in front of the hospital. And, we had to sit up there."[55] The hospital is one of about 500 beds. "An all Vietnamese hospital. We had two American patients while we were there. . . . We were treating all Vietnamese patients. And, we had one interpreter for [the] seven of us. . . . [There was] one lady also, who helped us out with a few words of English and so she would stay with one of us for the day."[56] But they soon learned to devise different ways of communicating. For instance, Miss Pojecky says, "We had one autoclave there that we couldn't figure out how to run . . . it was a Japanese autoclave. So . . . I wrote to the company [there was a tag on the autoclave with that information] and asked if they could please send some instructions in English . . . and, by golly, they sent pictures back and they sent a big translation back. . . . How we accomplished our communication with the people we had to work with, we typed up questions in English and then we had our translator put the Vietnamese right next to it, so that whether we were on the ward or whether we were in the emergency room, we could go and point to this question and then they could give us an answer [by pointing to] . . . the paper [with] our translation right next to it. . . .

"Almost all of the stuff we had, we had to jury-rig. We had traction for our [orthopedic] patients but all we had to start with was nylon cord. So, we had to use a bicycle [tire] innertube cut on the bias instead of mole skin [special twill-like material], you know how you taped it on the legs. Then we had to wrap that with ace bandages. Then for the pulley - we walked around the town and we saw some guy whittling."[57] They got hold of a book with a picture of a pulley and the man made pulleys for them. After that they had bags sewn to hold sand and these then became the needed weights for the traction and pulleys. Navy nurses are very, very versatile and innovative, especially when it comes to patient needs.

These two nurses spend one year at this duty. This is a normal tour of duty in Vietnam. They are in harm's way but they perform their duties well and come home safely, leaving the State Department assignment to return to the Navy Nurse Corps. (A total of "seven Navy nurses [are] assigned to AID between 1965 and September 1967."[58])

Meanwhile, Navy nurse Iris Stock is still aboard the MST ship, the *General Mann*. She informs us that, "Approximately the second week of February, 1965, we started on what seemingly was a routine trip. However, on reporting aboard for this trip, I noted that the gold ring normally on the stack of the ship had been painted over with gray paint and we no longer had the MST colors. This might not seem significant to many, but when a ship has become your home, you note any changes in a hurry. We were scheduled to sail to Hawaii, Okinawa, and then Taiwan. Shipboard life assumed its usual normal routine as we made our way across the Pacific, delivering passengers, picking up more, and continuing on our ports of call. The only thing really unusual was that from Okinawa to Taiwan, we picked-up no passengers for ports beyond Taiwan. . . .

"We arrived in Taiwan on February 27th, and found, to our consternation, that all liberties had been canceled and we would be allowed on the pier only. Our next information jolted us when, with the Dental officer, we met a friend of his stationed in Taiwan. His first words after they had greeted each other, were, 'Hey, I understand you guys are going to Vietnam.' None of us knew about this, as only the officers on a need-to-know basis had been informed. We stayed only four hours in Taiwan, no passengers were boarded, and all other passengers had been disembarked. We put to sea with only the ship's company. At 1400 hours, a meeting of the ship's company was held by the Commanding Officer who informed us of what was in store for the *Mann*. We would first sail into Sasebo, Japan, spending a week as the Korean troops we were to take to Vietnam were not quite ready to leave [over in Korea]. We would then sail to Inchon, Korea, pick-up the troops and sail for Vietnam.

"On the trip to Sasebo, the medical department was busy checking the crew's shot records, and then in addition to our usual immunization routine, we had to give everyone aboard immunization for the `plague.' . . . We had a good week in Japan, and then sailed for Inchon arriving one afternoon. Because of the tide we . . . anchored about a mile out. . . . Loading was started early the next morning, and late in the afternoon the troops came aboard, all with flowered leis about their necks. One young man was boarded with a massive second degree burn from having been scalded in some way with boiling water. We immediately hospitalized him on the ward and started treating his burns. Ordinarily, a person injured this seriously, in our armed forces, would have been immediately hospitalized . . . but the South Koreans apparently had felt his condition did not warrant medical attention. We were underway early the next day after a somewhat harrowing night. We had had reports that unfriendly agents had been seen swimming under the ship planting mines. An underwater demolition team, with numerous divers, was busy throughout our stay examining the hull of the *Mann*, searching for detonating devices. We were all relieved to be at sea again without incident. . . .

"On March 15, 1965, we arrived off the coast of Vietnam. . . . We arrived at 0600 in the morning. Everything was deadly quiet and the people who were expected to meet us were not in sight. It was an uneasy silence as even the ship's engines were still. Finally, around 0800 a small boat came out to the ship and activities were initiated to start landing our troops. The personnel aboard ship had been astir for hours. The troops were all on the deck in full battle dress, plus their weapons which were fully armed; empty ammunition boxes littered the deck. . . . A large barge with a flat platform atop had been anchored alongside the ship. The troops were going over the side on landing nets. Prior to the first troops disembarking, a flurry of activity suddenly started. We heard a helicopter gun-ship circling the ship and it appeared to be trying to land on the barge. Several attempts were made to land the helicopter, but without success. We found out that . . . South Korea's President was aboard and that he was trying to land and welcome his troops to Vietnam. This was the first time in over four hundred years that South Korean troops had been out of their country to fight. . . . Our Korean burn patient went ashore in full battle dress with his unit despite our Medical officer's objections. The man had a raging fever while he had been hospitalized and really required further treatment, but the Koreans were adamant about his accompanying his unit, so he went ashore. We had filled him with antibiotics, but his burns were such that I cannot think he would have survived long. . . .

"Following our departure from Vietnam, the Executive Officer had decided a cook-out for the ship's company would be a welcome interlude before we started our usual routine. . . . It was a fun evening everyone seemed to enjoy. As darkness fell, no one seemed to want to end the evening, and I remember we sat on deck watching a violent electrical storm in the distance, and enjoying the balmy night air. We all had another reason to stay up; about 2200 a small boat met us and we received our mail! . . . [Then] on home to Oakland. We had been cautioned that our whereabouts were to be kept secret, so we could not tell where we had been. The Golden Gate never looked so good as we sailed under her. We had been gone almost two months and everyone was eager to get home. Ironically, on my return call to my parents, my mother said, `Oh, by the way, Aunt Martha saw your ship on the evening news unloading troops in Vietnam.' So much for secrecy.

"We continued to make trips to South Vietnam with Army and Marine troops. . . . We made a total of four trips. On one trip we had a large Army Medical Unit of doctors, nurses and corpsmen. . . . On our arrival in Vietnam, we disembarked troops and portions of the medics at three different ports. My most vivid memory was of the apparent quietness of the shore and the vivid colors. . . . [Then] at our second stop . . . I looked over the side and saw a lonely female going ashore. She was a nurse anesthetist and was the only woman to go ashore at that stop. I cried inside for her, thinking of how I would have felt in that similar situation.

"I think, on our last trip to Vietnam, we took Marine units, and I remember, as we off loaded the last group that one day, that the ship's company, as usual, stood to and gave the last boat load going ashore, a farewell salute. They always did this, but as the boat pulled away . . . a lump came into my throat, wondering how many of these young men would ever see their country again, and in what condition they would be when and if they saw it again.

"We did, at times, see un-friendlies going up the hill sides when we were anchored off shore. We were always anchored far enough off shore that we did not have to be concerned too much about unfriendly fire.

"It was, at last, with relief that we finally heard that the ship [the *Mann*] was to be placed in mothballs. They were going to stop moving troops by ship and start flying them in. I was glad to call my [tour] over when I left the ship in late October. I had enjoyed my tour of duty, but the last few trips had not been good, having to leave Americans at war on a foreign shore."[59]

Navy Nurse Ruth Halverson is also aboard an MSTS ship that is diverted to carrying troops to Vietnam. She says, "we would pick up Marines and the SeaBee's from [the States] . . . and we would take them to Okinawa or to Vietnam. We took them to DaNang to build a hospital, we took the SeaBee's to Cam Ranh Bay to build the air strip and then we took a lot of troops generally to the fighting areas. . . . I think one of the hardest things was when we went into the mouth of the Saigon, in 1965 when the war escalated, and we took about 3,000 Marines in there and the monsoon was on. If you have ever been in a monsoon, you know what I'm saying. Anyhow, it was raining very heavily and we had to wait to get into the area to let the troops off. When we finally were permitted to move, we went in there under cover of night and destroyers on all sides of us. We sat there for about three hours, blacked out, with no radio communication. All of a sudden we heard this chopper hover over and flood lights flashing all over the ship . . . and over this microphone comes this big manly voice saying, 'you SOB's, if you don't identify yourself we're going to put a shell through your hull or your deck.!' . . . Finally, the lights went on. Our CO [Commanding Officer] had been told not to use any type of communication [but] he broke radio communication and the chopper went off. What they were doing was trying to identify us. We were just sitting there. The next day these young men [the troops] were permitted to go off the ship and I remember standing at the gangplank watching them. You could hardly see the gangplank it was raining so hard, and these young men were given their fighting pack and their rifle as they left and went down into the [boats] which were taking them right into the fighting that you could see about a mile or two up the river. . . . These young men would pick up their pack and their rifle and as they went down the ladder they handed in their next-of-kin cards to the company commander. It was raining and you knew that they were going to go off right into that fighting and some of them would never come back. I remember standing there and I had tears going down my face. I could see even the doctors had tears in their eyes. . . . We sat there for about a day or two and all during this period that we were there, night and day, every half hour the frogmen or UBT men would come and drop hand grenades all around the ship so that the Viet Cong couldn't come and put grenades under the ship."[60]

Navy Nurse Patricia J. Moris is also on an MSTS ship in 1965. She has just finished her tour of duty at Guam and is on orders to her next duty station. She says, "When I came back from Guam in 1965 . . . the ship was filled with dependents, wives and children, of the crew of two [Navy] ships that had been overseas for several years and [the ships] were being returned to the United States to be decommissioned because they were so old. As we steamed towards Hawaii, the [two old] ships passed us, but two days later we looked out and we saw both [of those] ships now headed in the opposite direction; towards the . . . [far east]. About a day out of Hawaii, it was announced to all the passengers on the [MSTS] ship that because of conditions in Vietnam, the orders to decommission the two Navy ships had been canceled and they were now headed back towards the Gulf of Tonkin [just off the coast of North Vietnam]. They then announced that those dependents on the ship who had planned to accompany their active duty members all the way to the United States, had the option of getting off in Hawaii, if they wanted, to await the outcome of whatever would happen in Vietnam. So, I knew then that there was a large build-up and that we needed to prepare for something more than just a little skirmish in Vietnam. I was very surprised to find out, when I got to the United States, nobody over here seemed to realize anything about that. There was no talk of any build-up, even among military personnel.

When I reported into St. Albans [Naval Hospital] and started questioning why the hospital wasn't making any preparations for an increased work-load, people acted as though I was just crazy. Several months later things got much busier, and in a period of what seemed to be just weeks, at the St. Albans Naval Hospital, our in-patient work-load increased from 400 to 800 in-patients. I was put in charge of Central Supply at the time, and the next year, for me, was one of the most harrowing years in my life. . . . At the time, we were trying to run the Vietnam War, and at the same time convince taxpayers that we had plenty of money for `guns and butter,' so the decision of the administration was that the hospital at St. Albans would have to get by on the same budget that we had the previous year for our 400 patients. Yet, most of our new patients were Vietnam casualties with horrible wounds. There I was in CSR [Central Supply Room] having to provide IV [intravenous] fluids, and the dressings, and suture sets, needles, and expected to do it out of my previous year's budget. I had to engage in incredible wheeling and dealing. For example, we had a number of [Navy] ships that would come into the New York area with corpsmen who had come to visit me to see if they could get supplies. They could not order open purchase supplies like disposable needles, which they desperately needed. I could order open purchase supplies, but I couldn't order anything expensive like the instruments that I needed. So, I would trade a corpsman fifty cents worth of disposable needles for one hundred dollars worth of instruments. . . .

"I was running CSR with four corpsmen, but I had 14 [convalescing] patients that we literally worked full-time; seven from the Orthopedic wards and seven from the Psychiatric wards. We would, the corpsmen and I, work from 6:00 a.m. until 9:00 p.m., six days a week. Sunday I would use to sleep and do my laundry and wash my hair, and we could just barely keep up with the work. . . . We had horrible casualties, so I worked-up a practice that whenever a patient was admitted, who would require extensive dressing changes, I would go up [to the ward] and the charge nurse and I would assess the patient's needs and what we would put into a dressing pack [just for that patient], and from then on the corpsmen and I would put up individualized dressing packs for these patients, and that worked very well. But, I reached a point where I felt like if I had to look at just one more horribly mangled casualty, I would start to scream and would never be able to stop. [You truly get that way when you see so many of the dreadfully appalling results of war. You wonder how the human body can sustain itself with such intolerable damage.] Fortunately, several days went by before the next casualty came in and by then my psyche had regrouped and I was able to continue to do what was necessary. I remember one evening, it was about 8:00 in the evening, a corpsman and I had been there all day, we were just exhausted, and I got a call from an angry doctor because we had run out of sutures, and I can still remember him telling me, `You know, there's a war going on and some of us are going to have to work a little bit longer than usual.' Again, I thought I would scream into the phone but I just said, `Yes, I know, I've been here since 6:00 this morning.' He said, `Oh.'

"One of the things that kept us going, the nurses and the corpsmen, was that we got tremendous support from our Commanding Officer . . . and our Executive Officer. . . . I don't think a week went by but what one or the other, or both, would come down to CSR, talk to the corpsmen and I about how things were going, and how proud they were of the work we were doing. Also, we got tremendous support from our Chief Nurse, Captain [Alice R.] Reilly. Captain Reilly was not the easiest Chief Nurse to work for, she expected a lot of her staff, she was known to be very demanding, but I thought the world of her because she was so good about backing-up her staff. I remember one time when the Chief of the Dental service went to Captain Reilly to complain because he had gotten some gloves from CSR [no disposable gloves at this time] and they were sticky, and before he could even finish his sentence, Captain Reilly said, `What? Do you mean to tell me that CSR is having to do gloves for you? CSR is there to take care of the wards, not the Dental service. You should be doing your own gloves!' Well, the poor man slunk out of her office and ended up coming and having to beg me to keep doing gloves for the Dental service. It was that kind of support that made a big difference."[61]

Meanwhile, the Nurse Corps is feeling the pressures of the country-wide shortage of nurses and with the increasing demands of Vietnam, it is decided that the length of the indoctrination course at Newport, Rhode Island should be shortened. In January, the U.S. Naval Women Officer School shortens the course to a four week program. In March, the Naval Medical Research Institute establishes "a Nursing Research Division of the

Department of Behavioral Sciences, Naval Medical Research Institute, Bethesda, Maryland."[62]

By the end of the fiscal year, July, the strength of the Nurse Corps is only 1870 so it is beneficial that on the 25th of August 1965, the Navy Nurse Corps at long last commissions the first male nurse. His name is George M. Silver and he is commissioned as Ensign. In October, he and four other commissioned male Nurse Corps officers report "to the Naval Schools Command [at] Newport, Rhode Island for a one month course of indoctrination to the Naval service."[63] The other four are "Lt(jg) Jerry McClelland, Ensign Charles Franklin, Ensign Israle Miller, and Ensign Richard Gierman."[64] In September, a tropical white uniform with long trousers was authorized for the male Nurse Corps officers. The rest of their uniform wardrobe is that authorized for all male Naval officers.

Speaking of uniforms, a review of all the female Navy Nurse Corps' uniforms of this period, seems appropriate here. The service dress blue and the service dress white uniform is a two-piece suit which features four gold buttons with the bald eagle design on them. The number and size of the gold-braid stripes on the sleeves of the jacket, tell the rank of the wearer, and the gold oak leaf above the strips indicates the Navy Nurse Corps. Since 1830 the oak leaf has been a symbol of the mighty oak ships of the U.S. Navy and denotes 'strength.' For the Nurse Corps, the insignia denotes strength in the healing arts. A short sleeved white blouse with a black tie is used with the service dress uniform. The black tie is a copy of the British sailor's neckerchief which was called a 'sweat rag' because the black color would hide dirt and sweat. The British sailors wore their 'sweat rag' both around the forehead and the neck. Some sailors used it to protect their jackets from the oil used in dressing their pigtails.

The combination hat or so called 'bucket hat' has separate covers; white, navy blue, or dacron light blue, for wearing with the service dress blue or white uniforms and with the light blue summer uniform. The 'bucket hat' has a navy blue brim rolled at the sides and two navy blue streamers attached to the back of the navy blue hatband. This hat is copied from the eighteenth century fore-and-aft cocked hat that Napoleon wore 'athwartships.' The insignia on the bucket hat is taken from the official seal of the U.S. government with an eagle, representing the Navy, and a shield with 13 stars representing the original 13 colonies.

The light blue summer uniform is a dacron cotton suit with short sleeves. The rank insignia is worn on the right lapel and the corps insignia is on the left lapel. Then there is the indoor white ward uniform made of polyester dacron with optional long or short sleeves, and a matching wide, white belt of the same material. All buttons are pearl buttons. The rank and corps insignias are worn on the appropriate lapels. With this uniform is the traditional nurses' cap with the gold stripes, denoting rank, on a black velvet ribbon across the permanently starched white cap. (Male Nurse Corps officers do not wear a cap with their male ward whites.)

On the 1st of January, 1965, all Navy nurses above the rank of Lieutenant were required to have the dinner dress uniform in both blue and white. It is worn for 'black-tie' occasions. The waistcoat length jacket has full length sleeves banded in velvet. The pleated ruffles of the round collared white blouse shows between the softly rolled jacket lapels. Three small gold 'eagle' buttons appear in a row on each front of the jacket. Collar devices are embroidered of gold and white silk and are placed on either side of the blouse's collar. A small, attached, black tie shows between the front edges of the blouse collar. The street length skirt is accentuated with an appropriate silk faille cummerbund. Matching shoes and handbag and white gloves are worn. A black velvet tiara embellished with the gold eagle device and rank adornment is worn with this uniform.[65]

To turn now to what is happening in space in 1965; the world and the space program sees a Russian cosmonaut become the first man to step into space. On 18 March 1965, he drifts from his spacecraft, with another cosmonaut aboard, and moves about for ten minutes by pulling on the line connecting him to his ship. In June the U.S. sends a spacecraft up with two astronauts aboard. On 3 June 1965, astronaut Edward White takes a twenty minute space walk. He moves about by firing oxygen from a rocket gun.[66]

1965 is the year Congress passes the Medicare legislation "and three bills to fund the war on poverty."[67] And, on the 6th of August, President Johnson signs "into law the historic Voting Rights Act of 1965, one of it provisions outlawing poll taxes. Five days later a race riot, triggered by a drunk-driving incident, exploded in the

Watts section of Los Angeles. Crowds chanting `Burn, baby, burn!' fire-bombed buildings and overturned cars; thirty-five persons were killed. `We were beset by contradictions-movement and progress alongside stalemate and retrogression,' reflected [President] Johnson. `Nowhere were these contradictions experienced more deeply than in the black community, where hopes aroused by the early victories were bright, but hostilities caused by the persistent gap between promises and fulfillment were deep.'"[68]

Outside the U.S. are further problems. In April and May, President Johnson sent military troops down into the Dominican Republic "to protect about 3,000 U.S. citizens there."[69] Rebel fighting had broken out. "He later sent in more troops to prevent communist rebels from taking over the Dominican government."[70]

Now, back to the Vietnam situation. "In July the President announced an increase in draft quotas along with the addition of 50,000 troops to bring strength in Vietnam to 125,000. Further additions brought the total to 200,000 by the end of 1965. . . . Belligerency was now a fact. United States soldiers were killing and being killed, United States pilots were diving through anti-aircraft fire and, when crashing, were being captured to become prisoners of war."[71] But, there is dissension. "A National Coordinating Committee to End the War in Vietnam was formed, which organized protest rallies and assembled a crowd of 40,000 to mount a picket line around the White House. Draft-card-burning spread. . . . In horrible emulation of the Buddhist monks, a Quaker of Baltimore burned himself alive on the Pentagon steps on 2 November 1965, followed by a second such suicide in front of the UN a week later. . . .

"While bombing [in Vietnam] resumed and the war grew harsher, the search for settlement continued. Talks in Warsaw with Polish intermediaries in mid-1966 seemed to be making progress until, at a delicate point, American air strikes, directed for the first time at targets in and around Hanoi, caused North Vietnam to cancel the contacts. . . . [Meantime] Progressive escalation bringing troop strength to 245,000 in April 1966 required a request to Congress for $12 billion in supplemental war costs. . . . Through the draft, required by repeated escalations [of troops], the war was now affecting the general public directly. In mid-1966, the Pentagon announced that the troop level in Vietnam would reach 375,000 by the end of the year."[72] This war is becoming extremely expensive, not only in American monies but in American casualties and lives.

To return to Nurse Corps matters, over in Vietnam itself, the U.S. Navy Station Hospital in Saigon is transferred to the U.S. Army in March of 1966. All Navy Nurse Corps officers from there are transferred to other assignments. A total of twenty Navy nurses served there between 1965 and 1966.[73]

Back in the States, Commander Alene B. Duerk NC USN, is the Senior Nurse at the Hospital Corps School at San Diego, California. The time is early spring in 1966. She tells us, "I was at Hospital Corps School and I got this phone call from Captain Erickson [Director of the Nurse Corps] and she asked me to please come to the Bureau [Bureau of Medicine and Surgery in Washington, D.C.]. They had a job they felt I might be able to do. She didn't tell me what it was. I was to get there in the next 24 hours. I had to drop everything and leave. I get to Washington and I'm told that they are looking for someone to represent the three military services [Army, Navy, and Air Force Nurse Corps] in the Department of Defense . . . [at the Pentagon and in the office of] the Assistant Secretary of Defense for Health and Environment. . . . I was to go, I thought, for an interview. I figured they had ten other people lined up.

"Anyhow, I get ready to go over there and Captain Erickson went with me. [We] arrive and there is the President of the ANA [American Nurses Association], and President of the NLN [National League of Nursing], and all the Directors and Chiefs of the Army Nurse Corps, the Air Force, and Captain Erickson and myself - not another soul. They're all talking about this need to have a nurse who represents military nursing in this department. Well, they didn't ask me a question. They didn't ask me what I did or what I thought. I didn't even know what they were talking about. So that afternoon, Captain Erickson told me to go back to my hotel, and I did. She called me and told me that I would be assigned to that job and that I had two weeks to go back and close up my stuff and report back to Washington. . . . I came back and I was assigned to the Department of Defense to the office of . . . [the Assistant Secretary of Defense for Health and Environment]. I arrived and they handed me this pile of information; it was letters and all this sort of thing about so and so being some place in Vietnam and they were doing this kind of a job and why were they there. There were letters about getting more nurses. This was the thing. All three military services [Army, Navy, Air Force] had problems recruiting nurses. The big thing was, they needed someone in the Department of Defense to keep [the Assistant for Health and Environment] up to date on how the recruiting was going and what they [the military services] were doing and what kind of programs they had.

"They finally found an office for me and a desk and I developed a job. But, to begin with I had to develop some kind of goals of what I was going to do. . . . Without very many guidelines it wasn't the easiest thing in the world to do. . . . But, it started out purely because of the lack of nurses in the three military services. That was the reason they put me over there. . . . [It was during this] time that [the Assistant Secretary for Health and Environment] wanted us to take the Associate Degree nurses into all military services because that was going to answer [supposedly] all our questions [and] take care of all our problems. . . . The Army and the Air Force did take the Associate Degree [people]; the Navy did not. . . . [The Assistant Secretary] said to me one time, `You will take the Associate Degree.' And I said to him, `Over my dead body.'"[74] And the Navy Nurse Corps never did take them in but the Army did and ran into many, many problems. The Associate Degree nurses are graduates of a two year nursing program at community colleges. Students are given an associate degree upon satisfactory completion of the course and are then able to take the State Board Examination for Registered Nurse. The problem is that they do not have practical experience as in the case of the three-year diploma graduate nurses and, of course, they have no where near the academics or practice of the baccalaureate nurses. In addition, during this period of time, three year schools of nursing are becoming less and less in number because the nursing profession is striving toward the collegiate level of education for graduate, registered nurses. The Navy Nurse Corps is also striving for an all-degreed Corps and foresees the problems that accepting the Associate Degree nurses would present, especially so since the idea is to have these nurses enter the military as Warrant Officers. And, since the Navy nurse's primary mission includes the special teaching of the Corpsmen, education is of particular importance. Commander Duerk responds to the Assistant Secretary in the only way a knowledgeable Navy nurse, and future Director, can. (This billet that Commander Duerk fills becomes a permanent and valuable asset to the three Nurse Corps. The billet becomes a one year term of duty and is alternated between the Army, Navy and Air Force in the coming years.)

As a possible source of nurses and because male nurses are now permitted in the Nurse Corps, the "Bureau of Medicine and Surgery requested a special Selective Service call for 200 professional nurses to report for active naval service."[75] This takes place in January 1966. (The Selective Service or 'Draft' pertains only to the male population.) The call was placed for 200 and we only obtained 31.[76] This was not a viable source for the Nurse Corps needs.

On 1 May 1966, Captain Ruth A. Erickson, Director of the Navy Nurse Corps, retires from active duty. During her career she "was awarded the Navy Unit Commendation, American Defense Service Medal with one star, the Navy Occupation Service Medal, the National Defense Service Medal, and the Asiatic-Pacific Medal."[77] Captain Erickson now resides in Rochester, Minnesota.

1   Erickson, Ruth A. Captain, Director Navy Nurse Corps, *Oral History Interview Tape Transcript*, Interviewer LCdr Alice Lech Laning Nurse Corps, 7 January 1990.

2   Ibid..

3   Information prepared by the Navy Nurse Corps Officers on the staff of the Director of the Navy Nurse Corps, circa 1990.

4   Updated *History of the Nurse Corps, U.S. Navy*, by the Navy Nurse Corps Officers on the staff of the Director of the Navy Nurse Corps, 5727.1, OONCA/np, revised 24 April 1991, p. 17.

5   Ibid..

6   Howard, Katherine A. Captain, Navy Nurse Corps, *Oral History Interview Tape Transcript*, Interviewer Captain Doris M. Sterner Nurse Corps, 19 February 1991.

7   Fritz, Barbara Ann LCdr Navy Nurse Corps, et al, editors, "History of the Nurse Corps, U.S. Navy," *75th Anniversary Nurse Corps Cookbook*, G&R Publishing Company, P.O. Box 238, Waverly, Ohio 50677, 1983.

8   Eberhardt, Marie CDR Navy Nurse Corps, *Oral History Interview Tape Transcript*, Self interview, 19 May 1990.

9   Gendron, Marie T. CDR, Navy Nurse Corps, *Oral History Interview Tape Transcript*, Interviewer CDR Lucy Ann Job Nurse Corps, 19 February 1991.

10   *The World Book Encyclopedia*, Field Enterprises Educational Corporation, Chicago, Volume 17, 1966 edition, p. 572f.

[11]   Pack, VaLaine CDR Navy Nurse Corps, *Oral History Interview Tape Transcript*, Self interview, 2 April 1990.

[12]   Martin, Kathleen LCdr, Navy Nurse Corps, *Oral History Interview Tape Transcript*, Interviewer LT Helen Barry Siragusa Nurse Corps, 26 March 1991.

[13]   Laird, LCDR Thelma NC USNR, Jones, LCDR Dorothy NC USN, Feeney, LCDR Elizabeth NC USN, Seidl, CDR Elizabeth NC USN (Ret.), Blaska, CDR Burdette NC USN, *Chronological History NAVY NURSE CORPS*, Prepared by: Nursing Division, Bureau of Medicine and Surgery, 1 August 1962, p. 47.

[14]   Covington, Margaret L. CDR Navy Nurse Corps, *Oral History Interview Tape Transcript*, Self interview, 30 July 1990.

[15]   Updated *History of the Nurse Corps, U.S. Navy*, op. cit., p. 17.

[16]   Root, Dorothy Eaton CDR Navy Nurse Corps, *Oral History Interview Tape Transcript*, Self interview, 1 January 1990.

[17]   Tuchman, Barbara W., *The March of Folly From Troy to Vietnam*, Ballantine Books, New York, 1985, pp. 299-310.

[18]   Twyman, Florence Alwyn CDR, Navy Nurse Corps, *Oral History Interview Tape Transcript*, Interviewer LCdr Dorothea Short Tracy Nurse Corps, 26 March 1991.

[19]   Barcott, Jan LCdr, Navy Nurse Corps, *Oral History Interview Tape Transcript*, Interviewer LCdr Linn Larson Nurse Corps, 1 April 1990.

[20]   Hovis, Bobbi LCdr Navy Nurse Corps (Ret.), *Station Hospital Saigon: A Navy Nurse in Vietnam, 1963-1964*, United States Naval Institute, Annapolis, Maryland, 1991, pp. 26-28.

[21]   Barcott, Jan LCdr, Navy Nurse Corps, op. cit.. Also, written material courtesy of LCdr. Jan Barcott.

[22]   O'Dell, Beverly Brase Captain Navy Nurse Corps, *Oral History Interview Tape Transcript*, Self interview, 22 May 1991.

[23]   Updated *History of the Nurse Corps, U.S. Navy*, op. cit..

[24]   *The World Book Encyclopedia*, op. cit., Vol. 11, p. 212h.

[25]   Ibid., p. 212g.

[26]   Wheeler, Marion Caesar CDR, Navy Nurse Corps, *Oral History Interview Tape Transcript*, Interviewer CDR Anna Corcoran Nurse Corps, 18 July 1991.

[27]   Copeland, Winifred L. Captain Navy Nurse Corps, *Oral History Interview Tape Transcript*, Self interview, 22 May 1991.

[28]   Pack, VaLaine CDR Navy Nurse Corps, op. cit..

[29]   Martin, Kathleen LCdr, Navy Nurse Corps, op. cit..

[30]   Hovis, Bobbi LCdr Navy Nurse Corps (Ret.), op. cit., p. 93.

[31]   *200 Years, A Bicentennial Illustrated History of the United States*, Joseph Newman, Directing Editor, Books by U.S. News & World Report, Inc., 2300 N Street, N.W., Washington, D.C. 20037, 1973, book, book 2, p. 344.

[32]   *The World Book Encyclopedia*, op. cit., Vol. 11, p. 120e.

[33]   Ibid., pp. 120g, 120h.

[34]   Ibid., Vol. 17, p. 572f.

[35]   Floyd, Candace, *America's Great Disasters*, Mallard Press, an imprint of BDD Promotional Books Company, Inc., 666 Fifth Avenue, New York, N.Y. 10103, p. 124.

[36]   Ibid..

[37]   Ibid. p. 126.

[38]   Updated *History of the Nurse Corps, U.S. Navy*, op. cit., p. 18.

[39]   Stock, Iris M. LCdr Navy Nurse Corps, *Oral History Interview Tape Transcript*, Self interview, 25 June 1990.

[40]   *200 Years, A Bicentennial Illustrated History of the United States*, op. cit., p. 269.

[41]   *The World Book Encyclopedia*, op. cit., Vol. 11, p. 120g.

[42]   Hovis, Bobbi LCdr Navy Nurse Corps (Ret.), op. cit., pp. 149, 150.

[43]   Ibid., p. 153.

[44]   Captain Ruth Mason Wilson Navy Nurse Corps supplied this information via telephone conversation with author on 5 September 1995.

[45]   Reynolds, A. Darby Captain, Navy Nurse Corps, *Oral History Interview Tape Transcript*, Interviewer CDR Patricia A. Warner Nurse Corps, 13 April 1990.

[46]   Ibid..

[47]   Ibid..

[48]   Ibid..

[49]   Erickson, Ruth A. Captain, Director of the Navy Nurse Corps, *Letter to LT Ruth A. Mason, NC, USN*, Bureau of Medicine and Surgery, Department of the Navy, Washington, D.C. 20390, BUMED-32-gd, 11 January 1965.

[50]   Mason, Ruth A. LT Navy Nurse Corps (now Captain Ruth A. Mason Wilson NC USN Retired), *Letter to Captain Ruth A. Erickson Director of the Navy Nurse Corps*, Station Hospital, Saigon, 29 January 1965.

[51]   Reynolds, A. Darby Captain, Navy Nurse Corps, op. cit..

[52]   McKay, Bernadette A. Captain, Navy Nurse Corps, *Oral History Interview Tape Transcript*, Interviewer Captain Bettye G. Nagy Nurse Corps, 10 May 1990.

[53]   Chow, Rita K. R.N. Ed.D., Hope, Gloria S. R.N. Ph.D., Nelson, Ethel A. LTC USAF NC, Sokoloski, James L. LTC ANC, Wilson, Ruth A. Captain NC USN Ret., "Historical Perspectives of the United States Air Force, Army, Navy, Public Health Service, and Veterans Administration Nursing Services," *Military Medicine*, Vol. 143, No. 7, July 1978, p. 463.

[54]   Pojecky, Ruth M. Commander, Navy Nurse Corps, *Oral History Interview Tape Transcript*, Interviewer Commander Joan McIntyre Nurse Corps, 10 May 1988.

[55]   Ibid..

[56]   Ibid..

[57]   Ibid..

[58]   Captain Winifred Copeland NC USNR (Ret.) supplied official documents confirming final date.

[59]   Stock, Iris M. LCdr Navy Nurse Corps, op. cit..

[60]   Halverson, Ruth E. Captain, Navy Nurse Corps, *Oral History Interview Tape Transcript*, Interviewer Captain Doris Sterner Nurse Corps, 10

July 1990.

[61] Moris, Patricia Joan Captain, Navy Nurse Corps, *Oral History Interview Tape Transcript*, Interviewer Tonya Emory - Clinical Nurse at the VA Medical Center in Boise, Idaho where Captain Moris was a patient until her untimely death, Interview dated 19 September 1990.

[62] Updated *History of the Nurse Corps, U.S. Navy*, op. cit., p. 19.

[63] Ibid..

[64] Ibid..

[65] From information distributed to Nurse Corps Officers in this period of time.

[66] *The World Book Encyclopedia*, op. cit., Vol. 17, p. 572g.

[67] *200 Years, A Bicentennial Illustrated History of the United States*, op. cit., p. 270.

[68] Ibid., p. 272.

[69] *The World Book Encyclopedia*, op. cit., Vol. 11, p. 120g.

[70] Ibid..

[71] Tuchman, Barbara W., op. cit., p. 325.

[72] Ibid., pp. 325, 331, 332, 339.

[73] *Navy Nurses in Vietnam between 1965 and 1970*, Information from BuMed, 1981, *op. cit.*.

[74] Duerk, Alene B. Rear Admiral, Navy Nurse Corps, *Oral History Interview Tape Transcript*, Interviewers Captain Doris M. Sterner Nurse Corps and Dr. Lynne Dunn of the Naval Historical Center of Washington, D.C., 12 July 1988.

[75] Updated *History of the Nurse Corps, U.S. Navy*, op. cit., p. 19.

[76] Sterner, Doris M. CDR Navy Nurse Corps, *Code 323 Planning*, BUMED-323-jg, 27 March 1969.

[77] Information prepared by the Navy Nurse Corps Officers on the staff of the Director of the Navy Nurse Corps, circa 1990, op. cit..

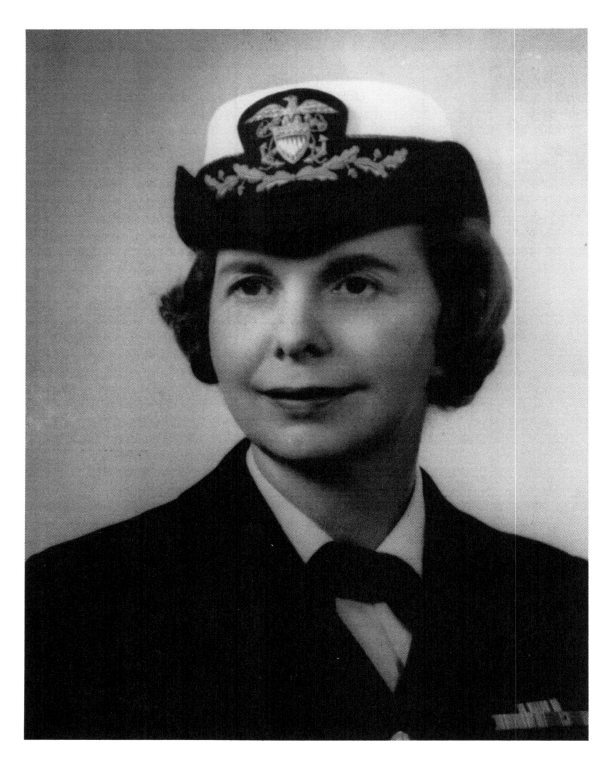

Director - Captain Veronica M. Bulshefski NC USN
(Official U.S. Navy photo courtesy of Nursing Division, Bureau of Medicine and Surgery, Navy Department.)

CHAPTER 12

Director - Captain Veronica M. Bulshefski
(1966 - 1970)

Captain Veronica Bulshefski takes the oath of office for Director of the U.S. Navy Nurse Corps on the 29th of April 1966. The Navy's Surgeon General, Vice Admiral Robert B. Brown, conducts the ceremony and delivers the oath. She begins her four year term in office on 1 May. Captain Bulshefski was the Chief Nurse at the Oakland Naval Hospital in California when she received notice of her selection for Director. "Captain Bulshefski brings to the Directorate a wealth of knowledge and experience in administration of nursing services, personnel management and research techniques. She has also authored and co-authored articles for the professional nursing bulletins."[1]

Veronica Bulshefski was born in Ashley, Pennsylvania on the 2nd of February 1916. She graduated from the University of Pennsylvania Hospital School of Nursing as an R.N.. Her Bachelor's degree in Nursing Education was from the University of Indiana and her Master of Science degree in Management was obtained at the U.S. Naval Postgraduate School at Monterey, California.

"After I completed nursing school, two of my classmates and I found an apartment near the hospital. I had to go find a dentist and I found one in my neighborhood. One day, when I went in to see him, he asked me what I expected to do in my life. That was when so much trouble was brewing in Europe [prior to World War II]. He suggested that I go in the Navy Nurse Corps. I knew nothing about the Navy Nurse Corps. So, a couple of weeks later . . . I had an appointment with him. His office nurse told me he was a patient at the Naval Hospital in Philadelphia and he wanted to see me. So, I went to see him the next day. When I went in there, he was so happy to see me and he called for the nurse to give me the address of the Bureau of Medicine and Surgery to whom I should write. Which I did. It wasn't very long before I was accepted into the Navy. But, unfortunately, the man died and he never knew I was a Navy Nurse. . . . He was in the Navy during WW I as a dentist. . . . He had so much respect and admiration for Navy Nurses that he really wanted me to be in the Navy. . . . I didn't even know there was a Navy Nurse Corps until I met him. . . .

"I had my physical [for the Navy] at the University of Pennsylvania because I was working at that time in research in diabetics at the metabolic unit of the University; the metabolic research unit with a specialist in diabetes and one in renal disease [both Doctors]. . . . I came in the Navy as a regular [v.s. a reserve]. I had to take my oath of office before I came so I had to go to the Justice of the Peace in my little town of Ashley, Pennsylvania. I had to have the oath of office on the day before traveling and I did that on a Sunday morning."[2] She traveled to her first duty station, the Brooklyn Naval Hospital in New York, reporting in on 8 January 1940.

Her promotions in the Navy are: Lieutenant(jg) in March 1943, Lieutenant in April 1946, Lieutenant Commander in January 1952, and Commander in October 1958. She was selected to Captain in September 1965 and was appointed Captain when sworn in as Director.

During WW II, Captain Bulshefski was stationed at the Pearl Harbor Naval Hospital and Base Hospital #8; both in Hawaii. At another time she was the Nurse Corps 'Detailer' (assignments officer) at the Bureau of Medicine and Surgery, Washington, D.C.. Also, she was "occupational therapy instructor at the Naval Medical School in Bethesda, Maryland. She served as Chief of Nursing Service at Naval Hospitals, Beaufort, South Carolina; Guam, Mariana Islands; Jacksonville and Pensacola, Florida and Oakland, California."[3] But now, Captain Bulshefski faces the greatest challenge of her professional career; the leadership of the Navy Nurse Corps.

Also, there is another happening on the 1st of May. A reorganization of the Navy Department becomes effective. "The Naval Material Command, Bureau of Naval Personnel, and Bureau of Medicine and Surgery are [now] . . . under the direct command of the CNO [Chief of Naval Operations]. All other bureaus placed under Office of Naval Material Command."[4] This does not have any direct or noticeable effect upon the Nurse Corps.

In June of 1966, a PCP (Program Change Proposal) is written by Code 323 of the Nursing Division of BuMed. This requires some explanation. First, Code 323 is one of the Nurse Corps officers on the staff of the Director of the Corps. This officer fills a billet (a job position) called 'Head, Personnel Planning and Accounting.' This person is responsible to the Director of the Corps for the accounting of all Nurse Corps billets, the number of Nurse Corps personnel at each Naval facility, worldwide, and responsible for the planning for both billets and personnel, including promotion plans. And, if you don't think that keeps one busy, think again. Especially, in this era without computers. Much work goes into the preparation of this PCP. The justification had to be dispassionate but cogent, and statistically powerful. It is, in essence, a request that goes through a long chain of command to the Secretary of Defense requesting that the end strength of the entire Navy be increased so that the Navy Nurse Corps can have an increase of 414 billets. And, that the billets be programmed into the Nurse Corps allowances beginning in Fiscal Year 1968 through Fiscal Year 1972. Remember, this (1966) is a time of an extreme shortage of nurses and here is a PCP requesting more billets when we couldn't fill the ones we already have. But, this is the whole purpose of Code 323, to propose planning to the Director and then to carry through on those plans approved by the Director. Because the Director, Captain Bulshefski, and Code 323, Commander Doris Sterner, are both graduates of the Naval Postgraduate School's Management course, this kind of planning and programming is possible. On 20 December 1966 the entire PCP, just as it was written, is approved by the Secretary of Defense! Now planning begins on how to find the nurses to fill those billets.

During this time, out at the University of Colorado's School of Nursing, Navy Nurse Phyllis J. Elsass is completing her Master's degree under Navy sponsorship. She says, "Shortly before I finished that program, it turns out that the Dean had a visit from Commander Upchurch [Head of Education and Training section of Director's staff at Nursing Division, BuMed] and I was given the opportunity to meet with her. She told me about her efforts to develop a new research organization, based at the Naval Medical Research Institute [NMRI] in Bethesda . . . of course, I had just completed a Master's Thesis and was heavily into the merits of research, so this all sounded very, very exciting. I told her that, yes, I would be very happy to come and work with her if that was what the Navy wanted me to do. But, at the end of three years at the University of Colorado, I felt obligated to do whatever the Navy asked me to do. I don't mean that to be corny, but that whole opportunity [at getting her BS and MS at Navy expense] shaped the rest of my life and career.

"I got orders to the Naval Hospital at Bethesda which was fine with me because I loved Bethesda. . . . I went to Bethesda and it turns out that, I guess, I had only been there about two weeks when I got orders to transfer to . . . [NMRI]. When I reported to the Research Institute in August 1966, I found myself with Commander Upchurch. We were the Nursing Research Division of the Behavioral Science Department. Ouida [CDR Upchurch] had a lot of big ideas of projects and their importance to the Nurse Corps, but we had no money and no employees. . . . To make a long story short, Ouida was a very astute lady who saw an opportunity to get some money attached to education and training, and she was able to re-orient the projects that she wanted to do . . . so they became education training problems, and money was available. We did apply for it and we got it. We then became our own department, the Education and Training Department at NMRI. . . . The two major efforts that I was associated with were the `Ward Manager Training Program' and the `Revisions to the Hospital Corps School Curriculum.' We trained about a total of twenty young hospital corpsmen. . . . We trained them at Bethesda. They worked on the wards at Bethesda and then, to get any kind of hard data on what the impact of this new person had on patient care, we transferred eight of the men to the naval hospital in Philadelphia where we did multiple measurements each month for a nine month period and came out with pretty significant results in terms of the nurses and the nursing corpsmen being able to re-direct more of their time towards direct patient care. Unfortunately, the bottom line came out to be that this was an additional person that was needed on the staff. Yes, we could demonstrate that the quality of care was increased, but people translate to money, and it just wasn't there. . . . I guess one of the most memorable of my experiences was having lunch with . . . [the former CO of Philadelphia Naval Hospital] when he came to Washington for briefings when he was enroute from the Naval Hospital Philadelphia to become the Commanding Officer of the Station Hospital of DaNang. He invited, I think then Captain, Upchurch and myself to have lunch with him. At that luncheon he admitted to us that he had been wrong, and in fact had proven our point and that he saw these people [ward managers] as very important members of the team. To me that was worth more than all of the hard data we got through our research project."[5]

Meanwhile, some of the stateside naval hospitals are beginning to receive some of the casualties from Vietnam battlefields. For instance, Navy Nurse Ruth Halverson says, "After I had gotten off MSTS, I went to the Naval Hospital at Philadelphia. It eventually became the largest Orthopedic center on the East Coast and, during the height of the war, we were averaging between 2,000 and 2,500 patients there. . . . Initially I worked on a medical ward . . . from there, because of my O.R. [Operating Room] experience, and at that point we were getting a lot of the casualties back, I was asked to go into the Operating Room and work there and also instruct on-the-job trainees, the corpsmen, in operating room technique. So we set up some classes just to get us through the heaviest part of that period."[6]

We turn now to the Naval Support Activity over in Naples, Italy where Navy Nurse Virginia M. Eberharter is the Senior Nurse. She notes that she arrived in November 1965 and that "Since NATO was in Naples, we received patients from all services and we served a population of ten thousand people.

"Shortly after reporting for duty, I was given the blueprints of the new hospital which was being built at the time. [Navy nurses have to be versatile and have a lot of knowledge with a wealth of common sense.] It was to be completed and dedicated seven to eight months after my arrival, so there were many meetings discussing plans and staffing for the new hospital. The old hospital had a gross area of 46,000 square feet; the new hospital a gross area of 85,600 so correspondence went to BuMed asking for additional personnel. One of my accomplishments in the old hospital was setting up an appointment system for all clinics. Heretofore they had walk-ins for each clinic. . . . The completion date for the new hospital was moved back several times. Finally a pink brochure with a picture of the new hospital on it was distributed to all staff and patients announcing the opening and dedication of the new hospital on July 21, 1966. It was built by the Italians so it could be converted back to an apartment building after the Navy's lease of one hundred years was up. . . . Captain Bulshefski, Director of the Navy Nurse Corps, and other officers from BuMed attended the dedication ceremony."[7]

On the other side of the world, in early 1966, another Navy nurse (Anne L. O'Connell) is arriving in Japan for duty at the U.S. Naval Hospital at Yokosuka, Japan. She arrives by MSTS ship in Yokohama. "I was met in Yokohama by four or five nurses with big banners [saying] `Welcome Anne.' That was exciting. . . . We had 29 nurses there, and the day I reported in to Yokosuka, we had around 230 patients in the hospital, and the day I left, two year later, we had over 700. While I was in Yokosuka, it was the real escalation of the Vietnam War. Although many things have been said about that war now, at the time we really thought we were supporting a good cause. Ninety five percent of our patients were Marines from Vietnam.

We worked very hard in Yokosuka, long hours, but we had such a professional staff, both nurse corps and medical corps, and corpsmen. Later on, when I was in other duty stations, when I would have trouble motivating people to work, I often looked back to Yokosuka as an example of how people in a difficult situation will pull together and really work hard. But, as hard as we worked in Yokosuka, we played just as hard. . . . We took leave, of course, more than once, and usually you went two places on one leave. One time we went to Taiwan and Hong Kong, and another time we went to Okinawa and Bangkok, and we took ten days to two weeks at a time [we were permitted a total of 30 days leave per year], we'd stay in a hotel and have clothes made, buy jewelry, and meet the fellows from the ships. . . . I think of my whole career, looking back now, and Yokosuka was the most adventuresome, the most professionally rewarding."[8]

Before we turn to the hospital ships, you might be interested in how the Navy names its ships. For instance:

Attack Aircraft Carriers; named after famous ships, battles or men.

Battleships; States.
Cruisers; Cities.
Destroyers; Naval heroes, Secretaries of the Navy or Congressmen.
Escort Aircraft Carriers; Bays or Sounds.
Transports; Flag or General officers and other historic figures.
Ammunition Ships; Volcanoes or explosive terms.
Hospital Ships; Words of comfort!!![9]

And speaking of hospital ships, we have the USS *Repose* back 'in harm's way' in 1966. After ten and a half years in the Reserve Fleet, she returned to active service when she was commissioned on 16 October 1965. She is supplied and staffed and departs San Francisco on 3 January 1966. After "refresher training and upkeep in Pearl Harbor and Subic Bay, she [arrives] in Chu Lai, Republic of Vietnam on 14 February 1966.

Vietnam marked the innovation of the concept of mobile hospital support offshore. In this war, *Repose* has stationed herself near the sites of the heaviest battles and has taken virtually all casualties aboard by helo [helicopter]. . . . Her mission is offshore medical support for United States and Allied Military Forces and her area of responsibility is the I Corps Tactical Zone from DaNang to the DMZ (17th parallel)."[10]

Now for some details about the ship: "Her length is 520 feet; her beam is 71 feet 6 inches. She has a cruising radius of 12,000 miles, traveling at seventeen and one-half knots. There are seven decks, with the clinical spaces being below the waterline so that the more desirable upper decks may be reserved for wards and recreation areas. . . . The entire ship is air-conditioned. In accordance with the Geneva Convention, the ship is painted white with red crosses on her sides. She is fully illuminated at all times and carries no armament, even when sailing in hostile waters. . . . She is also a floating medical store house carrying quantities of materials needed to run a 750 bed hospital. An additional role the *Repose* has in Vietnam is that of a consultation center. Problem cases from field hospitals ashore can be brought to the specialists aboard ship where the new diagnostic and therapeutic equipment can be utilized. When the work load permits, the medical personnel aboard the *Repose* are available to treat South Vietnamese civilians and other friendly nationals. In fulfilling this secondary mission, doctors, nurses and corpsmen may go ashore to help train and work with Vietnamese on a people-to-people basis. . . . [The] Surgeon General of the Navy states further, 'We will make our facilities aboard the *Repose* available for training selected South Vietnamese doctors and nurses when this can be done without interfering with our primary mission...'

"To carry out the multiple tasks assigned the *Repose* there are 22 Navy Doctors, 3 Navy Dentists, 29 Nurses, a Wave Medical Service Corps officer, 6 Medical Service Corps officers, two chaplains, 246 Hospital Corpsmen and 7 Dental Technicians. In addition, there are 18 officers and more than 200 men in the crew responsible for the operation of the ship. . . .

"Today, on the *Repose* another giant step has been taken in providing whole blood for transfusions to battle casualties and to surgery patients. It is a frozen blood bank which can hold up to 250 units of blood. . . . For the first time in the history of military medicine, an artificial heart can take over the functions of a damaged heart or major blood vessels within minutes of the time the patient has been wounded in action. The *Repose* carries such a machine. . . . This equipment, weighing less than 75 pounds, is instantly available. It can be used on the ship, or can be flown to a shore facility, if it is requested."[11]

Cdr Angelica Vitillo NC USN, was assigned as Chief of Nursing Service aboard the *Repose* and had reported aboard in November 1965 while the *Repose* was still in the States being prepared for the new assignment. In May of 1966, while the ship is at Subic Bay in the Philippines, Cdr Vitillo receives orders for reassignment in Washington, D.C., as Deputy Director of the Navy Nurse Corps. Cdr Mary T. Kovacevich, NC, USN, reports aboard, the end of May, as the new Chief Nurse, and Cdr Vitillo leaves in early June for BuMed.

In July, the *Repose* "proceeded north to Dong Ha and Phu Bai near the Demilitarized Zone in support of . . . the largest operation supported thus far. . . . Twelve hours later the influx of casualties began. The three major operating Rooms functioned continuously, without breaking, for three days, completing major surgery on 77 patients. Injuries involving chest and abdominal wounds, caused by multiple shrapnel fragments, necessitated several surgical procedures on one patient. It was not uncommon to find as many as three surgical specialists hovered over the operating table simultaneously at work mending head, extremity, and trunk wounds. During the months of July and August, the *Repose* remained on-station off the coast of Vietnam, perpetually steaming between Da Nang and Dong Ha, at the same time setting a new record of 43 days of on-station duty. After an extremely busy tour, breaking all previous records of patient admissions, the *Repose* left Vietnam on her first trip to Hong Kong for a much deserved rest. Three hundred and fifty-four patients accompanied her on the trip. . . .

"Hong Kong proved to be a most welcome diversion for the weary staff. The *Repose* anchored in the harbor bordered by Hong Kong on one side and Kowloon on the other. Water taxies called 'Walla Wallas,' piloted by the native Chinese, provided a novel form of transportation from ship to shore. The splendid five days spent here included the full gamut of activities from planned tours through Hong Kong and Kowloon (to view the Red Chinese border), to shopping and frequent visits to expert tailor shops."[12] After the short respite, they leave and return to their station off the coast of Vietnam.

(It should be noted that Navy nurses are also aboard the MSTS ships. As pointed out previously, some of these ships traveled in dangerous waters. Between 1965 and August 1966 there were 16 Navy Nurse Corps officers (female) aboard MSTS ships in the Pacific.[13])

In April 1967 the *Repose* is joined in harm's way, by the hospital ship *Sanctuary*. This ship had been recommissioned in November of 1966, supplied and staffed then sailed for Vietnam. Navy Nurse Claire M. Cronin is aboard and tells us that she and another Navy nurse "volunteered for duty in Vietnam. We were chosen to serve aboard the USS *Sanctuary*. [In] March of 1967 we were the first crew aboard the USS *Sanctuary*. We took the ship from San Francisco, we sailed under that Golden Gate Bridge with tears in our eyes as we said goodbye, and off we went to Vietnam. I guess I would have to say that was my most memorable experience in the Navy. I served thirteen months aboard the ship and I worked the Intensive Care unit the entire time. . . . We lived in very close quarters on the ship, there were 29 nurses and 2 Red Cross workers. Our quarters were on two decks. We had a little, tiny alcove area with a closed circuit TV and that was our recreational space. There were times when there were water restrictions and water hours; you could only take showers at a certain time of the day. We all got along well. Many of the wards had bunk beds but we did take them out of Intensive Care. Commander Sally Smith was our Chief Nurse and she was a tremendous role model to us. She never took a day off, she never went to bed at night before she made complete rounds, making sure everybody was taken care of and she frequently would come in and do things in patient care herself. These guys [the patients] were grubby, they were coated with sand and stuff, just coming off the battlefield, and she would give them baths and shampoo them, or she would help us mix-up the IV [InterVenous]; she was really great. One thing that happened that we never knew until we got back home, her mother had died during that tour and she did not leave the ship to go back, and she never even told any of us.

"One thing I want to mention, as people look back on history, people were not recognized at that time for any type of decorations; very few were. I think you saw more out of Da Nang on a land based operation than you did the ship. Unfortunately, there were very few people who received any recognition. My roommate and I, when we got back . . . [to the States], found a 'letter of appreciation' in our service record that we never knew we had. Commander Smith had come to Key West [Navy Hospital duty station] with us and when she found that out she was very upset. She made them pull the letters and give them to us at a 'presentation' [ceremony]. That was a big thing, that we got that letter of appreciation."[14]

At the end of July 1967, the *Repose* is called from Da Nang Harbor to the Gulf of Tonkin to give emergency assistance to the Aircraft Carrier USS *Forrestal*. A "Fire on the U.S.S. *Forrestal* killed 134 men . . . when a fuel tank fell from an A-4 Skyhawk [plane] warming up on the carrier's flight deck."[15] The *Repose* takes aboard 32 burn patients and 77 dead.[16] Aboard the *Repose* at this time, is Navy Nurse F. Carroll McKown who tells us, "We received word to proceed immediately to the DMZ, that the *Forrestal* was on fire. Information, of course, came in by bits and pieces. . . . I understand this was said on the ship, but of course, I don't have first hand knowledge of whether it was true or not, but I understand that President Johnson at that time had alerted Hanoi to let them know we were coming and why we were going there and basically threatened them that if anything happened to us while we were up there, he was going to level Hanoi. I don't know if that's a true story or not, but it made us feel pretty good, so we went up to Yankee Station [*Forrestal*'s assigned station in the Gulf of Tonkin]. Yankee Station is well past the DMZ up in the Hanoi vicinity and the U.S.S. *Forrestal* fell into a figure eight pattern behind the Repose. I have a picture of that and it was quite something to see—an aircraft carrier at a 30 degree list. Well of course we were supposed to be taking casualties from the *Forrestal*. The sad thing is we took very few casualties from the *Forrestal*. . . . We took on 77 bodies. It was bad. It was extremely demoralizing to all of us on the ship, that we were there and we could have helped so many and they were all gone. We certainly did take some on, shrapnel wounds and injuries and burns. We left the *Forrestal* after we had done all we could do and we went back to Da Nang."[17]

Navy Nurse Kathleen Martin is also aboard the *Repose*, working in the recovery room, and she tells us of a hazardous happening while refueling at sea, "We were . . . in the process of refueling from an oil tanker. When we refueled from most of the ships, they would come along side our starboard [right side of the ship] and throw over their . . . or shoot the gun . . . that would bring the lines [across] that eventually would carry the fuel line [to the *Repose*]. The line itself had been attached and [we] had taken on all the fuel that we could take at that time. They had just disconnected this fuel [line] and were allowing it to go back to the fueler. Suddenly, there was an announcement that came over the [ship's] loud speaker, `Stand by for collision! This is not a drill! Stand by for collision! This is not a drill!' The collision was, of course, on our starboard side; the side where the recovery room was.

"I had just stepped out to go to the blood bank to pick up some more units . . . when the announcement of collision came. . . . When I got back to the recovery room, they made the announcement that we were to be in the same holding position until further notice. No one knew exactly what was up, but we could hear the screech of the metal grinding against each other when the two ships hit. Later on, at the end of the day, after we'd been relieved from . . . [their shift], and had the evening meal, those who were interested were allowed to go forward and see what had happened. The two ships had remained together until the people in our damage control had gone in to the hole where the damage was and stuffed mattresses into the opening. . . . Then, gradually, our two ships had eased apart and we both remained afloat. . . . Apparently the steering mechanism on our ship had broken just as they had released the fuel line. This causing the starboard side of our ship to go into the port side of the fueling ship. The crash itself caused the mast of the fueler to fall, crashing the Captain's gig [small boat]. He was most unhappy about this. We were all very happy that there was only one injury—this was to the young man who tried to fix the steering mechanism, unsuccessfully, before we hit. When we went forward and looked at the damage, just about two feet back from the [bow] of the ship, it looked like a gigantic can opener had gone . . . completely down the side and underneath the water; it was gaping. We were making progress very, very slowly, but we didn't know the extent of the damage. We had to wait in that area until the frogmen could come out from the shore and go under water and inspect the damages there.

"Then the big question came up; could it be repaired at our usual port of Subic Bay [in the Philippines] or did we have to go to Sasebo, Japan? Everyone wanted to go there, see old friends and see many other places that we hadn't been able to. . . . The decision came down that they were going to take a chance on the [dry dock] located in the Philippines to see if we would fit aboard. So we made it as fast as we could down to Subic Bay. . . . We went directly to the pier. We off-loaded every single patient except the ambulatory ones. These patients were taken by ambulance either to the Subic Bay Naval Hospital [U.S. Navy] or to Clark Air Force Base [U.S. Air Force Hospital] and eventually flown back to the States. As soon as we had off-loaded all patients except the ambulatory ones, we then proceeded over to the ship yard and started to inch our way into the floating dock. When I say we had inches to spare, we had about a foot altogether; six to eight inches, perhaps, on each side. It took us several hours to go in, but we made it with only one casualty. Unfortunately, we were almost to the point of stopping and one of the cables forward broke and it whipped over and severely injured one of the sailors working on the dock. They brought him aboard our ship for emergency treatment, but we were only on generator power and we just were able to stabilize him and ship him out to Subic Bay Hospital for his surgery.

"Then, once we were in [the floating dock], they drained the ship. . . . We could see that, just like an iceberg, our ship had two thirds underneath the water and only one third showing."[18] Navy Nurse F. Carroll McKown finishes this saga, "They put us into dry dock. We were there, I guess about two weeks, maybe three. I think about two weeks. And, indignity of indignities, when we were released from Subic Bay and sent back home, the engineers, (there) in the shipyard, had slapped a huge band-aid across our bow!"[19]

Navy Nurse McKown also tells us, "On the ship we also had an international ward where we took care of Vietnamese and Thai (from Thailand) civilians. Now some of them had burns from napalm but most did not. Most of them had congenital abnormalities. . . . In the Vietnamese culture, if you had a deformity, you were ostracized, so this surgery really allowed some folks to be re-introduced into their society. . . . We also took care of some NVA's—the North Vietnamese soldiers. I think that the thing that I found most remarkable is that, of course they were prisoners, but we cared for them exactly the same as we cared for our own. Now maybe, if it got down to the last Band-aid and who would get it, we would give it to one of our own, but it never got that close. . . . The real hazards on the ship were the Koreans. Now, I have a lot of respect for Koreans; they are very tough. But, they hated the Vietnamese. We had one instance . . . where a Korean patient yanked out the chest tubes of one of our Vietnamese patients. So we had to watch them and keep them apart."[20]

Just one more 1967 item on the *Repose*, "On 19 August 1967, in ceremonies held while on station in Vietnamese waters, *Repose* was presented the Navy Unit Commendation by Rear Admiral N.G. Ward, Commander Service Group THREE, for exceptional service from 22 February 1966 to February 1967." And well they deserve it.

The next important topic for discussion is the Naval Hospital at Da Nang, Vietnam. "Sitting on a 50-acre site of sand dunes in Danang [sic] East, the hospital is located approximately 3 miles from Danang proper. Surrounded by a myriad of military components, it has frequently come under enemy attack either by design or otherwise. During initial construction stage, the hospital site was over-run in October 1965 by the Viet Cong who with satchel charges and mortars destroyed six of the buildings. Rebuilding began immediately and in January 1966 a 60-bed facility was opened. By June 1966 it had grown to 400 beds. . . . The Danang hospital is charged with the responsibility for providing emergency and definitive hospital care, primarily to Navy and Marine Corps personnel in I Corps Tactical Zone; for treating those patients with diseases or injuries requiring specialized care not available in other medical elements; and for furnishing dispensary services for personnel in the Danang area."[21]

The first chief nurse assigned to this facility is CDR Mary F. Cannon. She tells us, "The second challenging assignment that I had was my assignment to the Naval Hospital in Da Nang, Vietnam. This became an unusual assignment in that there was a hospital at Da Nang, a Naval Hospital . . . [that] was in operation and it was being run by the enlisted corpsmen and by doctors. There were not any nurses there. As you may realize, the Navy has never, to my knowledge, ever put nurses into a combat situation. In other situations of combat, the war came to the area and nurses were already there to begin with. Or, nurses were assigned out on ships but not on land. So there was a great deal of indecision from the military, from the Navy, as to whether would we go or wouldn't we be going. In fact, I think our orders were cancelled about twice before we finally received orders and the decision was made that we would go. So the four of us were selected to be the first to go over. We were to have a staff of eighteen eventually. They were going to be sent in three different increments with them following three to four weeks apart. So . . . [it] was in August 1967 that we [four] gathered on the coast of California to head off for Vietnam. There was Marie Lawrence, Nancy Sullivan, Dottie Effner, and myself. We flew out on a commercial plane from San Bernadino. We were the only four women on board, all the rest were men and were military. Our flight, including flying time and time on the ground was twenty-two hours. And it seemed that every place we were flying or all the time we were flying, it was night. . . . The stewardesses on the plane kept serving us breakfast. . . . So when we arrived in Vietnam . . . we had crossed the International Date Line and we arrived in Da Nang at 7:30 in the morning. We were met, as the plane landed, by . . . our CO and . . . our Administrative

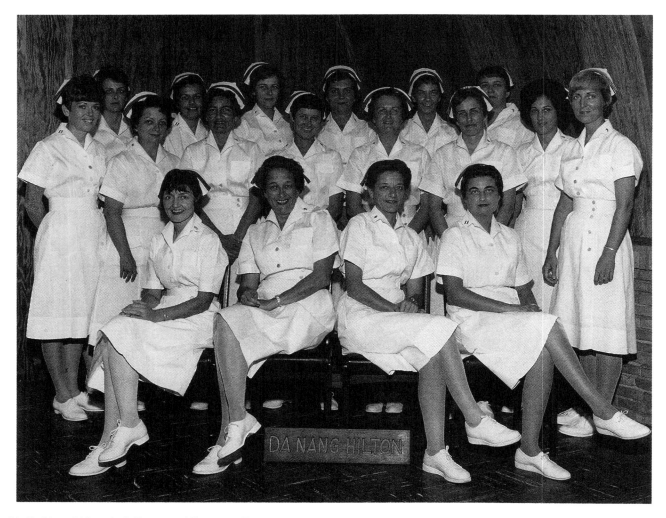

U. S. Naval Hospital, Danang Vietnam, December 1967. Chief Nurse Mary Cannon (Seated second from left.)
(Photo courtesy of Captain Mary F. Cannon NC USN (Ret.))

Officer. Since our plane was late getting in, I believe they had had quite a wait at the airport. . . . We were happy to see them and I hope they were happy to see us. We rode back to the hospital . . . [and] looking around at the country that we were to call home for the next year . . . it was sand, more sand [and] it was hot. . . . Since we had landed near downtown Da Nang we had a ride of about half an hour out to the Naval Hospital.

"We found our quarters to be very lovely. Each of us were to have a private room. There were two wings, each wing had eight rooms in it and we had a long corridor going down to a wing that had the showers, washbasins and the lavatories. And then a third wing coming off from that was a recreation room and three private rooms, two of the same size and one larger. All the quarters were air-conditioned; the floors were cement. . . . We were very impressed with it. It was new and the Seabees had done an excellent job. The hospital, which we saw very briefly on that day, was running at . . . about 275 patients, as I remember. But their capacity was 325 to 375. The hospital also was air-conditioned. It consisted of the triage area, intensive care unit, operating rooms, surgical wards, orthopedic wards, medical wards and up on the hill we had a ward for prisoners. We also had the various clinics; orthopedic, urology, etc.. . . .

"We settled in at an early hour that [first] evening and I don't think it took us long for sleep to descend upon us. Somewhere later that evening or somewhere in the night, I never did know what the time was, apparently there was quite a bit of mortar fire, machine gun fire going on outside. Our hospital was situated so that on one side of us was the perimeter, meaning the Vietnamese near-by, and on our other side was MAG-16 which was a helicopter strip. They were continually lobbing mortars over us trying to hit the chopper facility. . . . My phone rang and it was . . . [the CO] who was informing me that the fire that we were hearing and all the noise outside was friendly fire. It was our firing not the VC [Viet Cong] firing. He kept telling me about what was going on and I kept saying, `Yes, sir' and yawning and trying to appear coherent to talk to him. And finally he said, `Did I wake you up?' and I said, `Yes, sir. I was sleeping but I'll wake the others and tell them there's nothing to worry about.' That ended our conversation. The next morning when I saw . . . [the CO], he kind of looked up at me and said, `Well, I don't think that I'm going to have to worry too much about you girls, am I?' and I said, `No, I don't think so, sir. We certainly weren't bothered at all last night but it was nice of you to call us.' . . . We went to work that morning. We had decided and talked about, the previous night, . . . where in the world we were going to start and how we were going to start. We tried to remind ourselves that this had been an operation going along without us, so let us go slowly and see what was going on and change as things needed to be changed. But, let's not go in and decide everything is wrong and we are going to change it immediately. . . .

"[The CO] and I had had several discussions about the hospital situation and we determined it would be best for the four of us to stay on the day shift until we were able to have a full complement of nurses and to cover the more acute areas such as: the operating room, intensive care unit and the surgical and maybe an orthopedic ward. This was our plan. As we observed these various areas and, believe me, we did a lot of observing that particular day, we noticed the Vietnamese girls seemed to be functioning as aides. They were giving baths, which the patients certainly didn't seem to mind. However, the basin of water seemed to go from one patient to the other without being changed. And the wash cloths were used for various activities around the ward. The Vietnamese also seemed to be taking temperatures. . . . Corpsmen were overseers and showed us their systems and how they were doing things and they showed us their charting and how the wards were being run. The patients . . . in this type of hospital, weren't getting many medications but occasionally some were. Vietnamese girls seemed to be passing these out. We observed and noted what was going on and thought we'd have our big discussion and compare notes in the evening. Anything that was very drastically wrong, of course, was changed immediately. . . .

"We got back to the quarters that night and compared notes on our observations of the day. We found, generally, that some of the things that seemed to get lost along the way . . . were things like asepsis, techniques of changing dressings, or keeping areas clean or free from contamination, turning patients, coughing patients, elevating limbs, this type of thing. We realized patients that we had were not there for any length of time but still post-operative care did need many of the things such as turning, positioning, elevating limbs. We found that med cards just weren't used. There weren't a lot of medications given but, yes, there were some up on the medical wards. Of course [there was the] charting. Oh, my. This was unusual. So our attack was to work one nurse in the operating room, one in ICU, one of us on the orthopedic ward and one on the surgical ward.

"We were to have Vietnamese maids in quarters, our quarters, that would do the cleaning. . . . We had two assigned to us, sometimes three. . . . One of the other things I'd like to point out about our quarters, this was really our only head [toilet] facility. So from the hospital we had to come over and it took a little bit of time, of course, to walk from the hospital over to the quarters. It was a slight inconvenience and we learned not to drink a lot of fluids during the day. If things were desperate, there was a head facility around the triage area but, it wasn't conducive, really, for our use but, in an emergency, it could do. You had to have someone stand guard outside so this wasn't used too frequently. On one of these trips over to the facility in quarters, one of the [nurses] happened to notice all the girl-sans [maids] in the lavatory area laughing and having the best time. And what they found was, we had electric toothbrushes which we left by the washbasins in this area. All the girl-sans had the electric toothbrushes and they were trying them out. Now, you realize it's bad enough having somebody else using your toothbrush however . . . they chew some kind of beetlenut and they have all these `black' teeth! We were appalled when we realized what was happening. So that was the end of electric toothbrushes. . . .

"We started to have doctors asking when we'd be getting more nurses and if they'd have one up on their wards. We seemed to be making a dent. The corpsmen; some were a little bit irritated with our butting into their regime or their kingdom, but most of them took it pretty well in stride. There were a few bumps along the way but nothing too bad. . . . So you were continually balancing, in your mind and remembering, this had been going on for almost a year and nothing drastic had happened. Rome couldn't be changed or shouldn't be changed in a day. So, go slowly, don't be horrified but change and change as needed. This was the premise on which we tried to operate.

"One of the things we found we had to do in Vietnam was (many nights and always at night), we'd have alerts which meant there'd be incoming fire and incoming mortar rounds. We were to spend this time, once an alert was sounded, in . . . the nearest bunker to us. That was a good two hundred and fifty yard dash in the open area, across the sand from our quarters into the sandbagged bunker which was, well, we were in there with very young looking Marines carrying carbines. I might add, I was more afraid of the Marines because they looked so scared and I wasn't too sure they knew how to use those carbines if they had to. But, that was where we were to spend our time during any alert. Well, after a couple of times of this, I thought that the two-hundred-fifty yard dash we were exposed to . . . it's a long way and there's nothing protecting you. So, I asked . . . [the CO] one day, I said, `Sir, I wonder if there's any chance we could stay in our quarters when we have an alert because we have that three or four foot of concrete wall all around [the walls of the quarters are concrete]? Maybe, if we got under our beds and stayed there we'd be just as safe as if we were in the bunkers.' Well, he said, `No'. . . .

"The next big event was the arrival of our next . . . nurses; Joan McIntyre, Ruth Purinton, Bettye Nagy, Marjorie Warren, and . . . Ruth Morlock. . . . They were as tired as we must have looked the day we arrived. They had the same long trip that we had. . . . With our . . . additional nurses we continued to stay on the day shift and expanded coverage into other surgical wards and into another orthopedic ward and up into the medical ward. So we were able, pretty well, to cover the hospital at this point, at least during the day. And, we did not work an eight hour day. We worked until we felt that we could leave the area we were assigned in. Of course, we now had OR nurses and they certainly had their job to do. [We] tried to remind the girls that everything cannot be accomplished in one day and there was always tomorrow and the next day and not to wear one's self out because there was not going to be a day off coming up. Pace yourself and change what you can. What you can't do in one day, do the next day and that's how we tried to get along and keep thinking. . . .

"[Soon after,] we had one of our nights off to the bunker. And, it seemed, that particular night, many of us had chosen to wash our hair, put it up in curlers [and] do various beauty aids. So, when we hit the bunker that night, we were in rather strange attire. . . . It so happened, that particular night . . . [the CO] came to see how things were going in the bunker. He came in, took one look at us and left and didn't have much to say except to be sure that everybody was alright. The next day, when we had our usual [morning] eight o'clock discussion . . . he looked at me and said, `Well, I think you made your point. After looking at you girls in the bunker last night, I would say that you were going to be able to stay in the quarters, under the beds as you suggested.' I said, `Oh, thank you, sir. The girls will be happy to hear that.' We hadn't done this with any great intent of making our point but it certainly worked out to our advantage and everybody was most happy. We were able to get some litter pads from supply. Litter pads are just very thin mattresses that are used . . . on top of litters. We rolled these up, put them at the foot of our beds and when we had an alert or had to go under the bed, we just put those down and laid on that instead of the hard cement floor. And, it worked out very well. . . .

"Most of our patients were brought in by helicopter. Some were brought in by vehicle; via jeeps, carryalls or whatever was available. But, the majority were by helicopter. These [patients] were brought first into the triage area. . . . The wounds were multitudinous, horrible wounds, really. It was not unusual for someone to have limbs involved, abdomen, chest, all in the same patient. The types of injuries were so bad because of the claymore mines that were used, the booby traps and the punji sticks. . . . The corpsmen had some very difficult times over there because a lot of the time it was their `buddies' that they'd find coming in; that they'd known at Corps School. The corpsmen that were up on the line at the Aid Stations had tremendously tough assignments; tough job. There were many injuries of our corpsmen, many of them that were brought back [were] in body bags [dead]. It's a tragic loss of life in this war. And you all know, it made you realize how much the human body could take when you saw the terrible wounds that so many of these young men came in with and the hours of surgery and the days of recovery before they were able to be sent on back or out to the ships.

"Things that seemed important to the patients who were coming in to triage and into the operating room or wards or wherever they saw us, when they saw a Navy Nurse they felt they were in a safer place. They were also kind of glad to see a woman. There was a lot of security felt by them in seeing nurses. We were in our white uniforms and our caps. As time went on those white uniforms became a little more towards the off-white and then eventually to the beige because of the water used in the laundry. Incidentally, we did have our uniforms done in the hospital laundry. . . .

"It was soon time for our next contingent of nurses to arrive. We would have eight more and we looked forward to their day and arrive they did. In that group we had Shirlie Thomas, Joyce Kearns, Lois Butler, Nicki Nicora, Jean Peterson, Pat Harrington, Betty Matthewson, Kathy Reardon. . . . Our CO was extremely supportive of us. And, our corpsmen were mellowing as time went by. They'd run into some problems but none of them were gigantic ones. . . .

"One of the things that made us rather suspicious about our girl-sans [in the quarters] was sometimes when we'd come over and go to our rooms we'd find that our mattresses or litter pads were already under the bed. Sure enough, that night we'd have an alert and we'd be under the bed. Somehow they knew. We never did, at least I never did figure that one out but, the girl-sans were tuned [in] so we didn't know what side they might be on.

"With our complement now up to eighteen [nurses] we were able to cover all the wards. We were able to do it on three shifts; AM, PM, and night duty. One of the problems that the night people had was again going over to the nurses quarters for the use of the head. So, we had a ruling, if they could stick with it, that if one had to go, they both had to go, so they wouldn't be walking across this open area from the hospital to the nurses quarters by themselves or be alone at any time outside of the hospital area.

"The doctors were delighted and very happy to get nurses and more nurses and have them on their wards. [As] with anything else, it seemed the more they got, the more they wanted. It was ever thus and no different than it was at our stateside hospitals. `More nurses, we need more nurses,' always. `We need a nurse for the clinics, we need a nurse for here.' . . .

"We came into Christmas [1967] and we were remembered very well by our nurses in the States. We received a lot of Christmas presents and a lot of mail. It was nice to know that they were thinking of us and they were sending us things that were hard for us to get over there. So, it made for a good Christmas; as good as possible."[22]

Navy Nurse Bettye Nagy is one of the second complement of nurses that arrived at Da Nang and she says, "The hospital was a nice set up. . . . We had a triage area and when we arrived the corpsmen and the doctors did the triage. Then we got . . . the three OR nurses. If they had the duty, then they went into the triage area also and helped with the triage of the patients. The minor wounds were sent to the orthopedic clinic where the wounds would be debrided and dressed and they would come into the units; the major wounds would have to go to the operating unit. We admitted a lot of medical patients during the day that would come in and be seen. But, the casualties were usually in the evening or night time. We had a lot of encephalitis, Japan B encephalitis, and we had ulcers, gastric ulcers, bleeding ulcers, stress ulcers. We had hypertensives. We had some diabetics. . . . We had a lot of malaria even though we had the anti-malaria medication available. Everyone was supposed to take it once a week, but not everyone did. And It's not assured. So we had a lot of medical patients stop in. . . . I find when I'm watching TV now [1988] and they . . . try to defibrillate someone with the paddles, I think about a young man who died, and he had Japanese B encephalitis. He arrested on the ward. . . . He was about 18 or 19. He was a young Marine and we really didn't want him to die. They zapped him five or six times and every time I see that on TV, I think about him. They didn't revive him. They couldn't but they just tried so hard. . . .

"There are little things that you remember. We had a baby brought in to us; in fact, he was brought in right after we arrived and the Marines had found him in some village. He was malnourished. He was about three or four months old. He really was a baby; an infant. . . . The corpsmen were taking care of him. They built him a little crib out of plywood and the mattress was a pillow. They had cut bed-savers to make diapers for him. They didn't have a bottle so they put milk in a glove and they had a hole cut in the end of a finger so he could nurse. He thrived. They fed him some kind of mush that the galley [kitchen] made up for him. . . . They called him, `Ralph, the good guy.' I went to lunch one day and they had him on this medical ward; the medical ward I was first assigned to. I came back from lunch and I said, `Where's the baby?' They said, `Look in the ward.' Instead of using IV poles [the builders] had put up pipes (about one inch pipes) that ran the length of the ward. . . . [The pipes] ran the length on either side and then we had hooks and you just hooked your IV bottle up there [on the pipe]. We had slings, canvas slings that we put arms in to elevate the arms or for head injuries and arm injuries and they had that baby in one of these slings. His little head was sticking out the top and his legs out the bottom. They had laced him in and had hooked him on one of the hooks. He was sitting up there just watching everything that was going on, perfectly at peace. Every once in a while somebody would walk by and they'd give him a little tap so he'd rock; swing back and forth. When he got better . . . there was an orphanage in the area run by some Vietnamese; some Catholic nuns. So, we sent Ralph to the orphanage. . . .

"Then we had a large POW [Prisoner Of War] ward. We had a Marine company assigned to the hospital. They did guard duty around the perimeter of the hospital and they guarded the POWs. One of the strangest experiences that I had, early on; one day I was walking around the compound and I saw these people that were holding hands. They were led by a Marine and followed by a Marine. There were ten of them. They had paperbags over their heads. . . . I asked someone what they were. They were POWs that had been brought in from the prison camp, to be treated, and they had the bags over their heads so they couldn't see their surroundings. They used to use pillowcases, but they lost a lot of pillowcases that way so, they'd just gone with the paper bags and made them hold hands so they couldn't reach up and peek. That was so they wouldn't know what the compound looked like. Then they'd put them in the truck and take them back to the prison camp which was just a few miles down the road from us. . . . POWs were cared for by corpsmen. We would make rounds on the wards, but their facilities were very sparse. They were on cots. They received narcotics if they had severe pain. They received antibiotics, but they didn't receive the same treatment that our people did. And nobody wanted to give it to them."[23]

Turning now to another duty station; in early 1967, two Navy nurses are assigned as the first Navy nurses at a new duty station in Australia. Navy Nurse Ann Sheridan says, "I called it being a pioneer, to go to the Northwest Cape of Western Australia. Mary Jean Nelson and I went out there January of 1967 and we were there for the commissioning of the Station and all the attendant activities.

"It was wilderness. The Northwest Cape is located about 850 miles North of Perth, and there was nothing in the area where the Station was being built before they started building the Station. There was one Sheep Ranch in the area and there was a dirt landing strip . . . it just had a wind sock. That was the total expertise available at this landing strip, which is where we flew into when we arrived up there sometime around the middle of April and, at that time, we were required to live in the town site, that was being built, because the dispensary was not completed. . . . Our [temporary] dispensary was located in a three bedroom . . . [house]. The master bedroom was the examining room, the middle bedroom was the doctor's office and the small bedroom was the nurse's office - Mary Jean's and mine. The lounge area was the reception area and the kitchen was used for laboratory tests - whatever we could accomplish. We stayed there for about two-and-a-half months before we went into the supposedly modern dispensary that had been constructed on the base. We did have a few problems. . . . The electricians weren't used to American current which was 110 volt and theirs was 220 and it was on 50 cycles. . . . [All the machines were set for American current and took months to fix; i.e. autoclaves, EKG machine, dental chair, etc..] We were on the end of a long supply line and this was during the height of fighting in Vietnam and there were much more urgent needs in other areas than at this new, budding dispensary in Australia. We did get some of our medications, when we needed them, from the local nursing station, as it was called. It was a hospital staffed by two nurses who, when they needed medical advice, got on the radio telephone down to the nearest town, 250 miles away, to talk with a physician, but they did have some antibiotics and they had dressings that we could use and they were very nice to these foreigners who had come.

"They [the Navy] were in the process of building a radio communications station. . . . [The dispensary] was strictly for the personnel who were stationed there, and who would be running the communications end of things, and main support [personnel]. I think there was a total of 28 Officer Grade personnel, that would be civilian and military, when I was there. . . . It probably increased after that.

"We had two physicians aboard. . . . This was their first experience in the Navy. . . . One had had surgical training and was bitterly disappointed when he saw the finished operating room, knowing he couldn't do any surgery in it. It had been constructed with wooden cabinets inside the Theatre (as the English term is used for the actual surgical operating room) and there was no way it could be considered a sterile area with open cabinets for supplies. We used it as a sort of Emergency Room. . . . [They couldn't use it for the Delivery Room either, so] Six weeks prior to their due date they [the expectant mothers] were sent to Perth. A house had been rented that was used as a domicile for these women while awaiting delivery of their child at a local hospital and then they would be returned to the Cape after. Their children remained back at the Station and that posed a problem in that neighbors would have to take care of the children while the father was at work and it certainly wasn't the best situation . . . but, in the end, it worked out very well. We didn't have any major problems. We did rely on the people in the local nursing facility for some assistance and, fortunately, the majority of our personnel remained healthy. . . . We never had to do any surgery. I think we only sent one patient to Perth for a surgical procedure.

"One of the highlights of being there during this rather frustrating time, was getting ready for the commissioning of the Station. On the same day the Station was being commissioned, the Town Site (Exmouth, where all the housing was, about five miles from the Base) was to be dedicated by the Prime Minister of Australia. [He] was Harold E. Holt and the Australian Navy sent a couple of it's warships up. We attended a cocktail party aboard one of these ships, in our Dress Whites. It was an unusual thing to have a cocktail party on a commissioned Naval vessel but it's a practice in the Australian Navy. Then, the day of the commissioning, while the commissioning was in progress, the President of the United States, Lyndon Johnson, called and spoke with the Commanding Officer and Washington [D.C.] representatives who had come out for the commissioning. . . . [The President] also [spoke] with Harold E. Holt, a charming man. Unfortunately, about three months later he went swimming and his body was never recovered. We had a memorial exercise for him, on the base, a week after his death and, at a later time, the name of the Station, which had been . . . Northwest Cape Communications Station, was changed to the Harold E. Holt Communications Station."[24]

From Australia to France where, in February 1967 the Nurse Corps billet at Ville France is deleted. But, in the States, many Nurse Corps billets are assigned to a new Hospital. It is the naval hospital at Long Beach, California which is commissioned in February. On 1 March 1967, the USS Haven is struck from the Navy's listing of ships.[25] She had been decommissioned at Long Beach in 1957 but stayed at Long Beach, "'In Reserve, In Service' status until 1967. She [is] subsequently sold to Union Carbide Corp. and converted to an Ocean Chemical Tankship."[26] These last two events are both linked together and CDR Sue Smoker (Hummel),the first Chief Nurse of the new Long Beach Naval Hospital, tells us about it. "I was ordered to report to the USS Haven hospital ship berthed in Long Beach. This ship had not sailed for several years, but was a support activity for the Naval Dispensary [at the Navy Yard, Long Beach], and the ship sat in the harbor. There was a new hospital being built which was to be completed shortly and would move all of this from the ship over to the new facility. I was glad to arrive early to get settled. . . . I had the opportunity of working with the construction crew and the administrators in setting up this new facility with all new furniture and equipment. When this was all in place and the patients were moved out of the Haven, and the hospital was officially opened, the outpatient clinics were especially welcomed by the military dependents. It was a convenient location, as well as [having] the availability of all surgical and medical facilities. The nursing staff of 55 nurses and the [staff of] hospital corpsmen worked long hours to prepare these units for patient care. Civilian staff was soon in place for the food service and supply department. Patients were arriving from ships and the Navy base as well as other bases in California."[27]

In April of 1967 "Navy Nurse Corps officers [are] first assigned the the Naval Air Station at Albany, Georgia. [And,in June, a] Nurse Corps billet [is] first established at the Naval Air Station, Miramar, California."[28] Meaning, more demands for nurses.

Another type of job for the Navy Nurse, is the job as Recruiter. Navy Nurse Beverly Brase (O'Dell) notes, "I went on recruiting duty in 1967 in Philadelphia. There were a lot of anti-war protests, it wasn't a really safe place to be, anywhere alone in uniform. You had to be very careful of the demonstrations. Most of our school visits were tri-service visits, where the Army, Air Force and Navy would go into the Schools of Nursing or to the University, and present the program. The Army, of course, had two scholarship programs. They had collegiate scholarship programs, plus a hospital school scholarship program, and they could guarantee that they would send nurses directly to Vietnam without a previous duty station, after a short orientation, of course. The Air Force had flight nursing to offer, and a lot of people were interested in being flight nurses. The only thing that they didn't tell the students, was that yes, they would go to flight nurse programs, but they might never ever get a flying billet, or be able to be an actual flight nurse, although they could go through the training. Then the Navy had the two hospital ships, but the Navy could not offer people direct overseas [assignments] to Vietnam. It would have to be a second duty station, and this really put a crimp in the recruiting of nurses because many of them were interested in coming in and going directly to Vietnam.... I was very honest, when I was on recruiting, with the nurses that would ask questions. I wanted to make sure that those nurses that came into the Navy were truly motivated, fully understood what they were getting into and that they were not escaping from some unhappy situation.... I learned that I had moral courage, and that I could do what was correct, regardless of the effect on me personally. I did not make my quota of nurses. Each recruiting station was given a quaota to reach and my CO was not happy with me and I did receive an adverse fitness report from him.

"One of the greatest things available there, was support from the other Nurse Corps Recruiters. Some were having a little better luck, but a lot of them were having some problems too, so we did a lot of problem solving, a lot of support with each other. There were absolutely no problems getting enough applicants for the Navy Nurse Corps Candidate Program, in fact, they would beat down the door."[29]

Another Navy nurse tells us about her duty, "I went to [the Naval Hospital at] Philadelphia and by then, the Vietnam War was a huge concern for everybody. We had over 1,500 in-patients at Philadephia, including over 300 patients in our psychiatric unit, most of whom had come from Vietnam. We had over 300 amputees on our amputee wards. The nurses were extremely busy. I can't ever remember working anything less than a 6 day week. What was most depressing was that it seemed like there was absolutely no end to the war. ... When I was at Philadelphia, we had a very stable nurse group, but we had terrible press. Just no support from the local media, and it was increasingly discouraging because there was less and less support from the public. I remember one person whos stands out in my mind, who thought enough about the Vietnam veterans and active duty personnel, that she would come to visit. And, that was Martha Raye, and to this day I think of her with much affection."[30]

In Washington, D.C., in 1967, CDR Alene Duerk finishes her one year tour of duty in DOD (Department Of Defense). She has, literally, defined and set-up the position there and now turns it over to her relief. From there she has orders to BuPers (Bureau of Naval Personnel) where she is the Assistant Head of Medical Placement Liaison of the Nurse Corps. What this title means, in reality, is that she becomes the go-between for the Director of the Nurse Corps (and staff) and BuPers. All the Nurse Corps personnel records and fitness reports are kept in BuPers, therefore, when nurses are due to rotate to new assignments, a list is sent to CDR Duerk and she pulls their records in order to give the Nurse Corps' Assignments nurse the information she needs. Information which is needed to issue new assignments for orders to new duty stations. The Assignments Nurse Corps officer makes nominations for orders only with the approval of or at the direction of the Director; in this case, Captain Bulshefski. Of course, CDR Duerk has other duties there, but this is the main job. (Remember, this is a time of 'no computers,' so, archaic as it may sound, this really is the best way at this time.)

In June of 1967, naval hospitals are notified that a civilian position called 'Ward Clerk' had been established.

Now, hospitals can hire a civilian, train him/her for doing desk work on the busy wards. This would free both nurses and corpsmen for more compelling duties. The position is now one of the Civil Service jobs. However, the hospitals will have to pay the salary out of their funds; it would be at the discretion of the COs as to whether to utilize their monies for this new position description. This civilian position is the result of many weeks of work between the Nursing Division of BuMed and the Office of Civilian Manpower Management. Seldom (if ever) are innovations, programs or plans completed rapidly. Some things take years to see to completion. Many times what one Director sets in motion does not come to fruition until the next Director is in office.

Speaking of the Director, in November of 1967, Captain Bulshefski is present when President Johnson signs a significant piece of legislation into law; most significant to the Nurse Corps. "This legislation [gives] the Nurse Corps equal promotion opportunity with Line officers to the grades of Captain and Commander, [allows] for the possibility of a Rear Admiral [!!] for the Nurse Corps, [removes] age restrictions, [institutes the] `pass-over' system for the Nurse Corps, [allows] active duty enlisted time to be counted for retirement purposes, and [increases] Nurse Corps membership on Selection Boards."[31] As you can see, many steps forward within this new law. For one thing; heretofore, the Nurse Corps had been restricted to a mere six or eight Captains and the number of Commanders had also been severely small. Now, things will gradually begin to change with the equal opportunity with the Line officers. (This is how the legislation affected the Navy Nurse Corps, but this law also pertains to the Army and Air Force Nurse Corps. Because of this legislation, the Head of the Army Nurse Corps becomes the first female Brigadier General in June 1970. The Air Force and Navy Nurse Corps finally make it in 1972.)

At the end of 1967, the strength of the Navy Nurse Corps is 2,453 officers and the authorized strength is 2,563.[32] Still short.

To turn now to the Space Program; "On January 27, 1967, astronauts Virgil I. Grissom [LCol, USAF], Edward H. White [LCol, USAF], and Roger B. Chaffee [LCdr, USN] climbed aboard the Apollo I spacecraft for a simulation of a flight to the moon that was to take place on February 21. After they had been inside the capsule for five hours, one of the astronauts suddenly blurted out: `Fire in the Capsule.' Fifteen seconds later, all three were dead. Although the precise cause of the fire was never determined, some people believe that a spark ignited the pure oxygen inside the capsule."[33] The first major Space Agency disaster.

As for the U.S. as a whole in 1967, the nation is full of discontent and protest. From June through August there are race riots from the east to the mid-west and south to north. In October and November, there are protests and marches against the Vietnam war and the draft. In October, anti-Vietnam marchers storm the Pentagon.

In the rest of the world; in June, "Israel victor in war with Arabs. . . . Takes Sinai and Gaza from United Arab Republic. Old Jerusalem from Jordan and border areas from Syria."[34] In August, "Algeria seizes five U.S. oil companies, under state control since Arab-Israeli war in June."[35] Then in November 1967, the United Nations' "Security Council adopts British resolution calling for `eventual withdrawal of Israeli forces from Arab areas taken in June, and end of Arabs' state of belligerency with Israel.'"[36]

As for Vietnam, in "mid-1967, the level [of troops] reached 463,000 with [General] Westmoreland asking for 70,000 more."[37] The fighting, casualties, and deaths go on and on. "When the Tet offensive by the enemy exploded in Vietnam at the end of January 1968, the turn in American opinion against the war and against the President gathered force swiftly. Unlike the Viet-Cong's previous war against the rural villages, this was a massive coordinated assault against more than 100 towns and cities of South Vietnam at once. . . . Westmoreland at once demanded an emergency airlift of 10,500 troops."[38] In February, Walter Cronkite (renown and trusted newscaster) broadcasts his conclusions of what he witnessed. "On the political front, he said, `Past performance gives no confidence that the Vietnamese government can cope with its problems.' He said the Tet offensive required the realization `that we should have had all along,' that negotiations had to be just that, `not the dictation of peace terms. For now it seems more certain than ever that the bloody experience of Vietnam is to end in stalemate.'"[39] Then, in her book, *The March of Folly*, historian Barbara Tuchman states, "In dissatisfaction with the war, the public, if accurately reflected by press comment, was readier than the Administration to let go in Southeast Asia, and readier to acknowledge, according to *Time*, `that victory in Vietnam - or even a favorable settlement - may simply be beyond the grasp of the world's greatest power.'"[40]

At the end of March, "President Johnson orders end of North Vietnam bombing north of the 20th parallel and asks President Ho Chi Minh `to respond positively and favorably to this new step toward peace.' President Johnson also announces `I shall not seek and I will not accept the nomination of my party as your President.'. . . [In May] Vietnam War Peace talks open in Paris, France. . . . [In late September] U.S.S. *New Jersey* in Vietnam. World's only active battleship goes into combat off coast of North Vietnam. . . . Complete halt of U.S. bombings in North Vietnam ordered by President Johnson on November 1. . . . [A few days later,] Viet Cong delegation arrives in Paris, France. . . . [On November 26] South Vietnam ends boycott. Agrees to send delegation to Vietnam peace talks in Paris."[41] Even so, "the total number of Americans killed in action in 1968 reached 14,000. . . . [President Lyndon] Johnson's last year in office [1968], despite the bombing halt and Hanoi's agreement to talk, had brought the war no nearer to an end."[42]

Meantime, in another part of the Far East, on 23 January 1968, the U.S. Navy's "USS *Pueblo* . . . is captured by North Korean patrol boats. Four of the 83-man crew are injured and one dies later of those injuries."[43] President Johnson uses "diplomacy rather than retaliation in the Peublo incident. . . . Restraint paid off. The *Pueblo*'s crew was released at the end of the year. War on another front had been avoided."[44] It is on the 23rd of December that the "U.S.S. *Pueblo* crew [is] freed. The 82 surviving men cross Bridge of No Return to South Korea preceded by casket of . . . [crewman] wounded during seizure of ship."[45]

Last year,1967, when all the riots were taking place, "President Johnson appointed a commission to study civil disorders. Its report concluded, `Our nation is moving toward two societies, one black, one white - separate and unequal.' In April, 1968, a month after the report was published, a sniper shot and killed Martin Luther King as he stood on the balcony of a Memphis motel. Within hours of King's assassination, rioters were roaming the streets in the nation's capital. Breaking windows, flinging Molotov cocktails, they embarked on a three-day orgy of looting and burning. More that 11,000 federal troops were called in. . . . Now an army of occupation manned every intersection, ringed the White House, mounted a machine gun on the steps of the Capital."[46] It is appalling and frightening to drive home from BuMed into Virginia and see U.S. troops in battle dress standing on the bridge across the Potomac, with rifles at the ready. What is happening to my country?

Violence spreads across the country before it ends. Even so, the next month (May) "the Poor People's Campaign opens in Washington, D.C.."[47] Then on June 5th, "Senator Robert F. Kennedy shot three times in . . . Los Angeles. . . . The Senator dies 26 hours later. . . . [The end of June] `Resurrection City, U.S.A.' closed by police. It was campsite of Poor People's Campaign, near Lincoln Memorial in Washington, D.C."[48] The violence is still not over, in August "Chicago, scene of the Democratic [Presidential] convention, was an armed camp. Its streets became a battlefield. National guardsmen and . . . police . . . waded into mobs of young antiwar protesters."[49] Never-the-less, Vice President Hubert H. Humphrey is nominated to run against the Republican nominee, former Vice President Richard Nixon and his running mate, Spiro Agnew. In November, Richard Nixon is voted into the Presidency.

Turning to the state of professional nursing at this time, the nationwide shortage has already been mentioned, but the status of the student nurses is that, "Many highly motivated and well-qualified students [are] prohibited from pursuing a career in the health fields because of the expense involved."[50] This puts a crimp in the pipe-line leading to more nurses. "The Nursing Education Opportunities Grants (scholarships) had been authorized by a 1966 amendment and initiated in the summer of 1967. During the 2 years that the program lasted, grants were awarded to an estimated 15,900 students who could not otherwise attend a nursing school. . . . The Health Manpower Act of 1968 . . . established a new program of scholarship grants to nursing schools for full-time students of exceptional need. . . . The maximum annual amount of scholarship support a student could receive [is] $1500."[51] All of this helps explain why the Military Nurse Corps' student nurse subsidy programs are popular and serve as strong pipe-lines for Nurse Corps input. But, there are limits to these programs; certainly, they cannot be used as the sole source for needed nurses. Recruiting has to try to fill the gaps.

But, to return to the Navy Nurse Corps itself: on 5 January 1968 the first Male Nurse Corps officer,

Reserve, to augment to the Regular Navy is LT Clarence W. Cote. In May, a "Male Nurse Corps officer is assigned to the Military Assistance Command, Vietnam [and two] male Nurse Corps anesthetists are assigned to COMPHIBPAC [COMmander amPHIBian forces PACific]."[52] Also, in May 1968, Commander Phyllis Harrington (NC) USNR is selected for Captain. "My selection to Captain was the [**first**] for a Reserve Nurse Corps Officer, on active duty — as BuMed said, `history was made'!!"[53] At this time, Captain selectee Harrington is Chief Nurse of the Chelsea Naval Hospital outside Boston, Massachusetts. Speaking of Chelsea, in March of 1968, a Nurse Corps specialty Course in 'Operating Room Nursing' for Navy nurses is established there. (This is not the first time that a course in Operating Room Techniques is established for Navy nurses. Back in 1951 a three month course was set up at the Naval Hospital in Portsmouth, Virginia. These specialty courses are set up to meet a need for nurses in the specialty fields.) At the same time, in 1968, another specialty course (in 'Orthopedic Nursing') is established at the Philadelphia Naval Hospital in Pennsylvania."[54] Then in April a letter goes out to all Chiefs of Nursing Service and Senior Nurse Corps officers. The letter notes that two new short courses are being offered at George Washington University in Washington, D.C.; one course on Teaching Techniques and the other on Administration and Management Techniques. The letter states, "Two Nurse Corps officers from the larger Naval facilities will be considered."[55] This is all part of Director Bulshefski's planning for clinical nursing short courses of 6 months or less in order to expand opportunities for Nurse Corps officers to extend their clinical knowledge. Then in September of 1968, comes the news that the "Chief of Naval Operations [CNO] approved the Nurse Corps' request for [the] upgrading of billets to a total of 21 Captains and 162 Commanders."[56] Meaning that there can be a larger selection of Nurse Corps' Captains and Commanders at the next promotion boards, as long as it conforms to promotion regulations.

Back on 13 August 1968, a Chief of Naval Personnel Notice established the Navy Nurse Corps' Candidate Program (Hospital.)[57] This is a new program for students at three year Hospital Schools of Nursing. Its purpose is to help with the input of nurses to the Navy. It is a revision of the Nurse Corps' Candidate Program (Baccalaureate) "to include accredited Hospital Diploma School students. This program covered selection of qualified students from 3 year Hospital Schools of Nursing for participation in the Navy program during their senior year. Students are enlisted in E-3 [enlisted] pay grade and receive pay plus allowances but no tuition."[58] Earlier, in July, the CNO had "authorized 25 billets for FY [Fiscal Year] `69 and the out years"[59] for this program, as requested by the Nurse Corps. In December, as the result of a verbal presentation to a BuPers (Bureau of Naval Personnel) group, by Director Bulshefski and CDR Sterner, 50 students are allowed in the first year of the program, even though there are only 25 billets. This is because of the amount of time each student fills a billet; called 'manyear averaging of billets.' (You'll never need to know this term and never want to know it, but there it is, nevertheless.)

To return to other billets: in March 1968 a "Nurse Corps billet [is] first established at the Naval Station, Mayport, Florida."[60] Also, in Florida in July, the U.S. "Naval Hospital, Orlando . . . is commissioned."[61]

Now, what is going on in the 'field?' ('Field' is a term meaning Naval Medical facilities outside of BuMed.) Navy Nurse Anne Sheridan has finished her tour in Australia and is stationed at the Naval Hospital, Great Lakes, Illinois. "I got there in August of 1968 and we were still engaged, very heavily, in Vietnam and three times a week we were receiving Air-Evac planes with anywhere from 30 patients on up being admitted from the Air-Evacs. Many of the men were severely injured - some not so badly. One patient I will never, never forget was a young man by the name of . . . who had been hit by a land mine and had orthopedic problems and who had abdominal problems and was literally a mess. He spent about 12 months with us in the hospital and we nearly lost him on Thanksgiving Day, when he got about 20 pints of blood and [had] some emergency surgery. One time, when he was first starting to eat, after maybe 2 or 3 months of tube feeding, he was finding it difficult. When I was with him, one day, I said, 'Well, why don't you take one more bite?' That was just a comment that I made. I think it was a year and a half later when I was in the nursing office, one day, a young man came to the door and he said to the secretary, 'Could I speak to Ann Sheridan, please?' I looked up and he said, 'Just one more bite?' It was this huge, strapping young man who had gotten out [of the military], married and he had a picture of his baby and he wanted to show it to me. It was one of the most satisfying things that I can remember of that situation."[62]

Over the seas in Vietnam, 1968 is another rough year for the Da Nang Naval Hospital and its personnel. Chief Nurse Mary Cannon says, "As we came into the new year 1968, there was some conversation about the Vietnamese holiday `Tet' which . . . is their New Year. There were many rumors that this could be an active time with the Vietnamese; they might spring something. . . . It wasn't many days after that . . . maybe one or two when `Tet' descended upon us in full force. Of course, the one big clue was [that] none of the Vietnamese showed up for work and did not come to work for the whole time of `Tet.' We had a tremendous number of casualties. . . . The hospital had plans for expansion and there were wards to be opened but they were not ready. But, we had to open two of them. Two of them were opened and stocked and supplied and with patients in one day. God love those poor Seabees because they were out there under lights at night trying to hook up the plumbing and do everything they could to get those wards in operation. It was an unbelievable task for everybody concerned; the Seabees and for our staff and our nurses and for our corpsmen. But, we had the beds filled as soon as they were open. As a matter of fact, we had [patients] on litters until we were able to get beds onto the wards. . . . The operating rooms - all the tables were going full force. In addition to the business of the hospital, we had continually, at night, the mortars, the machine gun fires, the gunships going over. There was little sleep for any of us. . . . We had continual alerts night after night after night. There was a good possibility . . . during this time, that we could be evacuated; the nurses leave because of the danger of the situation. [The CO] and I talked about this several times and the idea was if we were going to leave, we'd have to get everybody together and ensure we all got out at the same time. Fortunately, this did not happen. . . . `Tet' lasted at least five to seven days. We were so busy that one didn't have too much time to think about it; to think about the terrible wounds that were received and the heavy, heavy numbers of patients. The neurosurgeons, we had two, were continually operating. The numbers of craniotomies that were done were staggering. And, of course, the shrapnel wounds. . . .

"We had a prisoner-of-war ward. This was always a coeducational ward but we rarely had any women. But, during `Tet,' we did have Vietnamese women as prisoners. And, there were quite a few prisoners. Prisoners meaning . . . ones that had some type of an injury. These patients during `Tet' were just left on the wards. There . . . were security MP's [Military Police] up there. We did have corpsmen assigned there. It was not a popular assignment for corpsmen, as one could understand. . . . As nurses we couldn't even get up to them. They were the lowest priority. . . . They'd be taken care of after the military was taken care of. We did get up there a couple of days later. We did manage to start some IV's . . . some had to be catheterized. We didn't have enough beds for all of them. We had patients on the floor on litters . . . but somehow we managed. Eventually those who had to have surgery were taken care of and you know, I don't have any recollection of where our POW's went; where we sent them back to. We must have sent them back somewhere because we didn't continue to have them. . . .

"The hospital was hit with a round of mortar during this time. Fortunately, it landed on the clinics. It was night . . . so there was nobody in the clinics. However, it did also hit one portion of our orthopedic ward. There was not a great deal of injury to any of the patients but one of our corpsmen was hit with a piece of shrapnel that had ricochetted from the metal medicine cabinet and hit his eye. He had to be evacuated . . . we were afraid he was going to lose his eye.

"We, of course, kept no hours at this time. One worked as long as there was work. There was no such thing as time off, 7-7, or 3-11, or whatever. I had a tremendous staff and a lot of effort was put in by all the girls. . . . So, we made it through `Tet.' We were happy that we did. . . .

"[A] request had gone in [to BuMed] around the time of `Tet,' for more nurses. The [Navy nurses] received very hurry-up orders. There were six of them. I believe they had something like forty-eight or . . . seventy-two hours notice to be out on the West Coast [Stateside] and be ready to fly off to Vietnam. . . . Our complement was now up to 24 nurses so we were able to cover the hospital and cover it well. . . .

"Many of the nurses going to the ships [hospital ships] or coming from the ships - all of them would land in Da Nang and if the ships were out, they would stay with us until the ship [came] in. We had a lot of nurses coming through that, maybe, spent a few days with us. I think many of them were glad to get out to the ship; they spent a night or two under the bed. I remember one nurse that was with us during the `Tet' period and when she left us to go out on the hospital ship, she said, `Well, I'm never going to see you all again; you're all going to be dead.' which was a very cheery goodbye. I haven't run into her since but I'm sure some of our girls did . . . and let her know we all survived. . . .

"I was very happy that I had that assignment and felt very privileged to be the Chief Nurse for that year."[63]

Navy Nurse Alicia Foley arrives in July 1968 for her year of duty at Da Nang and she tells us of another aspect of duty there. "Another thing that I don't know if many people know about, on your off duty time many of the [Navy] nurses would go out and work in the community. There were civilian nurses in Vietnam too, and they took care of the civilians in the civilian hospitals. Our people used to work very closely with them and with the hospital corpsmen group that used to work out in the fields; the nurses would go in, also. I think that's an aspect that not too many people are aware of. Sister Mary was a Vietnamese Nun who had an orphanage in downtown Da Nang. She used to come up and teach us Vietnamese; try to. She spoke some French, but very little English, and we used to try to help support her, too, as much as we could with donations. They used to make French bread so we used to buy our bread from her. She was a love, I often wonder what happened to her.

"I think there were about twenty-six of us [Nurse Corps officers], and we had [male Nurse Corps officers] in anesthesia. . . . [It] was a very wise move that the Navy made in assigning more mature nurses [at Da Nang]. The youngest ones we had, had at least one or two duty stations [prior to Da Nang] and, I think, that really was an asset to us - to have had that experience, not only professionally, but, I think, emotionally."[64]

Chief Nurse Mary Cannon finishes her one year tour at Da Nang. The new Chief Nurse, Helen L. Brooks, replaces her and tells us more; "Not all our patients were surgical. Malaria was the biggest thing we had. These patients were really sick and needed nursing care so much. Not to the extent . . . of the surgical wounds, but they were very, very sick cookies. There were other diseases that there was a tendency to forget about because the war wounds were more dramatic. But, we had two solid big wards, I think they were about 120 [beds] each, that were just for malaria. The nurse on the malaria ward found that whenever we had an alert, all the [patients'] temperatures went down. Come to find out, the coolest place in the ward was underneath the bed on the floor - these were dirt floors at the time, some had concrete which was cool too - so it wasn't long before, when a patient's temperature shot up, we'd just put him on the floor. It was a lot easier than getting ice out and trying to put them under it. We had some thermal blankets too, but it was a lot quicker and easier to put them on the floor under their beds if their temperature went up. A very good treatment for malaria.

"We had one ward of prisoners-of-war. They weren't easy patients. The VC's were not particularly happy about being with us. But, we had some altruistic young men among the corpsmen who did a very good job in taking care of these patients. It takes a very settled mind to take good nursing care of a POW. Some of the nurses resented having to take care of them. . . . Initially we had them in a quonset hut that had air conditioning and these patients hated it. While the Americans were all doing their very best to get any place that was air conditioned; out of the heat of Vietnam. Many wards didn't have it. . . . We decided to swap with the POW's and we did. The POW's were much happier after that."[65]

"Nearly 24,000 patients were hospitalized [at Da Nang] in the calendar year 1968 . . . approximately half were treated for combat wounds or injuries."[66] The hospital ship *Repose* is also accumulating some statistics at this time. "She achieved a new high for patient admissions in a single week, admitting 400 between 26 May and 1 June [1968], and established a new monthly high of 953 (of whom 630 were wounded in action), also in May. . . . By 1 November 1969, 22,610 patients had been admitted and over 34 thousand patients had been treated on an outpatient basis."[67]

From May 1968 to June 1969, the Chief Nurse aboard the *Repose* is Dolores Cornelius. "All the Navy nurses aboard the hospital ship and the corpsmen were volunteers. The doctors were not volunteers for the most part. It was interesting to see the change in a few of the doctors who were disgruntled about duty on the hospital ship; change their attitude and become a real member of the hospital team. There were 32 women assigned on the *Repose*, 30 nurses and 2 Red Cross workers. Since all the nurses were needed on the wards, I had no assistant and took care of orienting new nurses and making out the nurses schedule; everything that a supervisor would normally do, I did as Chief Nurse. . . . We did not have enough nurses so that I could assign one to triage, so I went there during the day and evening when flight quarters was announced [indicating incoming helo with patients]. Our triage was a rather small space in which four to six guerneys could be placed. I felt it was important for the casualties to see a nurse within a few minutes after arriving aboard ship. One or two of the doctors on triage duty objected to my being there, but our Chief of Surgery . . . wanted me in triage. . . . A number of patients told me how pleasantly surprised they were to see a nurse in triage. . . .

"One morning I was in my office with my two [enlisted] assistants when it was announced that the helicopter with our mail was arriving. We looked out the porthole and saw the helicopter preparing to land on the flight deck, then, to our horror, instead of going towards the flight deck, it fell into the water! There was our mail in the water! We didn't even think about the pilot. The ship's crew quickly got into action in boats and the mail bags were retrieved [the pilot was picked up, too]. Much of the mail had to be dried out and some of it 'autoclaved' before mail call could be called. Some of it had become too blurred to read. The contents of many of the packages were ruined. Mail call was so terribly important in Vietnam, so I will just never forget the day that we saw our mail go into the water.

"When a VIP [Very Important Person] came aboard, I would take them around the wards to visit any patients they wanted to see. I recall the day that Secretary of State . . . came aboard. His son was stationed on the *Repose*. I believe he was an Ensign. Anyway, when he came aboard, we were at the DMZ [DeMilitarized Zone] and I had never seen such an entourage of such high ranking officers and dignitaries accompanying him in my life. Mr. . . . wanted to see the patients in the intensive care unit and we saw about five when he motioned to me that he could not go on. He was too deeply moved by these terribly wounded patients. So we left the intensive care unit.

"Subic Bay [in the Philippines] was the place for us to unwind after three months on the line, and a place to recharge our batteries before we went back to Vietnam. Our stay at Subic Bay also gave me a chance to visit with the Chief Nurse at the [U.S.] Naval Hospital there and discuss mutual problems about nursing service. While one hospital ship was in Subic Bay, the other hospital ship, as I recall, stayed up at the DMZ the entire time and did not get back to Da Nang until the second hospital ship returned. . . .

"The year on the *Repose* was a year that I will never forget. There were depressing times when I saw some of the devastating wounds suffered by casualties. There were medical casualties, too. I recall one day that we had a large number of Marines admitted with malaria. They responded well to treatment and were ready to be med-evaced and some, perhaps, even ready to go back to duty. One young Marine in particular, I remember, was up and about and I don't remember whether he was going to be med-evaced or go back to duty, but suddenly he was in a coma and a few days later he died. This was such a shock to see someone respond so well and then suddenly he was gone. So there were depressing time, as I said before, but there were also happy times and rewarding times being there when you were needed. One thing that I wish is that some how we could capture the spirit of camaraderie and co-operation and giving that is found in war time and transfer these feelings to a peace-time atmosphere."[68]

Back to Da Nang and the hospital there. Navy Nurse Joan McIntyre tells us how it is in early 1969; "I was on p.m. duty in the surgical ward when I received a phone call from the Commanding Officer's office stating that a second 'Tet' offensive was about to begin and he was sending all of the nurses who were off duty, from the nurses' quarters to the hospital. We had enough staff on duty so he wasn't sending them for duty. He was sending them up there so that all the nurses would be in one area at the same time in case he felt he had to air evacuate all the nurses out of Da Nang and I was told to prepare beds at the back end of the ward for the nurses coming up. They were to bring their flak jackets, their helmets, no personal gear, be in uniform and I was to get cots ready for them to sleep . . . We got the beds ready and up came all the nurses and I can remember, as each one filed in, there was an awful lot of grumbling. They were very, very unhappy that they . . . had been ordered out of the nurses' quarters up to this area of the ward so that they might be air evacuated out, if possible. We were fortunate enough that the attack that night was not severe enough to warrant all the nurses being air evacuated. The next morning, the Chief Nurse with two or three other nurses went to the Commanding Officer and, very adamantly, told him we did not want this to happen again. That if the patients couldn't be air evacuated out then we didn't want to be air evacuated out and we all felt this way. No one in the group of nurses wanted to leave. They wanted to stay and do their job."[69]

On 25 August 1969, Da Nang's Chief Nurse Frances J. Jacobson writes a letter to Captain Veronica Bulshefski, Director of the Navy Nurse Corps. She says, in part, "Ward 1B was hit by a mortar shell about 0325 on Tuesday, August 12. It landed on the air conditioning equipment outside of the ward and blew a jagged hole on the inside of the ward. Patients were sprayed with flying fragments and fourteen required surgery. For most of the patients, the injuries were minor. The night corpsman was not hurt, neither was LCDR Joan McNair who was approaching the ward from outside after making rounds on another ward. She quickly summoned help from triage and within a few minutes, all of the patients had been checked for wounds and the injured had been transferred to Triage. The operating room was extremely busy for the next several hours caring for our wounded and casualties from other hostile action as well.

"A second mortar shell hit an operating room not in use, destroying a great deal of equipment with a great blast of bullet-like fragments. Fragments of metal passed through a wall . . . injuring two tecnicians, the one on the top bunk more seriously. A heavy door standing upright behind the bunk probably saved his life by absorbing some of the fragments around his head. Some fragments passed through the door into his arm and legs and he required extensive debridement and repair although no bones were broken. . . . LCDR Johnnie Bizzelle was walking on the ramp and saw the shells hit. They came in rapid succession and she was able to flatten herself out on the walkway for protection. Fragments rained down on the roof over the ramp but none came through so she was unhurt except for bruises. There were several air-bursts . . . one over the tennis courts in back of our quarters. Fragments from this air burst splattered against the sides and roof of our huts. Needless to say, every nurse was already under her bunk before I could get to each hut.

"There were eleven shells altogether, nine of them on or over the hospital and two just outside our perimeter. There seems to be little doubt that they were aimed at the hospital . . . particularly after the attack on the Convalescent Hospital at Cam Ranh Bay. . . .

"All of the staff responded very well and now that we are veterans, we are less complacent and realize how vulnerable we are. . . .

"On Saturday night about 2030, 23 August, an unidentified person tossed a canister of tear gas in the front door of the nurses' quarters. Fortunately, about 10 of the nurses had gone to a party earlier so only a few of us were left. It served one very useful purpose - we all tried out our gas masks and the experience probably seasoned us just a little bit more. . . . It's a little exasperating to know that one of our own people would do something like that just for the sake of harassment.

"All of the new nurses have reported aboard, the last two . . . on the day of the tear gas. I am sure they will remember the day for a long time."

Navy Nurse Alicia Foley has finished her tour in Da Nang and is on her way back home. "We had heard from people who had been back how poorly treated the military were when they got back to the States, and coming back to California we really were a little more anxious than we were in Da Nang, about how we would be treated. We had to travel in uniform. We stayed in a motel overnight and then we went to the airport and I was going to Bremerton to visit a friend of mine before I went back East. We were passing time looking in the gift shop. We were in our uniforms, and this woman kept looking at us and I said, `Nadine, something is going to come.' This woman came over and said, 'Are you Navy nurses?' We said, 'Yes,' we were. She said, 'Do you know anything about a hospital in Da Nang?' and we said, `Yes,' that's where we were stationed. She put her arms around us and she started to cry. She said her brother was wounded in Vietnam and they took him to the Naval Hospital in Da Nang and he often spoke about how wonderfully well he was treated. She said, `I'm so glad to have a chance to say thank you to somebody who might have taken care of my boy.' So, to me, that was a very pleasant surprise."[70]

A note here about the fact that from September 1967 and April 1969, three <u>male</u> Navy Nurse Corps officers are assigned to Marine Divisions in Vietnam.[71] And, on the other side of the world in October 1969, the one Nurse Corps billet at London, England is deleted.[72]

Back in Washington, D.C., at the BuMed Nursing Division, Captain Bulshefski and Commander Sterner make another verbal presentation on 10 January 1969, to an OP-NAV (NAVal OPerations) group requesting 100 enlisted billets for FY '70. (These billets to be for the Hospital Candidate Program to help obtain more nurses.) We had to place 100 of our Nurse Corps billets 'in hock' but we obtained the enlisted billets. The 100 'in hock' was not difficult because we had such a shortage of Navy nurses at this time, we knew we would have more than 100 Nurse Corps billets unfilled for FY '70, anyhow. At this time, OP-NAV recognizes our shortage problems and requests us to submit a Program Change Request for 125 enlisted billets beginning in FY '71 and through the out-years. Then in February 1969, the Chief of Naval Personnel approves another Nurse Corps' Candidate Program addendum which allows "selection of registered nurse student anesthetists into the Navy Candidate Program. Selected students from approved anesthesia schools [are] commissioned as Ensigns six months prior to graduation. Selectees [receive] pay and allowances but no tuition."[73] In March of 1969, a meeting is held with the CO of the Navy Medical School and with Navy Nurse Anesthetist CDR K. Wilson (stationed at the Medical School) to prepare an announcement of this new program to go to all approved Anesthesia Schools, Recruiting Nurses, and Nurse Corps Anesthetists. This is a program to help provide desperately needed nurse anesthetists for the Nurse Corps. The next Nursing Division action to help the shortage, is to request the Chief of Naval Personnel for a Continuation Board to retain selected LCdr Navy Nurse Corps officers. The 1967 Promotion Legislation makes it mandatory that LCdrs who have been 'passed over' (not selected for promotion) a certain number of times, must be discharged from active duty. So this request is for keeping these people on active duty, at least for another year, to help during the shortage. The request is approved and the first Continuation (retention) Board is held in September 1969. Yet another avenue of help is opened in the Augmentation Board route. This is the Board that meets to approve or disapprove requests from Reserve Nurse Corps officers to switch from being Reserve to Regular Navy. Heretofore, the Reserve nurse had to request selection and the Board would say 'yes' or 'no' based on the officer's record and recommendation. In October, Director Bulshefski's request for Augmentation Board changes, is approved. "The Board would not only consider forwarded requests but would now also review and select those best qualified and eligible and **invite** them to augment."[74]

The next event is in December of 1969 when a Nurse Corps officer is "first assigned to full-time duty as a member of the Naval Medical Inspector General's team."[75] Captain Anna Byrnes is the first nurse assigned this duty. She had already had some experience at this because, before this time, different members of the Director's staff (and, at times, the Director herself) had been given TAD (Temporary Additional Duty) orders to go on a trip with the IG's (Inspector General's) team. One Nurse Corps officer to go with the team for each trip and there were several trips made each year. Captain Byrnes says, "It was a great way to travel because all the arrangements were made by someone else. I never had to worry about plane tickets. I got the schedule that said we left at a certain time from Dulles or [National airport] Washington. The airplane tickets were procured and all that kind of thing. We visited the medical, not all the medical facilities in the world, but a good many of them. I was concerned with the nursing aspects in the hospitals or the clinics, the dispensaries. Usually, when we went in [the Navy medical facility], we had an orientation [briefed by the CO or his appointed representatives] and we went [through] the hospital [or facility]. Nurses were encouraged . . . to speak to me privately if they had problems. Then at the end of our week or three or four days, or whatever time we spent at the hospital, we had a critique [usually with the CO and Chief Nurse and/or other senior officers]. The good things about the hospital, nursing service or the administration were brought up, but also the parts that needed improvement or change. Sometimes we were welcomed and everybody was happy and sometimes we left under a cloud. But that was our job. . . . We tried to be kind and truthful."[76] But, the hospitals and medical facilities have to comply with all the rules set by the Navy and by JCAH hospital regulations and accrediting organizations. The Inspecting Team helps them in achieving and maintaining these standards. Anna Byrnes continues, "[At] another hospital that we went to, there were many problems. When we left, after the critique, the CO didn't say good-bye or anything. We just made our way to the front door . . . The CO wasn't very pleased with our critique. So we got in our cars and went off and said, `Well, that was what is known as a cold send-off.' But, almost every place we went, we were graciously received and whatever criticism we had was taken kindly. . . . After so many weeks or months, they [the inspected facility] had to send in a report that they had changed or [corrected] whatever it was that was a problem during inspection."[77]

Now, let's take a break and have a short run-down on the 'surroundings' of nursing in the 1960's. Intensive Care Units are just starting to emerge and in Obstetrics, rooming-in is starting (babies room-in with mother.) Medications are being added to the IV's on the wards, not in the Pharmacy. Narcotics are in vials, except for Demerol which comes in Tubex. Some narcotics are still tablets that nurses have to dissolve and even be able to figure out dosages from the resultant solution. Remember the formula? (What you want over what you have, times the amount you want to dissolve it in.) Penicillin is in powder form in vials and has to be mixed before administering. Not all wards have a 'crash' cart for emergencies. Navy nurses on night duty in hospitals can expect to cover 5 wards. RN's did not start IV's. RN's did not draw arterial blood. Circle electric beds are a rarity and Stryker and Foster frames are used. Central Supply Room personnel have to count thermometers, suture sets, glass syringes and a multitude of other items.[78] If you don't have a used suture set to turn in, you have to beg on bended knee and pledge your very existence to get a clean one. (I used to send the Senior Corpsman on the ward, down to CSR when the nurse wasn't there. The Senior Corpsman knew some of the CSR Corpsmen and so our ward got a couple of clean sets sometimes, when the need was dire.)

"The 1950's and 1960's were a revolutionary time for health care: `A sampling of major advances during the two decades includes the development of the heart-lung machine, open heart surgery, cardiac catheterization, renal dialysis, laser surgery, high frequency implements for blood coagulation, and new vaccines, pharmaceuticals, and monitoring devises. The expanding field of medical science had made nursing care increasingly more complex and had made demands of increasing gravity on nurses as well. To effectively give care, nurses needed to be able to identify very subtle changes in patients' status, learn new sophisticated treatment techniques, increase their ability to interpret laboratory data, recognize delicate physiological interrelationships, and closely monitor the efficacy of potent and sometimes experimental forms of drug therapy.'[79] "[80]

"In the 1950s and 1960s, 15 Black schools closed (Carnegie. 1964). There was a noticeable decrease in the registered Black nurse population during these years as the number of would-be admissions to the closed Black schools was not absorbed by the existing White schools. In fact, in 1969, while Blacks made up the largest minority group in the United States (more than 11%), the percentage of Blacks graduating from schools of nursing leading to registered nurse licensure was only 3.2."[81]

In other happenings; on the 20th of July 1969, "Former Navy pilot Neil Armstrong becomes the first man to set foot on the moon and places an American flag on the Sea of Tranquility."[82] And, on earth, some things are much less then tranquil. "The attainment of peace proved more elusive than the moon. In Paris peace negotiators bickered even over the shape of the conference table. Communist rockets again fell on Saigon; U.S. B-52s bombed near the Cambodian border; and the American death toll rose to nearly 40,000 - more than were killed in the Korean War. . . . [President] Nixon vowed he would not be swayed by antiwar protests, but he began to withdraw American troops from Vietnam. As the 1960's drew to an end, the nation was stunned by reports of American atrocities in Vietnam. Borrowing Viet Cong tactics, U.S. soldiers had massacred villagers in My Lai and Song My. `It has been an awful decade,' author Richard Rovere wrote in the *New York Times*, `a slum of a decade.'"[83]

Vietnam protest,"far from dormant, did not fade. An organized Vietnam Moratorium Day to demand 'peace now' was marked in October 1969 by demonstrations across the country, with 100,000 rallying on Boston Common to Hear Senator Edward Kennedy call for withdrawal of all ground forces within a year and all air and support units within three years, by the end of 1972. . . . A second Vietnam Moratorium Day, in November, mobilized 250,000 demonstrators in Washington."[84] On the 15th of December, "The President announces a 50,000-man reduction in Vietnam, bringing the total ordered home for the year to 110,000."[85]

"[In] April 1970, furor erupted when American ground forces together with ARVN invaded Cambodia.

To widen the war to another, nominally neutral, country when the cry in America was to reduce rather than extend belligerence was . . . the most provocative choice possible in the circumstances. . . . Nixon supposed that his previously announced schedule of with-drawing 150,000 troops in 1970 would cancel protest or, if 'those liberal bastards' were going to make trouble anyway, that he might as well be hanged for a wolf as a sheep. He announced the campaign in a combative speech as a response to North Vietnamese 'aggression,' with familiar references to not being a President who would preside over American defeat. . . . The overall result was negative: a weakened government in Phnom Penh [Cambodia] left in need of protection, land and villages wrecked, a third of the population made homeless refugees, and the pro-Communist Khmer Rouge greatly augmented by recruits. The North Vietnamese soon returned to over-run large areas, arm and train the insurgents and lay the ground for the ultimate tragic suffering of another nation of Indochina.

"Reaction in America to the invasion was explosive, antagonizing both political extremes, impassioning debate, kindling the hate of dissenters for the government and vice versa. . . . [Following] Cambodia, Americans killed Americans. On 4 May, at Kent State University in Ohio, the National Guard, called out by the Governor to contain what appeared to him dangerous campus violence, opened fire on the demonstrators, killing four students. . . . Protest blazed after Kent State. Student strikes, marches, bonfires caught up the campuses. An angry crowd of close to 100,000 massed in the park across from White House grounds, where a ring of sixty buses with police was drawn up like a wagon circle against the Indians. At the Capitol, Vietnam veterans staged a rally marked by each man tossing away his medals. . . . The antagonism was epitomized in physical clash when construction workers in hard hats attacked a march of student protesters in Wall Street, beating them with whatever they had at hand for use as weapons. It reached a peak in October at San Jose, where Nixon came to speak in the mid-term election campaign of 1970. He was greeted by a mob screaming oaths and obscenities and, when he left the hall, throwing eggs and rocks, one just grazing him. It was the first mob assault on a President in American history."[86] To top things off, "Paris peace talks end their second full year without progress toward peace in Vietnam."[87]

Meantime, in 1970, the costs of health care keep rising. "Hospital care costs in U.S. reach average of $81 per patient per day."[88] And, the costs of medical education keeps rising. Numbers of student nurses and would be student nurses find the prices prohibitive. This only tends to increase the shortage of nurses and, ultimately, it affects the Navy Nurse Corps. As a matter of fact, it is affecting all the Military Nurse Corps, to the extent that in some Congressional Hearings on Army Military Personnel, one of the subjects is: "Nurse Shortage. Plans to improve?"[89] In February 1970, a BuMed memo, signed by Captain Bulshefski, outlines the steps taken, during her regime, to help reduce the Navy Nurse Corps Officer shortage by increasing all the input programs:

The Hospital Candidate Program was increased from 25 to 150 billets; to start in FY '71.

The Collegiate Candidate Program was increased from 150 to 250 billets; to start in FY '71.

The Navy Enlisted Nursing Education Program increased from 40 to 70 billets; to start in FY '71.

The Nurse Corps Anesthesia Candidate program started in 1969.

This same memo then lists other steps taken:

Approval obtained for a special Continuation Board to continue selected LCdrs on active duty.

Approval obtained for a Continuing Augmentation Board to invite selectees to augment to Regular Navy.

Request submitted for a more equitable revision of service credit for nurses entering the Navy.

Full Time Duty Under Instruction billets increased from 45 to 90; to start in FY '71.

Clinical short courses (six months or less) increased to extend clinical specialty knowledge.

Last, but not least, recruiting efforts increased.[90]

In 1965, the year before Captain Bulshefski became Director, the end strength of the Nurse Corps was 1870 Nurse Corps Officers. In 1970, the year that Captain Bulshefski retires, the end strength of the Nurse Corps is 2273.

Captain Veronica M. Bulshefski, Director of the Navy Nurse Corps, retires on 1 May 1970. "Under her directorship, the Nurse Corps progressed to an unprecedented state of readiness and Nurse Corps requirements and billets were restructured to meet the current needs of nursing practice. . . . During her naval service she was awarded the American Theater Medal, WWII medal, the Asiatic Pacific Campaign Medal and the Legion of Merit."[91]

When asked what she felt was the highlight of her career, she answered, "I think being the Director of the Nurse Corps was my highlight . . . also, getting the Rank Bill passed for the Navy Nurse Corps. I think it was a legacy [for] the Nurse Corps because there were so many hurdles I had to get over. . . . After it was passed and signed by the President and when the bill came out, everybody stood in our way. They didn't want us to have the number of Captains or Commanders that we were allowed. I remember one incident; I had a memorandum on my desk stating that I'd have to agree that some Board would have to select the number of Captains and Commanders. . . . I didn't understand this but I knew that it was somebody's dirty work. After I read the memorandum and deliberated on it a little while, . . . I called . . . the Judge Advocate's Office. . . . I said, `I have this memorandum before me, does this mean we'll get more Captains and Commanders?' And he said, `Absolutely not. Hell no, you'll get less.' And I said, `Oh, is that right?' So I didn't sign that thing. Everybody was encouraging me to sign it but I didn't. Then later it came time for a selection board and we had to have the Surgeon General . . . sign that we [Navy nurses] would be included on the selection board. I couldn't get him to sign the papers. So one morning I went over there [to the Surgeon General's Office] and I sort of, in a back-handed way, . . . got him to sign the paper. And that's how our Nurse Corps Bill was enacted. . . . The Bill allowed for the Head of the Nurse Corps to be an Admiral and [allowed] for the additional Captains and Commanders. Without all this maneuvering we would never have had a Nurse Corps Bill. . . . There were so many stumbling blocks, I can't really enumerate them all. . . . Captain Doris Sterner was my billet officer and she would prepare the position papers. Because of those position papers, we [will] have an Admiral and increased Captains. . . . It's very difficult, you know, to get things."[92]

Captain Bulshefski retired to her home in Alexandria, Virginia until her death in May 1995. She was interred in Arlington National Cemetery with full military honors on 6 June 1995.

[1]   Information prepared by the Navy Nurse Corps Officers on the staff of the Director of the Navy Nurse Corps, 2 May 1966.

[2]   Bulshefski, Veronica M. Captain, Navy Nurse Corps, *Oral History Interview Tape Transcript*, Interviewers Captain Doris M. Sterner Nurse Corps and Dr. Lynne Dunn of the Naval Historical Center of Washington, D.C., 18 October 1988.

[3]   Information prepared by the Navy Nurse Corps Officers on the staff of the Director of the Navy Nurse Corps, September 1995.

[4]   "Chronology of the Sea Service, 1960 to the Present," All Hands, Magazine of the U.S. Navy, October 1975, Number 705, p. 52.

[5]   Elsass, Phyllis J. Captain, Navy Nurse Corps, *Oral History Interview Tape Transcript*, Self-interview, 5 May 1990.

[6]   Halverson, Ruth E. Captain, Navy Nurse Corps, *Oral History Interview Tape Transcript*, Interviewer Captain Doris M. Sterner Nurse Corps, 10 July 1990.

[7]   Eberharter, Virginia M. Commander, Navy Nurse Corps, *Oral History Interview Tape Transcript*, Self-interview, 5 August 1990.

[8]   O'Connell, Anne L. Commander, Navy Nurse Corps, *Oral History Interview Tape Transcript*, Self-interview, 1 September 1989.

[9]   The World Book Encyclopedia, Field Enterprises Educational Corporation, Chicago, Volume 14, 1966 edition, p. 80.

[10]   Pejic, Rade LT Medical Corps, et al, editors, *Cruise Book of the US Navy Hospital Ship Repose Republic of Vietnam 1969-1970*, Taylor Publishing Company [Yearbook Publisher], p. 5. Supplied through courtesy of Captain Rachel Fine NC USN (Ret.).

[11]   *Welcome Aboard U.S.S. Repose AH-16*, A pamphlet prepared for visitors and members of the press that come aboard the ship, Pamphlet contains the signatures of the Commanding Officer of the Ship and the Commanding Officer of the Ship's Hospital, circa 1966.

[12]   Kovacevich, Mary T. Captain Navy Nurse Corps, *U.S.S. Repose - Service In Vietnam*, circa 1966 and 1967, pp. 3, 4.

[13]   Information from BuMed, 1981.

[14]   Cronin, Claire M. Captain, Navy Nurse Corps, *Oral History Interview Tape Transcript*, Interviewer LT Helen Barry Siragusa Nurse Corps, 1 March 1991.

[15]   *The 1968 World Book Year Book*, Annual Supplement to The World Book Encyclopedia, Field Enterprises Educational Corporation, Chicago, 1968, p. 310.

[16]   "USS Repose in Vietnam - 1966-1970," *U.S. Navy Medicine*, Vol. 55, No.4, April 1970, p. 7.

[17]   McKown, F. Carroll Captain, Navy Nurse Corps, *Oral History Interview Tape Transcript*, Self-interview, 21 May 1991.

[18]   Martin, Kathleen LCdr, Navy Nurse Corps, *Oral History Interview Tape Transcript*, Interviewer LT Helen Barry Siragusa Nurse Corps, 26 March 1991.

[19]   McKown, F. Carroll Captain, Navy Nurse Corps, op. cit..

[20]   Ibid..

[21]   McClendon, Jr., CDR F.O. MSC, USN, "From The Annals Of Naval Support Activity, Danang, Republic of Vietnam," *U.S. Navy Medical Newsletter*, Volume 55, March 1970, p. 11.

[22]   Cannon, Mary F. Captain, Navy Nurse Corps, *Oral History Interview Tape Transcript*, Self-interview, 8 January 1990.

[23]   Nagy, Bettye G. Captain, Navy Nurse Corps, *Oral History Interview Tape Transcript*, Interviewer LCdr Margaret (Linn) Larson Nurse Corps, 15 July 1988.

24   Sheridan, Anne M. CDR, Navy Nurse Corps, *Oral History Interview Tape Transcript*, Interviewer CDR Barbara Ellis Nurse Corps, 11 March 1988.
25   Updated *History of the Nurse Corps, U.S. Navy*, by the Navy Nurse Corps Officers on the staff of the Director of the Navy Nurse Corps, 5727.1, OONCA/np, revised 24 April 1991, p. 20.
26   "A 1971 View of the Medical Corps Circa 1871," *U.S. Navy Medicine*, Vol. 57, No. 3, 1971, p. 52.
27   Hummel, Sue Smoker Captain, Navy Nurse Corps, *Oral History Interview Tape Transcript*, Interviewer LT Helen Barry Siragusa Nurse Corps, 29 January 1991.
28   Updated *History of the Nurse Corps, U.S. Navy*, op. cit., p. 21.
29   O'Dell, Beverly Brase Captain, Navy Nurse Corps, *Oral History Interview Tape Transcript*, Self-interview, 22 May 1991.
30   Moris, Patricia Joan Captain, Navy Nurse Corps, *Oral History Interview Tape Transcript*, Interviewer Tonya Emory, Clinical Nurse at the VA Medical Center in Boise, Idaho, 19 September 1990.
31   Updated *History of the Nurse Corps, U.S. Navy*, op. cit..
32   Department of Defense, "Health Personnel Manpower - Quarter Ending 31 December 1967," DAOSD (H&M), 27 February 1968.
33   Floyd, Candace, *America's Great Disasters*, Mallard Press, An imprint of BDD Promotional Books Company, Inc., 666 Fifth Ave., New York, N.Y. 10103, 1990, p. 168.
34   *The 1968 World Book Year Book*, op. cit., p. 10.
35   Ibid., p. 11.
36   Ibid., p. 12.
37   Tuchman, Barbara W., *The March of Folly From Troy to Vietnam*, Ballantine Books, New York, 1985, p. 339.
38   Ibid., pp. 348, 349.
39   Ibid., pp. 351, 352.
40   Ibid., p. 352.
41   *The 1969 World Book Year Book*, Annual Supplement to The World Book Encyclopedia, Field Enterprises Educational Corporation, Chicago, 1969, pp. 9-12.
42   Tuchman, Barbara W., op. cit., p. 357.
43   "Chronology of the Sea Service, 1960 to the Present," op. cit., p. 54.
44   *200 Years, A Bicentennial Illustrated History of the United States*, Joseph Newman, Directing Editor, Books by U.S. News & World Report, Inc., 2300 N Street, N.W., Washington, D.C. 20037, 1973, book, book 2, p. 273.
45   *The 1969 World Book Year Book*, op. cit., p. 12.
46   *200 Years, A Bicentennial Illustrated History of the United States*, op. cit., p. 272.
47   *The 1969 World Book Year Book*, op. cit., p. 9.
48   Ibid., p. 10.
49   *200 Years, A Bicentennial Illustrated History of the United States*, op. cit., p. 274.
50   Kalisch, Philip A., PhD, and Kalisch, Beatrice J., EdD, RN, FAAN, *The Advance of American Nursing*, J.B. Lippincott Company, Philadelphia, 1995, p. 435.
51   Ibid..
52   Updated *History of the Nurse Corps, U.S. Navy*, op. cit., p. 22.
53   Harrington, Phyllis Captain, Navy Nurse Corps, Handwritten notation on back of a signed Interviewee Agreement, dated 12 August 1991.
54   Updated *History of the Nurse Corps, U.S. Navy*, op. cit., p. 21.
55   Vitillo, Angelica Captain, Deputy Director Navy Nurse Corps, Letter to Chiefs, Nursing Service and Senior Nurse Corps Officers, BUMED-324-nr, 22 April 1968.
56   Ibid., p. 22.
57   Sterner, Doris M. CDR, Code 323, Nursing Division, BuMed, "Code 323 Planning," BUMED-323-jg, 27 March 1969, p.1.
58   Updated *History of the Nurse Corps, U.S. Navy*, op. cit., p. 22.
59   Sterner, Doris M. CDR, Code 323, op. cit..
60   Updated *History of the Nurse Corps, U.S. Navy*, op. cit..
61   Ibid..
62   Sheridan, Anne M. CDR, Navy Nurse Corps, op. cit..
63   Cannon, Mary F. Captain, Navy Nurse Corps, op. cit..
64   Foley, Alicia M. Captain, Navy Nurse Corps, *Oral History Interview Tape Transcript*, Interviewer Captain Doris M. Sterner Nurse Corps, 29 January 1991.
65   Brooks, Helen L. Captain, Navy Nurse Corps, *Oral History Interview Tapes Transcripts*, Self interview, 27 July 1990.
66   McClendon, Jr., CDR F.O. MSC, USN, op. cit., p. 13.
67   Code 15, BUMED, "Angel of the Orient," *U.S. Navy Medical Newsletter*, Volume 55, April 1970, p. 12.
68   Cornelius, Dolores Captain, Navy Nurse Corps, *Oral History Interview Tapes Transcripts*, Self interview, 28 December 1989.
69   McIntyre, Joan CDR, Navy Nurse Corps, *Oral History Interview Tapes Transcripts*, Self interview, 12 October 1989.
70   Foley, Alicia M. Captain, Navy Nurse Corps, op. cit..
71   Information from BuMed, 1981.
72   Updated *History of the Nurse Corps, U.S. Navy*, op. cit., p. 23.
73   Ibid., p. 22.
74   Ibid., pp. 22, 23.
75   Ibid., p. 23.
76   Byrnes, Anna Captain, Navy Nurse Corps, *Oral History Interview Tape Transcript*, Interviewer Captain Madeline M. Ancelard Nurse Corps, 11 May 1990.
77   Ibid..

78   Holmes, Sandra Captain, Navy Nurse Corps, Letter to author re recollections of the 1960's and 1970's., 1 October 1995.

79   This is footnoted as a quote from M.L. Fitzpatrick, *Prologue to Professionalism*, Robert J. Brady Co., Bowie, Maryland, 1983, pp. 34-35.

80   Donahue, M. Patricia Ph.D., R.N., *NURSING The Finest Art*, The C.V. Mosby Co., St. Louis, Toronto, Princeton, 1985, pp. 446, 447.

81 Carnegie, Mary Elizabeth, D.D.A., R.N., F.A.A.N., *The Path We Tread: Blacks in Nursing, 1854-1984*, J.B. Lippincott Co., Philadelphia, 1986, p. 44.

82   "Chronology of the Sea Service, 1960 to the Present," op. cit., p. 55.

83   *200 Years, A Bicentennial Illustrated History of the United States*, op. cit., pp. 275, 276.

84   Tuchman, Barbara W., op. cit., pp. 361, 362.

85   "Chronology of the Sea Service, 1960 to the Present," op. cit., p. 56.

86   Tuchman, Barbara W., op. cit., pp. 364-366.

87   Grun, Bernard, *The Timetables of History*, Based on Werner Stein's *Kulturfahrplan*, Simon & Schuster/Touchstone, New York, 1991, p. 568.

88   Ibid., p. 569.

89   Bulshefski, Veronica Director Navy Nurse Corps, Memorandum from Code 32 to Code 3, "Subject: Nurse Shortage; Plans to improve," 25 February 1970.

90   Ibid..

91   Information prepared by the Navy Nurse Corps Officers on the staff of the Director of the Navy Nurse Corps, circa 1990, op. cit..

92   Bulshefski, Veronica M. Captain, Navy Nurse Corps, *Oral History Interview Tape Transcript*, op. cit..

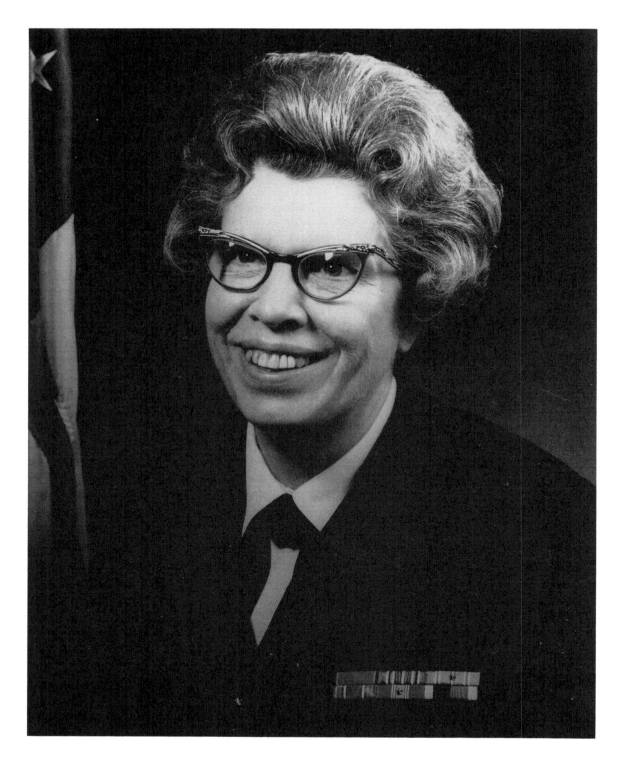

Director - Rear Admiral Alene B. Duerk NC USN
(Official U.S. Navy photo courtesy of Nursing Division, Bureau of Medicine and Surgery, Navy Department.)

CHAPTER 13

Director - Captain Alene Duerk
(1970 - 1972)
Rear Admiral Alene Duerk
(1972 - 1975)

☆ ☆ ☆

On the 11th of February 1970, the Secretary of the Navy announces "the appointment of Captain Alene Bertha Duerk as the next Director of the Navy Nurse Corps. Captain Duerk is presently serving as Chief of Nursing Service at the Naval Hospital, Great Lakes, Illinois."[1] Captain Duerk leaves Great Lakes, finds accommodations in the Washington, DC area then takes the oath of office and becomes the twelfth Director of the Navy Nurse Corps on 1 May 1970.

Alene B. Duerk was born in Defiance, Ohio in March 1920. She took her nurses training at the three-year diploma school of nursing at Toledo Hospital, also in Ohio, graduating in 1941. "I joined the Navy in 1943, I was in the Reserves at that time, so I served from March 1943 until January 1946 at which time I was released to inactive duty in the Reserves. Then, in the fall, I went back to school and . . . completed my degree in 1948."[2] Her Bachelor of Science Degree in Ward Management and Teaching, was earned at Case Western Reserve University in Cleveland, Ohio. "Then I taught for two years at Highland Park Hospital in Detroit and then, because I was still interested in the Navy . . . I joined one [of the Reserve Units] . . . I really enjoyed going [to the Reserve meetings]."[3] Then, in 1951, she was recalled to active duty because of the Korean Conflict. In 1953 she transferred to the Regular Navy, having decided to stay in the Navy Nurse Corps.

Her career pattern was wide and varied. "She was assigned to Naval Hospitals in Portsmouth, Virginia; Bethesda, Maryland; Philadelphia, Pennsylvania. She served aboard the hospital ship U.S.S. *Benevolence* in 1945."[4] Admiral Duerk says of this tour, "The mission that we had was that we were to join the third fleet for the invasion of Japan, that's what we were going out there for. I didn't know that at the time, but that's what it was. . . . Because we were going out to meet the fleet, we were not under way with a convoy. We were just sort of sailing out there on our own. We didn't join the convoy until we were in Eniwetok. . . . It was while we were on our way to Japan that the [atomic] bombs were dropped and the war was over. So we then came into Tokyo Bay at the end of August before the peace treaty was signed and we went in and rescued people from two prisoner-of-war camps. . . . General Wainright was on of those people in that prison camp. `Pappy' Boyington was another one who was in prison camp - those two camps that were liberated. It was a very tense and exciting time, really. . . . Mine sweepers were ahead of us as we went into Tokyo Bay. The Japanese had cut the mine nets and so the mines were floating all around us. And, the ships were along side shooting the mines out of the water so the area was clear."[5]

Her career also included, "Hospital Corps School instructor in Portsmouth, Virginia and recruiter in Chicago, Illinois. Rear Admiral Duerk was Assistant Chief Nurse, Naval Hospital Yokosuka, Japan and Chief Nurse at Navy Dispensary, Long Beach, California; Hospital Corps School, San Diego, California and Naval Hospital, Great Lakes."[6] Then there were the two special assignments: one with the Assistant Secretary of Defense for Health and Environment and the other as Nurse Corps Liaison at BuPers (Bureau of Naval Personnel).

"One of my biggest problems when I first came in [as Director] was to recruit enough nurses or to at least get some kind of program that we would be able to attract nurses to come into the Navy. We needed more people. . . . Vietnam was still going one and we had to have people in the pipeline. . . . So that was one of my goals; to increase the numbers. . . . [We had the] Navy Enlisted Nursing Education Program that had already started but,

. . . we were able to take more people in - it was increased and we set up boards for selection. We saw a really great need for people who had further education because a lot of our nurses were diploma nurses and we had, also, nurses who had Bachelor degrees who were interested in going for Masters and we saw that that was going to be a thing that we would have to do in the future. So our programs, our educational programs, became more active.

In order to get more nurses, we had the program for the student who was in the Bachelors program where we assisted them in the junior and senior year or in the last year and . . . we also had some assistance for students who were in a diploma program. . . . We never gave assistance to the Associate Degree program at that time, because what we were aiming for was an 'all-degree' Corps. So we felt that we should not assist the Associate Degree at that time. . . . The educational programs, I think, helped the Corps. [In 1952 only 1.4% had a Bachelor of Science degree, by 1970 51% of the Corps had a B.S. or higher degree.] And then, I'd also like to [mention] one other thing and that is that, during the time that I was Director, I was very fortunate. I had not only a Surgeon General who I could work with, and we were very compatible, but also the CNO [Chief of Naval Operations] who was very compatible. I was permitted to have direct contact with [Navy] nurses in the field. I was able to call them up and ask them whether they would be interested in taking an assignment. They could call me at any time; we broke down a lot of the barriers . . . that sort of thing. . . . For that period of time, it worked and I felt that I was much closer to the people in the Corps. That was a personal reward of mine. . . . Not only did I have more communication with my Corps, but I had better communication with other women in the Navy and . . . Line men [officers of the 'primary' Navy versus the Support Staff Corps such as the Medical Corps, Supply Corps, Nurse Corps, etc.]. . . . Of course, I also was at an advantage because I had had two years, earlier, in Washington; one [year] at the Pentagon and the other in BuPers. At that time I had met a lot of these people and had worked with them. And, also, that's when I had established some of the communications with people and found that they could talk to me and, I think, they felt I could talk to them. Then when [while Director] I used to go out to the hospitals, I made it a point of always having time, or trying to always have time, to be able to talk to people if they wanted to talk to me. If they didn't, that didn't make any difference, but if they had a problem, or if they just wanted to come in and talk, they did. And that was good."[7]

Meantime, back in February, the Chief Nurse at the Naval Hospital in Corpus Christi, is Captain Dolores Cornelius. She tells us, "I received a phone call from Captain Alene Duerk who was calling me from Great Lakes. Now, I knew that Captain Duerk was going to be the new Director of the Navy Nurse Corps in May of 1970 and I wondered why she was calling me in February. She asked me if I would like to be her Deputy Director. Well, I was stunned but, of course, said yes. So after just seven months at Corpus Christi, I packed my bags for duty at the Nursing Division at the Bureau of Medicine and Surgery in Washington, DC. During my short tour at Corpus Christi, I had been selected and promoted to the rank of Captain.

"Little did I realize, as I was packing out of my apartment at Corpus Christi, that it would be the last time that I would see my household goods that were being transferred to Washington, DC. . . . All my household goods, which were transferred, were destroyed in a warehouse fire in the Washington, DC area. They suspected that the fire was started by arson. The only things that I had left were what I was able to take in the car with me.

"Being stationed at the Bureau of Medicine and Surgery opened up a whole new world to me. I wish that more nurses in the Navy could have the experience of being stationed at BuMed.

"The years 1970 to 1971 were difficult for our country. The Vietnam war was very unpopular. Demonstrations were frequent and sometimes even violent. I lived in Arlington, Virginia and crossed the Lincoln Memorial Bridge to get to work. One morning, during a demonstration, there were bodies lying practically the entire length of the Bridge. The police were finally able, after a considerable amount of time, to clear the bridge so that traffic could pass through."[8]

One more item before we leave BuMed and Washington, DC; it is in 1970 that "pregnant women were permitted to stay in the military, though, curiously, their condition remained a 'service-connected disability' until 1975."[9]

At this point in time, with the shortage of nurses and the unpopularity of the war, the Nurse Corps

Recruiters are having a very complicated time. Pressure is on them to secure more nurses for the Corps while they also have to contend with the hazards and difficulties of the hostile and antagonistic atmosphere. Navy Nurse Anne L. O'Connell is a recruiter at this time and says, "I became the recruiter in Boston. . . . It was a difficult time. It was a very difficult time to recruit nurses into the Navy; into any branch of the military. The anti-military, anti-Vietnam war feeling was at its zenith. I can remember taking the insignia off my raincoat and taking my hat off and going out to lunch in Boston, because I would be heckled if I was seen [in uniform] on the streets in Boston. You could only go 'off-time' to the colleges and hospitals [to recruit]. They would not give us classroom time. We had to go in the evening. Sometimes I would drive hours to give a recruiting lecture, to have only three nurses show up. They [the colleges and hospitals] made it strictly voluntary for the students; it was very, very difficult. To show you how difficult recruiting was for the Navy in 1970 . . . the year that I was recruited into the Navy [1963], Navy Nurse Edith Principe recruited 83 nurses out of the Boston district. Seven years later when I was the recruiter, I recruited six, and I worked very hard to get those six nurses."[10]

Over in another part of the world in 1970, is Navy Nurse Ruth Halverson. "I went to become the Senior Nurse in . . . Morocco. I was asked if I would like to go there and I said yes. I was asked by [Captain] Duerk; she called me one day after she became Director. I was most happy because I loved eastern culture and I was real excited to go there. It was a small station hospital; we averaged about twenty to thirty patients. Actually, we were a support unit for a communication station. . . . We got out [off the Base] and shopped and ate frequently with the local people, and I loved them; they were great people. The Base was very adequate. The area we were in was rather hilly and lots of lovely trees. Our nurses' quarters (we had to live on Base) were excellent. It would get very hot in the summer months, the winters were kind of cool, and they also had a rainy season.

"One interesting experience I would like to relate; we were in an attempted assassination on the King's life. Apparently the head of his Air Force tried to kill him during one of his [the King's] birthday parties. He had invited all of our doctors to his golf course; they played golf for the day [since] it was his birthday. The soldiers somehow got into the compound and began to fire on all of them; the King and all of our doctors who were playing golf. Of course, everybody hit the sand dunes, and many of them [the doctors] came back later and showed us their golf bags; they were all riddled with holes. Fortunately, nobody was killed. The King was not killed either, otherwise we would have been evacuated out, immediately. But, the doctors were all stripped of their wallets, wristwatches, and their clothes at gunpoint and they had to come back . . . about twenty miles; they had to walk back in their boxer shorts. We were grounded for almost a month, behind machine guns, on the Base. Nobody was permitted off or anything, because the King was very upset about this and he wanted to make sure that it wasn't any American that had instigated this. The nice thing about it was that part of the 6th Fleet was sitting out in the Atlantic in the event that we would have to be evacuated out of there. We were told to have a little cosmetic kit packed, and, if we got orders, within five minutes to move and [leave] everything else. But . . . the King found out that it was one of his own soldiers who had attempted to assassinate him. [The soldier was killed] by a firing squad and the whole thing quieted down and then we were permitted off Base again."[11] In and out of harm's way, again.

In May 1970, the Dispensary at the Naval Air Station in Bermuda is opened and assigned Nurse Corps officers. Also, the Dispensary at the Naval Station Roosevelt Roads, Puerto Rico is "enlarged to assume total medical services upon closure of Rodriguez Army General Hospital. Additional [Navy] Nurse Corps officers were assigned."[12] (In January 1971 this facility is changed from a Dispensary to a Naval Hospital.[13])

Back in the States, in June of 1970, three Naval Air Station Dispensaries are closed; Olathe, Kansas; Minneapolis, Minnesota; Grosse Isle, Michigan. And, the "Nurse Corps billet at Vallejo, Mare Island, California [is] deleted."[14]

As for male Navy Nurse Corps officers in 1970, a total of seven served with COMPHIBWESTPAC (COMmander amPHIBian forces WESTern PACific) between October 1967 and June 1970. And, seven other male Navy nurses served with MACV in Saigon, Vietnam between May 1968 and December 1970.[15]

Now, once more we turn to the Naval Hospital at Da Nang in Vietnam. This time we hear from an operating room nurse, Lynne Agnew. "We had 12 operating rooms, most of them were going 24 hours a day. . . . Our job was to keep everything moving; coordinating triage with pre-op and the operating room. We had a 'squawk' box up in the corner of our tiny little office which was the voice of the communicator with all of the choppers, helicopters, that were bringing in the wounded. They would tell us how many wounded were coming on what flight and what type of injuries they had, which sort of gave us a good preparation as to what we needed to have on our [instrument] table and [what we needed to] be prepared for. There were four nurses assigned to the operating room. We had 18 units or crews of Navy operating room corpsmen, technicians, in addition to the number that was assigned to the supply unit, CSR. We had enough help as far as the corpsmen were concerned, but we really could have used two more nurses because of times when we were very, very busy and could have used many more hands. . . . Rare was the time when we worked just an eight-hour shift, usually it was ten hours, often twelve hours, and occasionally, once or twice, it was twenty-four hours. . . .

"For those of us in Da Nang together, we each had another person whom we conveyed vital information to so that in the event that we got hit and were killed, that other Nurse Corps officer would be responsible for going with us on our journey home; taking care of any of the personal kind of details that had to be cared for prior to reaching home. We all had our assignments and knew who we were responsible for. That, sort of, gave us a feeling of security in that we knew someone was going to accompany us and that our family wouldn't have to receive our bodies without someone else to sort of cushion the blow, so to speak. So, for the first time, I began to think of my own mortality.

"This now was spring of 1970. During this time . . . the quarters were gassed three times while I was there. That's ordinarily not a fun experience because it's terribly irritating to the eyes, nose and throat and, also, makes one very nauseated. . . .

"Working in surgery during that terrible conflict, was an experience I will never forget. . . . We had so many casualties coming at us, frequently and in big hordes. I remember one night we got in a whole village that had been hit by a sapper. We didn't know it at the very beginning, but they also brought in the Viet Cong person that lobbed in the charges. She was shot in the back as she ran away after setting off the charges. We didn't know that at the time. We had her in the operating room by the time it was determined which one she was. We took the bullet out of her back during that time. . . . She was pretty light under the anesthesia and as she came out of it, she came up off that table and went at the surgeon with the scalpel she grabbed off the Mayo table [small operating room instrument table]. Just about that time I came over to the OR table and grabbed her. The corpsmen, by that time, grabbed both of us because I had a `choke hold' on her. But, by that time the MP's were in the room and we completed putting the bandage on her back and she was escorted to wherever they sent the `brig' patients. . . .

"There were other times when we were in jeopardy as well. There were two specific incidents where we took out live shells; one from an abdomen . . . and the other one was a live shell in a young man's head. The first one was the large shell in the abdomen and none of us knew it was there. Often times we would get the patient before they'd have a chance to develop the x-ray films. He had gone through pre-op very quickly, to x-ray and then right into the operating room. When they brought in the x-rays, we realized that he had a very live shell in him. I was in the middle of prepping his belly at the time. I looked up and the doctor said, `Stop what you're doing right now!' We very, very cautiously moved everything we could away from the OR table, except for the gear that was absolutely needed. . . . There was a shield that was brought in for the doctors and the corpsmen and myself. It was strictly voluntary for us to remain in the room from then on because that shell was apt to go off at any time with any movement of instruments, or a touch, etc.. It really didn't impress upon me initially that this thing was extremely dangerous and could wipe out the entire operating room and perhaps half of the adjoining OR, until I saw the demolition crew coming in with their large box. They were wearing special gloves and gear and head dress and looking pretty serious about the whole situation. When the doctors removed the shell, it was given directly to the demolition squad. They put it in the box and immediately got it out of the OR. They took it out to the bunker and ignited it there. . . . The second incident was during a craniotomy and the shell was removed very quickly once the cranium was entered. . . . We did wear some protective gear, but this shell was considerably smaller than the one that was taken out of the abdomen. For some reason, we didn't feel quite as threatened, but it was still a potential hazard. Incidentally, both of those patients survived. . . .

"One of the doctors came in one day and started screaming. He kept saying he couldn't do it, he couldn't do it. He couldn't chop off another leg today. He just couldn't do it. We tried to get him to calm down but it was to no avail. He continued to scream and he just disintegrated right there in front of our eyes. We finally had to escort him out of the operating room and back to his quarters where he was sedated. Within twenty-four hours he was evacuated home. We all had our various ways of coping with the war, coping with the tragedies, the horrible consequences of war. Humor, of course, was the biggest one, but others withdrew. . . . Some others became very loud, boisterous and acting out. Sometimes you saw a personality or a portion of personality that you never saw under any other conditions, and certainly never saw State-side, if you knew them before. Their personalities changed and it was all in a reaction to the setting of war and the horrible things they had to witness and try to care for."[16]

Another Navy nurse (and future Admiral), Fran Shea (Buckley) tells us how she felt after caring for casualties aboard the hospital ship *Repose* out in Vietnam waters. She says, "From Vietnam I went into the operating room at Chelsea. I really didn't want to do that. I felt I had enough. I wasn't saying that I was worn out from it, but the situation had been so intense. I mean, I made decisions as an OR supervisor in Vietnam that no OR supervisor in the United States would ever make; what patient goes next into the OR, a general assessment of the wounds. You pretty much made your own decisions. You decided, well, OK, this kid goes in next. . . . I'm not saying you were the only one that made it, I'm saying that . . . you frequently did. You were the one that said, `OK, send in the choppers' or `we can do more cases.' And so, it was a very intense situation. I returned to the States where a big emergency was an appendectomy. . . . I had no patience. I had no patience with the group because I was used to a very intense working situation. When I got a chance to go into administration, I took it. . . .

"I did feel I had some problems that a lot of people had, coming back from Vietnam, that were never identified. One, we had never talked about our problems. We never talked about the situation or how we felt about it because it wasn't an acceptable thing to talk to other people about; you know, the whole Vietnam scene. And, you were made to feel guilty. But, I felt I had, in order to survive - I had distanced myself from the patients. I had to do that to survive. Otherwise, I'd have cracked up. I think that that distancing affected me in wanting to get out of the OR and wanting to get into administration where I didn't have to face the patient dying on me every time I turned around. And, it took awhile for me to realize that that was what was going on with me. I don't think I'm alone in that situation."[17]

From the after-effects, we turn to present effects. "This is Commander Florence Job aboard the U.S.S. *Repose* which is now sitting in Da Nang Harbor. These are days of great expectations for all of us. There is a certain amount of tension because we know we're being transferred; as yet we don't know where, and, to a certain degree, we don't know when. We don't have a definite commitment that we are leaving next Saturday, but we are anticipating that we are. Plans are being made for the departure ceremony, but, as of this date, everything is still very indefinite. We've been sitting here talking. We have a group of off-duty nurses gathered together. We're thinking about some of the memories we have of our tour aboard this ship. I think for all of us it's been a tremendous experience, probably, for most of us, the highlight of our careers. There are many things that we're going to remember, I'm sure, for the rest of our lives."[18] CDR Job relates her memories of reporting aboard the *Repose*, "[I] came aboard on a skimmer [small boat]. It was a beautiful day. We breezed right across the water . . . very rapid transportation. The [hospital] ship was sitting bright and lovely in the sunlight and, as we got up to the ship, I realized maybe I was going to have a little bit of difficulty. Because, [from] the skimmer to the accommodation ladder was a jump of about five feet straight up. I didn't have much time [to think] about how to get aboard . . . somebody reached down a hand and I was up before I knew it. The thing that I wrote home was that I think I was the only chief nurse, probably, in the Navy Nurse Corps who ever reported aboard on her hands and knees!"[19]

Navy Nurse Regina Humphreys is an operating room nurse aboard the *Repose*. She recalls, "When I first came, we were working eighteen hours a day all the time and it was not uncommon to do more than one case in a room at a time. In fact, in [operating] room 3 we set aside two tables. . . . We pushed a table near the wall and then we can operate on two [patients] at once. On one [patient] at one time there may be three operating surgeons. [There's] a corpsman for each surgeon and it really becomes quite crowded, but it's remarkable how things function very well. It's very evident, on the ship, that when you have an emergency, you have the people to do it. They're wonderful. They respond beautifully. Another interesting factor, while you're operating on the ship, is when it is rough you have to call the Bridge [of the ship] and tell them to please steer in a smoother course because you cannot do surgery when the ship is rolling and pitching. . . . They're quite nice about it. One time . . . we were doing a laparotomy [surgically opening the abdomen] and it was extremely rough. We were only operating on one patient in this room. `Please, call the Bridge and tell them to steer a better course. We can't operate.' So we call the Bridge and they steer a nice course . . . we were going north. Another hour passed and we're doing beautifully in the OR, but the Bridge is a little hesitant because they're going up north and there are some shoals coming on. [OR says,] `I'm sorry, please keep to the same course.' The operation lasted about three hours and the Bridge is having a fit because, `We're getting nearer Hanoi, Miss Humphreys. Could you please - - - could we turn?' So, due to the desperate voice of the man calling, I said, `Well, we might as well. We are nearly closing. Yes, please do as you think feasible.' There were some shoals up there, probably, and they weren't sure of where they were.

"Here's a drama that I think was quite unique and I hope I never experience it again. . . . We had an emergency . . . going to be in surgery; a through-and-through gunshot wound to the leg on a young twelve to fourteen year old Vietnamese. The x-rays were marvelous. They showed cradled in the fractured portions of the femur [leg bone], a metal object. The technique of the x-ray was so marvelous you could see that the pin was not engaged. It looked like a grenade, so [we] called down the liaison officer from the Marines . . . to identify this object. He wasn't sure what the object was or who owned the object. Therefore, we called the demolitions [people] from the beach. . . . While waiting for the demolitions expert to come, we set up damage control precautions. They were afraid it would explode and cause much damage to both personnel and the ship. . . . They couldn't send the patient back [to the beach] with this potential hazard because it would blow up the helicopter if it did explode.

"The damage control Chief came down with a six-foot lead shield which the anesthetist could stand behind while giving anesthesia. There were a very limited [number] of people in surgery who were to wear helmets, flack jackets and gas masks. I'd never worn a gas mask before, so I had a little difficulty, but the damage control Chief put it on. It was quite exciting. All I needed was some music in the background. It was quite evident that everybody wanted to volunteer. They were marvelous. You know, `I'll help. I'll help.' . . . Naturally, we had to limit the crew to six people; a surgeon, his assistant, a scrub [corpsman], circulator [corpsman], circulator nurse, and anesthetist. Naturally, the damage control Chief stood by with us. Other than the lead shield for the anesthetist, they brought in a huge suction pump so that if the object did explode, the gas in it would be exhumed from the ship via this portal. We did [the procedure] under aseptic precautions, as usual. The doctor was scrubbed. The patient was wheeled in, very gingerly, from X-ray [department]. Everyone was very careful. The patient was marvelous. These children are very stoic, can take very much pain. It's really remarkable. . . .

"The doctors were standing by, gowned and gloved, and in walks the two demolition experts who were really something out of TV . . . with their little black box in which they were going to put the metal object. They, too, had masks and gowns and cover boots. They walked in, Dr. . . . incised the wound, it was retracted by Dr. . . . very aseptically. The minute they found this cradled metal object spurred between [the two parts of the broken femur], one of the demolition experts, with his <u>bare</u> hand, reached in and pulled out the object. There go our aseptic precautions! It was done so quickly, it was quite nice. We were waiting with the gas masks on, ready to run in and put the gas masks on the doctors because they could not see very well to operate [with the gas masks on]. So, our drama ended with the men walking out with the metal object in the box and it did not explode. It was really quite interesting. Luckily, the patient did very well."[20]

Navy Nurse Irma Klaetke is also aboard the *Repose*, at this time, and describes a most recent event.

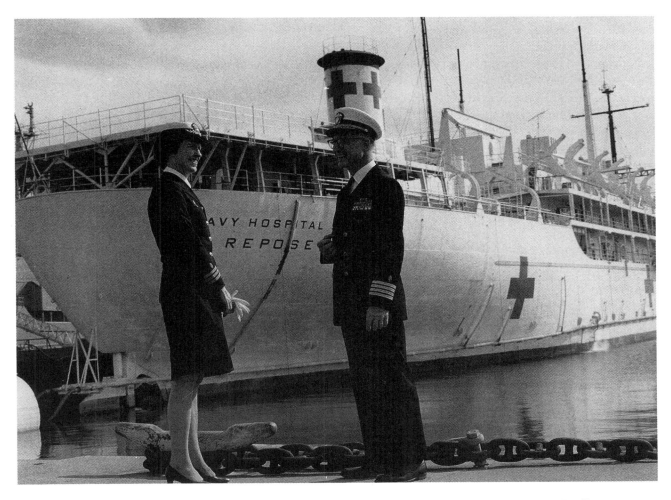

USS Repose at Long Beach circa 1971. (Photo courtesy of Captain Rachel Fine NC USN (Ret.))

"Yesterday a few of us were extremely fortunate having the opportunity to visit the British Military Hospital on the Kowloon side of Hong Kong. This hospital was built two and a half years ago. It has a capacity of two hundred and fifty beds, however, it is fifteen stories high, which seemed very strange to us. But, later, we found out that four stories are used for storage areas and the hospital probably could be expanded to a thousand or more beds, if necessary. . . . The hospital is extremely clean and they use colors more than we do, perhaps, at home; colored bedspreads, floral screens, colored tile on the bulk heads, and the view is extremely well worth seeing. The hospital is run by the British military and the chief nurse is a matron whose rank is Lieutenant Colonel. Lieutenant Colonel Parrish is an extremely attractive woman and very full of life; beautiful accent. Her assistant was a Major; Major Stark. Then they had a number of other Majors and so forth. The other nurses are called `Sisters.' They also employ Chinese-trained nurses and they have many men who are nurses but are of enlisted status. Besides touring the hospital, we were treated to a very nice luncheon which started off with sherry, which apparently is one of their usual noon-time treats. The young lady that I was talking to most of the afternoon, was a Captain who had been in the service now for two years. She was in charge of the pediatrics ward. She was extremely interested in coming over to the United States, not to join the Navy, but to see our country."[21]

Navy Nurse Glenda Dunn continues about the British hospital, "the only thing I can add . . . is to remark about the extreme graciousness of our hostesses. They were very, very friendly. It was a delightful lunch. The

Commanding [Officer] of the hospital joined us for lunch. The girls say he really enjoys coming over to visit with them and afterwards he took the time out to go on a complete tour of the hospital with us. He was very, very proud of this hospital, pointing out all the fine points. It was quite interesting; they have the same problem staffing, etcetera, that we have. The Colonel spent the entire afternoon with us and also provided us with a car to get back down to the Star ferry [renowned ferry that runs between Kowloon and Hong Kong]. It would have been lovely to have a much longer visit than we did. We thoroughly enjoyed talking to them and comparing notes about our various jobs and how we arrange our staffing problems; how we deal with basically the same problems you have in any hospital. . . . The one thing that is not remarkable, is the fact that hospitals are out-dated as soon as they are built and they were quite aware of this and we were talking about how they would have changed things if they had been able to be in on the planning stages of it."[22] What nurse hasn't often wondered why knowledgeable nurses couldn't be included in the planning process?

In May of 1970, the "Hospital Ship *Repose* departed [the] South China Sea and was decommissioned as AH-16 at Long Beach, California. It was then placed in reserve commission at Long Beach to serve as a shore-based Naval Hospital."[23] The ship is placed pier-side at the Long Beach Navy Yard and is an adjunct to the Long Beach Naval Regional Medical Center (Hospital). Navy Nurses from the NRMC staff the ship, along with other medical personnel, and the Chief Nurse of the Hospital is also responsible for the nursing service on the ship.

Meantime, aboard the USS *Sanctuary* is Navy Nurse Mary Lewis (Nester Conley) who started out the year being stationed at Da Nang Naval Hospital. "By January 1970 the war was winding down and plans for closing the hospital at Da Nang were underway. I was among five nurses who were sent to the USS *Sanctuary* to complete our [overseas] tour. That was another unique experience. We were still receiving battle casualties, but, again, we had wards full of malaria patients and some Vietnamese [humanitarian] cases. During the four months I was on the Sanctuary, we went to the Philippines for dry dock work. Although there was some work involved, it was also a much needed rest in pleasant surroundings. We returned to the line refreshed and with renewed vigor for our work. It was the tour of duty during which I felt the most needed and it was a humbling experience when you witnessed what so many of our fighting men gave for their country. I guess I would consider it the most challenging duty, but I never considered it hard. It was too rewarding."[24]

A few statistics about the USS *Sanctuary* during 1970; during calendar 1970, she "averaged a total on board [medical] staff of 59 officers, 236 corpsmen and eight dental technicians. . . . During the calendar year 1970, *Sanctuary* admitted a total of 6,354 patients and served 10,751 outpatients."[25] Also, during the period of December 1965 and 1970, 141 female Navy nurses served tours of duty aboard this ship.[26] Then, in 1971, the USS *Sanctuary* comes home and is decommissioned in July.

In another part of the world, Navy Nurse Lucille Emond is stationed at the hospital at Naval Air Station, Sangley Point in the Philippine Islands; right across the Bay from Manila. "It was unique for a variety of reasons. . . . There were very few [Navy nurses] there; there were only four. We took turns rotating call every night of the week. . . . We had a fair number of pregnant women that had to come to the base when they were ready to deliver. Some of them had to come by boat from Manila when they were in labor. The unique experiences that I had with pregnant women were: I had the opportunity to deliver a baby in one of these ladies' homes. We were called to the home to bring her back to the hospital in the ambulance, however, she delivered at home before we ever got there. I delivered a baby when I took the boat to Manila to pick up a pregnant woman to return to the hospital and she delivered on the boat. The third situation was, when some of our ladies in labor, labored too long, they were then flown to the Navy Hospital in Subic Bay, which was a twenty minute flight. On one of these flights, I assisted a doctor, and that's where this lady delivered in the plane. . . . Another aspect of my assignment there that was unique, was that after being assigned there for six months we were formally notified that the Base would be closing. That generated a series of instances that sometimes, even today, seem unbelievable. Our Navy Exchange was robbed, an ambulance was stolen when it was on the way to Subic Bay, fire trucks were stolen and, one of the saddest instances, our bank was robbed and a Marine guard was killed. Full scale thievery began to take place as many of the items on the Base, in the clubs, in the hospital, were removed . . . and many times we would come to work and find items completely missing. . . .

"The older Filipino nurses that were assigned to the hospital became very sad because they had been at that hospital since before World War II and had known many . . . Navy Nurses. . . . These Filipino women had been at the hospital when the Japanese invaded, and, in fact, worked at the hospital taking care of the Japanese soldiers and were still there when the Japanese left and the Americans liberated the hospital. . . . They were a part of the history of that hospital. . . .

"At the time [1971] there was no martial law, and the opposing political forces many times used violence to try to get their political person, that they were supporting, into office. This led to a lot of gun fire. . . . I had never really heard a gun or heard the sound of gun fire. One time, another nurse and myself were at a dressmakers and we were being fitted for gowns that we would be wearing as part of the Women's Chorale; a group that sang and entertained among many of the hospitals in Manila. While there [at the dressmakers], we heard what sounded like back-fire; a car back-firing. The Filipino dress-maker recognized the sound . . . and told us to follow her. . . . She ended up putting us on our hands and knees behind a brick wall, while still wearing the white gowns. Shortly after . . . a jeep filled with soldiers, or men in soldiers' uniforms, went by with machine guns and just shot, continuously shot, as the jeep moved down the street. A few minutes later, another truck came by doing the same thing. The dress-maker told us that living next to her was the Chief of Police. Apparently, there was a political faction that opposed him . . . and this shooting was, presumably, a warning to him. Not too long after that, there were a series of shootings as some of the various political leaders in the town were being shot and killed. This [caused] the Commanding Officer of the Base to move many [of the military] (particularly the medical personnel) onto the Base, because, he felt, it was no longer safe to be living outside in the city. Six months after I arrived, the Chief of Police was indeed shot, as were two or three policemen and their bodies were dumped at the gate of the hospital. Two of the men were not killed, they had not died at that time, but ultimately [they] did. So there were many times, when we left the Base, we almost felt like we had gone back in time to the times of the `Wild, Wild West.' In fact, there were many days when the Base was closed and we could not leave the Base at all. . . .

"The last month that the Base was open, it became, at times, `chaotic' as the dependents attempted to keep their personal things intact. The decision was made to collect all of the household effects of everyone on the Base, who was being moved back to the States, and send all of them on a ship to [the Naval Base at] Subic Bay. From there they [the household goods] would be shipped back to the United States. This sounded like a wonderful idea until I got back to the States and I began to open some of my boxes and discovered that, in some instances, total boxes were completely empty. They were broken into and probably 50 percent of my things were stolen. So the Philippines was truly a unique experience in many ways."[27]

In 1971, male "Nurse Corps officers [are] assigned and deployed with [the] newly established surgical teams [aboard] aircraft carriers in [the] Indian Ocean."[28] In March, the Secretary of the Navy approves and signs the Nurse Corps' request for a more equitable allowance for experience and education for nurses entering the Navy Nurse Corps.[29] In July, the Anesthesia section of the Navy Nurse Corps Candidate Program becomes official. This program is the attempt to recruit nurse anesthetist students for the Nurse Corps. Selectees in their last year at school, are commissioned as Ensigns and receive appropriate pay and allowances. After graduation, they are committed to two years of active duty. (Ten nurse anesthetists are the total result of this program over the next two fiscal years. This helps relieve the shortage of these specialists and the program is discontinued in June 1973.)[30] In October of 1971, "An OB/GYN Nurse Practitioner Program [is] established at the NRMC [Naval Regional Medical Center; Hospital], Portsmouth, Virginia."[31]

At this time, the Navy is experiencing a shortage of doctors. "As the Vietnam war continued, doctors were being sent overseas to tend the wounded, Naval hospitals in the United States were crowded, and large numbers of dependents were requesting health care. Rear Admiral Alene Duerk . . . depicted the urgency of the situation: `We just didn't have enough doctors...to go around. The doctors were asking for assistance, for help of some kind, that would relieve them of the tedious duties of taking histories and doing all of those preliminary things before they actually saw the patient, and so...the proposal was made from the Medical Department...[asking if it would] be possible for Nurse Corps officers to assist in a program which would be aiding the doctors in both outpatient and in the inpatient areas, especially in OB/GYN.' . . . The first class of six Nurse Corps officers graduated 16 June 1972 after completing the six-month course. . . . Upon graduation, the new nurse practitioners were sent for duty at Naval hospitals located in Portsmouth, Virginia; Newport, Rhode Island; Camp Lejeune, North Carolina; Charleston, South Carolina; and Orlando, Florida."[32]

So, as is evident, BuMed's Nursing Division received approval for this first Practitioner Program in 1971. It is noteworthy that at this same time, the civilian medical field professionals are beginning to move along these same lines. "In 1970 a committee of thirteen doctors, thirteen nurses and two hospital administrators was appointed by the Secretary of the Department of Health, Education and Welfare (HEW) to study possible extended roles of nurses. The committee's report in 1971 stated: `One of the most important opportunities for change in the current system of health care involves altering the practice of nurses and physicians so that nurses assume considerably greater responsibility for delivering primary health care services.' The committee used the term `primary care' to describe a patient's initial contact with a health care system; in this initial contact a plan of treatment would be determined, and responsibility assigned for the continuum of patient care, including maintenance of health, evaluation and management of symptoms, and appropriate referrals."[33]

On to other items; one of the shattering events in the U.S. during 1971, is the Los Angeles earthquake that "kills 60 and caused $1 billion in damage."[34] The nearby NRMC (Naval Hospital) at Long Beach and its adjunct, the pier-side *Repose*, suffer little damage except to the stress levels of patients and personnel.

1971 in Vietnam sees, "Anti-Americanism spread . . . Morale among the remaining American forces sank, with units avoiding or refusing combat, wide use of drugs, and - something new to the American Army - cases of `fragging,' or murder by hand grenade, of officers and NCOs. At home, polls showed a majority beginning to emerge in favor of removal of all troops by the end of the year, even if the result were Communist control of South Vietnam."[35] And, in Vietnam itself, on the 31st of December, "The U.S. Coast Guard ends six and one-half years of participation in Southeast Asia."[36] Then in January 1972, "President Nixon discloses a previous Vietnam peace proposal providing for pullout of U.S. forces in six months in exchange for a cease-fire and release of all American POWs."[37] (This proves to be premature.) In April, "The Navy withdraws its last combat force from Vietnam. . . .

"[Also, in April,] For the first time since 1968, hundreds of Navy and Air Force planes strike military targets in North Vietnam. . . . [In May] In response to the massive North Vietnamese offensive in South Vietnam, President Nixon announces the mining . . . [of some] North Vietnamese ports. . . . [On June 28] President Nixon orders that from this date forward, no draftees be sent to Vietnam unless they volunteer for duty there."[38] Meantime, President Nixon makes two trips to China and one trip to Russia with the emphasis on peace. At the same time he and the Vice President, Spiro Agnew, are running for re-election. The Democrats run Senator George McGovern and Sargent Shriver as their party's ticket. Earlier in the campaign, "District of Columbia police [arrested] five men inside Democratic National Headquarters in the Watergate complex - [this is the] beginning of the `Watergate' affair; Republicans deny Democratic charges that the raid was sanctioned by Nixon campaign officials . . . [the] cover-up continues as [the] trial of [the] original defendants begins."[39] Also, early in the Presidential campaign, "Gov. George C. Wallace of Alabama, a contender for the Democratic presidential nomination, is shot . . . and partially paralyzed."[40] Despite all of the turmoil, President Nixon and the Republican ticket wins by a landslide.

"After the election, [Vietnam] peace negotiations broke down. The week before Christmas, Nixon ordered a resumption of the bombing `until such time as a settlement is arrived at.' In round-the-clock raids F-52s battered the Hanoi-Haiphong area in the heaviest bombing of the war - or any war."[41]

In other U.S. happenings during 1972, after 27 years of American rule, Okinawa (in the East China Sea) is returned to Japanese control.[42]

But, to return to the Navy Nurse Corps; in February 1972, BuMed establishes its first Pediatric Nurse Practitioner Program. "Rear Admiral Duerk recalled how some pediatricians were training their own clinic nurses to help see patients: `The need for pediatric nurse practitioners was really quite acute, and so we found that in various areas...that the pediatricians were taking nurses from their pediatric clinics...and giving them some training to assist them...in the outpatient clinic areas...[I]n some of our outpatient clinics...we found that doctors were training their own nurses and they were being called pediatric practitioners. They really had not had any formal training at all except for on-the-job training.'

"In an apparent attempt to satisfy the need for more pediatric health care providers without resorting to on-the-job training that provided no academic credentials, the Navy turned to civilian pediatric nurse practitioner programs. The first program the Navy utilized was the pediatric nurse practitioner program at the Bunker Hill Health Center of the Massachusetts General Hospital in Charlestown, Massachusetts (R.A. Wilson, personal communication, 29 September 1992). Two Nurse Corps officers were assigned to be trained at the four-month certificate program beginning in February 1972. During the course they received clinical experience and supervision at Naval Hospital, Chelsea, Massachusetts (Outline History of the Navy Nurse Corps, updated 1989)."[43]

Also, in February, an enormous uniform change is authorized for Navy nurses. "An official BUMED Note will soon be forthcoming authorizing the optional wearing of a new work uniform designed by D'Armigene Inc., Long Island, N.Y. The attractive new pant suit is an optional work uniform to be worn by women officers in the Medical Department while actively engaged in patient care. (Not appropriate for those engaged in administrative duties) The uniform may be purchased at the officer's own expense, at an approximate cost of $32.00 per suit.

"The suit is made of white opaque 100% Dacron material which is machine washable and drip dry. The tunic style blouse has a back zipper and collar lapels to permit the wearing of grade and corps insignia. . . . Nurse Corps officers must wear their white cap, white stockings and white shoes with the uniform."[44] Director Alene Duerk says, "The pantsuit became a part of our uniform in the early `70s and one of the reasons for that was that at that time the mini-skirt was very popular. Our uniforms, the blue uniform . . . it came out in a paper that you could wear your blue uniform above the knee or at the knee cap. And so the white ward uniform got shorter and shorter. Finally, the doctors actually complained about the fact that the nurses were wearing such short ward uniforms. One of the Flag officers in the Bureau suggested that we wear pantsuits. So I got a couple of pantsuit models and modeled them for the Surgeon General. Between us, we selected a pantsuit that we thought would be suitable for the Navy Nurse Corps. That's how the pantsuit became a part of our uniform; because of the work that we did."[45]

In March, another uniform change is announced; the 'tiara' (head-piece) is declared optional for wearing with the dinner dress uniform.[46]

In late April 1972, one of the most historic events in Navy Nurse Corps history takes place. The Director of the Navy Nurse Corps, Captain Alene Duerk, tells us about it: "I had been in Akron, Ohio and I had talked . . to a Navy League group the night before, I think it was a Navy League. Anyhow . . . I'd had a couple of phone calls from the office [the Nursing Division at BuMed]. . . . I knew that the selection Board was meeting to select a woman [officer] for Flag Rank. I felt that . . . [a woman Line officer] was the person who was going to be selected; there was no question in my mind. . . . So, I had this phone call [from BuMed] and they said, `We've had some very peculiar questions asked but nothing has come out [about the selection]. So, I got on my way.

"I was going to my mother's home for the weekend then I was going on to Detroit because the American Nurses Association was meeting there for their annual meeting. . . . I was driving the car and as I'm wheeling along down the expressway, I hear on the radio the announcement that, `Alene Duerk was selected as the first woman Flag Officer in the Navy!' So there wasn't any `whoopee' or anything like that because I was all by myself and I just thought I was driving pretty fast and I thought I'd better slow down a little bit. Then I was amused because, when I went through the [toll] gate, I thought, `I'd like to tell that man what happened.' Then I got home and my mother came out to meet me and my stepfather came out on the steps of the house and they both looked stunned. . . . My mother said, `I'm so glad to have you home. That telephone is just driving us wild.' Of course, by that time people started to arrive and I had reporters and it was just a busy, busy, busy time. It was about midnight when the phone finally quit ringing and the people finally left. I could sort of relax a little bit and I thought, well, this was really an exciting period. Then, I thought, but it's all going to go past. Six weeks from now, nobody will know. Well, that didn't happen. Today [1988], here I am, sitting here talking to you people. It's still going on."[47] (And, even now, as this book is being written, it is still going on.) Rear Admiral Alene B. Duerk of the U.S. Navy Nurse Corps; the first woman Admiral in the history of the U.S. Navy.

On Thursday the 27th of April 1972, the Honorable Delbert L. Latta makes a speech in the House of Representatives. Part of what he says is, "Mr. Speaker, I am pleased to inform the House that the Navy today for the first time in its 197-year history named a lady admiral - Alene B. Duerk, an Ohio native, who joined the service 29 years ago. I am also honored to claim her as one of my constituents.

"Captain Duerk, head of the Navy Nurse Corps, was nominated for promotion to flag rank along with 49 men. The nominations were approved by President Nixon and are subject to Senate confirmation. . . .

"A Pentagon spokesman said Secretary of Defense Melvin R. Laird was `particularly pleased' that the Navy now has for the first time a lady admiral.

"I extend my heartiest congratulations to Admiral Duerk and commend the Navy on its choice."[48]

On 1 June, in a special ceremony, Secretary of the Navy John W. Warner pins the stars of her new rank, on the uniform collar of Admiral (selectee) Duerk while the Chief of Naval Operations, Admiral Elmo Zumwalt, looks on. She is officially 'frocked.' ('Frocked' means that the officer has been selected for promotion and can wear the new rank insignia and gold stripes of the new rank but does not receive the pay and allowances of the new rank until the actual date of promotion.) Admiral Duerk is fully promoted in July of 1972.

A Navy nurse on 'duty-under-instruction' at Indiana University (for her Masters degree) at this time, expresses the prevailing sentiments in the Nurse Corps, when she states, "During the time I was in graduate school . . . the first woman Admiral was selected for the Navy, and that was Alene Duerk. We all rejoiced over that. Not only the fact that we had an Admiral, but that Admiral Duerk was the one who was selected."[49]

On the other side of the country, the hospital ship USS *Sanctuary* is recommissioned in November 1972, and is "the first U.S. Navy ship to have women included in her crew."[50] On the 12th of December, the "USS *Sanctuary* (AH 17) steams out of San Francisco with a woman sailor in the bridge watch, ending a seagoing tradition dating back to the days of wooden ships."[51]

The Chief Nurse of the *Sanctuary*, Phyllis Butler (Fisher), tells us, "The ship was recommissioned at Hunter's Point in California and was then to go down and do `Project Handclasp;' a good-will mission. We did stop in Buenaventura, Colombia and go through the [Panama] Canal [to] Port-au-Prince, Haiti and stayed a month in both of those places [Colombia and Haiti], working with the locals. . . .

"[We] sailed to Buenaventura, Colombia, which is a seaport town. . . . It was small, dirty and poor. In fact, even in Colombia it was said that if you were going to give Colombia an enema, Ventura would be where you put the solution. That was the state of this tiny town. The people apparently knew we were coming. The first day they had to put guards on the gangway; there were such crowds waiting to come on board the ship. I swear to God they would have sunk the ship if they hadn't come on board! . . . The dock was full. We went down there thinking we were going to function as a clinic to help these people. . . . We thought our doctors would go out to the local hospitals (which they did do) and help them with surgeries. In actuality, though, we had to very quickly revise our thinking. I had to very quickly revise our Nurse Corps scheduling because we opened two wards. It seemed like overnight we did surgery on the ship, kept the patients there until they were able to move off, doubled and tripled the bunks, and acted just as a hospital.

"We went out and . . . toured one of the local hospitals. . . . [The] only ward that even had sheets on the beds was maternity. They had one sheet for each patient. . . . It was just a desperately poverty-stricken little town. Nobody had had any medical care. . . . [A] group of Nuns came on board and asked that we save all of our disposable syringes, I.V. tubing after use, so that they could clean and sterilize them. They didn't have any. They were treating not only the local people but the people out in the hills around the town and they had no supplies. We had taken, as part of the Project [Handclasp], a lot of medical supplies and necessities with us that we gave away to the local medical groups. Even this hardly made a dent in their needs. . . .

"We had children - battered, abused. We had middle-aged. We had elderly - the whole gamut. A

Colombian Indian came in one day . . . who had paddled someone with him for five days to get there. He was blind and he wanted to see if we could help him. There was nothing we could do for him - but, that man paddled for five days to get there. . . .

"The local hospital had a couple of problems. SeaBees [Construction Battalion naval men] were on the ship and they learned that the hospital's blood storage was on the fritz . . . so, the SeaBees went in and put a timer on the storage unit so that it wouldn't freeze. It would go down to a certain temperature and then click off for an allotted time so they could keep blood without freezing it. [Also, the hospital] didn't have enough water pressure to do their laundry . . . so the SeaBees rigged up something, I don't know what, so that they could get enough water pressure for their laundry facilities. . . .

"We basically changed our mission in mid-stream, from helping in the community and maybe running clinics on the ship, doing diagnostic types of things, minor type things, to being a hospital because there were so many needing help. . . . We started out with twelve or [thirteen] nurses to work in the clinic and suddenly I had to rearrange everything and staff two wards around the clock - plus, the clinic. That created more hardship on the nurses but nobody complained. They were working hard and having fun and learning a lot. They were seeing things they'll never see again. And the patients were so grateful. You know, you don't mind working hard for patients that are so very thankful you are there. They were getting free medical care - care they couldn't have gotten otherwise.

"We were there four weeks. Then we left there, went through the Panama Canal (another thing you might not do in a lifetime) then to Port-au-Prince, Haiti and spent four weeks there; another interesting tour. Not the same as Colombia. . . . There were the haves and the have-nots. This was . . . before Baby Doc was thrown out and the majority of the people there were the have-nots. We were not as well received in the community. They really were not too thrilled to have us. . . . I think they felt the *Sanctuary* was coming in as the `Great White Father' to cure all your ills and they weren't buying that. . . . But, we saw some very interesting things there, too. . . . [Probably], our most memorable patient there was a little boy called `Joseph.' When he was something like two years old, he got a chicken bone stuck in his throat. He was [now] somewhere around four. He had not been able to speak, but he could swallow. He was a healthy little kid. They brought him down from one of the Missions in the hills to the ship. Our doctors [operated] . . . took the chicken bone out, got his esophagus cleared and when he was healed up enough they closed [the tracheotomy they had done.] In time he became a pet [of the nurses and doctors.] . . . I'll never forget the expression on his face the first time he heard himself make a noise. . . . He was just an absolute darling little kid.

"Navy people. They go out and buy everything in sight [for souvenirs.] One of the big things bought were drums with goat-skin tops, pictures, goat-skin rugs. One of our female crew, not the hospital's but the ship's crew, came back to the States and got `anthrax.' [An infectious disease usually of cattle but can occur in humans.] Probably, her life was saved because one of our corpsmen, who had worked with a Dermatologist who had wards of Anthrax patients, recognized the lesion [that goes with the disease] and went with the girl to the hospital at Jacksonville, Florida where they'd never seen a patient with Anthrax. He [the corpsman] said, `I think you'd better test her for Anthrax.' She was in an Intensive Care unit for a long time. . . . You never think of it [Anthrax] when you buy a goat skin. . . . This girl was one of only twenty proven cases in the last twenty years. You just don't see Anthrax here [in the States] but they have it in Haiti."[52]

From the Caribbean, we cross over the Atlantic Ocean to the Mediterranean Sea area and Greece, in particular. Last year, 1972, a Navy Medical facility opened in Athens. Four Navy nurses were assigned there.[53] Navy Nurse Beverly Brase (O'Dell) is one of them and she says, "I . . . received dispatch orders to Athens, Greece to set up and open the Fleet Support Office Dispensary for the ships that were going to be home-porting in Greece. Someone had . . . selected a clinic space for us. . . . It was a street-level basement and balcony of an apartment building about two blocks up from the Hilton Hotel. It was not too well suited for a dispensary, but we made do the best we could. There was only one bathroom. It had a skeleton key for a lock. On OB [Obstetrics] days it was really wild trying to get both staff and patients in and out of the one bathroom. Of course, we would have kids lock themselves in and scream and cry and [we would] have to sit and talk to them about how to put the key back in the lock and turn it to get them out of there. So, that was not ideally situated, but we certainly managed and had a good time and worked well together.

"I have never been afraid for my own personal safety in any foreign country, but during the 1973 `coup' [coup d'etat] in Greece, I was out on the balcony of my penthouse apartment. I was watching the soldiers move from doorway to doorway. One shouted something at me in Greek, and I didn't answer. He knelt down and pointed his machine gun at me, so I slowly backed-up and went back into the apartment. I was a little shook after that because I could easily have been in the right place at the wrong time. [Another] experience I had . . . when I was stationed in Greece, was as the ship's nurse for a dependents' cruise to Rhodes [Rhodes Island, Greece] on the Aircraft Carrier the USS *Kennedy*. That was an enjoyable experience."[54]

From Greece to Spain where the Chief Nurse is Commander Phyllis Elsass. She tells us, "[Back] in August 1972, I received a call from Admiral Duerk asking me if I would go to the Naval Hospital Rota, Spain as the Director of Nursing Service. The idea was a little overwhelming, but Admiral Duerk was doing the asking and so I could say nothing but yes. I went to Rota, arriving there in January, 1973. . . . Probably, my most favorite memory came only a month or six weeks later when Admiral Duerk came to Europe on her first command tour of Europe. I remember it very vividly as it made a tremendous impression on me; having the opportunity to observe this great lady as she interacted with staff and all of the dignitaries of the base. The base in [Rota,] Spain, I found out when I got there, is not a U.S. Naval Base, it is a Spanish Base and the Commanding Officer is a Spanish Admiral. When we heard that Admiral Duerk was coming (she was to arrive . . . on a Sunday . . .), at my suggestion the Commanding Officer agreed that we would not plan any official activities for her until Monday, to give her a little time to catch-up. . . .

"I remember the CO graciously agreed to send me to . . . the airport to pick her up via official car, and he provided a driver. . . . The young enlisted driver took me in an official Navy car to the airport . . . where I met Admiral Duerk. . . . The Admiral had graciously agreed to be my guest in my apartment while she was in Rota. . . . Coming [back from the airport,] she was recounting all of her activities since she had left the States, and it was an exhausting schedule. . . . She was telling me how tired she was and how many official engagements she had had over the last few days, so when we got back to the apartment, the first thing I did was light the fire because it was chilly. . . . Kind of as an afterthought, I said to her, `Now, we can either have dinner here at home . . . or we can go out for dinner to a local restaurant.' . . . [She] said she would love to go out. . . . We went to a small place . . . . it was a favorite spot of both the Spanish and Americans, and it was just a small place, and it was very crowded, as it usually is, and there were no tables available so the Admiral and I sat at the bar and ate our dinner. Later on in the week, we were to have any number of people approach us . . . and recount having seen her at [the restaurant].

"While Admiral Duerk was there I had the opportunity to observe her in her encounters [with] everyone from the most junior hospital corpsman on the ward to the Spanish Admiral, and it was just a marvelous learning experience to watch her and see how she interacted with people; what actions she took in response to their questions and requests and then be able to go home in the evening and sit, leisurely, and talk with her and question her on why she did things and what her philosophy was. It was just a wonderful experience. . . . I remember one other encounter that we had; the Admiral wanted to go to the main Exchange and I remember taking her over to the Navy Exchange and we ran into a salty, old retired gentleman. I haven't any idea whether he was an officer or what, but he took one look at the Admiral and was just absolutely incensed that a woman should be wearing the rank of a Flag officer. Needless to say, he was the only one that we encountered that was anything more than absolutely and totally gracious to the Admiral."[55]

Now, back to the States and the Nurse Corps Indoctrination Program at Newport, Rhode Island. In May of 1973, the Nurse Corps Program is merged with the "Officer Indoctrination School, Naval Education and Training Command."[56] It is no longer a separate entity.

In the Nursing Division at BuMed, the position of Deputy Director of the Nurse Corps is deleted. The other Nurse Corps members of Admiral Duerk's staff assume the details previously assigned to the Deputy.

Admiral Duerk then appoints another Navy nurse to the job of detailing. (Detailing is the immense business of finding and assigning Navy Nurses for the world-wide Naval Medical facilities.)

In June, forty-eight Navy Nurse Corps officers, U.S. Navy Reserve, are released from active duty. This is the first involuntary release of Reserve Nurse Officers. These officers are Lieutenant Commanders who have been 'passed over' twice for selection to Commander.[57] It is the law for those twice failed. Also, in June, uniform changes are effected for the black and the white dinner dress uniforms. Gold braid is substituted for the black velvet used to indicate rank on the sleeves of the black dinner dress uniform and gold braid versus white braid is now official on the sleeves of the white dinner dress uniform. "Also, embroidered collar devices and [the] white skirt [are] eliminated from [the] dinner dress uniform; black skirt to be worn with either [the] black or white jacket."[58]

Another June event takes place when eight Nurse Corps officers are assigned to the Dispensary in Asmara, Ethiopia.[59] Actually, this had been an Army Communication facility with a dispensary and it is transferred to the Navy, the Navy nurses being sent to relieve the Army nurses. (As an aside; every time Ethiopia is mentioned, an order purported to have been given by the Emperor of Ethiopia comes to mind. Allegedly, Emperor Haile Selassie gave this order when Italy invaded Ethiopia in 1935. "Everyone will now be mobilized and all boys old enough to carry a spear will be sent to Addis Ababa. Married men will take their wives to carry food and cook. Those without wives will take any woman without a husband. Women with small babies need not go. The blind, those who cannot walk or for any reason cannot carry a spear are exempted. Anyone found at home after receipt of this order will be hanged." Sure beats having a draft.) Then in August 1973, two Navy nurses are assigned to the newly opened Naval Support office on the Italian island of Sardinia.

While all of this is going on, within the Navy "the physician shortage continued unabated. In fact, it was intensified by the reality that the physician draft was to end in July 1973. The Naval Regional Medical Center . . . San Diego, like most Naval hospitals in the United States, was faced with an increasing shortage of general medical officers, a situation the commanding officer considered critical (Ambulatory Care Nurse Practitioner Pilot Program, 1974). In response to this, the commanding officer appointed an ad hoc committee to study the outpatient health care delivery system; among the committee's recommendations was a proposal to institute a special program to educate Navy nurses to become providers of primary care to outpatients over the age of 13 years (Ambulatory Care Nurse Practitioner Pilot Program, 1974).

"CDR Angeline G. Liakos, a Navy nurse with experience in nursing education and program planning, was given the task of developing and implementing the Ambulatory Care Nurse Practitioner Pilot Program. . . . In May 1973 a formal announcement describing the new 'Continuing Nursing Education Program for Ambulatory Care Nurse Associate' was made (Ambulatory Care Nurse Practitioner Pilot Program, 1974, p. 10). . . . After the applicants were carefully screened, ten were selected, and on 9 July 1973 the first class convened (Ambulatory Care Nurse Practitioner Pilot Program, 1974). Among the students was CDR Liakos, the program director, who held a master's degree in nursing education but was not herself a nurse practitioner when she developed the nurse practitioner program (A. Liakos, interview 17 August 1992). Other members of the first class included LCDR Betty Thomas, LCDR Claire Cronin, LT Diane Sentinella, LT Lila Fillmore, LT Deborah Sherman, LT Judith Pattinson, LTjg Margaret Willey, LTjg Wendy Bregar, and LTjg Marilyn Stryker (Ambulatory Care Nurse Practitioner Pilot Program, 1974). The six-month course combined formal classes and supervised clinical experience.

"Formal graduation exercises for the students were held 11 January 1974 at NRMC [Naval Regional Medical Center; read Hospital] San Diego. The graduates, who were called Ambulatory Care Nurse Practitioners, were assigned to various dispensaries in San Diego and to the hospital Ambulatory Care Service to be preceptored by physicians. Although the original intention had been for them to see adults, they found themselves also caring for children. Because of this, weekly continuing education classes were established to further expand the capabilities of the Ambulatory Care Nurse Practitioners 'to include functions of the Family Care Nurse Practitioner' (Ambulatory Care Nurse Practitioner Pilot Program, 1974, pp. 5-6). . . .

"The nurse practitioners were generally well received in their new role. . . . However, not everyone would feel so eager about the new nurse practitioners. . . . [A] Senior Medical Officer noted some initial dissatisfaction. . . . There would be obstacles to overcome. . . .

"Although the Ambulatory Care Nurse Practitioner Pilot Program can generally be viewed as a success, it is important to note that it was a local NRMC San Diego continuing education program and that students received no academic credit for their six months of study. At the urging of Rear Admiral Duerk, then Director of the Nurse Corps, CDR Liakos approached the University of California, San Diego (UCSD) to explore the possibility of conducting a revised, expanded Family Nurse Practitioner program under the auspices of the University (Ambulatory Care Nurse Practitioner Pilot Program, 1974). As a result, UCSD's Department of Continuing Education agreed to award a nurse practitioner certificate and continuing education credit to each graduate, an agreement documented in a memorandum of understanding (O'Connell, 1978). . . .

"After NRMC San Diego's first class of Ambulatory Care Nurse Practitioners, then, the nurse practitioner program became a joint venture between the Navy and UCSD, known as the Primary Care Nurse Practitioner Program. By May 1974 it had gained official sponsorship from the Navy's Bureau of Medicine and Surgery (O'Connell, 1978). Subsequently, Navy nurses were sent to the program from other commands; it was no longer merely a local NRMC San Diego program. . . .

"The new Primary Care Nurse Practitioner Program, now one year in length, offered three areas of specialization—obstetrics and gynecology, pediatrics, and family practice. According to several nurse practitioners who attended the program, the obstetrics and gynecology component later became nurse midwifery. For the first six months of each class, all students took the same core curriculum. Instructors and facilities were provided jointly by NRMC San Diego and UCSD.

"The first class associated with UCSD convened in October 1974 and graduated in 1975 (Primary Care Nurse Practitioner Program, 1977). According to one nurse practitioner graduate of that class, after completing the classroom portion of the program, the nurses were sent to their next duty station for their six-month preceptorship. CDR Liakos indicated that prior to their arrivals, she had traveled around the country to set up the preceptorship programs at various Naval hospitals."[60]

Other Naval Hospitals are also feeling the difficulties of the physician shortage and are finding their own answers to the problem. For instance, at the new Navy Hospital in Millington, Tennessee, a male Nurse Corps Officer, Ensign Lynn Day, reports aboard in July 1973. He says, "I was first assigned to the SICU [Surgical Intensive Care Unit] and recovery room. After six months, I was called to the Chief Nurse's office. . . . [She] had been reviewing personnel records for nurses who could be trained as Nurse Screeners since the Navy was short on physicians. After accepting the assignment, I spent six months in a training/preceptorship program with a general practice physician. At the end of my training I opened a 'stand-alone' [separate] walk-in clinic and was assigned one corpman and one corpswave. I was to see all walk-in patients 12 years and older; [those who were] not assigned to the newly established Family Practice Clinic. I could consult with and refer patients to any of the specialty clinics on an . . . urgent or follow-up basis. The program was successful and within the next year, two more nurses were selected and trained for the clinic. The clinic's name was changed to the Acute Minor Illness Clinic and a Physicians Assistant [corpsman specifically trained in the Physicians Assistant Program] was also assigned. . . .

"I was working 12 to 14 hour days, five days a week. I also met with various physician groups for training and continuing education in my off time. Additionally, I provided training for the corpsmen in the area medical clinics."[61] Nurse Corps officer Lynn Day is a graduate of the Navy Nurse Corps Candidate Program program and before that he was a Navy corpsman. To demonstrate and acknowledge the very special background and dedication of the Navy's hospital corpsmen, Lynn Day's own account of his experience is well worth recounting: "In February 1964 I received the traditional 'greetings' from Uncle Sam to join 'his' Army. I was determined to be a Navy Hospital Corpsman. In April 1964 that dream was realized when I was sent to Great Lakes for Boot Camp and Corps School. In January of 1965 I reported to NNMC [National Naval Medical Center], Bethesda, Maryland. While there, I participated in President Johnson's inauguration. Later, I was assigned a special watch when he was admitted for a possible heart attack. It turned out to be a `bad case of indigestion.' He wanted a hot mustard plaster; they finally found someone with the skill who could make one. The only problem was that it was `hot' and his skin turned out to be more red than his red silk pajama's. . . .

"I became senior corpsman of an Orthopedic/Neurosurgery SOQ [Sick Officers Quarters - an officers' ward] within four months of arriving at Bethesda. (I had worked four years as an orderly in a hospital at home before joining the Navy.) However, it was LT Skyler, my supervisor [Nurse Corps officer], who set the standards for quality nursing care and inspired me to provide the best nursing care.

"In September 1965 I was one of 28 corpsmen shipped to Field Med School in Camp Pendleton, California. We finished training and were sent to Vietnam via Okinawa. In February 1966 I joined the First Reconnaissance Battalion, received further training and then [was] sent to Chu Lai, Vietnam. The saying was, `if you could make it past your third patrol, and you remained in the rear area for the last thirty days in-country, you had a good chance to make it [make it back to the States].' On my third mission in NAM [VietNAM], just the morning after making Hm3 [Hospitalman third class], we got into an early morning fire fight. . . . The Viet Cong tried to break through our parameter by tossing a grenade into our position. The explosion injured the three of us, one seriously. After getting the other two safely aboard a helicopter and giving report, I got off. The LT ordered me back on the helicopter, much to my resistance. It was not until I arrived at the hospital and looked in a mirror that I realized why he was so insistent about me leaving. I was covered in blood; some from the injured, the rest was my own. I was very angry to leave my platoon because that left them without a corpsman. As a corpsman my duty was to protect the injured and provide medical care to the best of my ability. Everyone in the company had their responsibilities as I did, so when they presented me with the Purple Heart and Bronze Star, I was embarrassed; `I was just doing my duty.' There were many more patrols and many fire fights over the next 13 months. Each had its own special story but, luckily no one else in my platoon was killed. . . .

"In November 1966 we moved our company from Chu Lai to Danang. . . . I would watch the medical staff as they triaged and transferred the injured to special care areas. There were no nurses assigned to the Medical Battalions so the corpsmen had to utilize the knowledge and skills they obtained from their hospital experiences. I believe the nurses would have been very proud to see the dedicated services their corpsmen were providing. We would sit on the beach and watch as the USS *Repose* would cruise just off shore and we were reminded of the quality of care available if our time came.

"After Vietnam I was assigned to VP-26 in Brunswick, Maine. . . . Six months after arriving at Brunswick, November 1967, we were transferred to Sangley Point, Philippines; the first east coast patrol squadron to be sent on a West Pac in support of our troops in NAM. I was responsible for 350 men and their records. . . . While standing duty at the clinic, I went up to the ward on the second floor [of the medical facility at the Sangley Air Station]. The first person I saw was LCDR Skyler, my supervisor at Bethesda. What a great experience."[62]

His, Lynn Day's, enlistment time was up shortly thereafter, so he got out of the active duty Navy, but he continued to keep up his reserve status. He wanted to become a Navy Nurse. He states, "In April 1968, I moved to Texas and began my education at . . . Junior College. The $125.00 per month did not go far in supporting a wife and a son while attending college [on the G.I. Bill]. I worked full time and went to school full time. But, in my sophomore year I had to cut back to one or two courses per semester and work more hours to make enough money to continue. . . . In 1970 I went to see the Army to apply for their educational assistance program. I was told I was too old for their program but maybe I should check out the Navy's program. I was surprised and elated to hear about the `Navy Nurse Candidate Program.' [Lynn had been completely unaware that the Navy had such a program.] It was like a prayer had been answered. The next step was to apply for and be accepted into the program. . . . The greatest day was when I was notified that I had been selected and could enter the Bachelors of Nursing Program at Texas Christian University. Without the NNCCP [Navy Nurse Corps Candidate Program] I probably would have finished with an associate's degree and sought employment in a civilian hospital. After graduation in May 1973 I reported to OIS [the Officer Indoctrination School] at Newport."[63] From there he went to Tennessee.

To return to 1973 and the Director of the Nurse Corps; in November 1973 history is made again when Rear Admiral Alene Duerk attends the <u>first</u> NATO Conference for senior military women.[64]

One more military happening, that is of interest, occurred in May of 1973: "The Supreme Court rules that women members of the armed forces are entitled to the same dependency benefits for their husbands as servicemen have always received for their wives."[65]

As for affairs of State, "On January 15, 1973, five days before his inauguration, the President [Nixon] directed that `the bombing, shelling, and any further mining of North Vietnam be suspended.' Kissinger returned to Paris `for the purpose of completing the text of an agreement' to end the war. After a few days of bargaining, an accord was reached, and on January 27 - at last - the cease-fire went into effect.

"The coming of peace found Americans strangely silent, as if troubled by the thought that they had paid an enormous price in blood and money for an uncertain outcome. . . . Unlike the riotous celebrations that took place in New York's Times Square at the end of World Wars I and II, people went about their business quietly in the square. . . .

"The terms of the Vietnam peace settlement provided for the withdrawal of American forces from Vietnam within sixty days and the return of all American prisoners of war. In the twelve years of the war, the United States military had suffered 45,033 men killed, 303,616 wounded, 587 captured, and 1,335 missing. . . .

"The public's quiet acceptance of the Vietnam cease-fire was followed by emotional scenes when the prisoners of war began coming home. Some of them had been away for eight years; it was a new world they entered. Nearly all of them, especially those held captive longest, had been sustained by old ideas of God, flag, and country during the months and years in prison. President Nixon's `peace with honor' found favor with the returning men. . . . The newly freed men were much interested in learning who won the war. American officials assured them that South Vietnam did not lose and North Vietnam did not win. The ex-prisoners seemed virtually unanimous in opposing amnesty for draft evaders and deserters, saying such men should not be allowed to enjoy the privileges of an America for which they were not willing to fight. . .

"Many thousands of Americans were directly involved in the amnesty question. During the Vietnam War the rate of desertion from the military reached the highest point in our history, with upwards of 32,000 men listed by the Pentagon in 1972 as deserters `at large.' About 10,000 other men had evaded the draft, some of them having fled to foreign lands."[66] Actually, the draft ended on 27 January 1973 "and the era of an all-volunteer force begins."[67]

On the 15th of August 1973, "All American offensive operations in Southeast Asia end. [On the 1st of September] The last squadron of Marine F-4 Phantoms on the Asian mainland flies out of Thailand, The unit is also the last U.S. Marine combat force to leave after an 11-year commitment in Indochina."[68]

1973 is the year that the Vice President of the U.S. "resigns and pleads `nolo contendere' [no argument] to one count of income tax evasion. Gerald Ford, Republican leader in the House of Representatives, named vice president."[69] Then there is the 'Watergate' scandal: "the five original defendants plead guilty. . . . [On April] 17 President Nixon, who has previously maintained that there is no official involvement in the affair, announces 'major developments' arising from his own investigation; his aides H.R. Haldeman and John Ehrlichman are forced to resign; the Senate Watergate committee . . . hears former White House and campaign officials, one of whom, John Dean, attempts to implicate the president. . . . Attorney-General Elliot L. Richardson resigns; serious talk of impeachment begins."[70]

In 1974, "several former White House aides are convicted and sentenced in Watergate cover-up and related matters; President Nixon agrees to pay $432,787 in back taxes; it is revealed that a grand jury secretly named Nixon as an unindicted co-conspirator; when made public, tapes of White House conversations damage the President's cause; the U.S. Supreme Court decides, unanimously, that the President must turn over additional tapes to the Special Prosecutor; the House Judiciary Committee recommends three articles of impeachment for consideration by the full House of Representatives; additional tapes reveal early Presidential involvement in the cover-up; Nixon resigns Aug. 9 and Vice President Gerald R. Ford becomes 38th U.S. president."[71] Then, later on this year, "President Ford grants former President Nixon a pardon for any criminal offenses committed while in office; widespread protest develops."[72] Then on 16 September 1974, "President Ford announces establishment of a clemency program for draft evaders and deserters of the Vietnam War."[73]

Let's turn now to the subject of the civilian side of professional nursing in the 70's. "In an effort to improve access to and restrain costs of health care, Federal legislation of the 1970s encouraged educational programmes to prepare nurses for expanded roles, such as nurse practitioner, and practice settings, such as HMOs and community care. . . .

"Federal efforts to eliminate the still perceived nursing shortage included, in addition to assistance to all levels of nurse training programmes, traineeships for preparation of nurse faculty and administrators, school building construction, leadership development through research grants and the nurse scientist programme. Professional autonomy was undoubtedly advanced by this expansion of educated, university-based leadership and also by the requirements in practice for more specialisation and technical competence and for more personalised patient care. However, achievement of the political goals of creating a large supply of relatively inexpensive nurses fostered expanding associate degree and continuing diploma education which was problematic for those nursing leaders promoting professional autonomy."[74] This is of interest because the Navy Nurse Corps continues on its course in aiming for an all-degree Corps and the 'Sacred Twenty,' as well as every Director of the Nurse Corps, would undoubtedly approve.

The Nurse Corps historical events for the year 1974 begin in March with a change in uniform regulations; the wearing "of [a] black beret as substitute for [the] 'bucket' hat [is] authorized for female officers. [In April the] Augmentation Board [discontinues the] process of inviting Nurse Corps officers to augment into the Regular Navy."[75]

In June 1974, for the first time, a Navy Nurse Corps officer participates in the Personnel Exchange Program (PEP). Admiral Duerk tells us that the women Line officers of the Navy had PEP for a while but this is a first for the Nurse Corps. The Navy nurse is assigned to England to teach at Queen Alexandra's Royal Navy Nursing Service's School of Nursing at Hassler, England.[76] Also, in June, three elderly Naval Hospitals are decommissioned; one at St. Albans, New York; one at Chelsea, Massachusetts; one at Quonset Point, Rhode Island. Then the Navy Nurses at the dispensary in Ethiopia return home as the Communication Station there closes in July.[77]

Also in July 1974, the 'Education and Training' position of Admiral Duerk's staff at BuMed, is moved out to Bethesda into the newly established Naval Health Sciences and Training Command (HSETC.) This new command is physically located in the 'Towers' of the old Naval Hospital. All of the Corps in BuMed (Medical Corps, Nurse Corps, Dental Corps, Medical Service Corps, and Hospital Corps) have their 'Education and Training' transferred to the new Program Directorate of the new command (HSETC.) Navy Nurse Ruth Mason (Wilson) was the nurse in 'Education and Training' of Admiral Duerk's staff, and she is now the Program Directorate of this new organization. (CDR Ruth Mason Wilson was the Nurse Corps' representative on the Board that developed this new command's organizational plan.) But, she still takes care of the Nurse Corps' various education and training programs. It is just that all of BuMed's education and training and the funds are now centered in one location. Each of the Corps has their education and training officer at Bethesda, in the Towers, all in one area. Program Directorate Ruth Mason (Wilson) has a Nurse Corps assistant who takes care of the continuing education and short courses at Bethesda. There are, in addition, Nurse Corps officers for the Anesthesia Program, and instructors in the Operating Room Technicians' program as well as the NeuroPsychiatric Technicians' program.

In another July 1974 change, the Navy Nurse Corps Candidate Program for senior students in Diploma Schools of Nursing, is discontinued. The reason for this is that the BS degree Candidate program, has candidates sufficient to meet the projected needs of the Nurse Corps, retention of Nurse Corps Officers is good, and with the Nurse Corps emphasis on an all-degree Corps, the Diploma program is halted and the last students graduate in September 1974.[78]

One last education event for 1974 is in October when the six month course in Operating Room Techniques and Management, for Navy nurses, is "moved from Naval Hospital, Chelsea, Massachusetts to NRMC, Long Beach, California."[79] (Due to the closure of Chelsea.)

On the 2nd of December 1974, the "Navy confirms that [the] USS *Sanctuary* (AH 17) will be decommissioned and with it the women-at-sea [women in the ship's crew] would be discontinued in the spring of 1975."[80] And, as Chief Nurse of the *Sanctuary*, Phyllis Butler (Fisher) says, "In January 1975 I left the ship as it sailed off to Philadelphia to the shipyard to be decommissioned."[81] The ship is officially decommissioned on 31 January 1975.[82]

In April 1975, Vietnam again fills the news when Communist forces take over South Vietnam. "U.S. helicopters . . . land on Saigon rooftops and at . . . air base to evacuate all but a handful of the 900 Americans still in Saigon."[83] Then the "U.S. Congress approves $405 million for Vietnamese refugee aid and resettlement in [the] U.S."[84] Some "Navy Nurse Corps officers [are] sent TAD [Temporary Additional Duty orders] to Guam to assist with PROJECT NEW LIFE for Vietnamese refugees. Additional nurses [assist] in stateside locations when refugees [are] evacuated to CONUS [CONtinental United States]."[85]

Now, just a few notes on some of the changes affecting Navy Nursing in the early half of the 1970s; there are mandatory requirements for continuing education for registered nurses to keep their RN licenses active. In 1972 I.V. certification began and nurses had to be certified to start I.V.'s. I.V.'s are coming in plastic, versus glass, bottles and medications no longer are mixed in the I.V. container but are given in a 'piggy-back' system. There are new nursing journals on the market and electronic thermometers are replacing the old glass ones. Night duty for Navy Nurses is coming down to one week versus the two week stretch or the earlier one month assignments.[86] And, many, many other rapid changes are being made in this electronic, computer age.

Speaking of changes, it is during Admiral Duerk's regime that Navy Nurses with children are allowed to stay on active duty. Admiral Duerk says, "it was during this time that we also brought [nurses with children] into the Navy and kept [nurses with children] in the Navy. Before that . . . we had a few who had made application. . . . It was during that time [the time when the Nurse Corps began the Nurse Practitioner Programs], I can't tell you the dates, but . . . [nurses] then began to stay in the Navy. But after I left [retired] that became much more prevalent than before. But, the ground work was there; that they could remain in the Navy with dependent children. And, I think the fact that we had men in the Navy who had dependent children, had something to do with it."[87]

Another giant step is taken in 1975, when, for the very first time, the Navy Nurse Corps is included in the screening of Medical Department officers for command positions; screening of all the officers in the rank of Commander and above. The first two officers selected and their respective commands are:

1. Captain Bernadette A. McKay as Director of Administrative Services (formerly called the 'Administrative Officer) at the Naval Submarine Medical Center, New London, Connecticut.
2. Captain Harriet A. Simmons as Officer-In-Charge at the Branch Clinic, Mayport, Florida.

Captain McKay tells us, "My role then, was to direct the activities of the administrative people who were all Medical Service officers, and really just had no direct responsibility to the Director of Nursing Service. My direct responsibility was to the Commanding Officer. I think that there were 21 Medical Service officers at that time, and I think there was division about who was this funny lady coming, not only a lady but a nurse. . . . I think there was some opposition, it was never blatant, but always an undercurrent. Yet, there were five or six of those . . . officers, the rank of LT or LCdr, who were just absolutely tremendous; whose support and advice I would not have been able to function without. They were extremely generous with their knowledge. . . .

"Submariners are a different breed of cat. They weren't used to dealing with females. . . . One time, somebody called me on the phone . . . [and asked for] 'the Director of Administrative Services.' (I knew he was reading [the title] from the phone book.) I said, 'I am she.' and he hung up. He called back, reading [the title] again from the phone book. I said, 'This is Captain McKay. I am the Director of Administrative Services.' He hung up again. The third time he called back, he said to me, 'Look, you don't understand, lady, I want to talk to a Naval officer.' I said, 'Do you have a blue book [register of all active duty Naval officers]?' He said, 'Yes, ma'am.' I said, 'Then open it up to the index, look under McKay, B.A., and you are talking to a Naval officer, because,' I said, 'when you find that name, that's me.' And, he said, 'What's your rank?' I said, 'Two above you. Now, would you like to continue this conversation?' They were so unused to talking to a female who identified themselves as Captain, that they thought I was saying 'Cathy,' so they would say, 'Cathy, may I talk to Captain McKay, please?' . . . First of all, there weren't that many female Captains in the Navy in 1975 . . . line or staff, and to turn up in a place that was such a male-oriented place, and to turn up in a position that was not nursing, was very difficult for a lot of people to get used to. It wasn't that they were opposed to it, but it was just hard to get used to."[88]

Another occurrence, in 1975, is a first. CDR Julia O. Barnes becomes the first black nurse to receive an assignment as a Director of Nursing Services. Her assignment is Director of Nursing Services at the Naval Hospital, Guam.[89] (Later on in her career she is selected and promoted to Captain. But, the first black Navy nurse to be selected and promoted to Captain is Captain Joan Bynum, U.S. Navy Nurse Corps, in the year 1978. In 1983, the first male Nurse Corps officer to be a Director of Nursing Service is assigned to the naval hospital at Groton, Connecticut, in September 1983. His name is CDR Clarence W. Cote, U.S. Navy Nurse Corps. Then in November 1983, CDR Cote is selected and promoted to the rank of Captain; the first male Navy Nurse Corps Captain.

"In May of 1985, Captain Cote, Navy Nurse Corps, becomes the first male Nurse Corps officer to be assigned as the Commanding Officer of a Naval Hospital, Guantanamo Bay, Cuba. Then in July 1986, Captain Julia O. Barnes, Navy Nurse Corps, becomes the first black Nurse Corps officer to become the Commanding Officer of a naval hospital; Naval Hospital, Great Lakes, Illinois. The first Nurse Corps officer to ever be assigned as a Commanding Officer is Rear Admiral Frances T. Shea Buckley, Director of the Navy Nurse Corps. In 1980, in addition to being Director of the Nurse Corps, she is assigned as Commanding Officer of HSETC. These Commanding Officer positions, particularly in the larger medical facilities, had previously been the function of Medical Corps officers. But, in October 1982, Nurse Corps officers are included in the Medical Department's major Command Screening Board and three Nurse Corps officers are selected for Commanding Officer assignments: Captain Phyllis J. Elsass as CO of the Naval School of Health Sciences at Bethesda; Captain Mary O. Fields Hall as CO of Naval Hospital, Guantanamo Bay, Cuba; Captain JoAnn Jennett as Commander of the Naval Medical Command, Northeast Region.)[90]

To return to events in 1975, the first Navy Nurse anesthetist to be assigned to an operational aircraft carrier is LCdr Jimmie Cothern. He is assigned aboard the USS *America* in February. In March, at Long Beach, California Naval Hospital, the Operating Room course for Navy Nurses is discontinued. But, also in March, a six week TAD course in basic operating room techniques is started at Navy Regional Medical Centers in Charleston, South Carolina and Camp Pendleton, California. Both courses are funded by HSETC with the purpose of providing junior Nurse Corps officers with the fundamentals of being an Operating Room nurse.[91] (Most civilian nursing education curriculums of these days, carry very little education in this subject and very little practical experience. Aseptic techniques knowledge is vital to this specialty, as well as other areas.) Also, in March, the first Navy Nurse is assigned to the Naval Medical Research Unit #3 in Cairo, Egypt.

Now, back to BuMed. As 1 July 1975 approaches, so does the retirement of the Director of the Nurse Corps. In the discussion of her time in office, she speaks of her staff in BuMed; "When I was promoted [to Rear Admiral], I had Jan Emal, Ruth Wilson, Jean Miller, Anna Byrnes, and later, Bettye Nagy. Those were the people I worked with. And, if it hadn't been for those people, I could never have done all the things I did. They were the people who, when I was gone, took over and ran the show. When I was there, they were there to help me. . . . You know, I might dream all kinds of things, but to get it on paper and to present it as a project, takes a lot of paper work and that's what they did. Ruth Wilson worked very hard on the education programs. Anna Byrnes was with us for a long time with the Reserves and with Recruiting and with the extra sections that we had there. We worked very hard with those things. Jean Miller worked long, long, long hours on planning and she finally got it into the system, but she didn't get that right away. It was hard work and she worked at it 20 hours a day."[92] "Jean Miller was the assignment officer. She researched each assignment so that the individual that she felt was best qualified would be assigned. She did it in order that the Nurse Corps officers could do their best. Not only that, but the individual officer was consulted regarding their assignment.[93]" Jan [Emal]; I just couldn't get along without her because she was the person who helped write my speeches. She was the person who did a lot of the research. She was the billet lady as far as my 'bodies and billets' were concerned. And, without a staff like I had, I could never have accomplished what I did. So they really should be given a lot of credit.

"I'd also like to explain one other thing . . . and that is 'why did I stay [in office] five years.' I was selected [for Rear Admiral] in 1972. At that time, if you remember . . . [the Army] had selected Brigadier General . . . as the first woman Flag Officer in the Army and she stayed one year. The next [Army Nurse Corps Brigadier General] . . . also, only stayed a short time. The third one was [also] like this. [This was because] once they made Brigadier General, I think they could only have a two year tour, or something like that. They could not be promoted to Major General. When [the Director of the Air Force Nurse Corps] . . . was promoted, she was promoted to Brigadier General and then in three years [their laws] . . . made it possible for a woman to be promoted beyond the 07 level; she could go to 08. [Rank structure in the military carries a name plus a number; Lieutenant is 03, Lieutenant Commander is 04, Commander is 05, Captain is 06, etc..] So, in order to be promoted or even considered for promotion, you had to complete three years in grade [in your rank]. My three years [as Rear Admiral, grade 07], was not up until 1975. In order to be promoted you had to prepare paper work that was unbelievable to change Title 10 [the laws] so that women in the Navy could be considered for an 08. Now, I wasn't even considered. It wasn't until Fran Shea [Director in 1979] came in, that they did consider for 08 and she was promoted to 08. . . . You see, it takes years for the wheels to turn and unless somebody starts it, it never turns. So that was the reason that I stayed - - I requested another year beyond the four years."[94]

The Nursing Division's Biography notes that "During her [Directorship] as the first woman [Admiral], she traveled over 150,000 miles and presented nearly 200 speeches relating to women in the Navy. She was the recipient of several honorary degrees which included: Doctor of Human Relations, Bowing Green State University, Ohio; Doctor of Humanities, Mary Mount College, Arlington, Virginia; Doctor of Science, Iowa Wesleyan College and Doctor of Science, Medical College of Ohio. Additional civilian awards included the Ohio Payne Bolton, Case Western Reserve in 1974. Military honors included the Legion of Merit, Asiatic-Pacific Victory, National Defense and Japanese Occupation Medals.

"Rear Admiral Duerk retired on 1 July 1975 and is currently a resident of Longwood, Florida."[95]

(As you can see, vast changes are occurring in the Navy Nurse Corps and in the profession of nursing itself. It is a new generation and your author is of the old generation. Because of this, the in-depth history of the Navy Nurse Corps ends here. Somewhere, somehow, someone else can now take up the gauntlet and carry on the in-depth history of the U.S. Navy Nurse Corps.)

[1]   Public Affairs Officer, "Captain Alene B. Duerk Appointed Director Of Navy Nurse Corps," Bureau of Medicine and Surgery, Navy Department, 11 February 1970.
[2]   Duerk, Alene B. Rear Admiral, Navy Nurse Corps, *Oral History Interview Tape Transcript*, Interviewers Captain Doris M. Sterner Nurse Corps and Dr. Lynne Dunn of the Naval Historical Center of Washington, D.C., 12 July 1988.
[3]   Ibid..
[4]   Information prepared by the Navy Nurse Corps Officers on the staff of the Director of the Navy Nurse Corps, circa 1990.
[5]   Duerk, Alene B. Rear Admiral, Navy Nurse Corps, *Oral History Interview Tape Transcript*, op. cit..
[6]   Information prepared by the Navy Nurse Corps Officers on the staff of the Director, op. cit..
[7]   Duerk, Alene B. Rear Admiral, Navy Nurse Corps, *Oral History Interview Tape Transcript*, op. cit..
[8]   Cornelius, Dolores Captain, Navy Nurse Corps, *Oral History Interview Tape Transcript*, Self-interview, 28 December 1989.
[9]   Schwartz, Linda Spoonster, R.N., M.S.N., "Our Unknown Veterans Emerge From The Shadows," *Yale Medicine*, Alumni Bulletin of the School of Medicine, Yale University School of Medicine, Editor - Dr. Michael Kashgarian, New Haven, Connecticut, Volume 26, Number 3, Summer 1992, p. 17.
[10]   O'Connell, Anne L. CDR, Navy Nurse Corps, *Oral History Interview Tape Transcript*, Self-interview, 1 September 1989.
[11]   Halverson, Ruth Captain, Navy Nurse Corps, *Oral History Interview Tape Transcript*, Interviewer Captain Doris M. Sterner Nurse Corps, 10

July 1990.

[12] Updated *History of the Nurse Corps, U.S. Navy*, by the Navy Nurse Corps Officers on the staff of the Director of the Navy Nurse Corps, 5727.1, OONCA/np, revised 24 April 1991, p. 23.

[13] Ibid., p. 24.

[14] Ibid., p. 23.

[15] Information from BuMed, 1981.

[16] Agnew, Lynne A. LCdr, Navy Nurse Corps, *Oral History Interview Tape Transcript*, Self-interview, 12 September 1993.

[17] Buckley, Frances T. Shea Rear Admiral, Navy Nurse Corps, *Oral History Interview Tape Transcript*, Interviewers Captain Doris M. Sterner Nurse Corps and Dr. Lynne Dunn of the Naval Historical Center of Washington, D.C., 13 July 1988.

[18] Job, Florence K. Commander, Navy Nurse Corps, Chief Nurse aboard U.S.S. Repose (and a number of Navy Nurse Corps officers also aboard during this taping), *Tape Transcript* of two tapes, *Homeward Bound I* and *Homeward Bound II*, Taped while in Da Nang Harbor, Vietnam, 1970.

[19] Ibid..

[20] Humphreys, Regina B. CDR, Navy Nurse Corps, ibid..

[21] Klaetke, Irma E. CDR, Navy Nurse Corps, ibid..

[22] Dunn, Glenda M. Captain, Navy Nurse Corps, ibid..

[23] Updated *History of the Nurse Corps, U.S. Navy*, op. cit., p. 23.

[24] Conley, Mary Lewis Nester Captain, Navy Nurse Corps, *Oral History Interview Tape Transcript*, Self-interview, 16 June 1991.

[25] "A 1971 View of the Medical Corps Circa 1871," U.S. Navy Medicine, Vol. 57, No. 3, March 1971, pp. 53, 48.

[26] Information from BuMed, 1981, op. cit..

[27] Emond, Lucille G. Captain, Navy Nurse Corps, *Oral History Interview Tape Transcript*, Self-interview, 1 May 1990.

[28] Updated *History of the Nurse Corps, U.S. Navy*, op. cit., p. 24.

[29] Ibid..

[30] Ibid., pp. 24 and 25.

[31] Ibid., p. 24.

[32] Lukasik, Susan Diana Mahsman LCdr, Navy Nurse Corps, "Nurse Practitioners In The U.S. Navy: A Historical Perspective," A special project submitted in partial fulfillment of the requirements for the degree of Master of Nursing, University of Washington, 1993, pp. 10-12.

[33] Liakos, Angeline G. CDR NC USN, "Ambulatory-Care Nurse Practitioner Program," U.S. Navy Medicine, Vol. 63, No. 5, May 1974.

[34] Grun, Bernard, *The Timetables of History*, Based on Werner Stein's *Kulturfahrplan*, Simon & Schuster/Touchstone, New York, 1991, p. 571.

[35] Tuchman, Barbara W., *The March of Folly From Troy to Vietnam*, Ballantine Books, New York, 1985, pp. 368, 369.

[36] "Chronology of the Sea Service, 1960 to the Present," All Hands, Magazine of the U.S. Navy, October 1975, Number 705, p. 57.

[37] Ibid..

[38] Ibid., pp. 57, 58.

[39] Grun, Bernard, *The Timetables of History*, op. cit., p. 570.

[40] Ibid..

[41] *200 Years, A Bicentennial Illustrated History of the United States*, Joseph Newman, Directing Editor, Books by U.S. News & World Report, Inc., 2300 N Street, N.W., Washington, D.C. 20037, 1973, book 2, p. 279.

[42] "Chronology of the Sea Service, 1960 to the Present," op. cit., p. 57.

[43] Lukasik, Susan Diana Mahsman LCdr, Navy Nurse Corps, "Nurse Practitioners In The U.S. Navy: A Historical Perspective," op. cit., pp. 14, 15.

[44] "Notes and Announcements," U.S. Navy Medicine, Vol. 59, No. 2, May 1974, p. 53.

[45] Duerk, Alene B. Rear Admiral, Navy Nurse Corps, *Oral History Interview Tape Transcript*, op. cit..

[46] Updated *History of the Nurse Corps, U.S. Navy*, op. cit., p. 25.

[47] Duerk, Alene B. Rear Admiral, Navy Nurse Corps, *Oral History Interview Tape Transcript*, op. cit..

[48] "Alene B. Duerk, First Lady Admiral," Congressional Record, Vol. 118, No. 68, Friday, April 28, 1972, pp. E 4409, E 4410.

[49] Pack, VaLaine CDR, Navy Nurse Corps, *Oral History Interview Tape Transcript*, Self-interview, 2 April 1990.

[50] "Chronology of the Sea Service, 1960 to the Present," All Hands, op. cit., p. 58.

[51] Ibid..

[52] Fisher, Phyllis Butler Captain, Navy Nurse Corps, *Oral History Interview Tape Transcript*, Interviewer CDR Joan McIntyre Navy Nurse Corps, 8 May 1988.

[53] Updated *History of the Nurse Corps, U.S. Navy*, op. cit..

[54] O'Dell, Beverly Brase Captain, Navy Nurse Corps, *Oral History Interview Tape Transcript*, Self-interview, 22 May 1991.

[55] Elsass, Phyllis J. Captain, Navy Nurse Corps, *Oral History Interview Tape Transcript*, Self-interview, 5 May 1990.

[56] Updated *History of the Nurse Corps, U.S. Navy*, op. cit..

[57] Ibid..

[58] Ibid., p. 26.

[59] Ibid..

[60] Lukasik, Susan Diana Mahsman LCdr, Navy Nurse Corps, "Nurse Practitioners In The U.S. Navy: A Historical Perspective," op. cit., pp. 16-23.

[61] Day, Lynn LCdr, Navy Nurse Corps, *Written History Interview*, Self-interview, 10 October 1995.

[62] Ibid..

[63] Ibid..

[64] Updated *History of the Nurse Corps, U.S. Navy*, op. cit., p. 26.

[65] "Chronology of the Sea Service, 1960 to the Present," All Hands, op. cit., p. 59.

66   *200 Years, A Bicentennial Illustrated History of the United States*, op. cit., pp. 279-281.
67   "Chronology of the Sea Service, 1960 to the Present," *All Hands*, op. cit., p. 58.
68   Ibid., p. 59.
69   Grun, Bernard, *The Timetables of History*, op. cit., p. 574.
70   Ibid..
71   Ibid., p. 578.
72   Ibid..
73   "Chronology of the Sea Service, 1960 to the Present," *All Hands*, op. cit., p. 60.
74   Maggs, Christopher, Editor, *Nursing History: The State of the Art*, Croom Helm of London, Sydney, and New Hampshire, 1985, p. 166.
75   Updated *History of the Nurse Corps, U.S. Navy*, op. cit., pp. 26, 27.
76   Ibid., p. 27.
77   Ibid..
78   Ibid..
79   Ibid..
80   "Chronology of the Sea Service, 1960 to the Present," *All Hands*, op. cit., p. 60.
81   Fisher, Phyllis Butler Captain, Navy Nurse Corps, *Oral History Interview Tape Transcript*, op. cit..
82   "USS Sanctuary Joins Ranks of Reserve Fleet," *Regional Reflections*, Paper published monthly for personnel of the command, Naval Regional Medical Center, Philadelphia, Pennsylvania, Vol. IV, No. 8, February, 1975, front page.
83   "Chronology of the Sea Service, 1960 to the Present," *All Hands*, op. cit., p. 61.
84   Grun, Bernard, *The Timetables of History*, op. cit., p. 580.
85   Updated *History of the Nurse Corps, U.S. Navy*, op. cit., p. 28.
86   Holmes, Sandra Captain, Navy Nurse Corps, Letter to author re recollections of the 1960's and 1970's., 1 October 1995.
87   Duerk, Alene B. Rear Admiral, Navy Nurse Corps, *Oral History Interview Tape Transcript*, op. cit..
88   McKay, Bernadette A. Captain, Navy Nurse Corps, *Oral History Interview Tape Transcript*, Interviewer Captain Bettye G. Nagy Navy Nurse Corps, 10 May 1990.
89   Updated *History of the Nurse Corps, U.S. Navy*, op. cit., p. 28.
90   Ibid., pp. 28, 31, 33, 35-38.
91   Ibid., pp. 28.
92   Duerk, Alene B. Rear Admiral, Navy Nurse Corps, *Oral History Interview Tape Transcript*, op. cit..
93   Duerk, Alene B. Rear Admiral, Navy Nurse Corps, Telephone conversation with author, 11 November 1995.
94   Duerk, Alene B. Rear Admiral, Navy Nurse Corps, *Oral History Interview Tape Transcript*, op. cit..
95   Information prepared by the Navy Nurse Corps Officers on the staff of the Director of the Navy Nurse Corps, circa 1990, op. cit..

"[I] came aboard on a skimmer [small boat].
It was a beautiful day. We breezed right across
the water . . . very rapid transportation.
The [hospital] ship was sitting bright and lovely
in the sunlight and, as we got up to the ship,
I realized maybe I was going to have a little bit of difficulty.
Because, [from] the skimmer to the accommodation ladder
was a jump of about five feet straight up.
I didn't have much time [to think] about how to get aboard
. . . somebody reached down a hand
and I was up before I knew it.
The thing that I wrote home was that I think I was
the only chief nurse, probably, in the Navy Nurse Corps
who ever reported aboard on her hands and knees!"

☆ ☆ ☆

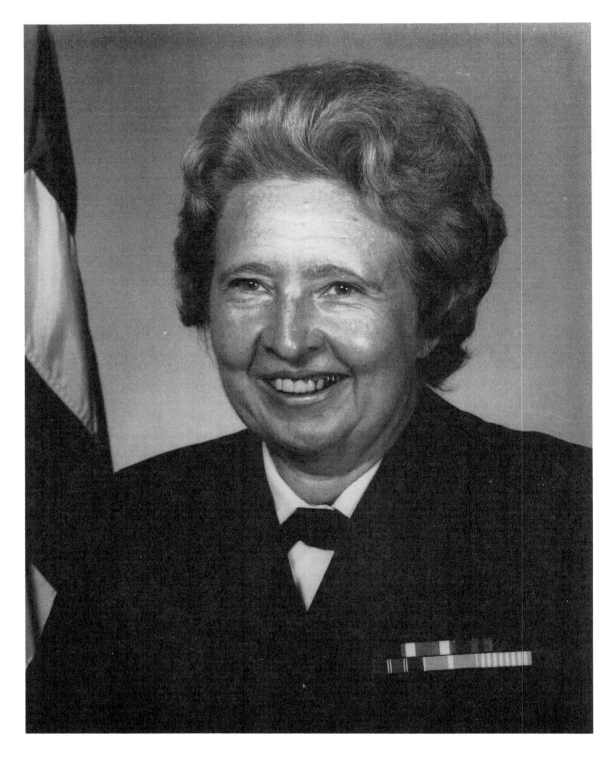

Director - Rear Admiral Maxine Conder NC USN
(Official U.S. Navy photo courtesy of Nursing Division, Bureau of Medicine and Surgery, Navy Department.)

EPILOGUE

☆☆☆

(This portion of the Epilogue covers only the highlights <u>for each Director</u> up to October 1987.)

REAR ADMIRAL MAXINE CONDER
(1975 - 1979)

On 1 July 1975 Captain Maxine Conder is promoted to Rear Admiral and is appointed Director of the U.S. Navy Nurse Corps. She tells us, "In late 1974 . . . the Navy Nurse Corps was led to believe that when Admiral Duerk retired . . . there would not be an Admiral to replace her as Director of the Navy Nurse Corps. . . . I, for one, had certainly accepted that as a sure thing. It was in January [1975] that I received a phone call from someone in BuPers [Bureau of Naval Personnel], who told me there was, in fact, going to be a selection board for a new Nurse Corps Admiral that would take place . . . the latter part of January and early February, and that I was in the [promotion] zone. . . . I was in competition with some fantastic senior nurses, and I knew that. I had not much hope of ever being selected. But, while down in Puerto Rico with my parents (I had taken them to Puerto Rico to celebrate their 50th wedding anniversary,) I was notified that I had . . . been selected for Admiral.

"I had . . . mixed feelings about this honor and it truly was an honor and I knew that. . . . Political climate at that time was such that . . . [there] was great mistrust of anything connected with the government. We had just . . . finished with the Vietnam War; the military was certainly not trusted in any way. We knew that a great amount of the military budget would be cut and there were continual talks of closures and discontinuing of programs . . . . Then we were being threatened with what was known as a 'Purple Suit' - - a combining of all the military medical departments into one unit or department and we would all wear purple suits rather than our individual Army, Air Force or Navy Nurse Corps uniforms. . . . I did not want to be present, certainly not the leader, at the demise of the Navy Nurse Corps as we had known it since its beginning in 1908. . . .

"I came to the realization that in all likelihood I would be the first Director of the Navy Nurse Corps to be able to serve my complete tour in time of peace. . . . I felt that I had at least four years . . . of peace time and so I looked at what I wanted to accomplish during my tour as Director of the Navy Nurse Corps. . . . I decided I wanted to look at the overall needs of the Navy Nurse Corps throughout the world; to look at every billet. . . . So, this was one of my goals; to evaluate every nurse corps billet . . . and . . . to identify the experience of every Nurse Corps officer so that we could computerize both of these and see if we couldn't make a better match [of the two, for assignments,] than we had in the past. . . . Along the same lines, I wanted to identify career ladders for Nurse Corps officers. We had dedicated a large number of nurses to education, . . . [in] Corps School, [in] Newport, continuing education, [and] HSETC [Health Science Education and Training Command]. All . . . required nurses in the educational field. We had a large number of nurses with educational backgrounds and, I felt, that this area was going to continue to grow. . . . We had a continuing need for nurses . . . in administration. We had . . . a great need for nurses to be able to progress through the clinical [pathway] and still be eligible for promotion without leaving the clinical field. . . . This took us a great deal of time but I felt this was absolutely required. As a result . . . it certainly helped to identify our education needs . . . [and] helped us identify our recruiting requirements. We wanted to work on budget and be able to justify [the need for] larger budgets. We could do this if we computerized all the information that we had. . . . All of this material was [eventually] computerized . . . it was a long, long assignment. . . .

"One other . . . of my objectives, was to be fair [in dealing] with all Nurse Corps officers . . . the only thing

I could really and truly guarantee to the Nurse Corps officers in the field, was that I would be as fair as possible to each and every one of them and that was my philosophy during the four years that I served. I truly am very proud of what we accomplished.... Most of what we did was within the Bureau itself, but it had to be done before it would impact out into the field. I don't know if they're using the billet structure and educational requirements today, but I hope so....

"I received an invitation from the American Nurses Association to be with the first group of nurses, representing American nurses, to make a trip into the Peoples Republic of China.... I went to the Surgeon General... and he informed me he could see absolutely no reason why I should go to China.... The next day or two, I went to Bethesda for my annual physical. The policy [at Bethesda] is that they do three or four `Flag' [Flag officer] physicals every Wednesday. On this day, Admiral ..., the Chief of Naval Personnel, was one of those whose [flag] physical was being done. After our blood work and such, we went to the dining area where we ... had breakfast and he asked about the Nurse Corps; wanted to know about recruiting. I told him how well it was going and he wanted to know why, because the rest of the Navy was having such difficulty. I told him that we had always been an all volunteer Corps; from 1908; our numbers had never been driven by the draft; that we had established our civilian contacts over all these years and it was paying off; ... we were very selective in our [assigning of Nurse Corps] recruiters, and we were doing exceptionally well. And, I said, `As an example, this week I received an invitation from the American Nurses Association to accompany them on a trip to the Peoples Republic of China.' And his words were, and I quote, `Oh, my God! Go!' I told him that the Surgeon General didn't feel it was in the best interest of the Medical Department. And he said, `Well, it is. You just keep trying.' In a couple of days, the Surgeon General called and said that my invitation had been discussed ... and it was felt that I should go.... In discussing my trip, it was felt that I must not hide the fact that I was an Admiral or that I was on active duty, but not to play it up big. And so I never lied about it.... I feel that I did help get Americans in there. The three of us [the Directors of the Army, Air Force, and Navy Nurse Corps] ... were the first active duty military allowed into China since 1941, except those that went with President Nixon....

"I also worked very closely with the Chiefs of the various Federal Nurse services; the Army, Air Force, Public Health, and the VA nurses. Fortunately, we were able to work together and able to maintain unity because of the threat from so many sources, especially from Congress, to lower standards for [the nursing profession]. There were threats of institutional licensure.... Some Congressmen wanted us to lower our standards so that we would accept the two-year graduates.... We were able to stick together and withstand these and I'm grateful for that. They were fabulous women to work with....

"I'm very pleased at what we accomplished [during her four years as Director]. I feel, at times, that people in the field thought we were moving too slowly and they really could not see results. But, when you start making changes such as we did, and trying to get it all approved, all the way up the line.... It took us [nearly the entire] four years."[1]

Rear Admiral Conder retired in July 1979.

REAR ADMIRAL FRANCES T. SHEA BUCKLEY
(1979 - 1983)

On 1 July 1979 Captain Frances T. Shea is promoted to Rear Admiral and is appointed Director of the U.S. Navy Nurse Corps. As to what she considers her greatest achievements during her tour, she says, "some to the things we were able to accomplish from an educational point of view and from an assignment point of view. . . . I think that we were able to get [Navy nurses] into programs other than strictly nursing, and get them into policy decision making jobs that could affect nursing and the Nurse Corps.... For example; we were able to get them into Monterey [the Naval Postgraduate School at Monterey, California] ... in [the] Computer [course].... We had a male nurse who had been an aerospace engineer ... and then decided to give that up and go into nursing. We

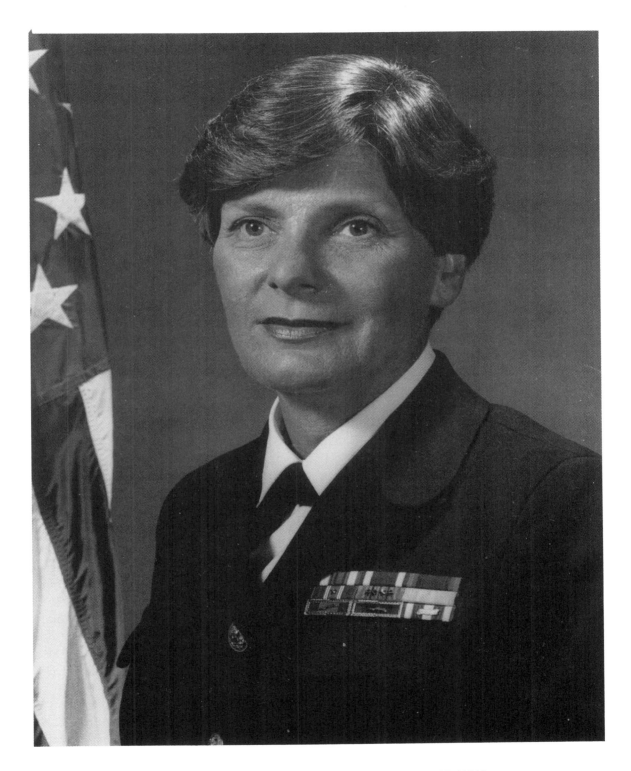

Director - Rear Admiral Frances Shea Buckley NC USN
(Official U.S. Navy photo courtesy of Nursing Division, Bureau of Medicine and Surgery, Navy Department.)

knew he could do the mathematics [required at Monterey]. . . . We sent him there so that when computer people were telling us [the Nurse Corps] how we were going to do our computer programs, we could say . . . `We're going to do it for [Navy] nursing, the way we want it done.' We sent some people for education to George Washington [University]. . . . We also sent [nurses] to Baylor University to get a degree in Health Care Management. . . . Nursing [the profession itself] feels that only the degrees in `nursing' are important. We didn't feel that way because [in the Navy] we're not just dealing with nurses; we were dealing with Line [officers], physicians [Medical Corps], Medical Service Corps. . . . The [Navy nurses] who were sent to these [educational] programs . . . did exceptionally well. They were the top students in their classes. . . . [They] couldn't take three years to get a degree, they had to have had enough education so that they could finish in two years. . . .

"We developed an officer career plan for nurses. They could go into an administrative route, they could stay in a clinical route, [or] they could stay in an educational route. Consequently, what's happened is that when they needed . . . people to take on educational programs, . . . they chose nurses to do this. In many Navy Hospitals you will find that the Command Educational Officer . . . [and the] Quality Assurance Officer are nurses because these were people that the Navy Nurse Corps had trained or educated. Some people may not agree with this, but I think that it was important for Nursing that we got nurses in the positions of Commanding Officers and . . . Executive Officers . . .; they [the Nurse Corps officers] have a better understanding of what patient care needs are. . . . Those nurses who have gone in as Executive Officers or as Commanding Officers, have done . . . [the Corps proud]. I think it proves . . . that nurses can do this sort of thing. My feeling was that if you're in a policy-making . . . job, then you can affect the situation so that it improves the working conditions for nurses . . . and not [just] for nurses but for [the] patients. The nurse is the patient advocate. . . .

"We were able to get eleven nurse anesthetists on board [Aircraft] Carriers. We had some fights as to whether they'd be male or female. . . . But, we could put [the female Nurse Corps officer anesthetists] on a Carrier for three weeks at a time [as long as the Carrier was not] `in harm's way,' which is ludicrous because you could be on a Hospital Ship or in Da Nang [hospital] `in harm's way.' But, that wasn't the point. The point was, that they [the Line] gave up eleven Aviator billets to get eleven Nurse Corps billets. . . . The billet [system]; most nurses don't understand. . . . There . . . [are a given number of billets in the Navy] and the Line was willing to give up their piece of the pie. They gave up eleven Aviator billets to get eleven nurse anesthetists.

"The FSSG [Force Service Support Group], a Marine Corps component [field hospital] that . . . [supports Marines in] battle, asked for nurses to go along with them, on a training mode, to teach their corpsmen. We said, 'OK, we'll do it if we can send females.' The Marines said, 'Yes.' . . . Marines have taken those nurses with them on their operations to Korea and all over. . . . We had three of those billets and they were Marine Corps billets that they gave up for the nurses. . . .

"The Secretary of the Navy . . . wanted the Navy Medical Department reorganized, based on what some of his appointees . . . had decided needed to be done. . . . But, what they did . . . [was to create] another layer of bureaucracy . . . [without an] increase in the number of billets. . . . So you had more people . . . in the administrative arena, and fewer people doing the actual work. . . . One of the [decisions made] was that the Flag officers could have different assignments, including the Director of the Nurse Corps. . . . I do give [the Surgeon General] credit. He said, 'OK, I'm going to make Fran Shea the Commanding Officer of the Naval Health Science Education Training Command [HSETC].' [This is in addition to being Director of the Nurse Corps. In the Navy this, having two jobs, is called wearing 'two hats.'] [HSETC] is the Command that manages all Navy Medical Department programs [not just the Nurse Corps]. . . .

"Under the new reorganization [the Surgeon General] was designated as OP 093. We were supposed to meet weekly or every other week. This did not always happen. Instead of having direct access to him, I had to go through the Commander of the Navy Medical Command as Deputy Commander for Personnel Management. As Director of the Nurse Corps, I was supposed to have open access to the Surgeon General but he was physically located at the Pentagon. So it was not that easy. . . . Nobody really liked it [the reorganization]. . . . I think that the Nurse Corps probably benefited more than anybody. . . . But, nobody was that enthusiastic about the change because they felt that it was mandated. Any study would have shown that it wouldn't have worked. . . .

"I was talking to [the woman Line Admiral] who said, 'You really ought to get [the Navy nurses] out of [the white ward uniform].' . . . So I went to the Uniform Board and I said we would like our nurses to look like everybody else in the Navy and that means no white [ward] uniforms and no [nurse's] cap. They [should] dress like every other Naval officer . . . [and to] do it on a trial basis. So they said, 'Go ahead and do it; try it for a year.' . . . The decision, according to the law, was the Director of the Nurse Corps' decision . . . but, you had to sell it. . . . So we picked four or five hospitals . . . we told them that whatever the Area Commander said was the `Uniform of the Day' would be what they [the nurses] could wear on the wards. We got some static from the physicians, not from the nurses. . . . At the end of the year, we had a Director of Nursing Services Conference and we had all the Directors of Nursing Service there. . . . Every single one of those senior nurses said that they wanted to go with [the Uniform of the Day] because it identified them, clearly, as a Captain or as a Commander; that physicians had to look at them as a person with equal rank, not with that `angel of mercy' kind of look. . . . I think that we made them feel as Naval officers who happen to be nurses; just as Naval officers who happen to be lawyers or doctors. I think that's important for the nurses to feel that way; their identity with the Navy. . . . Not that there's anything wrong with just being a nurse but, [the Navy nurse] has a dual responsibility. . . .

"We started a Patient Classification System. Our hope was that we could develop a . . . system whereby you could classify the acuity of patient care, put it through a computer and that computer would tell you how many people you needed on the ward [daily, to provide the patient care]. . . .

"We did get the Nurse Corps up to about 80 percent with Bachelors degrees. . . .

"The other thing that we were able to do . . . we were able to get a nurse . . . as Deputy for Reserve Nurse Corps Affairs. Up to this time . . . we had clusters of places where . . . a Reserve nurse could do her [two weeks of] active duty training. Many of the Reserve nurses left and joined the Army . . . [or] the Air Force Reserve Units or the National Guard because there were no Navy billets. . . . Well, the Marines came up with a bunch of billets. So, the nurses were assigned to the Marines, in the Reserves and did their drilling with the Marines. During that time, after . . . [the Deputy] came in . . . we were able to focus on the Reserve Program and to put it into the budget cycle . . . for Reserve nurses. . . .

"I went [into the Director's position] on July 1st 1979 and I retired in October of 1983. I was on active duty an additional three months. One of the reasons [for that] . . . was that because of DOPMA[2], the Chief of Naval Personnel . . . asked several Flags [Flag officers] to stay on for three months and I agreed. In addition, I was anxious to stay on because a bill had been passed . . . (through the efforts of other women Flag and General officers) that would give us our second star [promotion from Admiral (lower half) to Admiral (upper half); from grade 07 to grade 08]. . . . I was anxious to have that done, not so much for myself, because I would only have it only for a couple of months, but because I wanted the precedent set. . . . If we could get the precedent set, that women had two stars . . . that would open the doors. . . . That's why I stayed on."[3] She did indeed set the precedent. She had to wait the extra time because there was no opening in the 08 ranks until one of the present 08's retired. When that opening occurred, Rear Admiral Shea then became the first Navy nurse to become a Rear Admiral (Upper Level); grade 08. She then retired, on 1 October 1983.

COMMODORE MARY J. NIELUBOWICZ
(1983 - 1985)
REAR ADMIRAL MARY J. NIELOBOWICZ
(1985 - 1987)

Captain Mary J. Nielubowicz is promoted to the rank of Commodore [which was the rank between Captain and Rear Admiral] and is selected as the fifteenth Director of the Navy Nurse Corps. She relieves Rear Admiral Shea on 1 October 1983. Commodore Nielobowicz says, "During Admiral Conder's tenure, I was her

Deputy Director and, also, the Senior Nurse Corps Detailer [assignment officer]. That was from 1974 to 1979 . . . . I think having had that previous Washington tour was a blessing when I became the Director. You were still fighting many of the same battles . . . and, I think, it made you aware of political ramifications; it made you well aware of the shenanigans that people tried to pull if you were a neophyte in that arena. That previous Washington tour was a real blessing, especially when . . . Navy Medicine went through a tremendous restructuring; when we went from the Bureau of Medicine and Surgery to the Navy Medical Command. . . .

"As Director of the Corps, I had two hats [meaning two jobs']. I belonged to the Office of the Surgeon General (as Director of the Nurse Corps) and to the Navy Medical Command (I was responsible for Code 05 . . . Personnel Management for Navy Medicine was the proper title.) After a year, I was transferred to Code 03, which was Health Care Operations, where I stayed for three years. Health Care Operations was a very difficult job because it involved the running of all medical treatment facilities ashore, both at home an overseas. It also included beneficiary services and Champus. . . . We had health benefits, health promotion, quality assurance . . . contracting for personal services; that all came under Code 03."[4] "It was the first time a non-physician held this position at Health Care Operations."[5]

"At that time, as Director of the Corps, I had two Assistants, a Captain, and one Lieutenant Commander. We worked very, very hard. Then . . . the Reserves [Reserve Nurse Corps officers] were being increased in numbers. . . . I was instrumental, at that time, in bringing a Reserve Captain [Nurse Corps officer] on active duty to handle Reserve affairs because it was too much for the three of us. Captain Margaret Armstrong [a Reserve nurse] was brought in on July [of 1987] . . . to handle Reserve issues. The numbers [of Reserves] were increasing dramatically and we needed someone skilled in Reserves to assist. . . . I think one of the greatest achievements was the spirit of camaraderie . . . that was developed between the active forces and the reserve forces. Not only did we increase the numbers in the Reserves, but we also tried to make things better when they came into the hospitals. They were welcomed. They were given meaningful jobs. Many came on active duty with the specialties that we needed; anesthesia, critical care, operating room. . . . Reserve nurses need to have meaningful jobs or they are not going to remain in the Reserves. We recruited many reserves with advanced educational degrees; [even] Ph.d's have come into the Navy. . . . Our Reserves are an extremely well-educated group and we utilized their talents in many ways. . . . Nursing Professors at Universities were willing to give of their time and effort to assist the Director in major projects. . . . We had submitted [the plan] to have a Flag officer for the [Nurse Corps] Naval Reserve. This was in my second year [as Director]. . . . [It] finally [happened in 1990] . . . a Reserve nurse was selected for Flag officer. . . . It's disappointing when you don't see the results of things you try to accomplish and it may take several years [to occur] but at least you're very happy when you find that something you've [planned] has come to fruition. . . .

"We brought a lot of the [Reserve nurses] on two weeks of [active duty training] into [the Naval Medical Command] to work in the Nursing Division. They worked in other codes also; in education, in training. They helped us develop some of our contingency planning. It was this acceptance of them (bringing them into the fold) that really started . . . an active, viable Reserve Nurse Corps that we didn't have before."[6]

In 1985, the rank of Commodore is deleted and all Commodores are designated Rear Admirals (lower rank.) Commodore Nielubowicz becomes Rear Admiral Nielubowicz with one star; grade 07. Further she is the first and the last Navy Nurse Corps' Commodore.

"In 1986, Nurse Corps members of the Association of Military Surgeons of the United States (AMSUS) established the Mary J. Nielubowicz Essay Award in recognition of her outstanding support and encouragement of active and reserve nurses."[7]

Rear Admiral Nielubowicz retired on 1 October 1987

(At this point, the author discontinued the practice of personally conducting oral history interviews with the Directors of the Nurse Corps. This was done in order to - at long last - bring the book to publication. Therefore, the epilogue format is changed here, to give merely the general background of the succeeding Directors through 1996. Also, included will be the background of the first Reserve Navy Nurse Corps flag officer.)

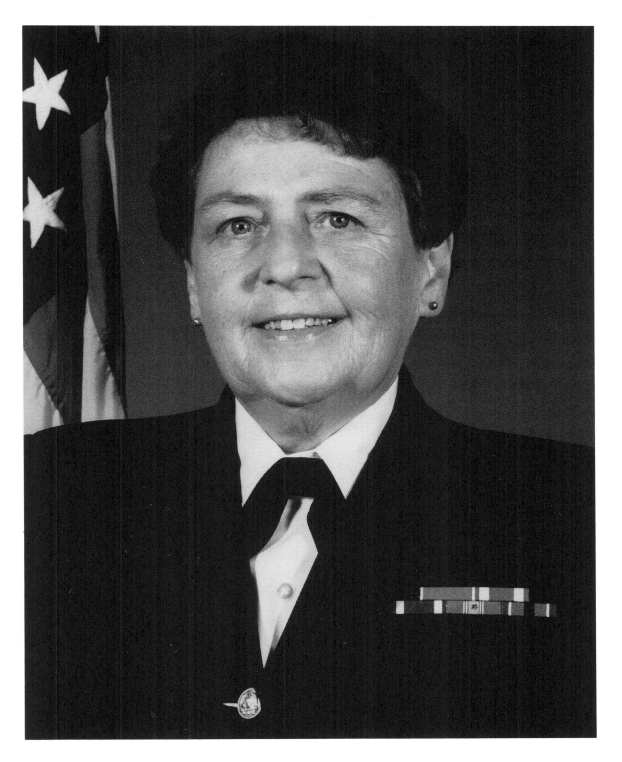

Director - Rear Admiral Mary J. Nielubowicz NC USN
(Official U.S. Navy photo courtesy of Nursing Division, Bureau of Medicine and Surgery, Navy Department.)

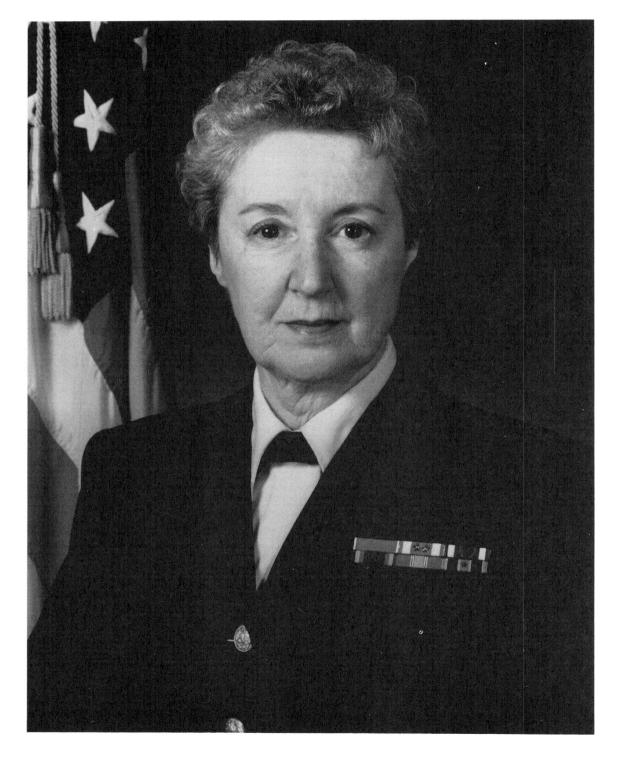

Director - Rear Admiral Mary F. Hall NC USN
(Official U.S. Navy photo courtesy of Nursing Division, Bureau of Medicine and Surgery, Navy Department.)

REAR ADMIRAL MARY A. FIELDS HALL
(1987 - 1991)

On 1 October 1987, Rear Admiral Mary Hall is appointed Director of the U.S. Navy Nurse Corps and Deputy Commander for Personnel Management, Naval Medical Command.

Mary Alice Fields (Hall) was born in the town of Clear Ridge in Pennsylvania. After high school, she entered nurses' training at the Episcopal Hospital School of Nursing in Philadelphia where she graduated in 1955. In 1959, she joined the Navy Nurse Corps. Her first duty station was the National Naval Medical Center at Bethesda, Maryland. In 1966 she received her Bachelor of Science degree in Nursing from Boston University in Massachusetts. In 1973 she was awarded a Master of Science degree in Nursing Service Administration at the University of Maryland. In 1983, she is the first Navy Nurse Corps officer to be selected and appointed as a Commanding Officer of a naval hospital. She is selected for flag rank in October of 1986. Then, in 1987, Rear Admiral Hall assumes her new assignment as Director of the Corps and Deputy Commander for Personnel Management.[8] Rear Admiral Hall retires at the end of her term in office in September 1991.

It must be mentioned that Rear Admiral Mary A. Fields Hall is the first Navy Nurse Corps officer ever to be awarded the Distinguished Service Medal. A portion of the summary of action for the Distinguished Service Medal awarded to Admiral Hall refers to a particularly stressful period of her term in office; the time of Desert Shield and Desert Storm. This excerpt from the summary for the medal states: "Recognized a disparity between war-time requirements and active duty Nurse Corps strength. Appointed a Deputy Director for Reserve Affairs who facilitated and monitored the use of recruitment incentives to increase the Reserve Nurse Corps from fifty-six percent manning in FY [Fiscal Year] 1987 to one-hundred-nine percent manning in FY 1990, an on-board strength increase from eleven-hundred to twenty-seven-hundred-fifty. Over fifty percent of these Nurse Corps Reserve assets were called up during Operation Desert Shield and Storm as they supplied the largest number of Reservists recalled for service. Only because of her foresight and program management successes was the Medical Department able to provide adequate support to our deployed forces and maintain State-side medical capabilities."[9]

Rear Admiral Mary F. Hall retires in September 1991. But, just one year before her retirement, another first occurs; the first Reserve Nurse Corps flag officer is selected, Rear Admiral Mary-anne T. Gallagher Ibach.

Rear Admiral Ibach was born in

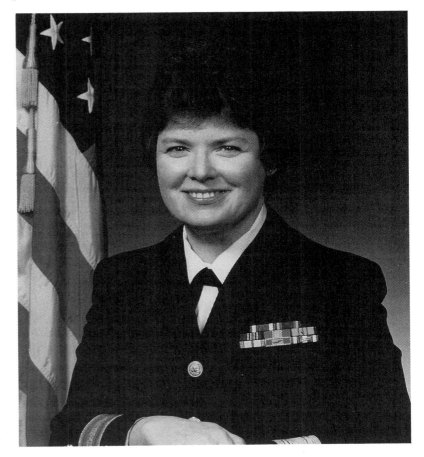

Rear Admiral Maryanne T. Ibach NC USNR
(Official U.S. Navy photo courtesy of Nursing Division, Bureau of Medicine and Surgery, Navy Department.)

Philadelphia, Pennsylvania. She graduated in 1962 from the Misericordia Hospital School of Nursing in Philadelphia. In 1964 she joined the Navy Nurse Corps. During the next eleven years she is assigned duty at several naval hospitals and one tour of duty "aboard the hospital ship, USS *Repose* (AH-16) at sea in the Viet Nam combat zone. . . . In 1975 she resigned her regular commission and transferred to the Naval Reserve."[10] Some of her early Reserve assignments were at some of the California Naval Medical clinics. "From 1981-1984, she served in a variety of [Reserve] assignments of increasing responsibility in the Washington, DC area. . . . In November 1984, she affiliated with . . . [Reserve Headquarters] and spent more that eight month on active duty at Naval Hospital, Bethesda where she was responsible for establishing the Reserve Liaison Office and developing the command's Reserve Integration Program. . . . [Later, in 1988] she was assigned to . . . [Reserve Headquarters in the] Office of the Surgeon General. She assumed her flag duties in September 1990. . . .

"Rear Admiral Ibach holds a Bachelor of Science Degree in Nursing from the University of Pennsylvania, 1972; a Master of Arts Degree in Higher Education from George Washington University, 1975; and a Master's Certificate in Gerontology from George Mason University, 1985."[11] Rear Admiral Ibach retires on 1 October 1995.

REAR ADMIRAL MARIANN STRATTON
(1991 - 1994)

Rear Admiral Mariann Stratton becomes Director of the Navy Nurse Corps and the Assistant Chief for Personnel Management in Navy Medicine, in September 1991.

She is originally from the Houston, Texas area. She graduated from high school in 1962 and attended the Sacred Heart Dominican College in Houston. In 1966, "She earned a Bachelor of Science in Nursing and a Bachelor of Arts in English from"[12] this institution. "She holds a Master of Arts in Human Resource Management from Webster College. . . . [She] attended the University of Virginia, completing a Master of Science in Nursing with a Major in medical-surgical nursing and certification as an Adult Nurse Practitioner in 1981."[13]

"In September, 1964, Rear Admiral Stratton joined the Navy as a Navy Nurse Corps Candidate and was commissioned [as an Ensign] in September 1965."[14] Her first duty station was the Naval Hospital at St. Albans, New York. Besides other stateside Naval Medical facilities and one tour in Navy Recruiting, she has had overseas duty in Japan, Ethiopia, Greece, and Naples, Italy.[15]

She was selected to flag rank in November 1990 and became Director of the Nurse Corps and Assistant Chief for Personnel Management in 1991. "Since September 1991, RADM Stratton has served as Chair of the Health Care Committee for the Interservice Training Review Organization; Chair of the Working Group on the Prevention of Sexual Harassment on the Standing Committee on Military and Civilian Women in the Department of the Navy; and Chair of the Federal Nursing Chiefs Council, a council composed of the Chiefs of the five Federal Nursing Services and the American Red Cross. As Director, Navy Nurse Corps, she conceptualized and implemented the *Navy Nurse Corps Strategic Plan-Charting New Horizons*. At the request of the Minister of Defense, RADM Stratton provided consultation on military nurse functions and training programs in the Arab Republic of Egypt."[16]

Rear Admiral Stratton retired in September 1994.

It must be noted here that on May 25, 1994, a most noteworthy Navy Nurse Corps historical event took place in Bremerton, Washington. On that day, six Navy Nurse Corps Rear Admirals (flag officers) met together to hold a panel for the staff of the Bremerton Naval Hospital. Five were former Directors of the Corps and one was the active Director of the Corps. It was another 'first' for the Navy Nurse Corps. The Panel members were: RADM Alene Duerk (retired), RADM Maxine Conder (retired), RADM Frances Shea Buckley (retired), RADM Mary Nielubowicz (retired), RADM Mary Hall (retired), and RADM Mariann Stratton NC USN. The Program

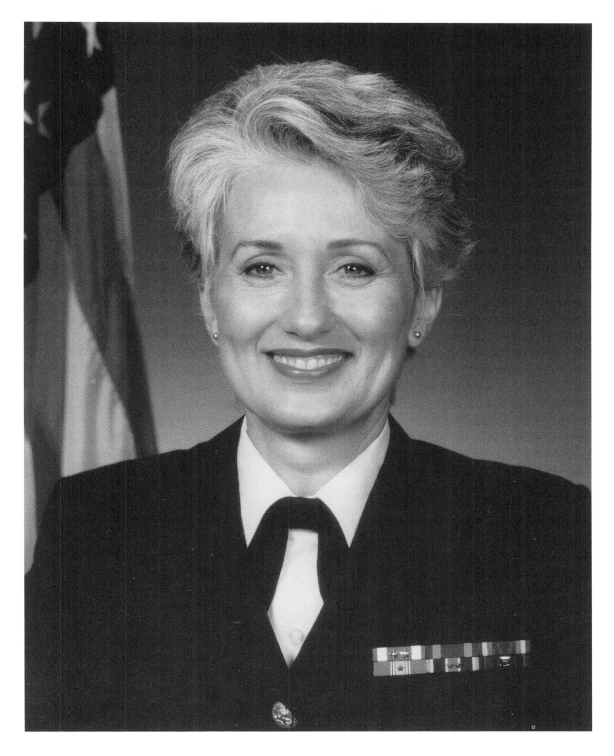

Director - Rear Admiral Mariann Stratton NC USN
(Official U.S. Navy photo courtesy of Nursing Division, Bureau of Medicine and Surgery, Navy Department.)

Committee of the Northwest Chapter of the Navy Nurse Corps Association planned and sponsored this event in conjunction with the 1994 NNCA Reunion being held in Seattle, Washington at this time. Each of the Admirals had the opportunity to speak to the group.

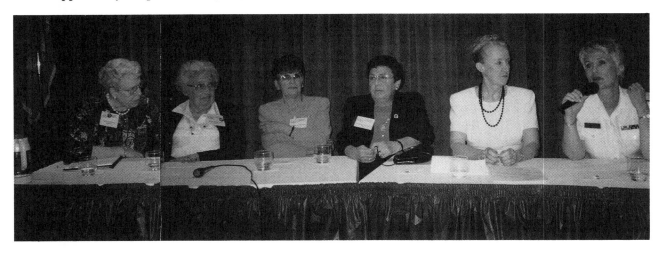

First Admiral's Panel (Photo courtesy of Public Affairs Office, Naval Hospital, Bremerton, WA.)

REAR ADMIRAL JOAN M. ENGEL
(1994 - Present)

In September 1994, Rear Admiral Engel becomes Director the Navy Nurse Corps and then Assistant Chief for Education, Training, and Personnel in the Bureau of Medicine and Surgery. It is now January 1996 and her term of office continues. But, her term is of the here and now; it is not yet history. When Rear Admiral Joan M. Engel's term becomes history, only then can she be initially portrayed in the chapters of the next 'History of the United States Navy Nurse Corps.'

☆☆☆ Carry on! ☆☆☆

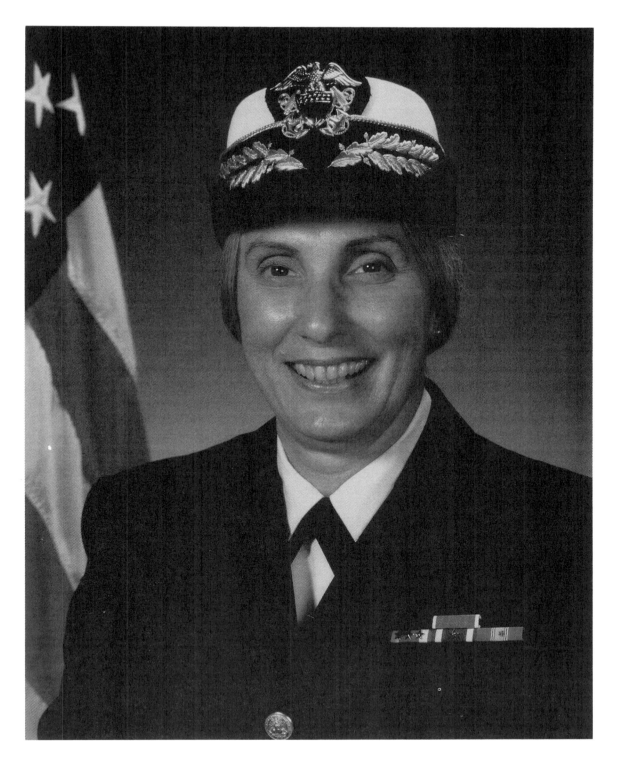

Director - Rear Admiral Joan M. Engel NC USN
(Official U.S. Navy photo courtesy of Nursing Division, Bureau of Medicine and Surgery, Navy Department.)

1   Conder, Maxine Rear Admiral, Director of the Navy Nurse Corps, *Oral History Interview Tape Transcript*, Self-interview, July 1991.
2   In September of 1981, "Title 10, United States Code: Defense Officers' Personnel Management Act (DOPMA) enacted. One of the primary objectives of DOPMA was to provide reasonably consistent career opportunity among the services [Army, Navy, Air Force]. To achieve this, DOPMA standardized the laws governing appointment, promotion, separation and retirement of active duty officers. . . . The most significant impact of DOPMA on the Nurse Corps was its mandate regulating the number of officers in the 04-06 [Lieutenant Commander to Captain] grade levels based on the size of each of the Service's officer corps. Prior to DOPMA, Nurse Corps officers were promoted with their lineal [Line] running-mate regardless of requirements or authorizations. With the enactment of DOPMA, all communities were given a defined number of 04-06 authorizations. When DOPMA became effective, the Nurse Corps exceeded grade authorizations. This led to a grade imbalance problem which gave nurses a lower promotion opportunity than that available to their counterparts." Quoted from the updated *History of the Nurse Corps, U.S. Navy*, by the Navy Nurse Corps Officers on the staff of the Director of the Navy Nurse Corps, 5727.1, OONCA/np, revised 24 April 1991, p. 33, 34.
3   Buckley, Frances T. Shea Rear Admiral, Director of the Navy Nurse Corps, *Oral History Interview Tape Transcript*, Interviewers Captain Doris M. Sterner Nurse Corps and Dr. Lynne Dunn of the Naval Historical Center of Washington, D.C., 13 July 1988.
4   Nielubowicz, Mary J. Rear Admiral, Director of the Navy Nurse Corps, *Oral History Interview Tape Transcript*, Interviewer Captain Doris M. Sterner Nurse Corps, 8 May 1990.
5   Nielubowicz, Mary J. Rear Admiral, Navy Nurse Corps, *Transcript of Navy Nurse Corps Admirals' Panel*, Bremerton, Washington, 25 May 1995.
6   Nielubowicz, Mary J. Rear Admiral, Director of the Navy Nurse Corps, *Oral History Interview Tape Transcript*, op. cit..
7   Information prepared by the Navy Nurse Corps Officers on the staff of the Director of the Navy Nurse Corps, circa 1990.
8   Information prepared by the Navy Nurse Corps Officers on the staff of the Director of the Navy Nurse Corps, circa 1993.
9   From the summary of action for the Distinguished Service Medal awarded to Rear Admiral Hall at the end of her tour as sixteenth Director of the Navy Nurse Corps. Said summary as it appears in the: Hall, Mary Fields Rear Admiral, Director of the Navy Nurse Corps, *Oral History Interview Tape Transcript*, Interviewer Captain Margaret Armstrong Nurse Corps, 14 October 1992.
10   Pamphlet issued for the 'Change of Command Ceremony' when Rear Admiral Stratton retired and Rear Admiral Engel becomes the eighteenth Director of the Navy Nurse Corps, Washington, D.C., 2 September 1994.
11   Ibid..
12   Ibid..
13   Ibid..
14   Information prepared by the Navy Nurse Corps Officers on the staff of the Director of the Navy Nurse Corps, circa 1993.
15   Ibid..
16   Pamphlet issued for the 'Change of Command Ceremony' when Rear Admiral Stratton retired and Rear Admiral Engel becomes the eighteenth Director of the Navy Nurse Corps, op. cit..

"IN AND OUT OF HARM'S WAY"

A Navy Nurse Corps History
By Capt. Doris M. Sterner USN (Ret.)

"In and Out of Harm's Way" is a compilation of first-hand historical experiences of Navy Nurses. A unique perspective of achievements of those forerunners of the Corps. It is history. It is the US Navy Nurse Corps' heritage.

Order Form

Send with payment to: NNCA, P.O. Box 1229, Oak Harbor, WA 98277-1229

Ordered by: Name _____   Telephone # _____

Street _____

City _____   State_____   Zip _____

Ship to: Name _____

Street _____

City _____   State_____   Zip _____

Number of Hardback Books _____ @ $39.95 each = _____

Number of Paperback Books _____ @ $24.95 each = _____

(Washington Residents Add 8.1%)   Sales Tax   = _____

Shipping & Handling   = _____

Total   = _____

Shipping & Handling:

Add $3.50 for 1 copy.
Add $1.50 for each additional copy shipped to the same address.

Share this order form with your family and friends.